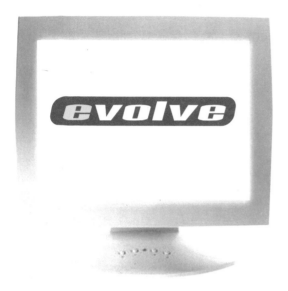
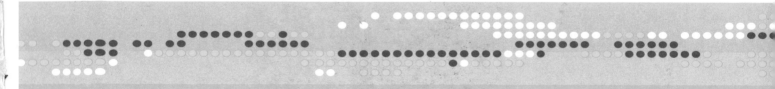

Mosby's

Pharmacy Technician

PRINCIPLES & PRACTICE

evolve

To access your Student Resources, visit:

http://evolve.elsevier.com/Hopper/

Evolve Student Learning Resources for *Hopper: Mosby's Pharmacy Technician: Principles & Practice* offer the following features:

The Latest Evolution in Learning

Evolve provides online access to free learning resources and activities designed specifically for the textbook you are using in your class. The resources will provide you with information that enhances the material covered in the book and much more.

- **Animations**
Chapter-specific animations provide students the opportunity to see various procedures and body functions in action.

- **English/Spanish Audio Glossary**
Audio pronunciations in both English and Spanish help students master key terms, while also reinforcing word meanings.

- **Additional Math Exercises**
Self-grading math exercises will provide students additional practice in conversions, dosing, and basic math skills—all of which are vital to providing accurate pharmacy service.

- **Mosby's Essential Drugs for Pharmacy Technicians**
Detailed drug monographs, including full-color pill photos, for the top 200 dispensed drugs in the United States.

Mosby's Pharmacy Technician

PRINCIPLES & PRACTICE

TERESA HOPPER, BS, CPhT

Instructor of Pharmacy Technology
San Joaquin Valley College
Rancho Cordova, California

Second Edition

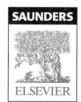

SAUNDERS

ELSEVIER

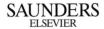

11830 Westline Industrial Drive
St. Louis, Missouri 63146

MOSBY'S PHARMACY TECHNICIAN: PRINCIPLES &
PRACTICE, 2ND EDITION

ISBN 13: 978-1-4160-3940-2
ISBN 10: 1-4160-3940-6

ISBN 13: 978-1-4160-3940-2
ISBN 10: 1-4160-3940-6

Publishing Director: Andrew Allen
Executive Editor: Loren Wilson
Developmental Editor: Lynda Huenefeld
Publishing Services Manager: Julie Eddy
Senior Project Manager: Rich Barber
Designer: Andrea Lutes

Working together to grow
libraries in developing countries

www.elsevier.com | www.bookaid.org | www.sabre.org

ELSEVIER   BOOK AID International   Sabre Foundation

Printed in Canada

Last digit is the print number: 9 8 7 6 5 4 3

Preface

YOU ARE ABOUT TO EMBARK on an exciting journey into one of today's fastest-growing fields in health care. Whether you will end up working in a hospital pharmacy, a community pharmacy, one of the large pharmacy chain stores, or another location, the knowledge you will gain from this textbook and its supplements will prepare you well for your new career. The authors and publisher have made every effort to equip you with all of the background knowledge and tools you will need to succeed on the job. To this end, *Mosby's Pharmacy Technician: Principles & Practice* was designed as a fundamental yet comprehensive resource that represents the very latest information available for preparing pharmacy technician students for today's challenging job environment.

Who Will Benefit From This Book?

Pharmacy technicians are increasingly called upon to perform duties traditionally fulfilled by pharmacists. This is because of new federal regulations that now require pharmacists to spend more time with patients providing patient education. As the number of pharmacy technicians in the United States continues to grow, the need to outline a scope of practice for the pharmacy technician profession across all 50 states has become more urgent. *Mosby's Pharmacy Technician: Principles & Practice* provides students a solid coverage of information needed to be successful, while also giving the instructor the tools needed to present the information effectively and easily.

Why is This Book Important to the Profession?

Although there is no standardization for the qualifications and job descriptions for pharmacy technicians at this time, this textbook covers all the theory and skills set forth by several national certifying bodies, including the Pharmacy Technician Certification Board (PTCB), the National Healthcareer Association (NHA), the American Society of Health System Pharmacists (ASHP), and the American Pharmaceutical Association (APA), the last two of which created the criteria for the Pharmacy Technician Certification Board's certification exam. These criteria are designed to help pharmacy technicians work more effectively with pharmacists, provide greater patient care and services, create a minimum standard of knowledge across all 50 states, and help employers determine a knowledge base for employment.

Organization

Mosby's Pharmacy Technician: Principles & Practice is a reliable and understandable resource written specifically for the pharmacy technician student and for those technicians already on the job, including those who are preparing for the National Pharmacy Technician Certification exam (PCTB), or the Certified Pharmacy Technician exam (CPhT). The writing style, content, and organization guide the student to a better understanding of anatomy and physiology, diseases, and, most importantly, drugs and agents used to treat these diseases. Pharmacologic information is presented in a thorough, yet basic and concise, manner. The text is divided into five sections—**General Pharmacy, Body Systems, Classifications of Drugs, Basic Sciences for the Pharmacy Technician,** and **Starting Your Career as a Pharmacy Technician.**

Section One, General Pharmacy, provides an overview of pharmacy practice as it relates to pharmacy technicians. Highlights of Section One include history, law and ethics, drug calculations and dosage forms, abbreviations, routes of administration, filling prescriptions, over-the-counter medications, and the differences in the roles of pharmacists and pharmacy technicians. *Mosby's Pharmacy Technician* is the only book on the market that devotes an entire chapter each to alternative and complementary medicine and psychopharmacology.

Section Two, Body Systems, provides a brief overview of each body system and the medications used to treat common conditions that afflict these systems. Unique to this section are detailed discussions of anatomy and physiology, as well as photographs of a number of drugs used to treat various conditions of each body system.

Section Three, Classifications of Drugs, discusses each major drug classification. A description of every drug classification helps the pharmacy technician student understand how similar agents work. Section Three also includes a chapter on vitamins and minerals.

Section Four, Basic Sciences for the Pharmacy Technician, includes two chapters—on microbiology and chemistry—that are indeed unique to this textbook.

Section Five, Starting Your Career as a Pharmacy Technician, provides materials to assist the student in preparing for the Pharmacy Technician Certification Board (PTCB) examination.

Distinctive Features of this Edition

DRUG NAMES AND PRONUNCIATIONS

A list of the drugs (generic and trade names) discussed within a chapter, along with the pronunciation, appear at the beginning of each chapter. This helps familiarize students with the spelling and pronunciation of drugs that they need to be familiar with on the job. It is essential that students be proficient in this area.

RESPIRATORY MEDICATIONS

Trade Name	Generic Name	Pronunciation	Trade Name	Generic Name	Pronunciation
Antitussives			**Analgesic/Antitussives**		
Benylin DM	dextromethorphan	(dex-troh-meh-**thor**-fan)	Tussionex	hydrocodone/	(hi-droe-**koe**-deen/
Robitussin DM	guaifenesin/	(gwi-**fen**-ah-sin/dex-troe-		chlorpheniramine	klor-fen-**air**-ah-meen/
	dextromethorphan	me-**thor**-fan)			
Tessalon Perles	benzonatate	(ben-**zoe**-na-tate)			

RESPIRATORY MEDICATIONS—cont'd

Trade Name	Generic Name	Pronunciation	Trade Name	Generic Name	Pronunciation
Expectorant			Adrenalin	epinephrine	(ep-i-**nef**-rin)
Hycotuss	hydrocodone/ guaifenesin	(hye-droe-**koe**-done)	Isuprel	isoproterenol	(eye-so-pro-**tear**-in-all)
			Alupent	metaproterenol	(met-a-pro-**tear**-in-all)
Robitussin	guaifenesin	(gwi-**fen**-ah-sin)	Maxair	pirbuterol	(pur-**bu**-ter-all)
			Serevent	salmeterol	(sal-**met**-er-ol)
Antihistamines					
Benadryl	diphenhydramine	(dye-fen-**hi**-dra-meen)	**Xanthines**		
Chlor-Trimeton	chlorpheniramine	(klor-fen-**air**-ah-meen)	Phyllocontin	aminophylline	(am-in-**off**-eh-lin)
Claritin	loratadine	(lo-**rat**-ah-dean)	Theo-Dur	theophylline	(thee-**off**-ah-lin)
Mucolytic			**Leukotriene Receptor Antagonists**		
Mucomyst	acetylcysteine	(a-sea-till-**sis**-teen)	Singulair	montelukast	(mon-tea-**lu**-cast)
			Accolate	zafirlukast	(zay-**fur**-lu-cast)
Decongestants			Zyflo	zileuton	(zi-**leu**-ton)
Sudafed	pseudoephedrine	(sue-doe-e-**fed**-dren)			
Neo-Synephrine	phenylephrine	(fen-ill-**ehf**-rin)	**Corticosteroids**		
Afrin	oxymetazoline	(ox-e-met-**taz**-o-leen)	Beclovent	beclomethasone	(beck-low-**meth**-the-sewn)
			Azmacort	triamcinolone	(try-am-**sin**-oh-lone)
Antituberculosis			AeroBid	flunisolide	(flew-**nis**-oh-lide)
Laniazide	isoniazid	(eye-soe-**nye**-a-zid)			
Myambutol	ethambutol	(e-**tham**-byoo-tole)	**Bronchodilator/Steroid Inhaler (Combination)**		
Rafadin	rifampin	(rif-**am**-pin)	Advair Diskus	fluticasone/ salmeterol	(flu-**tick**-ah-sewn/sal-**met**-er-ol)
	streptomycin	(strep-toe-**mye**-sin)			
Bronchodilators			**Anticholinergics**		
Proventil, Ventolin	albuterol	(al-**bu**-ter-all)	Atrovent	ipratropium bromide	(ih-prah-**trow**-pea-um **bro**-mide)
Tornalate	bitolterol mesylate	(bye-**tole**-ter-ole **mess**-ah-late)	Intal, Nasalcrom	cromolyn	(**krom**-oh-lin)

TECH NOTES

Helpful pharmacy technician notes appear interspersed throughout the chapters, providing interesting historical facts, drug cautions, hints, and safety information. These notes enhance students' knowledge of practical information that they will need to know in a pharmacy setting.

TECH NOTE!

Remember: You must place the proper units (such as mL, L, mg, or g) next to the number amount. This cannot be stressed enough, especially because you will be working with various systems. Putting the units on all numbers is the only way to help avoid mistakes.

Metric System

The metric system is used throughout pharmacy because of its accuracy. The units used in the metric system include the milliliter (mL), cubic centimeter (cc), and liter (L) for volume; kilogram (kg), gram (g), milligram (mg), and microgram (mcg) for weight; and millimeter (mm) and meter (m) for distance. A technician must know the difference between each unit given. For example, if a prescription were filled with 1 g of drug when only 1 mg was ordered, the patient would overdose by 1000 times the ordered dose. A 1000-unit difference exists between each measurement. This means that 1000 mcg equals 1 mg.

The use of millimeters is reserved for drug calculations that are based on body surface areas and would be calculated by a physician or pharmacist using a surface area calculation chart. For most technicians, knowing the basics for volume and weight conversions is adequate.

MINI DRUG MONOGRAPHS

Drug monograph information with pill photos is provided in every body systems and drug classification chapter. These monographs include drug class, generic and trade names, strength of medication, route of administration, dosage, and photos of drugs, providing students with quick, easy to understand information about specific drugs

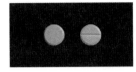

GENERIC NAME: haloperidol decanoate
TRADE NAME: Haldol
INDICATIONS: psychoses; Tourette's syndrome
STRENGTH: 50-mg injection, 100-mg injection; 0.5- to 5-mg tablets
ROUTE OF ADMINISTRATION: injection, oral
COMMON DOSAGE: 10 to 15 times the normal daily dose every month (maximum dose should not exceed 100 mg). Most daily oral doses range between 5 and 20 mg per day in divided doses
AUXILIARY LABELS:
- Do not drink alcohol.
- May cause dizziness and drowsiness.

PHARMACIST'S PERSPECTIVE

Written by a practicing pharmacist on specific topics related to content, these boxes provide students with more information on content from the point of view of the pharmacist, making the content more interesting by relating the content information to on-the-job situations.

Pharmacist's Perspective
BY SUSAN WONG, PharmD

In recent years, there has been a national shortage of medical professionals, especially pharmacists and nurses. In some states, recent legislation has been approved to help pharmacies deliver better service in a timely manner. This allows pharmacists to spend more time counseling patients. As an example in California, more technician support for pharmacists is allowed (up to two technicians to work with each pharmacist in certain situations—the technician-to-pharmacist ratio.) Now the challenge will be to find enough qualified technicians to work in the pharmacies. More emphasis will be placed on competency, communication, and ethics/professional behavior as the growth and expansion of the pharmacy technician role continues.

As mentioned in a previous chapter, the technician role has evolved from a clerical role to a more technical one behind the scenes, helping pharmacists provide medicines to those who need it. The technician is part of the team, not an individual practitioner. The technician must be willing and competent to work anywhere from the front line helping customers to working behind the counter with the pharmacist answering phones, assist in filling prescriptions, preparing intravenous admixtures, and so on. Being competent in as many skills as possible is what sets the technician apart as a valued team member. Together, under the guidance and supervision of licensed pharmacists, this team functions as a well-oiled machine. This allows efficiency on the job, delivery of world-class pharmaceutical care, and personal job satisfaction. ■

TECHNICIAN'S CORNER

Technician's Corner boxes appear at the end of each chapter, providing critical thinking questions to help students prepare for on-the-job experiences.

TECHNICIAN'S CORNER

Dr. Beth Golden writes an order for the following prescription:
DEA#BG1958366
Disp: hydrocodone/acetaminophen tablets #50
Sig: Take 1 tablet q8h prn severe pain
10 refills
Determine whether this DEA number is correct, and explain each step of the checking process. List how many mistakes, if any, you find on all parts of this order.

New to This Edition

NEW CHAPTER! CHAPTER 31—REVIEW FOR THE PTCB EXAMINATION

This new chapter presents a 125-question practice exam formatted in the same fashion as the PTCB exam with multiple choice questions, assisting students as they prepare for taking the PTCB exam, which is now a requirement in some states.

TECH ALERT! BOXES

This feature appears throughout each chapter and provides critical reminders to the pharmacy technician, helping the pharmacy technician focus on specific warnings and avoid common pharmacy errors.

TECH ALERT!

Not all generic drugs are bioequivalent to the trade/brand drugs. Even if a generic drug has the same active ingredient, it may vary in additional additives, making it different. An example is albuterol inhalant; although all generics contain the same main ingredients and propellants, they differ in types of additives. Also the size of the valve differs between trade/brand that may alter the amount of medicine being dispensed.

BIOEQUIVALENCE

Bioequivalence is the comparison between drugs from different manufacturers or in the same company but from different batches of drug. This is an important aspect of a drug because patients assume that every tablet they take is exactly the same as the one before and that all are the exact strength as listed on the label. Generic drug manufacturers strive to achieve the same equivalence as brand name manufacturers so that they can compete with the original manufacturer. Another reference to use in order to see whether the generic drug is rated as bioequivalent is the *Orange Book*. This book lists the approved drug products with therapeutic equivalence and evaluations.

Most of the final metabolism of a drug takes place in the liver. This is the final processing center of the body that extracts toxins and unwanted chemicals from the body and forwards them onto the excretion process (in the kidneys). The liver works hard but can process only so much within a given time. Persons suffering from any type of liver damage must be monitored closely when taking various medications to ensure that toxic levels are not present in the liver.

ADDITIONAL PILL IMAGES

Approximately 100 new pill images have been added to the second edition, assisting the pharmacy technician in identifying pills on sight and avoiding pharmacy errors.

ADDITIONAL MATH EXERCISES

Additional math exercises have been added to the textbook, as well as to the Evolve site, and student CD-ROM. These additional math exercises will help students strengthen their math skills in the appropriate areas.

ANSWERS TO REVIEW QUESTIONS

Answers to odd-numbered review questions now appear in Appendix G. This will allow students to check their own progress while working through the review questions, and still allow instructors to assign even-numbered review questions as graded assignments.

OVERALL CONTENT UPDATE

Mosby's Pharmacy Technician provides the student with the most up-to-date pharmacy information available. New drugs added, including indications and pill photos, provide pharmacy technicians with the most current information.

Learning Aids

FOUR-COLOR DESIGN

The colorful design, figures, and pill images help to present a difficult subject in an inviting and unintimidating manner.

EXTENSIVE VISUAL AIDS

Mosby's Pharmacy Technician contains over 500 line drawings and photos in full color, helping students see concepts and procedures in visual form, while greatly enhancing learning of this new information that can be difficult to learn.

CHAPTER OBJECTIVES

Chapter objectives appear at the beginning of each chapter, clearly outlining key concepts covered.

KEY TERMS

Key terms with definitions appear at the beginning of each chapter, identifying new terminology for the student and making it easier to learn.

DO YOU REMEMBER THESE KEY POINTS?

This review of key points appears at the end of each chapter, providing students the opportunity to quickly revisit the main concepts of the chapter before attempting to answer the review questions.

DO YOU REMEMBER THESE KEY POINTS?

■ The basic measurements of the metric, apothecary, and avoirdupois systems
■ That the primary system used in pharmacy is the metric system
■ How to convert metric numbers from kilograms all the way to micrograms
■ That all measurements must have units attached to keep them straight
■ How to convert pounds into kilograms and vice versa
■ That double-checking calculations is important before preparing medications
■ How to determine how long an intravenous solution will last
■ When to use ratio/proportion and the steps involved in both methods shown
■ When to use alligation and how to set up the equation
■ How to convert Roman numerals to Arabic numbers

ENGLISH/SPANISH GLOSSARY

A comprehensive glossary containing both English and Spanish terms appears at the end of the text and on the student CD-ROM. This makes it convenient for students to look up the meaning of new terminology. Spanish terms and definitions are added for both Spanish-speaking students, and students who will be working in an environment where they will interact with many Spanish-speaking customers.

Ancillaries

Considering the broad range of students, instructors, programs, and institutions for which this textbook was designed, we have developed an extensive package of supplements designed to complement *Mosby's Pharmacy Technician: Principles & Practice,* second edition. Each of these comprehensive supplements has been thoughtfully developed with the shared goals of students and instructors in mind: producing students who are well prepared for a career in pharmacy, as well as for earning their National Pharmacy Technician Certification. These supplements and their inventive features include:

FOR THE INSTRUCTOR

Instructor's Electronic Resource
This CD-ROM product, included with *TEACH for Mosby's Pharmacy Technician,* includes:

• All textbook review question answers
• Answers to the workbook exercises
• Nearly 1,000 test bank questions programmed into the ExamView platform.
• Chapter-specific PowerPoint presentations
• Electronic image collection

TEACH for Mosby's Pharmacy Technician

TEACH for Mosby's Pharmacy Technician is designed to help the pharmacy technician instructor prepare for class by reducing preparation time, providing new and innovative ideas to promote student learning, and helping to make full use of the rich array of resources available. This completely revised manual includes:

- Detailed lesson plans
- Class activities
- Chapter-specific PowerPoint presentations, and more. *TEACH for Mosby's Pharmacy Technician* also incorporates full line of Elseviers pharmacy technology products into the lesson plans, including Neville: *Mosby's Pharmacy Technician Lab Manual* and DAA: *Pharmacy Management Software for Pharmacy Technicians*. The Instructor's Electronic Resource (IER) is bound into the back of the manual, providing easy access to additional instructor materials.

TEACH Online Pharmacy Technician Program Guide

The TEACH Online Pharmacy Technician Program Guide assists instructors seeking to start or expand a pharmacy technician program. The Program Guide is accessible via this textbook's Evolve web site at http://evolve.elsevier.com/Hopper/.

FOR THE STUDENT

Student CD-ROM

The Student CD-ROM, bound into the back of this textbook, provides students with:

- Self-grading chapter-specific quizzes,
- An English/Spanish audio glossary,
- Additional self-grading math exercises,
- Procedural and anatomical animations.

Student Workbook

The student workbook includes:

- Exercises designed to reinforce cognitive content,
- Lab worksheets to reinforce performance skills,
- Internet research activities to teach students how to keep current with an ever-changing industry,
- Case scenarios to assist students as they develop critical thinking and decision-making skills.

Online Resources

EVOLVE COMPANION WEB SITE
(http://evolve.elsevier.com/Hopper/)

For the Instructor

The Evolve Companion Web Site includes all content from TEACH, the TEACH Curriculum Guide, chapter-specific PowerPoints, test bank questions, an electronic image collection, exercise answer keys, and more.

For the Student

Student resources on the Evolve Companion Web Site include self-grading, chapter-specific quizzes; procedural and anatomical animations; web links to related material; and an English-Spanish audio glossary.

MOSBY'S ESSENTIAL DRUGS FOR PHARMACY TECHNICIANS

Mosby's Essential Drugs for Pharmacy Technicians is an online resource that includes detailed drug monographs for the top 200 drugs dispensed in the United States. The drug monographs will include:

- Full-color drug images
- Brand and generic drugs names of the drug
- Description of the drug
- Mechanism of action
- Pharmacokinetics
- Indications and dosage, including off-label uses
- Administration guidelines
- Contraindications/precautions
- Interactions
- Adverse reactions
- Therapeutic classification
- Patient information

This new resource is powered by Gold Standard, the leading developer of drug information databases, software, and clinical information solutions.

Each new copy of Hopper: *Mosby's Pharmacy Technician*, 2nd edition, includes a passcode providing students access to this valuable information. Mosby's Essential Drugs for Pharmacy Technicians can be accessed through this text's Evolve web site at http://evolve.elsevier.com/Hopper/.

Acknowledgments

TO ENSURE THE ACCURACY of the material presented throughout this textbook, an extensive review and development process was used. This included evaluation by a variety of pharmacy technician instructors and experts in anatomy and physiology and pharmacology. We are deeply grateful to the numerous people who have shared their comments and suggestions. Reviewing a book or supplement takes an incredible amount of energy and attention, and we are glad so many colleagues were able to take time out of their busy schedules to help ensure the validity and appropriateness of content in this new edition. The reviewers provided us with additional viewpoints and opinions that combine to make this text an incredible learning tool.

We wish to thank the following Editorial Review Team:

Karen Davis, CPhT
Consultant
Lyons, Georgia

Danny Lame, CPhT
Platt College
Tulsa, Oklahoma

Michael C. Melvin, BS PHARM, RPh
Griffin Technical College
Griffin, Georgia

James J. Mizner, Jr., BS, MBA, RPh
Applied Career Training
Arlington, Virginia

John J. Smith, EdD
Corinthian Colleges, Inc.
Santa Ana, California

Marsha L. Wilson, BS
Clarian Health Partners
Indianapolis, Indiana

Contents

SECTION THREE Classifications of Drugs

SECTION FOUR   Basic Sciences for the Pharmacy Technician

SECTION FIVE   Starting Your Career as a Pharmacy Technician

APPENDICES

SECTION

one

General Pharmacy

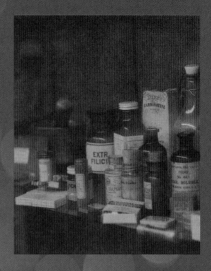

History of Medicine and Pharmacy

Objectives

UPON COMPLETING THIS CHAPTER, YOU SHOULD BE ABLE TO
DO THE FOLLOWING:

- Discuss ancient beliefs of illness and medicine from 440 BC through AD 1600.

- List common ancient treatments that prevailed in Western civilization.

- Describe nineteenth-century medicine, and identify influences that major wars had on medicine.

- Describe the wide use of opium and the problems surrounding them.

- Differentiate between opiates and opioids.

- Describe how the first pharmacies came about in the United States.

- Identify the role that early pharmacists played in society.

- Describe the first technicians in pharmacy.

- List major ways pharmacy has changed over the past 100 years.

- Identify the need for protocol in the pharmacy profession and its relation to formulary drugs.

- List important current trends in pharmacy in relation to pharmacy technicians.

- Identify the resistance to technicians that parallel historical resistance to pharmacists.

Ancient Beliefs and Treatments (Early Western Civilization)

Medicine has been practiced for thousands of years. Archaeological discoveries have unearthed civilizations that have documented the use of minerals, animals, and plant parts to heal the sick. However, it is difficult to know exactly what people of that time believed to be true concerning death and disease. Some remedies, such as herbals, have been used throughout history. Various herbs were used for minor ailments such as intestinal problems, arthritis, and gout.

However, many of the popular beliefs of the past have mostly disappeared. A belief surrounding healing the sick was the idea that severe illness was caused

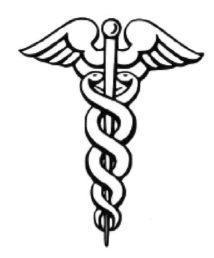

FIGURE 1-1 Medical staff.

by evil spirits. To rid oneself of an evil spirit, a cut was made into the skull to give the disease a portal through which to leave. This type of treatment was called trephining and often was performed by a tribal shaman (a spiritual person in a tribe who cares for the spiritual, medicinal, and physical health of the tribe). Tribal shamans were believed to have the gift of being able to communicate with spirits. Other shamans believed that they were connected with a special spirit who helped them render the evil spirits harmless through the use of prayer, herbs, or potions. Shamans were prevalent throughout societies in ancient times. Some still exist in various societies throughout the world. In North America, various Eskimo and Native American tribes held shamans in high esteem.

The Medical Staff

Aesculapius was the Greek god of medicine. His symbol—still used today to signify medicine—was a staff with snakes wrapped around it. Because snakes shed their skin, they signify new life (Figure 1-1). Treatments for illness were based on the dreams or visions of the believers. A dogma, such as gods being able to cause and cure illness, is based on a set of beliefs (e.g., church doctrines) set forth by authoritarians. These beliefs are based on writings from prophets rather than on hypotheses based on scientific methods.

Medicine in Its Infancy

The infancy of medicine was not a smooth road. Throughout the ages, many plagues killed thousands of persons. The existence of microbes, unseen by the eye, was not known to be responsible for many of the diseases that caused death and despair. Despite advancements made through early history, most remedies for physical ailments tended to be extreme. Other ancient remedies have been used for hundreds of years. Prevalent thoughts included, for example, that sickness was an entity within the body that needed a means to leave the body. Another was that spirits were responsible for illness. The most common form of treatment, prayer, still has remained in many cultures as the only way to cure illness.

Hippocrates (460-357 BC) was born on the small island of Cos near Greece, and he was a third-generation physician. He taught at Cos School of Medicine, which was one of the first medical schools established. He believed in the prevailing concept of that era, that life consisted of a balance of four elements that were linked to qualities of good health. They consisted of wet, dry, hot, and cold.

In addition, he believed that illness resulted from an imbalance of the four humors of the body system: blood, phlegm, yellow bile, and black bile. These four humors were linked to the four basic elements: blood is air, phlegm is water, yellow bile is fire, and black bile is earth. Methods used to treat imbalance of the humors included bloodletting and laxatives to help rebalance the humors. Hippocrates was responsible for much advancement in the world of medicine. Some of his observations included the effects of food, climate, and other influences on illness. He was one of the first physicians to record his patients' medical illnesses. This new way of viewing the causes of illnesses eventually led to the belief that sickness originated from something other than the supernatural.

Hippocrates believed that the spirit of the patient should be as important as the condition being treated, and he promoted being kind to the sick. He also believed in letting nature do the healing and promoted rest and eating of light foods. He taught that doctors needed to bring the four humors back into balance. Most of his teachings have been documented in a collection of books called the *Corpus Hippocraticum*. Although many of the writings are believed now to be from different authors, they still reflect the teachings of Hippocrates.

Today's medical schools still use the Hippocratic Oath as part of their graduation ceremony. This oath, taken from the book of *Ancient Greece and Rome* by Moulton, states, "Doctors act only for the good of their patients and keep confidential what they learn about their patients." As the book explains, the Hippocratic Oath outlines the physician's responsibility to the patient. Hippocrates practiced what he preached with respect to exercise, rest, diet, and overall moderation in one's lifestyle. Various records have his death at 377 BC, whereas others record his death in 357 BC. Considering that the average human life span was no more than 40 years at that time, living between 83 and 103 years was astonishing. Because of the advancements he promoted in the world of medicine, it is not surprising that Hippocrates is known as the Father of Medicine.

Before Hippocrates and other innovative scientists, people believed that they were at the mercy of the gods or supernatural forces. One such god was Aesculapius, the god of healing, to whom temples and shrines were built to pray for health.

Later in history, the Greek philosopher and scientist Aristotle (384-322 BC) was responsible for many advancements in the areas of biology and medicine. His main area of interest was biology and the study and classification of various organisms. He classified human beings as animals. Because the belief system in those times did not allow dissection of the dead, he described much of human anatomy from observations he made from dissections of other animals. This included in-depth descriptions of the brain, heart, lungs, and blood vessels.

Claudius Galen (AD 129-210) began to study medicine at the age of 16. He attended medical schools in Greece and the famous Alexandria school of medicine in Egypt. He later resided in Rome and was the personal physician of the Roman imperial family. Although he was born nearly 600 years after Hippocrates, he followed many of the same beliefs, such as eating a balanced diet, exercise, and good hygiene. He contributed greatly to the study of medicine, writing more than 100 books on topics such as physiology, anatomy, pathology, diagnosis, and pharmacology. Many of his books were used in medical schools for 1500 years. He proved that blood flowed through arteries rather than air.

Philosopher and alchemist Roger Bacon (AD 1214-1294) further refined and explained the importance of experimental methods, moving even further away from the dogmatic beliefs of the era.

Paracelsus (AD 1493-1541), a Swiss physician and alchemist, believed that it was important to treat illness with one medication at a time. At that time it was a common practice to give multiple remedies or large quantities of agents that had not been tested previously. Through the use of documentation of the effectiveness of each individual agent, Paracelsus was able to produce many

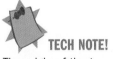

TECH NOTE!

The origin of the term *black humor* stems from the belief that too much of the black bile humor resulted in a person showing signs of melancholy.

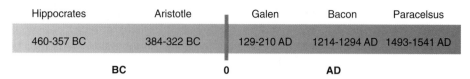

FIGURE 1-2 Time line. Persons who had a profound influence on medicine between 460 BC and AD 1500.

nontoxic medications. He introduced one of the most popular tonics of that time—laudanum, which was used to deaden pain. Figure 1-2 lists major figures in early medical history.

Ancient Herbal Remedies

Over the millennia, some prevalent treatments consisted of multiple mixtures of plants, roots, and other concoctions. Digestion of the type of plant that resembled the organ affected by disease also was believed to cure illnesses. For example, those with liver problems ingested a plant called liverwort (named because the leaves were shaped like a liver). Other popular treatments included using garlic for inflammation of the bronchial tubes, wine and pepper for various stomach ailments, onions for worms, and tiger fat for joint pain. It was difficult to detect which, if any, of the ingredients administered actually worked because many concoctions contained a multitude of ingredients. As strange as many of these archaic remedies seem, there were many people who were "cured" because of their strong belief in the treatment or person treating them. This outcome is called the *placebo effect* and is still evident today; there is still no conclusive explanation of why or how it works.

Throughout history, popular religious beliefs revolved around the idea that evil spirits were the cause of illness in a person who had sinned. This belief may have persisted partially because no one had the slightest idea about germs or genetics. Many times, through trial and error (error sometimes causing death), certain treatments were found to be fairly effective.

Any time new theories are proposed, they may be met with some skepticism and disbelief. A new hypothesis should be treated as a possible answer that has not been disproved. As new scientists emerge and new methods are devised to test hypotheses, their results give way to advancements. This was especially evident throughout the golden age of microbiology (see Chapter 29).

Nineteenth-Century Medicine

During the nineteenth century, religious leaders of the church became active in researching medicinal remedies to treat the sick. During this period, a famous scientist and monk, Gregor Mendel, documented experiments on plants. He was born in Austria on July 22, 1822. Mendel's research on generations of pea plants and other species helped determine the mechanism of how more hearty plants could be propagated. He founded the basis of current understanding of genetics and how genes are interwoven into heredity. Not until a decade after his death did Mendel become known as the father of genetics for his research papers. This ultimately led us into the study of genetics and more currently, genetic engineering.

Medicine in America

In early America, as new immigrants brought their families from England and other parts of the world, disease followed. Doctors were responsible not only for diagnosing the conditions but also for preparing the necessary remedies to cure patients in early times. Therefore the first druggists were doctors. Disease was widespread in the colonies; many persons did not survive the voyage across the sea from Europe, succumbing to diseases such as scurvy and severe intestinal infection. Patients were at a disadvantage throughout the colonies as doctors were few, and hospitals were fewer.

The main remedies used in early American history included cinchona bark (quinine), used to treat malaria, and more unconventional and dangerous treatments such as the use of mercury to treat syphilis. Many persons died of mercury poisoning because of its toxicity. Hundreds of persons also died of typhoid fever, malaria, diphtheria, and dysentery. The need for doctors and treatments increased dramatically. The average life expectancy was around 40 years, and many families lost several children to childhood diseases such as chickenpox, for which there were no vaccines available. Most treatments were concoctions handed down through family tradition. If a person were to use a doctor, he or she most likely would be treated at home or in a doctor's office, with treatments ranging from minor procedures to surgery.

Another popular treatment that originated in Europe was bloodletting. This became a standard treatment for thousands here in early America, and lasted many decades. The belief was that poisons causing illness could be eliminated through bleeding patients. A well-known victim was George Washington, who suffered from an infection and died of complications from this treatment, as did many others. It was not until the early 1900s that this type of treatment was declared quackery.

OPIUM AND ALCOHOL

One of the most popular tonics made for medicinal use in early America contained opium and alcohol. Its effectiveness was surpassed only by its addictiveness. This tonic was given as a sedative and to dull the sensation of pain. Paracelsus (as mentioned before) introduced the opium-alcohol mixture called laudanum in the sixteenth century, and laudanum was used as a medicinal remedy. Laudanum was used widely during the Civil War not only to treat painful wounds from the battlefield but also found its way into households throughout the United States for less severe problems and even for depression. Individuals became addicted at an alarming rate. Even though it was well known by the eighteenth century that opium and alcohol were addictive, alternative remedies were hard to find. Another alcohol-based liquid was absinthe. This herb *(Artemisia absinthium)* was mixed with alcohol and other additives. Absinthe was served with water and sugar to rid oneself of tapeworms.

Origin of Opium and Opiates
Opium has a long history in the relief of pain and unfortunate addictiveness (Chapter 2). Opium is a by-product gathered from a plant named *Papaver somniferum*, commonly known as the opium poppy. The sap is taken from the head of the poppy. The raw opium then is precipitated from the sap. The result from this process is a potent drug that causes the analgesic effect. Another form of analgesic is called an *opioid*. However, an *opioid* differs from opium because it is made in a laboratory rather than being taken from the plant. Opioids and opiates react on the same receptor sites in the nervous system (Chapter 17). The effects associated with the opioid receptors include analgesia, respiratory depression, pupil constriction, reduced gastrointestinal motility, euphoria, dysphoria, sedation, and physical dependence. Opioid and opiates share many of the same side effects. These include nausea and vomiting (Chapter 20). When used properly, the opium/opioid drugs are effective and help many patients who otherwise would suffer extreme pain. Not until 1909 did prohibition of opium importation (except for medicinal purposes) begin.

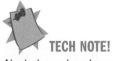

TECH NOTE!
Alcohol use has been dated back to 3500 BC in Egypt, and opium made its appearance in Europe about 5000 BC.

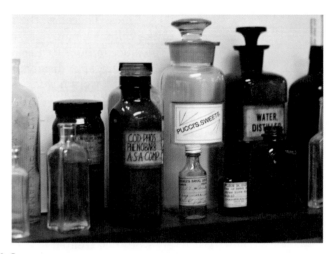

FIGURE 1-3 Medications were compounded by hand using a variety of compounds.

BOX 1-1 TYPICAL REMEDIES OF THE 1800S

To stop earaches	Blow tobacco smoke into the ear.
To treat a cold	A mixture of sugar, mineral oil, sulfur, ginger, lemon, and whisky in 8 oz. of water: drink and go to bed.
For baldness	Rub the head with an onion in the morning and at night before bed until the skin becomes red and then rub it with honey.
For worms	Take a tablespoon of molasses and mix it with tin rust and ingest.

EARLY PHARMACISTS

The need for specialists such as veterinarians, eye doctors, and pharmacists was caused by the growing population and the need for more trained medical personnel. In addition, the shipping of medicines to America from England was becoming difficult as the colonies separated from England. After the Civil War, apothecaries (pharmacies) began to spring up in towns across America, manufacturing plants were built, and persons were trained to prepare medications accurately. As the physician's role moved away from distributing drugs to diagnosing disease and surgery, pharmacists moved into the role of druggist. The first pharmacy school opened in 1821 at the College of Pharmacy and Sciences in Philadelphia. The school now is called the University of the Sciences in Philadelphia. Through the 1800s the pharmacist compounded nearly every drug ordered by physicians (Figure 1-3). Various sizes of ornate apothecary jars were used to store herbs and ingredients. The remedies were contained in medical books and read like a recipe book. Ingredients such as chalk for heartburn; rose petals for headaches; and oils, herbs, and spices filled containers in the apothecary. Some of the remedies of the 1800s are listed in Box 1-1.

Another type of interesting container associated with the pharmacy are show globes. These globes have been the beacons for pharmacy dating back as far as the early 1600s. Although there are many theories on what their original meaning was, a common one is that they were placed in the apothecary stores of the town to let visitors know the status of the health of the town. Red meant there was illness or that the town was in quarantine because of disease, whereas green meant the town was healthy and thus that it was safe to come into the town. These types of jars can be seen today in many pharmacies for show along with other artifacts from the past (Figure 1-4).

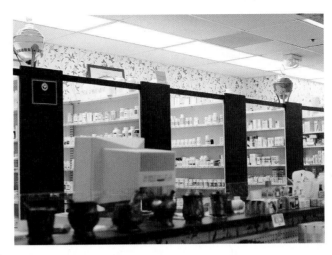

FIGURE 1-4 Large show globes *(above)*. An assortment of different mortars and pestles *(below)*.

EARLY PHARMACY TECHNICIANS

The first pharmacy technicians were those enlisted in the military because of the high demand for medications to treat injuries and illness. These individuals were trained on the job not only to fill prescriptions but also to do all the functions of a pharmacist. To this day, military technicians have a broader scope of training than a civilian technician. Technicians also were used by pharmacists who owned the corner drugstores. Family members helped behind the counters, filled stock, and waited on customers. These early clerks then moved on to become what we now call pharmacy technicians. Although the transition from clerk to technician is fairly recent in history, forecasts indicate that the pharmacy technician will play a critical role in the future pharmacy setting.

THE SODA FOUNTAIN/PHARMACY IN AMERICA

Early pharmacists played a minimal role in health care. In the mid 1800s and early 1900s the soda fountain became an extension of the town drugstore. As mineral water became known as a treatment for many different ailments, the soda fountain was the natural place to store and prepare the beverages. Many of these drinks, such as carbonated drinks, required chemicals that the pharmacist had in supply. Some of the many conditions mineral water was supposed to cure were obesity, upset stomach, depression, and nervous disorders. Pharmacists sold phosphate sodas and ice cream favorites, worked the lunch counter, and filled the prescriptions for the day. The first 7-Up drink was made with lithium and was sold from soda fountains for conditions such as gout, uremia, and rheumatism. By the late 1800s the soda shop/pharmacy was so popular that persons came to drink the sweet concoctions whether they were ailing or not. This type of pharmacy setting undoubtedly added to the image of the friendly neighborhood pharmacist that one could trust. The stereotypic local neighborhood pharmacist who wore a white jacket, packaged medications, and sometimes worked the soda machine has all but disappeared except in a few small towns in America, where a person may still get an old-fashioned malt or shake while waiting for a prescription to be filled.

TABLE 1-1 Important Advancements in Medicine

Name of scientist	Year of discovery	Disease identified	Vaccine/treatment found
Edward Jenner (England)	1796 (acknowledged in 1800)	Smallpox	Smallpox vaccine
Robert Koch (German)	1876	Anthrax, tuberculosis, cholera, malaria	
Albert Neisser (what is now Poland)	1879	Gonorrhea, syphilis, leprosy	
Louis Pasteur (France)	1877-1887	Staphylococcus, streptococcus, pneumococcus	Rabies, chicken cholera, anthrax vaccines
Paul Ehrlich (German)	1910	Syphilis	Chemotherapy
Alexander Fleming (Scotland)	1928		Identified penicillin
Gerhard Domagk (German)	1932		Discovered sulfonamides
Howard Florey (South Australia)	1938		Produced penicillin in large enough quantities to treat soldiers during World War II

Advancements in Drug Therapy and Vaccinations

Many of the most famous chemists, biologists, and doctors who contributed to science were from other countries, such as Germany, England, France, and Poland. Louis Pasteur (France) (most well known for the pasteurization process) was also responsible for inventing vaccinations such as the anthrax vaccine. Also in 1932, sulfonamide was invented by Gerhard Domagk (Germany), a bacteriologist/pathologist. Sulfa drugs are bacteriostatic, which means that they inhibit growth; they do not kill the microbes that already exist (see Chapter 29). Because of many resistant strains to sulfa drugs, they now are used primarily for urinary tract infections. Table 1-1 gives a list of the diseases that were discovered along with vaccines to prevent those diseases.

Changing Pharmacy

Times have changed and so have the requirements of today's pharmacist. All states now require new pharmacists to obtain a doctor of pharmacy degree (PharmD), which requires 6 years of education in an accredited school of pharmacy. Those pharmacists who received a bachelor of science in pharmacy before this change have been allowed to work in pharmacy without attaining a doctor of pharmacy. Required grade point averages for pharmacy school admission are rising, as is the cost of a pharmacist's education. Today's pharmacist also needs in-depth and broad communication skills with doctors and with customers. Today's typical pharmacy technician (an emerging profession) is required to do an array of tasks, all of which require competency in many areas . Thus in some states, today's technicians are required to get education in addition to on-the-job training. Currently, there are no nationally standardized requirements for pharmacy technicians. With the increase in available medications, the fear of interactions or wrong dosing also increases in the pharmacy setting. Technicians help the pharmacist by preparing prescriptions and compounding. In a hospital setting, also known as an inpatient pharmacy, tasks include supplying floor stock to the hospital floors, preparing parenteral medications, transcribing doctors' orders, and filling them in patients' medication cassettes. Other specialized technicians may do all the ordering of drugs and supplies. As always, filtering phone calls and the need for strong communication skills are required by the technician in the hospital or inpatient pharmacy and community or outpatient pharmacy (see Chapter 3).

Pharmacists can specialize in a field. For example, some pharmacists read patients' laboratory results to determine the level of a drug (e.g., anticoagulants or aminoglycosides) that should be dosed. These pharmacists then are allowed to write the necessary change in medication strength based on the laboratory results. Other specialty duties include oncology pharmacists and compounding pharmacists.

Protocol

Protocol is a set of standardized rules that are agreed on within a pharmacy setting. All medical personnel must abide by the protocol of their workplace. In the same sense, all pharmacies have a formulary. Some hospitals have specialty pharmacists called drug education coordinators. These individuals meet to discuss various new medications that have become available. The drug education coordinators are part of a hospital committee along with physicians, dietitians, and other medical staff. Each new drug is reviewed, and the committee determines whether the drug is better and more cost-effective than current medications being used. These types of pharmacists can be considered clinical pharmacists. Other information that the committee takes into consideration is any new literature that drug companies produce concerning the best use of their medication. The best medication then is placed on the formulary or list of medications that can be prescribed. For example, if a doctor writes a prescription order for ceftriaxone every 6 hours (normally given once or twice daily), the pharmacist on duty will call the doctor to find out whether the patient had the proper diagnosis for this dosing regimen. In another institution the pharmacist may have the ability to change the doctor's orders when necessary as long as the change is predetermined per protocol and adheres to the formulary. Special codes can be used to bypass certain formulary medications if the patient's needs require them.

Trust in Pharmacists/Trust in Technicians

Over the decades, pharmacists have become known as persons who can be trusted to provide truthful information, and someone with whom a person can be comfortable confiding. Although some traditions live on, times have changed concerning the role of the pharmacist. The most prevalent change can be seen in the inpatient setting of the hospital. As the competency of a pharmacist has become more "clinical," pharmacists are becoming more involved alongside doctors in the appropriate prescribing of medications and their dosages. These clinical pharmacists are found in the community pharmacy as well as hospital settings. An important change in pharmacy concerns the laws governing patient consultation. All patients who are prescribed new or changed medications must be offered consultation. This is meant to enlighten the patient about the medication he or she is taking. Because of these changes in the way pharmacies function, virtually every pharmacy employs pharmacy technicians. Therefore, it is important that the patient can trust a technician to provide the best care by filling the correct medication and referring the patient to the pharmacist for appropriate counsel. This takes a true commitment to the profession of pharmacy on the part of the pharmacy personnel to continue the trust that has existed between patient and health care provider. Through education, training, and good communication skills, technicians will gain the trust of the patients whom they serve.

Technicians of the Twenty-First Century and Beyond

TECH ALERT!

When applying for a state license, a complete background check will be performed on you. Any felony drug-related offense or other offense may cause a delay or decline of your application. Each person's application is determined case by case by the board of pharmacy. The board will require all court documents in order to make its decision. You should attach a letter with your application explaining the reason for your felony or criminal action and let the panel know the specifics of the crime. Although you should not assume that your application will be denied, the most important part of applying is not to lie or withhold any information. The board will find out.

In the new millennium with the roles of pharmacists, technicians, and clerks becoming more clearly defined, new concerns arise: We must be aware that just as the advancement of medicine through the ages met with much resistance, so has the profession of pharmacy. The changing roles of pharmacists, technicians, and even clerks have had their share of blockades, mostly from within the medical community. Some doctors are not eager to have pharmacists writing orders, even if the medications are simple. Likewise, technicians have been perceived as posing a threat to pharmacy. Some pharmacists believe that technicians may take jobs away from pharmacists or increase the liability to the pharmacist if someone who is not properly trained makes a mistake. Therefore there is disparity across the United States regarding the duties of a pharmacy technician. In some states, pharmacies limit technicians' duties to a clerk level. In other states, technicians are required to be certified as pharmacy technicians before they are employed. All technicians must be aware of what is happening legislatively within their state. To find out more information on what your state laws are pertaining to pharmacy technicians, visit the website *www.nabp.gov.* The federal government has not yet intervened to a high degree in the regulation of technicians (Chapter 2).

Clerks' duties also are expanding and changing. In some pharmacies, clerks regularly enter new prescription orders into the computer. This task previously was done exclusively by a pharmacist or technician. The pharmacist is moving into a more highly clinical role, not only counseling patients but also working with medical staff. To a degree, the technician has become what the traditional pharmacist once was—one who transcribes orders, pulls medications, and fills prescriptions. Finally, the clerk has replaced the early technicians. Some colleges are offering specialized training programs for pharmacy clerks. The introduction of trade/generic drug names and billing are some of the curriculum taught specifically for future pharmacy clerks. To learn more about future pharmacy, see Chapter 3.

DO YOU REMEMBER THESE KEY POINTS?

- Terms and definitions used within this chapter
- Common ancient beliefs, including the dogmas of those eras
- Common treatments used for conditions in earlier times
- Major persons who influenced the changes of dogmas in medicine
- The beginnings of pharmacists and pharmacy technicians
- How the roles have changed for pharmacists, pharmacy technicians, and pharmacy clerks
- New standards being required of today's technicians
- The use of protocol in setting standards in medicine and pharmacy

MULTIPLE CHOICE QUESTIONS

1. _____ is known as the father of genetics.
   A. Hippocrates
   B. Paracelsus
   C. Mendel
   D. A pharmacist

2. Which of the following choices best describes sources of materials for remedies in ancient times?
   A. Chemicals, minerals, vitamins
   B. Minerals, animals, prayer
   C. Minerals, animals, plants
   D. Plants, seeds, leaves

3. The best definition for dogma would be _____.
   A. A system of beliefs that is considered the absolute truth whether it is truly wrong or not
   B. A type of herbal remedy used in ancient times
   C. A certain way of treating patients
   D. A belief that only certain treatment is proper based on religion

4. Taking new prescriptions and entering them into the computer are tasks a _____ can do.
   A. Pharmacist
   B. Pharmacy technician
   C. Pharmacy clerk
   D. All of the above

5. The time when pharmacies were owned and run by pharmacists was _____.
   A. After the sixteenth century
   B. After the Civil War
   C. After World War I
   D. After World War II

6. Doctors used to perform all of the following tasks except _____.
   A. Mend farm animals
   B. Dispense drugs
   C. Prepare drugs
   D. Use prayer for healing

7. Opium and alcohol were once used to _____.
   A. Desensitize a person from pain
   B. Help ease depression
   C. Sedate patients with minor pain
   D. All of the above

8. Apothecary means _____.
   A. Pharmacist
   B. Pharmacy
   C. Doctor
   D. Drug

9. _____ is known as the father of medicine.
   A. Hippocrates
   B. Paracelsus
   C. Mendel
   D. Aristotle

10. Trephining was the technique of _____.
    A. Bloodletting to rid the body of toxins
    B. Prayer to rid the body of sickness
    C. Making an incision into the skull to release poison and/or evil spirits
    D. The making of opium and alcohol

TRUE/FALSE **If a statement is false, then change it to make it true.**

_____ 1. In ancient times, plants were the only available remedies for illness.

_____ 2. Bloodletting was a short-lived treatment because of many deaths.

_____ 3. Sometimes families of the "early" pharmacists assisted behind the counter.

_____ 4. Shamans were medicine men who communicated with the spirits.

_____ 5. The roles of pharmacy technicians have changed little since their beginning.

_____ 6. Plants given to ill patients in early times resembled the organ being treated.

_____ 7. Pharmacists have little contact with patients in today's pharmacy.

_____ 8. Only pharmacists can fill prescriptions.

_____ 9. Over the years, the pharmacy technician's job description has remained the same.

_____ 10. The concept of the four basic elements of life (air, water, fire, and earth) was created by Hippocrates in the late fifth century BC.

TECHNICIAN'S CORNER   Write a brief summary on the new types of advancements that are occurring in medicine today. Do any of the dogmas that plagued ancient civilizations affect current beliefs?

BIBLIOGRAPHY

Anderson MJ, Stephenson KF: *Scientists of the ancient world,* Springfield, NJ, 1999, Enslow.

Ballington DA: *Pharmacy practice for technicians,* ed 2, St Paul, Minn, 2002, EMC/Paradigm.

Moulton C, editor: *Ancient Greece and Rome,* vol 3, New York, 1998, Simon & Schuster.

Narcto D: *The complete history of ancient Greece,* San Diego, 2001, Greenhaven Press.

Suplee C: *Milestones of science,* Washington, DC, 2000, National Geographic.

WEBSITES

FOR MORE INFORMATION ON TOPICS COVERED

http://nobelprize.org/nobel_prizes/medicine/laureates/
www.nida.nih.gov
www.pasteur.fr/english
www.thinkquest.org

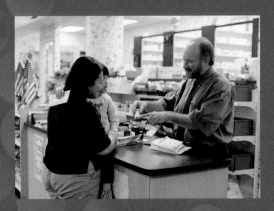

Law and Ethics of Pharmacy

Objectives

UPON COMPLETING THIS CHAPTER, YOU SHOULD BE ABLE TO DO THE FOLLOWING:

- List the history of federal law in chronological order.

- Explain which law prevails among state, federal, and local laws.

- Define the functions of the Food and Drug Administration (FDA) and Drug Enforcement Administration (DEA).

- Describe the FDA reporting process of adverse reactions.

- Explain the necessary forms and regulations used for controlled substances.

- List the current laws pertaining to ordering stock and required record keeping.

- Explain the difference between technicians' tasks and pharmacists' responsibilities.

- Identify the major laws within which technicians need to work when performing nondiscretionary functions in a pharmacy.

- Explain how to verify a DEA number.

- List who can prescribe medications/devices.

- Define the responsibilities of pharmacy personnel as they apply to morals, ethics, and liabilities.

- Describe the implications of the new Health Insurance Portability and Accountability Act laws that are in effect as of 2003.

Adulteration *The mishandling of medication that can lead to contamination and cause injury or illness to the consumer*

Board of pharmacy *State board that regulates pharmaceutical practice*

Controlled substance *Any substance that is similar to the structures of drugs in schedule I or II, primarily stimulants, depressants, and hallucinogens*

Drug Enforcement Administration *Federal agency within the Department of Justice that enforces laws against the misuse of controlled substances*

Drug Facts and Comparisons *Reference book found in all pharmacies containing detailed information on all medications*

Food and Drug Administration *Federal agency within the Department of Health and Human Services that regulates the manufacture and safeguarding of medications*

Health Insurance Portability and Accountability Act of 1996 *Federal act for protecting patients' rights*

Legend drug *Drug that requires a prescription for dispensing*

Misbranding *Deceptive or misleading labeling of a product that may lead the consumer to believe that the product will cure an illness*

Monograph *Medication information sheet provided by the manufacturer that includes side effects, dosage forms, indications, and other important information*

Narcotic *A drug (such as opium) that in moderate doses dulls the senses, relieves pain, and induces profound sleep but in excessive doses causes stupor, coma, or convulsions. This may include drugs such as marijuana or LSD (lysergic acid diethylamide). Opium, opiates (derivatives of opium), and opioids are included.*

Over-the-counter medication *Medication that can be purchased without a prescription; nonlegend medications*

Pharmacy Technician Certification Board *National board for the certification of pharmacy technicians*

Physician's Desk Reference *Reference book of medications*

T HE PRACTICE OF PHARMACY is governed by a series of laws, regulations, and rules enforced by federal, state, and local government. Pharmacy is also subject to rules made by institutions and/or pharmacy management at each pharmacy site. The number of rules and regulations is staggering, and most of us cannot easily decipher the legal tangle of words; however, we are required to follow these rules and regulations. Therefore, this chapter presents the most basic of these laws and regulations as they pertain to pharmacy, pharmacists, and especially the technician. A good understanding of these laws is necessary to pass the Pharmacy Technician Certification Board examination, and more important, it is necessary to know your responsibilities when working in pharmacy. The laws are described in chronological order along with a short description of how and why each one was put into place. Common record-keeping practices are covered. The legal liabilities of pharmacists and technicians are explained. Morals and ethics are discussed at the end of this section because they play a vital role in the decisions that technicians will make in pharmacy.

Following is a list of well-known federal laws in chronological order that will be explained in detail within this chapter:

1906 Federal Food and Drug Act
1912 International Opium Convention
1914 Harrison Narcotic Act
1938 Food, Drug, and Cosmetic Act
1951 Durham-Humphrey Amendment
1962 Kefauver-Harris Amendments (thalidomide disaster)
1970 Comprehensive Drug Abuse Prevention and Control Act
1970 Poison Prevention Packaging Act
1983 Orphan Drug Act
1987 Prescription Drug Marketing Act
1990 Anabolic Steroids Control Act
1990 Omnibus Budget Reconciliation Act (OBRA '90)
1996 Health Insurance Portability and Accountability Act (HIPAA)
2005 Combat Meth Act

Description of Laws

What is an *act?* An act is defined as "a statutory plan passed by Congress or any legislature which is a "bill" until en**act**ed and becomes law." (www.law.com) An *amendment* is a change in the original act or law. The following examples of description are brief because the various acts and amendments encompass broader descriptions. Further reading is suggested to gain a deeper insight into the laws that pertain to pharmacy and patient rights.

1906 FEDERAL FOOD AND DRUG ACT

The 1906 Federal Food and Drug Act was one of the first laws enacted to stop the sale of inaccurately labeled drugs. All manufacturers were required to put truthful information on the label before selling their drugs. Although this act was well intentioned, there were many drugs that still made their way onto the market because of continued false claims regarding their effectiveness. Additional changes were made to this act that ultimately required manufacturers to prove the effectiveness of the drugs through methods such as scientific studies. These changes are summarized in the listed acts that follow. In 1970 the Federal Food and Drug Act was rewritten to incorporate all the changes.

1914 HARRISON NARCOTIC ACT

By 1912, international meetings were being held to curb the rise in controlled substances trafficking. The International Opium Convention of 1912 was one of these meetings. Limitations on opium transport and use were attempted. The Harrison Narcotic Act of 1914 was enacted because of the excessive number of opium addicts in the United States. Individuals could no longer obtain opium without a prescription, and it became harder to get.

1938 FOOD, DRUG, AND COSMETIC ACT

The 1938 Food, Drug, and Cosmetic Act was enacted because the earlier Federal Food and Drug Act of 1906 was not worded strictly enough and did not include cosmetics. Two important terms were *adulteration* and *misbranding.* For example, false or exaggerated claims commonly were placed on a drug label and often misled the consumer. This was a breach of misbranding. All controlled substances were required to be labeled "Warning: May be habit forming." This act also provided the legal status for the Food and Drug Administration (FDA). Adulteration deals with the preparation and/or storage of a medication. Mishandling of the food or drug may cause injury or even death to a consumer. This act defined the exact labeling for products and defined misbranding and adulteration as being illegal. The new law also required drug companies to include package inserts and directions to the consumer regarding use.

1951 DURHAM-HUMPHREY AMENDMENT

The 1951 Durham-Humphrey Amendment added more instructions for drug companies and required the labeling "Caution: Federal law prohibits dispensing without a prescription." Under this amendment, certain drugs require a doctor's order and supervision. This amendment also made the initial distinction between legend drugs (by prescription only) and over-the-counter medications that do not require a physician's order (nonlegend drugs).

1962 KEFAUVER-HARRIS AMENDMENTS

The Kefauver-Harris Amendments were enacted in 1962 in an attempt to ensure the safety and effectiveness of all new drugs on the market. The burden was put on the drug manufacturing companies as good manufacturing practices were put into place. One example of the effectiveness of the FDA is illustrated by its role in preventing the sale of thalidomide in the United States. In Europe, persons were taking this new medication to help them sleep. In Europe in 1962, women who had taken thalidomide while pregnant gave birth to children with severe defects including the absence of limbs. In the United States, however, few cases occurred because of the FDA ban on thalidomide. Consumers became aware that drug companies were not doing enough to test the drugs they were marketing. More laws ensued after the thalidomide tragedy to better safeguard the public and greatly increase the time and money spent on testing a drug for its safety and effectiveness.

1970 COMPREHENSIVE DRUG ABUSE PREVENTION AND CONTROL ACT

The Drug Enforcement Administration (DEA) was formed to enforce the laws concerning controlled substances and their distribution. A stair-step schedule of controlled substances was introduced. The stair-step schedule of controlled substances requires stricter rules as the drug rating increases. Therefore a schedule V drug requires less documentation than a schedule II drug.

1970 THE POISON PREVENTION PACKAGING ACT

This act requires manufacturers and pharmacies to place all medications with childproof caps. This includes both over-the-counter and legend drugs. The standard specifies that medication should not be able to be opened by at least 80% of children under the age of 5 and that at least 90% of adults should be able to open them. Exceptions to this act include physician requests for non-child proof caps for their patients, certain legend medications, hospitalized patients, or at the specific request of the patient.

1983 ORPHAN DRUG ACT

The 1983 Orphan Drug Act allowed drug companies to bypass the lengthy time requirements of testing a new drug and the costs that accompanied testing to provide a medication to persons who had a rare disease. Before this act, companies had no incentive to find medications and spend millions of dollars and many

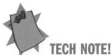

years of trials to treat a disease that affected a small portion of the population. Therefore, many of the restrictions were waived for diseases that affected fewer than 200,000 persons in the United States. The act also covered diseases that affected more than 200,000 persons if it could be proved that the cost of developing and testing a drug could not be recovered by the eventual sales.

1987 PRESCRIPTION DRUG MARKETING ACT

One of the main labeling changes required by the 1987 Prescription Drug Marketing Act controlled the use of drugs in animals. Until 1987, many drugs were sold over the counter (OTC) in feed stores for use in animals without any restrictions. This new act required the labeling "Caution: Federal law restricts this drug to use by or on the order of a licensed veterinarian." Therefore, veterinarians now must write prescriptions before persons can buy drugs for their animals.

1990 OMNIBUS BUDGET RECONCILIATION ACT

Passed by the U.S. Congress, OBRA '90 deals specifically with practicing pharmacists. The law came about because of reimbursement regulations for persons who are covered under Medicaid or Medicare insurance. OBRA '90 deals with the specifics of reimbursement for medications, the bottom line that has affected pharmacy. This act states that a pharmacist must offer to counsel (at the time of purchase) all patients who receive new prescriptions. This requirement was to ensure that all medications being prescribed to patients would be investigated for any problems, interactions, possible allergic reactions, and so forth. All patients must be given information on the drug that they are taking, its name, when to take it, how long to take it and any side effects or possible interactions. If these provisions are not met, the board of pharmacy that oversees the compliance of OBRA '90 can fine pharmacies and pharmacists.

1996 HEALTH INSURANCE PORTABILITY AND ACCOUNTABILITY ACT

The Health Insurance Portability and Accountability Act of 1996 (HIPAA) is a bill that has been implemented only partially. Specifically, this bill deals with a patient's right to continuance of health insurance even when changing employers. Recently, however, Congress has placed a date on many new regulations that will affect almost all areas of medicine, including pharmacy. As of April 14, 2003, major changes became required of pharmacies to ensure the privacy rights of patients. HIPAA will affect pharmacy technicians in many ways because technicians have direct knowledge of patients' medical information each day. Most of the changes are related to implementing consent forms that will need to be signed by patients before any information can be accessed. This pertains to releasing patients' information outside the pharmacy or hospital and requiring consent forms within the hospital.

The effects of having to implement computer programs, generate forms, and code sensitive information relating to the patient's medical history are just some of the many changes that will shape pharmacy operations of the future. Not all changes that need to be made have been completed, and many have not begun. Also, the impact on the cost to health care is not fully known at this time. For technicians to keep abreast of all new laws such as HIPAA that come into effect in the future is important because they can be held liable if they do not work within these guidelines.

2005 COMBAT METH ACT

Until 2004, the drug pseudoephedrine was sold OTC as a decongestant and was not limited in quantity for purchase by the consumer. Several different manufacturers produce this drug, and it was stocked outside the pharmacy on shelves of every store that carried cold remedies. The OTC status of pseudoephedrine has changed since the U.S. government has become aware of its use as an ingredient in the preparation of methamphetamines.

Congress passed a bill named the Combat Meth Act of 2005 in response to this problem. This bill addresses all areas of the manufacturing, law enforcement, and sale of this drug. Although pseudoephedrine still is labeled as a "no controlled substance," it has several strict guidelines. According to these guidelines, only a licensed pharmacist or technician may dispense, sell, or distribute this drug. The maximum amount a person may have in possession is 9 g within a 30-day period. Beyond these guidelines, each state has responded by enforcing controls over the sale of pseudoephedrine. Drug enforcement also is taking place worldwide in countries such as Canada, Germany, and the Netherlands. Many of the pharmacy regulations range from requiring seeing a picture identification and having the consumer sign a log book for the amount bought to requiring a prescription. Even so, the court systems are battling over the final judgment of this drug because it is a popular antihistamine. Drug companies are sure to be affected adversely if more constraints are placed on the purchase of pseudoephedrine. For a quick overview of other Pharmacy-Related Acts, see Table 2-1.

Food and Drug Administration/Drug Enforcement Administration

Two government agencies that are important with respect to pharmacy are the FDA and DEA. The FDA was created under the Department of Health and Human Services. The main functions of the FDA are to enforce the guidelines for manufacturers to ensure the safety and effectiveness of medications. Under the Food, Drug, and Cosmetic Act are standards that prohibit misbranding and adulteration or misleading labeling of any products before they are given to consumers. Any food, drug, or product that contains any avoidable, added, poisonous, or deleterious substance is unsafe and is considered adulterated. The term *misbranding* includes the following provisions. The Food, Drug, and Cosmetic Act (section 502) ensures that the following information is given to the public:

1. Mandatory food labeling
2. Standards of identity
3. Imitation foods
4. Nutritional information for special dietary foods
5. False or misleading statements about product

A few examples of misleading labeling would be the following:

1. Incorrect, inadequate, or incomplete identification
2. Unsubstantiated claims of therapeutic value
3. Inaccuracies concerning condition, state, treatment size, shape, or style
4. Substitution of parts or material
5. Ambiguity, half-truths, and trade puffery
6. Failure to reveal material facts, consequences that may result from use, or existence of difference of opinion

The other enforcement department is the DEA. This entity was created later under the Department of Justice. The function of the DEA is to prevent illegal distribution and misuse of controlled substances. The DEA also issues licenses to practitioners, pharmacies, and manufacturers of controlled substances. Each agency plays a different part in law enforcement, but the agencies work together

TABLE 2-1 Additional Pharmacy-Related Acts

Date	Act	Abbreviation	Brief description
1967	Fair Packaging and Labeling Act	FPLA	Label must show net contents; name and place of business of the manufacturer, packer, or distributor; and net quantity of contents in terms of weight, measure, or numerical count. Measurement must be in metric and U.S. units.
1972	Drug Listing Act	DLA	The act provides the commission of the Food and Drug Administration accurate list of all drugs manufactured, prepared, propagated, compounded, or processed by a drug establishment regulated under the administration. This act amends the Food, Drug, and Cosmetic Act and prevents unfair or deceptive packaging and labeling.
1990	Anabolic Steroids Control Act	ASCA	The act helped to stiffen regulations on abuse problems because of misuse by athletes.
1990	The Humanitarian Device Exemption-Safe Medical Devices Act	SMDA	The act encourages the discovery and use of devices intended to benefit patients in the treatment and diagnosis of diseases or conditions that affect fewer than 4000 individuals in the United States.
1990	Nutrition Labeling & Education Act	NLEA	This act covers food items and their labeling; vitamins, minerals, or other nutrients are on the label and in some cases are highlighted.
1994	Dietary Supplement Health and Education Act	DSHEA	The act better defines the term *dietary supplements* to include herbs such as ginseng, garlic, fish oil, psyllium, enzymes, glandulars, and mixtures of these. Consumers must be informed of health-related benefits. The manufacture of these supplements is held under the same regulations. Labels cannot mislead the consumer. Labels must include nutritional values.
1997	Food and Drug Administration Modernization Act	FDAMA	New drugs are being reviewed and released into the public faster. Millions of persons have a wider and more timely access to information on new medications.

when the DEA must get a determination on new drugs and the level at which they should be controlled.

FDA REPORTING PROCESS AND ADVERSE REACTIONS

The FDA has a toll-free number (1-800-FDA-1088) for reporting any defect found in OTC medications or any drug problem of which persons become aware.

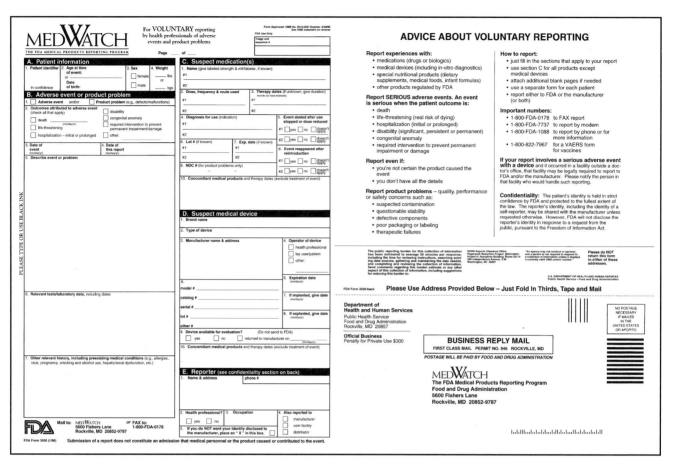

FIGURE 2-1 Drug Enforcement Administration MedWatch form.

A technician or pharmacist also has this number available to report any problems with a drug, whether it is OTC or legend (prescription). A product that looks different from its normal package should be reported. Adverse reactions also should be reported to the FDA and to the state poison control center. Any medication reaction that may cause disability, hospitalization, or death should be reported along with any less disabling type of reaction such as fainting or other types of reactions that may not have been covered in the drug monograph. MedWatch is the program under the FDA that allows consumers and health care professionals to report discrepancies or adverse reactions with medications. The form for such reports may be found in the *Physician's Desk Reference* (also known as the PDR) and in *Drug Facts and Comparisons*. The patient's identity is kept confidential (Figure 2-1).

Controlled Substances

Controlled substances, more commonly known as narcotics, are substances that are addictive and have a potential to be abused. Controlled substances are derived from opium or opium-like substances. Opium comes from the poppy plant and is well known for its analgesic effects and its effects on mood and behavior. Opiates, such as codeine and morphine, are substances created from opium, whereas opioids are controlled substances that are produced synthetically in a laboratory. All opiates and opioids are addictive. When consumed over time, a person can build up a tolerance to their effects and require increased doses. Each type of controlled substance is assigned a rating that depends on its addiction potential. Figure 2-2 gives an example of a labeled narcotic.

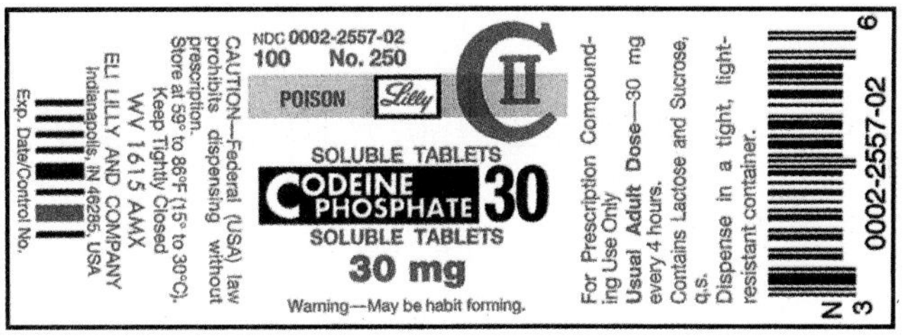

FIGURE 2-2 Codeine label showing C-II imprint.

TABLE 2-2 Three Methods of Filing Controlled Substances and Legend Drugs

System	Drawer I	Drawer II	Drawer III
1	C-II separate	C-III, C-IV, C-V	All other prescriptions
2	C-II separate	C-III, C-IV, C-V* and all legend drugs	
3	C-II, C-III, C-IV, C-V*		All other prescriptions

*If any C-III, C-IV, or C-V controlled drugs are kept with noncontrolled drugs (System 2) or mixed with C-II drugs (System 3), they must be stamped with a red "C" for easy identification. All records must be kept on site for no less than 2 years. Many states, however, have longer requirements for keeping records; remember that the strictest law is the one that must be followed. When taking inventory, one must have exact counts of C-II substances at all times. The final count can be inventoried only by a *licensed pharmacist.*

RATINGS OF SCHEDULED (CONTROLLED) SUBSTANCES

The letter *C* (meaning controlled substance) is used in addition to Roman numerals to indicate the addictiveness or abuse potential of controlled substances. In 1970 the U.S. Congress established five levels of control based on the potential for abuse. The strongest in terms of abuse potential are C-I drugs. These include such drugs as D-lysergic acid diethylamide (LSD) and heroin. Pharmacies do not stock drugs in the C-I class because they have not been determined by the FDA to have any medicinal use in the United States. Therefore, doctors cannot prescribe C-I drugs for their patients. All medicinal controlled substances are placed in the following four categories: C-II, C-III, C-IV, and C-V. Table 2-2 shows the schedule, types of medications, and abuse potential for each level of controlled substances.

In some states, C-V medications (referred to as exempt controlled substances) are kept OTC because of the low potential of abuse, whereas all states are required to lock up C-II drugs because of their high potential of abuse. However, for these exempt controlled substances there are specific rules governing the quantity kept on hand and records that need to be retained by the pharmacy on their purchase by consumers. The U.S. attorney general has the authority to decide under which schedule a drug should be placed. The decision is made after careful consideration is given to scientific findings and input from various authorities on the possible dependency potential of each agent. Some drugs may be labeled under two different schedules because the dose may alter the dependency of the drug. Sometimes, controlled substances can be reevaluated; for example, dronabinol previously was rated as a C-II drug but is now a C-III drug. In contrast, Percodan (a combination of oxycodone hydrochloride, oxycodone terephthalate, and aspirin) previously was rated as a C-III and has been upgraded to a C-II.

Certain narcotics are used for procedures in hospitals, such as opium (morphine) in its natural form and cocaine. Cocaine has the ability to vasoconstrict and is used to stop bleeding.

REGISTRATION REQUIRED FOR MAINTAINING NARCOTICS

The DEA has three main registration forms used in the regulation of controlled substances. Only Form 224 is needed by the pharmacy to dispense controlled substances. Uses of other forms are as follows:

1. To manufacture or distribute controlled substances: Form 225
2. To run a controlled substances treatment program or compound controlled substances: Form 363
3. To dispense controlled substances: Form 224

REFILLING CONTROLLED SUBSTANCES

Strict guidelines control the amount of controlled substances that can be refilled. Drugs with a rating of C-III or C-IV can be refilled if indicated by the physician or authorized prescriber but only to a maximum of 5 times or within 6 months from the original order, whichever comes first. In addition, the amount ordered on the refills may not exceed the original order. A record must be kept of controlled substance refills indicating the pharmacist's initials and the date it was dispensed.

ORDERING CONTROLLED SUBSTANCES

A pharmacy has two ways to obtain schedule II controlled substances from a distributor. A DEA Form 222 (Figure 2-3) must be filled out by the receiving pharmacist. This form must be filled out only with a pen, typewriter, or an indelible pencil. The top copy and the middle (DEA) copy with the carbon paper are sent to the supplier or manufacturer by the pharmacy receiving the drugs. Filing electronically is also possible. This electronic order can be done online. Digital signatures are issued by the DEA and include a unique number that the purchaser assigns to track the order. The number is in a nine-character format—the last two digits of the year, X, and the six characters as selected by the purchaser. An electronic order can include controlled substances that are not in schedules I and II and noncontrolled substances. The purchaser must create a record of the quantity received and the date received. This record must be linked electronically to the original order and archived.

The pharmacy retains the bottom copy. When the medication is shipped to the pharmacy, the middle (DEA) copy is forwarded to the DEA to prove that the medication is accounted for properly. When the pharmacy receives the controlled substances, the pharmacist compares the pharmacy's copy of Form 222 with the invoice and signs both. The invoice and the form are stapled together and retained for 7 years. If any error is made, the form becomes invalid but must be retained for reference; therefore, you cannot erase mistakes or throw away the form. When returning any C-II drugs, the pharmacy must have the manufacturer or wholesaler fill out the same form (Form 222) to request the controlled substance, and the pharmacy then is the provider who retains the top copy and sends the middle copy to the DEA. Other controlled substances (C-III, C-IV, and C-V) are ordered on normal invoice forms, but invoices must be filed and retained for possible DEA or state board of pharmacy inspection. These should be kept separate from other nonscheduled drugs for easy retrieval. Once the scheduled drugs are received, the invoice forms for schedules III to V must be kept for no less than 2 years.

RECORD KEEPING

A pharmacy has three methods of filing controlled substances and legend drugs, as shown in Table 2-3. Although federal law allows any one of these three

See Reverse of PURCHASER'S Copy for Instructions	No order form may be issued for Schedule I and II substances unless a completed application form has been received, (21 CFR 1305.04).	OMB APPROVAL No. 1117-0010

TO: *(Name of Supplier)*   STREET ADDRESS

CITY and STATE   DATE   **TO BE FILLED IN BY SUPPLIER**
SUPPLIERS DEA REGISTRATION No.

L I N E No.	No. of Packages	Size of Package	**TO BE FILLED IN BY PURCHASER** Name of Item	National Drug Code	Packages Shipped	Date Shipped
1						
2						
3						
4						
5						
6						
7						
8						
9						
10						

◄ **LAST LINE COMPLETED** *(MUST BE 10 OR LESS)* SIGNATURE OF PURCHASER OR ATTORNEY OR AGENT

Date Issued **20010101**   DEA Registration No. **DEAREGNO**   Name and Address of Registrant
VOID VOID VOID
Schedules **XXXXXXXXXXXX**   VOID VOID VOID
VOID VOID VOID
Registered as a **XXXXXXXXXXXX**   No. of this Order Form **000000005**   VOID VOID VOID
VOID VOID VOID

DEA Form -222 (Oct. 2004)   **U.S. OFFICIAL ORDER FORMS - SCHEDULES I & II**
DRUG ENFORCEMENT ADMINISTRATION
SUPPLIER'S Copy 1   **107051797**

FIGURE 2-3 Drug Enforcement Administration Form 222.

methods to be used, a state board of pharmacy may require a specific one. In addition to the filing of controlled medications, every time a controlled substance is issued to a patient or nursing station, it must be logged out of the pharmacy stock (Figure 2-4). Levels are first counted, the amount of each drug must be correct. Then the technician or pharmacist will subtract the amount taken. Again, the remaining stock is double checked for accuracy. This same standard holds true for returning items or adding new stock to the inventory.

Monographs

Under the FDA labeling regulations, the following information must be available in monographs, also known as package inserts, because of the lack of room on the drug container. Doctors refer to this information in the *Physicians' Desk Reference,* and it also is contained in the *Drug Facts and Comparisons* reference book in the pharmacy (see Chapter 6). All information is required to give the date of the most recent revision. As new information is found or reported, new monographs are written. Thus it is important to have an updated copy of the *Physicians' Desk Reference* and *Drug Facts and Comparisons* in the pharmacy. If you do not have one available, you always can read the package insert from the medication container to find the most recent information. The type of information contained in a package insert follows.

TABLE 2-3 Typical Controlled Substances

Drug level	Type of medication Generic name	Trade name	Potential for abuse
C-I		LSD Crack Mescaline Heroin	Drugs that have no accepted medical use in the United States and have a very high abuse potential
C-II	Meperidine Codeine Morphine Oxycodone/APAP Oxycodone/ASA Amphetamines Hydromorphone Methadone Opium Methylphenidate Fentanyl	Demerol Percocet Percodan Dilaudid Ritalin Duragesic	High potential for abuse; used for medicinal purposes; abuse may lead to severe psychological or physical dependence

C-III	Hydrocodone/
	  APAP
	Acetaminophen/
	  codeine
	Hydrocodone/
	  ibuprofen
		Vicodin
		
		Tylenol/
		  Codeine
		Vicoprofen
			The potential for abuse under this schedule is less than that of controlled substances under C-II; abuse may lead to moderate or low physical dependence or high psychological dependence. Most of the schedule III drugs are combination narcotics.

C-IV	Diazepam Lorazepam Pentazocine Chlordiazepoxide Chloral hydrate Flurazepam Phenobarbital	Valium Ativan Talwin Librium Dalmane	The potential for abuse is low compared with that of C-III drugs; abuse may lead to limited physical or psychological dependence compared with C-III drugs.

C-V	Diphenoxylate/
	  atropine
	Guaifenesin/
	  codeine
	Promethazine/
	  codeine
		Lomotil
		
		Robitussin
		  AC
		Phenergan/
		  Codeine
			Low potential for abuse in relation to C-IV drugs; abuse may lead to limited physical or psychological dependence compared with C-IV drugs.

APAP, Acetyl-*p*-aminophenol (acetaminophen); *ASA,* acetylsalicylic acid (aspirin).

DESCRIPTION

The basic description of the medication indicates the basic chemical structure, including pH, and may show the chemical structure in picture form. Additional information on chemicals, including pH, can be found in Chapter 30.

CLINICAL PHARMACOLOGY

The clinical pharmacology section lists the drug action, drug interaction, and any other information related to the action of the medication.

INDICATIONS AND USAGE

The indications and usage section describes the specific conditions that the medication is used to prevent or treat. Some medications cannot treat the condition

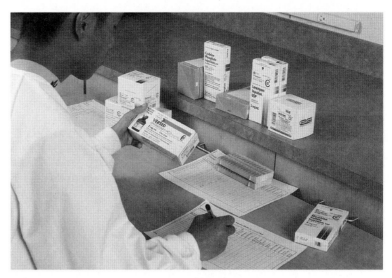

FIGURE 2-4 All controlled substances must be counted and logged in or out in ink or other nonerasable pen.

but are used to relieve the symptoms of the condition. Side effects of some medications are used for treating some diseases.

CONTRAINDICATIONS

The section on contraindications explains the types of persons who should not use the medication. Studies have shown that certain patients such as diabetic patients or patients taking certain medications have a severe reaction if they take the medication. Many times contraindications include a class of drugs to be avoided rather than one specific drug that a patient might be taking.

WARNINGS

The warnings heading lists serious side effects of the medication and what should be done if the patient experiences such side effects. Warnings are not necessarily contraindications but fall close to that heading. The prescriber must be aware of potential problems of the drug before prescribing it to a patient.

PRECAUTIONS

The precautions section gives a list of information about possible side effects that the patient should know when taking the medication. Cautions such as "Do not operate any heavy machinery" or "Do not drink alcohol while taking this medication" are the types of information provided on auxiliary labels.

DRUG ABUSE AND DEPENDENCE

If patients have shown any tendency to become addicted to the medication or if the medication has been found to be abused by patients, the information is listed in this section.

ADVERSE REACTIONS

An adverse reaction is an unexpected and possibly life-threatening reaction to a medication, such as an allergic reaction. A side effect is a possible reaction caused by the action of the drug, such as drowsiness. All possible adverse reactions to the medication are listed. In addition to listing of specific reactions, such as nausea, the percentage of persons affected by the reaction (from reported studies) is included.

DOSAGE

The recommended dosing is indicated in this section. The section usually specifies by age and/or weight the most common strength of drug to administer or prescribe to the patient, along with the dosing time and interval or length. The section also gives suggested dosing regimens for patients with specific conditions.

HOW SUPPLIED

Information about how the medication is supplied often is given in chart format because it lists the varying strengths, amount of drug per container, dosage form, and whether it should be given any special considerations such as protection from light or storage in a refrigerator.

Prescription Regulations

WHO CAN PRESCRIBE?

The FDA and DEA have no authority in determining prescribers. Doctors and other medical prescribers are licensed by their governing bodies. The scope of practice is determined by their degree. For example, a podiatrist, a doctor of feet, can prescribe medications and devices that are used in treating foot conditions; a podiatrist would not and should not be prescribing heart medication. The same is true for dentists, veterinarians, and optometrists because each is an expert in a specialty and not in others. The prescribers can vary from state to state (Box 2-1); therefore the specific laws governing them are not covered. However, more states are allowing professionals such as nurse practitioners and physician assistants to prescribe a limited number of medications and/or devices. These practitioners are required to be supervised by a physician who assumes

---

BOX 2-1 PRESCRIBING AUTHORITY

Except for the footnoted prescribers, each state varies on whether prescribing is authorized, specific exceptions, for use only, in requirements, and limitations

Advanced registered RN	Neuropathic MD	Medical doctors*
Certified RN anesthetist	Nurse practitioner	Chiropractors[†]
Clinical RN specialist	OB/GYN RN	Dentist[†]
Doctor of homeopathy	Optometrist	DVM (veterinarian)[†]
Doctor of osteopathy	Pediatric RN practitioners	Doctor of podiatry[‡]
Emergency medical technician-paramedic		Physicians assistants
Midwife, nurse midwife		Psychiatric RN practitioners

*Have unlimited, independent prescribing authority in every state.
[†]Have no prescribing authority in any state.
[‡]Have independent prescribing authority limited to their specific course of practice in every state.

For a list of specifics, refer to National Board of Pharmacy 2006 Survey of Pharmacy Law.

responsibility for their prescribing methods and scope of knowledge. Each state also regulates whether it will accept out-of-state prescriptions written by practitioners who are not licensed within the state. Persons who are able to prescribe controlled drugs must be registered as a midlevel practitioner with the DEA Form 224.

WHO CAN RECEIVE A PRESCRIPTION?

Clearly, a pharmacy technician takes in prescriptions, interprets them, and fills them; the pharmacist is responsible for reviewing the prescription before dispensing. However, it is not within the scope of the pharmacy technician, at this time, to take phone orders. Often prescriptions are called in by the doctor's office. A pharmacist must translate verbal orders into written form. Also, if a patient wants a prescription transferred to another pharmacy, this must occur between licensed pharmacists or pharmacy interns. A pharmacy intern also can receive prescriptions by phone.

RECEIVING PRESCRIPTIONS FOR CONTROLLED DRUGS

Pharmacists can receive an oral prescription for a controlled drug over the phone by reducing it to written form. If the drug is a C-II substance, the pharmacist is allowed to take the order and fill the prescription following strict guidelines. The guidelines are as follows:

1. The doctor must determine that the patient needs the C-II drug and considers it to be an emergency with no alternative treatment possible.
2. The doctor cannot give a written prescription to the pharmacist. This may be because the doctor is away from the office.
3. The pharmacist must obtain all information from the doctor, including the drug name, strength, dosage form, and route of administration. The doctor's name, address, phone number, and DEA number are required.
4. The amount of the drug can be only enough to sustain the patient through the emergency period. The pharmacist should indicate on the prescription that it is being filled because of an emergency.
5. The pharmacist must make every effort to verify the doctor's authority unless he or she knows the doctor personally.
6. The prescriber has only 72 hours to produce the written prescription covering the filled prescription. If this is not done, the prescriber must be reported to the DEA.

PRESCRIPTION LABELS

The information on a prescription label differs from what is required on a prescription order. Two necessary components for the prescription label are the pharmacy information and patient information. Samples of these are given in Figure 2-5. The two different components are listed as follows:

Component 1
1. Name of pharmacy
2. Address of pharmacy
3. Name of prescriber
4. Date prescription was filled

Component 2
1. Name of patient
2. Directions
3. Any cautions described or provided on auxiliary labels
4. Refill information

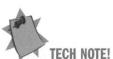

TECH NOTE!

Many states are adopting a new type of controlled substance prescription, which has several security features designed to stop forgery or fraud with a doctor's intended order. For example, the word *void* will appear if scanned, photocopied, or faxed. Watermarks appear when held up to light. Any exposed surface to ink solvents causes a void pattern to appear. These are a few of the many features states are beginning to adopt. The DEA must approve the printer, but there is no specific format because each state may adopt its own features, colors, or size. Check with your state's Board of Pharmacy for more information.

Thomas Pharmacy
519 Barney Lane
Clarksville, TN 03542
Phone: 931-555-1122

Patient: Christopher Gilbert
RX # G03011984

Dosage: Clonazepam 1mg tablets   Quantity #30

Take 1 tablet by mouth at bedtime

Refills 0
Filled: 12/12/07   Expiration date: 09/25/09 *th*
Dr. Ronald Belham

A

Dr. Tracy Crum   **11287 E Villanova Drive**
DEA#AC1243170   **Aurora, CO 30358**
                                                         Phone: 303-555-1212

Date: *12/12/07*

Patient's name: Billie Jones   Age: *83 yrs*
Address: 125 Grand Canyon Drive, Tucson, Arizona 85707

Rx:
                  K-Dur 20 mEq tab
                  1 qd   #90

Substitution permitted Y N
Refills 1 2 3 4 5 6 7 8 9   Signature____Tracy L Crum
MD_____

B

FIGURE 2-5 **A,** Sample of information necessary on a patient prescription label. **B,** Sample of information on a doctor's prescription order.

BOX 2-2 DRUGS REQUIRING ADDITIONAL INFORMATION

Estrogens
Injectable contraceptives
Intrauterine devices
Oral contraceptives
Progestational drugs
Retinoids

Special Labeling

Certain drugs require that additional information be given to a patient because of the possibility of teratogenicity (genetic harm) to an unborn fetus. These instructions are given out by the prescriber or the pharmacy dispensing the medication (Box 2-2).

DRUG ENFORCEMENT ADMINISTRATION VERIFICATION

All prescribers must be registered with the DEA to write prescriptions for controlled substances. When approved, the prescribers are given a nine-character identification code. This code is different for each prescriber. There is a method

BOX 2-3 DRUG ENFORCEMENT ADMINISTRATION VERIFICATION PROCESS

Dr. Tom Johnson writes an order for Tylenol #3. The doctor's DEA number is AJ1234892. To verify physician's DEA number:

Step 1 Make sure the first letter is either A, B, or M.
Step 2 The second letter must be the first letter of the prescriber's last name (in this case, J for Johnston).
Step 3 Add the first, third, and fifth number in the DEA set (1 + 3 + 8 = 12).
Step 4 Add the second, fourth, and sixth number and then multiply by 2: (2 + 4 + 9 = 15; 15 × 2 = 30).
Step 5 Add the two sums together (12 + 30 = 42).
Step 6 The last digit "2" from your total must match the last number in the DEA set. In this case all steps match; therefore the number is good.

TABLE 2-4 Drugs That Can Be Packaged in Non–Child-Resistant Bottles

Drug	Dosage form	Restriction on strength of drug
Betamethasone	Tablet	X
Cholestyramine	Powder	X
Colestipol	Powder	X
Erythromycin (E.E.S.)	Tablet, granules	X
Isosorbide dinitrate (less than 10 mg)	Sublingual, chewable tablets	X
Mebendazole	Tablet	X
Methylprednisolone	Tablet	X
Nitroglycerin*	Sublingual	
Prednisone	Tablet	X
Sodium fluoride	Package	X

*Nitroglycerin is the only medication that does not have a strength limit on filling it without a childproof cap.

of verifying DEA numbers. The first two characters are composed of letters. The first is an A, B, or M followed by the first letter of the prescriber's last name. For example, for Dr. D. Wong the DEA number could begin with AW or BW. The next seven digits are composed of numbers that are added together. Following the six steps laid out in Box 2-3, one can verify a DEA number.

CHILD-RESISTANT CAPS

The Poison Prevention Packaging Act of 1970 addressed the issue of accidental poisoning of children. Most medications are required to be packaged in containers that are exceptionally hard for children to open. Hence, childproof caps were created. Unfortunately, the caps can be difficult for some adults to open as well. Therefore, some exceptions to this regulation were made because of the necessity of patients to access their medications easily (Table 2-4). In addition to these exceptions, medications can be packaged in non–child-resistant containers if certain requirements have been met. Either the prescriber, such as a doctor, will order the medication to be filled without a childproof cap, or the patient will request that the medication be filled without a childproof cap. Usually this information will be put into the patient's medical record for future reference. Some pharmacies may require the patient to sign a release form that is kept in the patient record.

TABLE 2-5 Required Patient Information

Type of facility	Patient's full name	Prescriber's name	Name and strength of drug	Date of issue	Prescription number	Expiration date	Lot and control number of drug	Manufacturer	Name of drug dispensed
Hospital	X	X	X	X	*	X	*	*	X
Community	X	X	X	X	X	X	X	X	X
Home health	X	X	X	X	X	X	X	X	X

*These areas represent information not transcribed onto the patient's computer record.
Each medication sent to the floor has manufacturer name, lot number, and expiration date on each unit dose medication. Hospital patients are not given prescription numbers but are listed in the computer under their medical record number, and a hard copy is made daily of all their medications.

MAILING PRESCRIPTION DRUGS

A common practice is to mail medications through the post office or other authorized mailing system. This option will always be available for patients with the introduction of online pharmacies and mail-order pharmacies. Rules govern the way in which drugs are mailed. When drugs are sent to the patient's home, they must be unmarked on the outside as to what the contents are. Manufacturing mailing differs between pharmacies and the manufacturer. In this case, all medications and controlled substances are allowed to be mailed as long as the recipient (pharmacy) is registered with the DEA.

RECALLED DRUGS

The manufacturer must recall items that have been found to be defective or somehow tainted. In pharmacies, there are forms used for such events. All stock must be pulled from the shelves following the guidelines of the manufacturing company. The three classes of recalls are as follows:

Class 1: The highest level of recall dealing with products that could cause serious or even fatal harm
Class 2: The next level dealing with products found to cause serious but reversible harm
Class 3: The lowest level used for products that may have a minor defect or other condition that would not harm the patient, but the drugs cannot be resold

Records and Labeling Requirements

Hospitals and community pharmacies differ in the length of time that patient records are to be kept. Both institutions are required to keep complete and accurate records of patients. For the purpose of simplicity, Table 2-5 lists outpatients (community, home health) separately from inpatients (hospital).

REPACKAGING

Unit dose medication that is prepared in the pharmacy requires the following record-keeping rules. Technicians traditionally make most of the unit dose medications in a pharmacy setting. Any medication taken from bulk packages and placed into blister packs must have the following information on each individual label:

1. Drug name (trade/generic)
2. Strength

3. Dosage form
4. Manufacturer
5. Lot number
6. Expiration date

All information must be logged into a binder or a system in which such information can be retrieved easily. For more information on repackaging, refer to Chapter 12.

State Laws

Each state has its own set of laws that pharmacists, interns, pharmacy technicians, and clerks must follow when working in the pharmacy. You must know the regulations of your state. All pharmacy personnel should become familiar with the laws by obtaining the regulations booklet from their state board of pharmacy. You will notice that many states have laws that differ from federal law. Remember that the strictest law is the one you follow. Therefore, if the FDA states that you must keep records for no less than 2 years but your state regulations require 7 years for inpatient records, then you would follow the strictest regulation, in this case your state regulation. To learn more about your specific state regulations and laws, go to your state board of pharmacy website.

Liabilities

You also should be aware of federal and state liability laws pertaining to pharmacy technicians. A patient can make various charges against a pharmacy technician if the pharmacy technician caused damage because of negligence or intentional action in the workplace. A tort is causing injury to a person intentionally or because of negligence. The word *negligence* may describe an action taken without the forethought that should have been taken by a reasonable person; a mistake was made. For an intentional mistake, the penalty can range from criminal charges to the awarding of damages, which usually means that money is paid to the person or persons who were wrongly affected. A negligent mistake can affect a person's ability to continue to work as a technician and also may result in punitive damages (i.e., money).

Mistakes happen for many reasons. Some are because of excessive workload or possibly staffing shortages that can lead to a mishap and could be classified as a negligent tort. Criminal behavior, such as false insurance claims or diverting drugs, could be called an intentional tort and could result in imprisonment. One of the questions you should ask your employer is whether you are covered under the company legal department. If a lawsuit were to be filed with you as the plaintiff, do you know who would represent you? Many companies have lawyers that represent the company, although you should not assume that they would represent you. If you are not covered by your employer, you may want to purchase malpractice insurance. Most technicians do not have such insurance, and it is a personal preference. At the very least, be aware of what your rights and responsibilities are, including legal considerations, before entering a workplace. Based on the state in which the technician works, laws vary as they pertain to the liability of the technician. Therefore, you must check your state laws as they pertain to you. If any incidents should happen at work that you might be involved in or witness to, you should follow these guidelines:

1. Review your state's regulations
2. Understand employer's rules and practices
3. Define scope of employment

TECH ALERT!

More states are enacting laws to make technicians accountable for their actions in the pharmacy. Previously, pharmacists would have to take the responsibility for any mistakes even if the mistake were caused by the technician. This is not true any longer; a technician can lose his or her license, certification, and job and may have to pay court fees. This of course is in addition to the possibility of having to spend time in jail if the crime is bad enough. Such cases are listed in pharmacy journals and on the FDA website.

In case of an "event" that takes place in the pharmacy,

1. Know who your attorney is
2. Always be careful of what you say and to whom you say it if you are ever questioned by state or federal investigators pertaining to a mishap
3. Write down in-depth notes on the facts of the event and keep them for reference

Morals versus Ethics in the Workplace

One important factor that the pharmacy technician must remember is that he or she has a clear responsibility to the patient on many levels. Patients are consumers, and as consumers they have the right to receive goods that have been handled properly and are in good condition. They also trust the pharmacy personnel with their personal information, expecting that their information will be treated as confidential and will not be discussed. Many times within a pharmacy or any work setting, employees will voice their beliefs concerning various medical procedures such as abortion, surgery, or a type of treatment. These are controversial topics, and the opinions that each person has are a part of personal morals or beliefs. Although each person has his or her own set of morals, many morals tend to coincide with others' beliefs, such as that stealing is not good.

In a workplace, however, technicians, pharmacists, and other health care workers are faced with patients who come in for help and who might have different morals. In these situations, the type of professionalism that must be shown to the patients is one's ethics. Ethics are morals in the workplace and in the public domain. When you take on the responsibility of serving the public in a setting such as the pharmacy, you take on work ethics that will guide your behavior. For instance, in a hospital setting there may be a need for medication that is used in abortions or other controversial treatments. The responsibility of the pharmacy staff is to provide services for all patients. If you have a deeply rooted belief that you believe prohibits you from participating in servicing patients, you must bring this to the attention of your supervisor.

On a lighter side, just keeping small matters in perspective can help you decide what the right choice is in many decisions. Keeping patients' information confidential and working within pharmacy laws and guidelines, including policies and procedures, will ensure that patients are getting the best service possible. One should remember that pharmacists, technicians, and clerks are there to serve the patients and customers in a professional manner at all times.

DO YOU REMEMBER THESE KEY POINTS?

- Terms and definitions covered in this chapter
- Major federal laws affecting pharmacists and pharmacy
- The differences between functions of the DEA and FDA
- Filing systems required for stock and controlled substances inventory
- Filing requirements for patients' information
- Who can write a prescription
- The legal limitations of pharmacy technicians
- Labeling requirements for repackaged medications
- How to decipher a DEA number
- Types of recalls and how to handle them
- The functions and authority of the state board of pharmacy
- The difference between morals and ethics and the importance of them
- Which medications require package inserts when dispensed

MULTIPLE CHOICE QUESTIONS

1. The amendment that required the labeling "Caution: Federal law prohibits dispensing without a prescription" was the _____.
   A. Durham-Humphrey Amendment
   B. Kefauver-Harris Amendment
   C. OBRA '90
   D. None of the above

2. What does the Orphan Drug Act do?
   A. Puts into effect stricter rules concerning controlled substances sales and distribution
   B. Allows drug companies to bypass lengthy testing to treat persons who have a rare disease
   C. Stops the use of drugs without a prescription in animals
   D. Ensures safety and effectiveness of manufacturing practices

3. The law that requires pharmacists to counsel patients on new medications is _____.
   A. OBRA '90
   B. Comprehensive Drug Abuse Prevention and Control Act
   C. Prescription Drug Marketing Act
   D. Durham-Humphrey Amendment

4. The main purpose of the FDA is to _____.
   A. Make arrests
   B. Ensure that safety and effectiveness of medications is met by manufacturers
   C. Prevent distribution and the illegal use of controlled substances
   D. Make sure all laws pertaining to physicians and pharmacists are met

5. A pharmacy that will be dispensing controlled drugs must have which one of the following forms on file with the DEA?
   A. Form 222
   B. Form 224
   C. Form 363
   D. Form 225

6. All adverse reactions should be reported to the _____.
   A. FDA
   B. DEA
   C. CIA
   D. Pharmacy management

7. The five categories of controlled substances are rated based on _____.
   A. Cost
   B. Strength
   C. Conditions that they treat
   D. Potential for abuse

8. Of the information contained in a monograph of a medication, which of the following statements best describes the information related to the action of the drug?
   A. Description
   B. Clinical pharmacology
   C. Adverse reactions
   D. Indication and usage

9. Of the types of health care providers who follow, which one is not one of the standard practitioners that all states accept?
   A. Doctors of podiatry
   B. Dentists
   C. Chiropractors
   D. Veterinarians

10. Which of the components listed is not required on a prescription label?
    A. Name, address, and phone number of the pharmacy
    B. Name, address, and phone number of the prescriber
    C. Date prescription was filled
    D. Any auxiliary stickers and/or warnings

TRUE/FALSE **If a statement is false, then change it to make it true.**

_____ 1. The thalidomide tragedy of 1962 resulted in the United States banning the drug.

_____ 2. DEA Form 222 is used to obtain controlled substances from the manufacturer or distributor.

_____ 3. Scheduled drugs such as LSD and heroin are C-I drugs and are used only in extreme cases.

_____ 4. Monographs can be found with the drug and in the *Physician's Desk Reference*.

_____ **5.** The contraindication section of the monograph explains the abuse and dependence dangers of the medication.

_____ **6.** Physicians should order only medications within their scope of practice.

_____ **7.** Pharmacy technicians can take oral prescriptions as long as there is a pharmacist on duty who gives permission for them to do so.

_____ **8.** Only pharmacists can fill out Form 222 required by the DEA in pencil.

_____ **9.** Isosorbide and nitroglycerin can be dispensed without childproof caps.

_____ **10.** A recall that is classified as Class 1 means that it is the lowest level of a recall and is used for products that contain only a minor defect.

TECHNICIAN'S CORNER

Dr. Beth Golden writes an order for the following prescription:
DEA#BG1958366
Disp: hydrocodone/acetaminophen tablets #50
Sig: Take 1 tablet q8h prn severe pain
10 refills
Determine whether this DEA number is correct, and explain each step of the checking process. List how many mistakes, if any, you find on all parts of this order.

BIBLIOGRAPHY

Ballington DA: *Pharmacy practice for technicians,* ed 2, St Paul, Minn, 2002, EMC/Paradigm.

Gray Morris D: *Calculate with confidence,* ed 4, St Louis, 2005, Elsevier.

National Association of Boards of Pharmacy: *Survey of pharmacy law*, Mount Prospect, Ill., 2005, The Association.

Nielsen JR, James JD: *Handbook of federal drug law,* ed 2, Philadelphia, 1992, Williams & Wilkins.

Potter PA, Perry AG: *Fundamentals of nursing,* ed 6, St Louis, 2004, Elsevier.

Shargel L, Mutnick A, Souney P et al: *Comprehensive pharmacy review,* ed 5, Baltimore, 2003, Lippincott Williams & Wilkins.

www.law.com

WEBSITES

www.bacteriamuseum.org
www.fda.gov
www.fda.gov/cder/
www.nabp.org

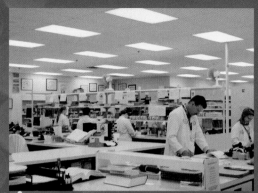

Pharmacy Associations, Certification, and Settings for Technicians

Objectives

UPON COMPLETING THIS CHAPTER, YOU SHOULD BE ABLE TO DO THE FOLLOWING:

- Discuss historical data on technicians.

- Describe current qualifications of technicians.

- Explain the term *nondiscretionary duties*.

- Explore various settings for technicians.

- Describe various pharmacy setting requirements as they apply to technicians.

- Describe how pharmacy has expanded onto the Internet.

- List the new position openings for technicians that are available in the health care field.

- Explain how networking is important in the search for a pharmacy position.

- List the organizations available to technicians.

- Determine which attributes each pharmacy organization has that are important to the technician.

- List the positive attributes of joining a pharmacy association.

- Describe the various aspects of the National Certification Examination.

- Determine the ways to approach job searching.

- Explain how the Internet can be used for research and information pertaining to pharmacy.

Certified pharmacy technician *A technician who has passed the National Certification Examination; the technician can use the abbreviation CPhT after his or her name*

Continuing education *Education beyond the basic technical education, usually required for license renewal*

Hyperalimentation *Parenteral nutrition for patients who are unable to eat solids or liquids*

Inpatient pharmacy *A pharmacy in a hospital or institutional setting*

National Association of Boards of Pharmacy *National organization for members of state boards of pharmacy*

Outpatient pharmacy *Pharmacies that serve patients in their communities; pharmacies that are not in inpatient facilities*

Parenteral medications *Medication administered by injection, such as intravenously or intramuscularly*

Pharmacy Technician Certification Board *National board for the certification of pharmacy technicians*

BECAUSE OF OUR RAPIDLY CHANGING health care system, job descriptions and educational requirements of pharmacy technicians are rapidly changing. Among the changes are increased responsibilities, the need for higher education, more legal responsibility, and even continuing education. This trend can be seen across the United States as more states require a high school diploma or general equivalency diploma in order for a person to become a registered technician, and more states have accepted the National Certification Board as their measure of the knowledge base of pharmacy technicians. Positive aspects of these changes include a wider range of jobs available, bonuses, raises in pay, and better benefits for technicians.

Each of America's 50 states has not standardized the qualifications and job descriptions for the pharmacy technician. This is also true for pharmacists because each state has different laws to which pharmacists must adhere, although the laws do not vary as much as technicians' requirements do. Therefore, each state board of pharmacy determines what the standards are and how they must be met by technicians. This one area of discrepancy is an issue that will become more defined through the continuing efforts of the boards of pharmacy over the next decade.

This chapter begins with a brief overview of the history of pharmacy, and then explores each area in the health care field pertaining to pharmacy, along with the necessary job qualifications and expectations. We also take a look at national pharmacy organizations and the benefits of pharmacy technician certification, the importance of preparing to search for a job, and the possible future roles of the pharmacy technician. This will help the student technician determine the best road to follow and the various positions the student can hold.

Historical Data

Historically, technicians have answered to a variety of titles. These include pharmacy clerk, pharmacist assistant, pharmacy aide, pharmacy technician, and pharmacy helper. Technicians have held a variety of positions. Some of the job responsibilities have been billing, ordering, stock clerk, typist, phone receptionist, troubleshooter, cashier, and errand runner. Technicians have been a part of the pharmacy field since the beginning of pharmacy, even though they were not always called pharmacy technicians (see Chapter 1). However, more recently, pharmacy managers and their respective state boards of pharmacy have been attempting to classify and clearly define the role of the pharmacy technician as the needs of pharmacy change.

Current Qualifications

Each state in the United States has its own board of pharmacy that is overseen by the National Association of Boards of Pharmacy. Each state board of pharmacy serves many functions besides registering technicians and licensing pharmacists. The board also provides consumers with a way to complain or report any problems or illegal actions they have experienced in a pharmacy. The board of pharmacy also reviews and updates current rules and regulations pertaining to pharmacy practice (see Chapter 2). The National Association of Boards of Pharmacy currently is looking into the expanded use of technicians in the pharmacy field. This examination of the current uses of technicians no doubt will reveal the skill level necessary for various types of pharmacy tasks, and ultimately changes will be made throughout each state board of pharmacy. Boards of pharmacy also may change technician-to-pharmacist ratios in pharmacy settings.

Nondiscretionary Duties

All technicians, regardless of their title, can and do perform many types of nondiscretionary duties in the pharmacy setting. As the job classification of pharmacy technicians expands, so will their duties and their knowledge of pharmacology. Nondiscretionary simply means that the final approval for any task completed in a pharmacy setting must be checked and approved by a pharmacist. This limits technicians from interpreting scientific studies, counseling patients about their current or adjunct medications, and conferring with other medical personnel about proper treatments.

Inpatient Setting Requirements

Inpatient pharmacy usually refers to those located in hospitals in which patients stay overnight or longer, depending on the procedures they require. Most departments in a hospital have medication and supplies that are specific to their department. This is supplied by the inpatient pharmacy. Therefore, inpatient pharmacies traditionally have a wider range of stock than outpatient pharmacies so that they can provide all the necessary supplies required of each department. For example, the labor and delivery unit stocks a large amount of the drug oxytocin (induces labor), whereas the intensive care unit and coronary care unit require a wide variety of cardiac medications in their stock areas. The cancer units may stock high amounts of morphine and other analgesics, whereas the pediatrics department stocks many drugs in liquid form for children. Stocking all of these areas is just one of the responsibilities of an inpatient pharmacy technician.

In addition to knowing all of the various drugs, strengths, and dosage forms, the technician must be able to react on a moment's notice when emergency (stat) orders are received by the pharmacy. The dynamics of an inpatient pharmacy can fluctuate minute to minute depending on the flow of patients into and out of the hospital. Stat doses are to be delivered within 15 minutes to the station

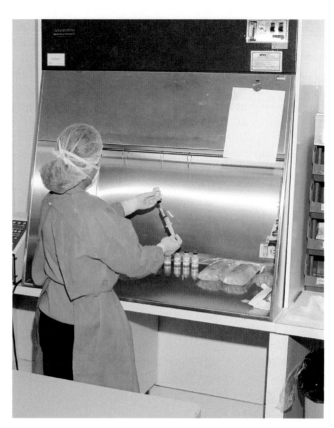

FIGURE 3-1 Room for preparing intravenous solutions for inpatients.

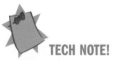

TECH NOTE!

The bottom line in working any area of pharmacy is "Always make sure the pharmacist has checked all drugs and/or devices before they leave the pharmacy." If this step is taken, the technician is working within the scope of practice and fewer mistakes will result.

requesting them, such as the emergency room, operating room, intensive care unit, cardiac care unit, and other departments. This duty includes preparing any intravenous solutions (Figure 3-1).

An aspect of the inpatient pharmacy is the ability to prepare parenteral medications, hyperalimentation medications, and chemotherapy. Helping the pharmacist answer phones, preparing first doses, and loading the medication drawers for patients are other tasks that the technician must be able to do competently. All patient medications are loaded into medication drawers in amounts to complete a 24-hour cycle. All documentation in the inpatient pharmacy is usually based on a 24-hour cycle for each patient. One must be quick, but more importantly, thorough when distributing medications to patients. Another aspect of the inpatient pharmacy is the preparation of unit dose medications (see Chapter 12). Medications need to be repackaged because:

1. The drug companies do not have the medication available in unit dose.
2. The hospital has chosen to prepare its own medication for cost-saving reasons.

Following are common job descriptions of inpatient technicians, along with some new responsibilities that are new additions in the pharmacy setting. The jobs listed do not require any additional educational training other than the training provided by each pharmacy setting. Most inpatient pharmacy technicians who are interested in the following areas in pharmacy will receive additional on-the-job training to prepare them for these additional tasks:

- Inventory technician: Orders all stock, takes care of billing, talks to drug representatives, and may be responsible for ordering lowest-cost items

- Robot filler: Many pharmacies are installing robots to fill patient medication drawers each day. Technicians must be trained to load these million-dollar mechanical robots and to keep them running smoothly
- IV technician: Interprets orders and prepares all parenteral medications, both large and small volumes, including controlled substance drips, hyperalimentation, insulin drips, and any other special-order intravenous or intramuscular drugs
- Chemotherapy technician: Interprets orders and prepares all chemotherapeutic agents and their adjunct medications, such as antiemetics
- Anticoagulant technician: Helps assist the anticoagulant pharmacist in contacting patients to alter their warfarin doses
- Clinical technician: Helps assist the clinical pharmacist with tracking patients' medications; the pharmacist contacts physicians who may not be ordering formulary drugs or drugs used for specific conditions
- Supervisory technician: Schedules other technicians and may even hire prospective technicians by reviewing their skills and backgrounds

Outpatient Setting Requirements

Working in outpatient pharmacy is one of the most difficult tasks in pharmacy because of the front-line interaction with patients. This job tests communication skills and stress levels of the technicians who work with the public. The job has a high volume of interaction on the telephone, taking in refill prescriptions, and answering questions pertaining to various insurances. Computer skills are often necessary to look up specific patient information to assist the customer over the phone or in person. Many neighborhood pharmacies fill a high volume of prescriptions daily (Figure 3-2). For a midsize pharmacy to fill 300 prescriptions in

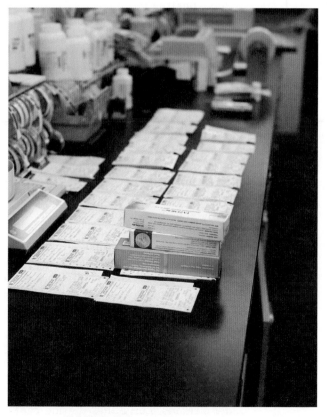

FIGURE 3-2 Outpatient filling station.

a day, answer phone calls, and take care of patients' problems is not uncommon. In addition to filling prescriptions, the outpatient technician must be able to order stock in a timely manner. Smaller community pharmacies may keep minimal stock because of limited space and the limited variety of drugs prescribed by physicians in the area. Billing various insurance companies is another skill the outpatient technician must master. This includes knowing all of the various rules, regulations, and special codes that may accompany each prescription.

Following are the job descriptions of outpatient pharmacy technicians and a few new positions being filled by technicians in community pharmacies. In addition, larger drug companies that are community based have seen the positive aspects of hiring technicians to fill certain positions:

- Insurance billing technician: This person must know the guidelines of Medicare, Blue Cross, Medicaid, and other insurance companies.
- Retail technician: This person must have excellent communication skills, phone skills, and prescription-filling abilities.
- Stock inventory technician: This person must know contacts for fast service, be able to get products and drugs as soon as possible, and perform proper billing functions for the pharmacy, including processing returns, recalled drugs, and controlled substances.
- Technician recruiter: Some outpatient pharmacies and/or temporary agencies employ these technicians to recruit other technicians into their company.
- Technician trainer: Various outpatient pharmacies employ technicians to train newly hired technicians on computer programs and to master other necessary skills relevant to their specific pharmacy.

Home Health Settings Requirements

A home health pharmacy fits somewhere between inpatient and outpatient pharmacy. On one hand, the technicians usually are processing prescription medications for patients weekly or monthly, which is similar to an outpatient setting. They prepare the drugs with the same type of labeling required for patient use. On the other hand, there are no patients, doctors, nurses, or other health care providers in the facility. Most home health pharmacies are based away from hospital sites and are not open to the public (Figure 3-3). Couriers deliver the medications to the home health clients. In addition, the prescriptions usually are packaged differently. Flat cardboard blister packs are prepared by technicians for use by nurses who administer the drugs in the home health setting (see Chapter 12). Other technician responsibilities include preparing parenteral medications. Usually a few days' to a month's supply is filled each time instead of only 24 hours' worth. A licensed pharmacist checks all medications filled for a patient at home before they are delivered. Home health clinics also provide services for patients who are taken care of by nurses in the patient's home. Home health nurses may receive supplies from the pharmacy clinic, or the patient's family may pick up or have supplies delivered. Patients who may receive care at home include kidney dialysis patients receiving peritoneal dialysis and hospice patients.

Mail-Order Pharmacy/E-Pharmacy

The mail-order pharmacy and E-pharmacy are growing as the "baby boomers" reach maturity. The need to fill prescriptions expeditiously increases with more medications becoming available to treat commonly acquired illnesses specific to older persons. Large distribution centers process new prescriptions and refills. Technicians are used in these settings as well. This is a relatively new area of

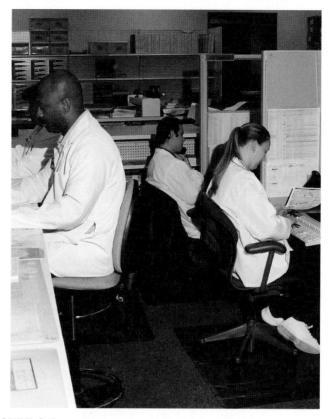

FIGURE 3-3 Home health and long-term pharmacy industry setting.

pharmacy that is growing steadily. This growth is occurring partially because many aging Americans are living longer and are taking multiple medications that can be costly. By using mail order, they normally receive drugs at lesser cost.

National Certification for Technicians

The infancy of any profession sees a lack of regular guidelines and standards, or continuity. Pharmacy technicians work across the United States and in all types of pharmacy settings under different rules determined by the individual states, which makes this profession challenging. At some point in the near future a national minimum standard for the profession must be met and agreed on across the United States. Although there will always be some variations from state to state, the overall skill level of a pharmacy technician should be a well-known standard. Currently, the range of skill levels, experience, pay, and belief systems is wide. One of the most basic aspects is the lack of a common title. Pharmacy technicians also are known as pharmacy clerks and pharmacy assistants. Other variances from state to state include pay, benefits, job description, and latitude of skill range.

The Pharmacy Technician Certification Board (PTCB) is an organization founded in 1995 by four organizations (Box 3-1) with the intent to implement an examination that would certify that a technician has met a basic skill level. These organizations are the American Society of Health-System Pharmacists, American Pharmacists Association, Illinois Council of Health-System Pharmacists, and the Michigan Pharmacists Association. These four entities created the PTCB and created the following goals for pharmacy technicians:

BOX 3-1   HISTORY OF THE PHARMACY TECHNICIAN CERTIFICATION BOARD

Founding Associations
American Pharmacists Association
American Society of Health-System Pharmacists
Illinois Council of Health-System Pharmacists
Michigan Pharmacists Association

Goals
To work more effectively with pharmacists
To give greater patient care and service
To create a minimum standard of knowledge of pharmacy technicians
To help employers determine knowledge base of pharmacy technicians

- To work more effectively with the pharmacist
- To provide greater patient care and service
- To create a minimum standard of knowledge
- To help employers determine knowledge base

Eligibility requirements to take the exam include the following:

- A high school diploma or general equivalency diploma
- Never been convicted of a drug-related felony

The PTCB examination is given 3 times per year on the same days nationwide and at many different locations. Different versions of the examination are used; therefore the results are weighted differently. The test is divided into three specific areas of pharmacy by percentage:

- Assisting the Pharmacist in Serving Patients is 64%.
- Maintaining Medication and Inventory Control Systems is 25%.
- Participating in the Administration and Management of Pharmacy Practice is 11%.

The scoring is done by an independent group that grades the various areas of pharmacy knowledge based on the difficulty of the question. Because of the variance in examinations, the examination is described as being relatively easy to difficult to pass. The student must have a passing score of 650. The test uses modified Angoff method test questions. This means each question is evaluated separately. The exam has no raw score because of the various difficulties of each question. All sections are combined for an overall score. The results are mailed 30 days after the end of the examination. Technicians also can access their test results online. The types of pharmacy knowledge that are tested include the following:

- Pharmacy math
- Pharmacy law (federal only)
- Pharmacy operations
- Drug names (trade/generic)
- Drug classifications

Once certification is attained, technicians are required to obtain 20 hours of continuing education every 2 years. Continuing education can be obtained through pharmacy organizations that offer free continuing education to members, journals that include continuing education units, or seminars. Technicians who meet these requirements may use the initials *CPhT* on their identification tag, indicating that they are a certified pharmacy technician. Continuing education is less expensive for association members, and many drug

BOX 3.2 DUTIES OF A CERTIFIED TECHNICIAN

- Handling of ongoing pharmacy telephone calls from members, pharmacy providers, and physicians daily under the supervision of a pharmacist
- Troubleshooting third-party prescription claims questions with an understanding of online rejections and plan parameters
- Developing and maintaining an electronic service log on all telephone calls with complete follow-up history
- Developing a trending report on the aforementioned service calls with an eye toward forecasting possible trends in pharmacy service
- Providing as-needed telephone and administrative support for the department

BOX 3.3 QUALIFICATIONS OF A CERTIFIED TECHNICIAN

- Strong organizational, prioritization, communication, and mathematical skills required
- Pharmacy Claims Processing Computer System experience preferred
- Minimum 2 years' experience in a retail pharmacy setting and/or managed care/pharmacy benefit environment is beneficial
- Comprehensive understanding of third-party pharmacy benefit plan parameters is necessary
- Ability to understand the importance of and to respect the confidentiality of all patient information
- Computer literacy with proficiency in general word processing and data entry is necessary

This information was obtained from the Pharmacy Technician Certification Board website *(www.PTCB.org).*

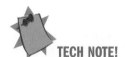

TECH NOTE!

Visit *www.PTCB.org* to get statistics on certified technicians and to access your state board of pharmacy for the latest laws pertaining to technicians.

TECH ALERT!

The PTCB examination may be repeated if one fails it. The cost of $120 per exam is required before taking the exam again. Also, the PTCB previously allowed students and technicians to take a sample 125-question exam on the Internet free of charge. Because of the growth of the exam, the PTCB now charges $29.00 for a 60-question sample exam. Chapter 31 provides a practice exam.

companies offer free continuing education units to pharmacists. Technicians can use the same continuing education units as pharmacists, although certain courses can be difficult to understand. Independent pharmacists and other small businesses offer low-cost continuing education credit on the Internet.

Many pharmacy technicians receive a raise in pay after completion of the PTCB examination, although some pharmacies do not recognize the examination, possibly to keep technician wages low. As time passes and federal and state regulations stiffen with respect to qualified personnel, the necessity of skilled technicians undoubtedly will rise to the top of pharmacy issues, and the examination will be accepted as a basic requirement.

Many states still do not require certification of their technicians but have different guidelines for their capabilities in the pharmacy practice. Certain states require licensing but not national certification. States such as Texas require certification of all new technicians but do have exemptions for certain pharmacy technicians. Alabama does not require certification, but the state does require that all pharmacy technicians receive continuing education each year. Not all states' requirements are standardized. However, most, if not all, now require technicians to have a high school diploma. Each student must visit the website of his or her board of pharmacy to become familiar with the current state laws pertaining to pharmacy technicians.

Box 3-2 lists common duties, and Box 3-3 lists qualifications for technicians according to the PTCB.

According to the current statistics, there are more than 200,000 technicians nationwide. Many states are beginning to recognize the importance of certification to guarantee that the technicians hired are competent in all areas of pharmacy. More information about this credential, and schools that offer it, can be obtained at *www.nhanow.com.* Employers increasingly are using these credentials as a requirement for hiring technicians.

Opportunities for Technicians

Pharmacies use computers daily; therefore, software must be developed for pharmacy personnel. Some pharmacy-related fields do require more education in specific areas such as computers. With the proper educational training such as an associate in science or bachelor of science degree in computer science, the pharmacy technician is well equipped to write software or supply support. Also, as many technicians move into the area of training technicians, their expertise may help them write curriculums, articles, and even books for pharmacy technicians. Many vocational schools hire experienced pharmacy technicians to teach students the necessary requirements to be a competent pharmacy technician. Completion of such training programs offers different degrees, such as certificates, an associate's degree (AA, AS), or a bachelor's degree (BA, BS).

Pharmacy technicians can fill many other (not well-known) positions. The following is a list of various nontraditional jobs:

- Pharmacy business management operators—Pharmacy business management companies are beginning to realize the importance of knowing not only the trade and generic names of drugs but also the classifications of drugs. They are hiring technicians, rather than registered pharmacists, to help pharmacy customers over the phone, which is a cost savings for the company.
- Computer support technician (PYXIS, SUREMED)—Large companies that supply hospitals, community pharmacies, and other facilities with automated medication dispensing systems are employing technicians as support personnel.
- Software writer—Some pharmacy software writers are using technicians with additional computer background and/or training to prepare software services. Technicians use their terminology and drug knowledge in creating new software programs.
- Authors—Technicians with additional education background and extensive knowledge of pharmacy can participate not only in preparing and presenting continuing education credits but also in writing supplemental books for pharmacy technicians.
- Poison control call center operator—Some poison control centers are using technicians to triage calls coming into the 911 stations. If the call is in regard to something life threatening, then technicians transfer the call to a pharmacist or poison specialist. If the call is something less critical, technicians are authorized to take the call.
- Nuclear pharmacy technician—The technician may assist the pharmacist with handling and preparing doctors' orders for radioactive medications used in diagnosis and treatment.
- Director/instructor—Pharmacy technicians can oversee technician training programs and/or instruct in schools around the country. Some require a bachelor of science degree or vocational education teaching credentials.
- Corporate pharmacy analysis—Working through an independent management service, a technician surveys the efficiency in all areas of the pharmacy and recommends changes to help the pharmacy work more productively and efficiently. The analyst may travel and even work on Joint Commission on Accreditation of Healthcare Organizations standards to prepare pharmacies for inspection.
- Pharmacy supervisors—Supervisors oversee as many as 20 to 30 technicians and pharmacist interns within the pharmacy. They are responsible for training them on all software and may organize work schedules.

- Clinical coordinator—Responsibilities include monitoring patients who are taking specific medications and those who have conditions such as asthma. They may schedule patients for educational classes or refer them to the pharmacist or doctor if necessary.

In addition to the positions listed, new positions are being developed by different pharmacy settings. Although these positions currently may be nontraditional, their numbers are growing. It would not be surprising if these positions became commonly held positions for future technicians.

Incentive Programs

Pharmacies sometimes have an incentive program for employees who want to further their careers in pharmacy. Many pharmacists once began their careers as technicians. Many pharmacy employers usually give incentives for returning to school to become a pharmacist. They may reimburse tuition costs or give pay incentives. Whether a company does support and partially fund a school program is something one should consider when inquiring about a pharmacy position.

As the geriatric community increases in number over the next millennium, so will the need for qualified medical personnel. Pharmacy technicians know much about the challenges and benefits that pharmacy has to offer. The future of technicians still is being determined, but judging from the ground currently being broken by technicians, their only limitations are self-imposed. Many pharmacy companies reimburse their technicians after they pass the PTCB examination. This is more likely to take place in states in which certification is not mandatory but preferred. Attaining increased skill levels, including becoming certified pharmacy technicians, opens more doors for technicians in pharmacy.

Two Sides of the Story

If pharmacy technicians are not required to have a more in-depth knowledge of pharmacology and other aspects of pharmacy, then wages, benefits, and variety of skills will not increase. However, errors in pharmacy are increasing partially because of the shortage of pharmacists. Because of this shortage, pharmacists cannot perform all the tasks necessary, including overseeing technicians. If this continues, errors will continue to increase and pharmacies will be in direct noncompliance with the new laws requiring a decrease in error rate.

However, if the minimum requirement should include national certification or college degrees, then the current supply of pharmacy technicians would be in jeopardy because most seasoned technicians do not want to return to school to continue performing their jobs. In which case, a national pharmacy technician shortage could rival the current pharmacist shortage. Wages would rise sharply, and errors again would become a problem with a shortage in workforce. What is the answer to this problem? The answer lies somewhere in the middle. Each state is researching the levels of training that it will require of its technicians and will allow a transition period for their current technicians. When the state of Texas required national certification, it allowed more than 1 year for all technicians to become certified. In addition, many pharmacies subsidized the cost of the examination if the technician passed, and small raises have been given to technicians who were willing to reach the higher level of knowledge. However, many states do not require any type of skill level or even registration for their technicians.

The Professional Technician

Many websites are available to learn tips for preparing resumes and cover letters and about the interview process. Remember that as a student, your work experience is not a strong point because this is a new vocation for you. Instead, you must focus on your educational background. It is important that the program you attend supplies you with an adequate knowledge base to prepare you for this important vocation in pharmacy. The importance of attitude, attendance, and punctuality in pharmacy cannot be stressed enough. Arrive early for interviews and a few minutes early every day to work. This shows your dedication to your profession.

The following is a list of websites that help with resumes and letters of interest:

> *www.resume-help.org*
> *www.jobstar.org/tools/resume*
> *www.resume.monster.com*

Organizations

Four main associations are concerned with the practice of pharmacy:

> American Society of Health-System Pharmacists
> American Association of Pharmacy Technicians
> National Pharmacy Technician Association
> American Pharmacists Association

Each association has a state-run organization that can be accessed through its website. The only way to determine whether the organization in your state has the benefits that you require is to visit the website and to learn about its resource areas for technicians. Many different resources will benefit the career-oriented technician; they are as follows:

- Continuing education
- Legislative movement toward promoting technicians
- A pharmacy technician division
- Journals, books, and other educational references
- Seminars for continuing education and networking capabilities
- Message boards for communicating with other technicians
- A good website that has links to other important technician sites

Table 3-1 lists the websites for each of the organizations. It would be good to visit each site and read the mission statement to find out the level at which pharmacy technicians participate in the association. Each state chapter may operate differently than other state chapters. Therefore, it is important to check out the specific chapter in your state to find the differences. As pharmacy technology increases in qualifications, responsibilities, and benefits, it is necessary to join an association that will provide continuing education specific to technicians and advocate for the profession.

Less Is More . . .

Pharmacy is predominantly a conservative profession. Dressing professionally includes proper clothing; shoes; hairstyle; and the lack of off-colored hair, facial jewelry, visible tattoos, or any other feature that detracts attention from your personality. Medical personnel should appear to be professional, knowledgeable, competent, and not scary looking to the patients. You will not find many doctors with strange haircuts or nurses with pierced noses popping bubble gum at the

TABLE 3-1 National Organizations of Pharmacy

Organization	History	Benefits	Resource areas	Specific to technicians	Miscellaneous	Fees*
American Society of Health-System Pharmacists www.ashp.org	Founded in 1925 to meet the needs of hospital pharmacy. Changed name in mid 1990s from *Hospital Pharmacists* to *Health-System Pharmacists* to expand information and services to a wider range of pharmacies.	Monthly journal includes continuing education. Biannual seminar meetings. Influences laws concerning pharmacy practice. Other benefits: credit card, insurance coverage, member loan program, product line for sales.	Information on acute care, practice management, ambulatory care, clinical, home care, long-term care, managed care, students, technicians, and patient safety.	Accreditation process for pharmacy technician training programs provides course curriculum, aseptic technique videos, books, and links to other websites of interest.	Each state has own association headed by pharmacists. Many have technician divisions. 30,000 members nationally.	$65.00 annually (no journals); $170.00 includes journals. No student rates available.
American Association of Pharmacy Technicians www.pharmacytechnician.com	Annual seminars include continuing education units; possible networking capabilities.	Message board on Internet (to communicate with others); pharmacy technician products such as books, patches, bags, miscellaneous items.	Links to websites	Promotes pharmacy technicians; provides continuing education specific to technicians.	This organization is run by pharmacists and technicians. It has all seminars in Midwest to East Coast only, no West Coast coverage.	Active: $50 ($47.50 if applying online) annually. Student: $25 ($23.75 online) annually.

Continued

TABLE 3-1 National Organizations of Pharmacy—cont'd

Organization	History	Benefits	Resource areas	Specific to technicians	Miscellaneous	Fees*
National Pharmacy Technician Association www.pharmacytechnician.org	Founded in 1992 by Mike Johnston; based in Houston, Texas.	Journal: *Today's Technician*. Includes continuing education, annual seminars that include continuing education for technicians and possible networking capabilities.	Links to websites	Promotes pharmacy technicians; provides continuing education specific to technicians.	This organization is run by and promotes only technicians. It is the newest organization of pharmacy technicians and has more than 25,000 members.	$54 includes journal (includes free continuing education). No student rates available.
American Pharmacists Association www.aphanet.org	Founded in 1852. First established pharmacy group in United States.	Journal: *Pharmacy Today*. Provides various insurance to members and discounts on cars, phones, and other things.	Links to websites	Some state branches allow technicians to join. Most do not have technician divisions and do not stress the vocation of technicians.	N/A	$57 annually includes monthly journal. No student rates available.

*Fees are current at the time of printing this book.

patient's bedside. It is just as important that the pharmacy technician show the public that he or she is professional and does not view the vocation as just a job. You show this directly and immediately by appearance and demeanor.

The Possibilities . . .

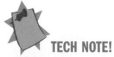

TECH NOTE!

Each year pharmacy technicians celebrate the profession. National Pharmacy Week is held every October 20 to 26.

Although it is impossible to foresee the future of any profession, there are clear indications regarding the direction a profession is taking. Reviewing the history of pharmacy, one can see a trend. The education requirements of pharmacists have increased from a bachelor of science degree in pharmacy (requiring 5 years of college) to a doctor of pharmacy degree (requiring 6 years) because of the necessary skill level needed in today's pharmacy practice. The pharmacist's role is more clinically oriented to patient consultation and to providing information services to medical staff. The roles of pharmacy technicians are changing as well. The technician's role has evolved from a clerk, cashier, and shelf-stocker to a clinical technician, chemotherapy technician, nuclear medicine pharmacy technician, and inventory specialist technician. In addition to the change in duties are the changing guidelines that all states are researching to provide a base level of training for pharmacy technicians in the future.

DO YOU REMEMBER THESE KEY POINTS?

- The major pharmacy associations and their resources for technicians
- Nontraditional jobs that pharmacy technicians can perform
- Where technicians can find the current state requirements necessary to work as a pharmacy technician
- The differences between the functions of inpatient (hospital), outpatient (community), and home health pharmacies
- New expanding areas of pharmacy, such as mail order and E-pharmacy, that are incorporating pharmacy technicians
- Various duties that pharmacy technicians can perform under the supervision of a pharmacist
- The type of information on which the Pharmacy Technician Certification Board tests technicians
- The importance of national certification and the benefits for technicians
- Additional degrees for pharmacy technicians that can lead them into other areas of pharmacy
- The requirements of national certification after passing the examination

MULTIPLE CHOICE QUESTIONS

1. The pharmacy association run for and solely by technicians is _____.
   A. National Pharmacy Technician Association
   B. American Association of Pharmacy Technicians
   C. American Society of Health-System Pharmacists
   D. American Pharmacists Association

2. Certified technicians must meet which of the following Pharmacy Technician Certification Board standards?
   A. Continuing education
   B. State registration requirements
   C. Membership in a pharmacy association
   D. All of the above

3. All of the following statements are true concerning national certification except _____.
   A. All 50 states have the examination the same day
   B. All 50 states have the examination 3 times per year
   C. All 50 states are aware of the certification examination results
   D. All 50 states give raises to technicians who pass the Pharmacy Technician Certification Board examination

4. All of the following statements are true concerning pharmacy technicians in general except _____.
   A. Dressing professionally can increase chances of being hired.
   B. Punctuality is important in working in pharmacy.
   C. The pharmacy technician is expected to take the Pharmacy Technician Certification Board examination prior to employment.
   D. Communication is an essential skill for pharmacy technicians.

5. The following reasons to become involved in pharmacy organizations are true except _____.
   A. For networking possibilities
   B. For new information on the future of pharmacy technicians
   C. To increase knowledge about new pharmaceuticals through continuing education
   D. For the tax deduction

6. Boards of pharmacy serve what function?
   A. Licensing and registration of pharmacists and technicians
   B. Writing and enforcing the rules and regulations of pharmacy practice
   C. An avenue for consumer complaints
   D. All of the above

7. All pharmacies in their perspective states are overseen by _____.
   A. Each state National Association of Boards of Pharmacy
   B. Each state board of pharmacy
   C. Pharmacy managers
   D. Consumer advocacy groups

8. Nondiscretionary duties of a technician include all of the following except _____.
   A. Requiring all work to be checked by a pharmacist
   B. Duties that do not require interpretation of reference materials
   C. Duties that assist the pharmacist in preparing and dispensing medication
   D. Counseling patients on all nonprescription medications

9. All of the following duties are required of an inpatient technician except _____.
   A. Supplying stock to emergency clinics
   B. Repackaging medications into unit dose packages
   C. Helping customers with insurance claims
   D. Preparing chemotherapy

10. Important aspects of outpatient pharmacy are the need to keep lower levels of drugs on the shelf but in stock at all times. This is caused by _____.
    A. Lack of shelf space
    B. The need to keep employee hours down
    C. Changes in medication usage by physicians
    D. A and C

TRUE/FALSE **If the statement is false, then change it to make it true.**

_____ 1. The National Association of Boards of Pharmacy determines regulations in each state pertaining to technicians.

_____ 2. Technicians currently hold the same positions that they have held historically.

_____ 3. Most pharmacies that hire technicians require the same basic skills.

_____ **4.** Most companies that use pharmacy technicians outside of the pharmacy require a college degree.

_____ **5.** Most prescription orders filled in a hospital pharmacy are for 24 hours, whereas a community pharmacy fills the full length of the prescription order.

_____ **6.** Inpatient technicians assist inpatient pharmacists to monitor patients who are taking certain medications.

_____ **7.** Stat doses are to be delivered within 3 minutes.

_____ **8.** Technicians giving advice to a nurse on what dosage form to use for a patient in the hospital is nonjudgmental.

_____ **9.** Most states require technicians to be certified.

_____ **10.** Certification renewal for a pharmacy technician requires 30 hours of continuing education per year.

TECHNICIAN'S CORNER

Internet assignment: Log onto the Internet, and visit the National Association of Boards of Pharmacy *(www.nabp.org)*. List the board objectives, and find the listing for your state and another state. Visit the two boards of pharmacy sites, and find the current requirements for technicians. Print out your findings and submit them to your instructor. Write a one-page summary on the differences between the two states as they pertain to the description of a pharmacy technician.

BIBLIOGRAPHY

Harteker LR: *The pharmacy technician companion,* Washington, DC, 1998, American Pharmacists Association.
www.ptcb.org PTCB Guidebook to Certification 2005

WEBSITES

www.ptcb.org
www.nabp.org

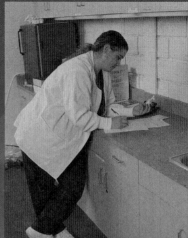

Conversions and Calculations Used by Pharmacy Technicians

Objectives

UPON COMPLETING THIS CHAPTER, YOU SHOULD BE ABLE TO DO THE FOLLOWING:

- Describe the differences among the following measurement systems:
  - Apothecary system
  - Avoirdupois system
  - Metric system
  - Common household measurements

- Convert Arabic numbers into Roman numerals.

- Demonstrate the ability to convert between the following measurement systems commonly used on prescriptions:
  - Metric system
  - Apothecary system
  - Household system

- Use mathematical calculations to determine dosage:
  - Ratios/proportions
  - Fractions
  - Percentages
  - Demonstrate the ability to set up equations and solve problems for the following:

- Determining day's supply

- Pediatric dosages

- Drip rates

- Alligation

- Percent dosages

TERMS
AND
DEFINITIONS

Alligation *A method of determining the needed amounts of two different concentrations to prepare a needed concentration*

Apothecary system *A system of measurement used in pharmacy*

Avoirdupois system *A system of measurement used for determination of weight*

Household system *A system of measurement commonly used for weight, volume, and length in the United States*

International time *A 24-hour method of keeping time in which hours are not distinguished between AM and PM but are counted continuously through the entire day*

Metric system *A system of measurement based on multiples of 10*

Volume *The amount of liquid enclosed within a container*

THE ABILITY TO MANIPULATE CONVERSIONS is a required competency of pharmacy technicians. This skill is also a foundation for filling orders and calculating doses in the pharmacy. This chapter covers the basics in conversions in pharmacy along with common mathematical problems that a technician may encounter. Although a pharmacist needs to check all transcriptions and calculations, it is important that the technician have a good understanding to avoid medication errors. As you move through this chapter, make sure that you learn each basic step before moving on to the next. Once you have a good knowledge of the basic conversions, then you can begin to work out the calculations that follow.

Pharmacy has a long history (see Chapter 1), and many of the old forms of measurement are still in use. These measurements come from different regions of the world; therefore, not all units are converted easily or exactly. For example, many equivalencies are rounded to a more usable number. The pharmacy technician must be well versed in all of the different measurements. The four most common types are as follows:

1. Metric system
2. Household measurements
3. Apothecary system
4. Avoirdupois system

All of these systems are used in a pharmacy at one time or another.

A good way to become familiar with common pharmacy measurements is to start with what you know and then slowly build on that knowledge. For example, most persons are familiar with the measurement of a teaspoon. In fact, most persons could gauge a teaspoonful by eye alone. Some doctors may prefer not to write instructions for 1 tsp when ordering a prescription; instead, you will see the measurement for a teaspoonful in one of the other three systems. The pharmacy technician must translate the doctor's orders into layperson's terms. Remember always to read what will be printed on the label to see whether it makes sense. Do not assume that a person understands what a milliliter or an ounce is. You must make the instructions easy enough for a child to understand. This will decrease the chance of any misreading of the instructions.

TABLE 4-1 Common Household Measurements

Household measurements (volume)	Metric (volume)	Household equivalent
1 tsp	5 mL or cc*	1 tsp
1 tbsp	15 mL or cc	3 tsp
1 cup	240 mL or cc	8 oz
1 pt	480 mL or cc	2 cups
1 qt	960 mL or cc	4 cups
1 gal	3840 mL or cc or 3.84 L	16 cups

*Remember that 1 mL and 1 cc contain the same amount of liquid.

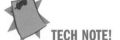

TECH NOTE!

Remember: You must place the proper units (such as mL, L, mg, or g) next to the number amount. This cannot be stressed enough, especially because you will be working with various systems. Putting the units on all numbers is the only way to help avoid mistakes.

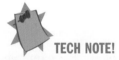

TECH NOTE!

If you have measuring cups and spoons in your kitchen, pull them out and convert them into milliliters and ounces. Do the same for food items on your kitchen shelf.

Metric System

The metric system is used throughout pharmacy because of its accuracy. The units used in the metric system include the milliliter (mL), cubic centimeter (cc), and liter (L) for volume; kilogram (kg), gram (g), milligram (mg), and microgram (mcg) for weight; and millimeter (mm) and meter (m) for distance. A technician must know the difference between each unit given. For example, if a prescription were filled with 1 g of drug when only 1 mg was ordered, the patient would overdose by 1000 times the ordered dose. A 1000-unit difference exists between each measurement. This means that 1000 mcg equals 1 mg.

The use of millimeters is reserved for drug calculations that are based on body surface areas and would be calculated by a physician or pharmacist using a surface area calculation chart. For most technicians, knowing the basics for volume and weight conversions is adequate.

Household Measurements

The most common measurement system that still is used extensively in the United States is the household system. You probably already know this system. Measurements come in a variety of units. For instance, volume refers to liquids, weight refers to dry ingredients, and length refers to distance. If you want to bake a cake, you must use utensils to measure dry and liquid ingredients. If you carpet a room, you need to multiply width by length to get the square footage or distance. Let's review some of these measurements. The most common household measurement is probably the teaspoon. Other common measurements include tablespoons and cups. Table 4-1 lists these common household measurements next to some of the most common volumes written (in metric) by physicians.

Apothecary System

Although the apothecary system originated in Europe, it is used throughout the medical field in the United States. The units used in this system are the grain (gr) and scruple (℈) for dry weight, and ounce (℥), dram (ℨ), and minim (♏) for volume. More common measurements include ounces and pounds. The apothecary conversions are shown in Box 4-1. When using the apothecary system, place the measurement before the amount; for example, 1 gr is written as gr 1. How do you write $\frac{1}{2}$ gr? The most common way is gr $\overline{ss}$ ($\overline{ss}$ means $\frac{1}{2}$) gr vii $\overline{ss}$ thyroid qd = $7\frac{1}{2}$ gr daily.

The most common pharmacy units are converted into metric and household measurements (Table 4-2). Be sure to learn these conversions before continuing. See Figure 4-1 for examples of conversions between household, metric, and apothecary systems.

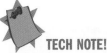

TECH NOTE!

The weight of a grain in the apothecary system may vary between 60 mg, 64 mg, and 65 mg. Why? When the grain was used in ancient times to determine weight, real grains of wheat were used, and the weight depended on that year's harvest. If the crop was good, then it took fewer grains because each one weighed more. If the crops were bad that year, then it may have taken more grains to equal the same weight. Therefore, be aware that some medication labels will say that there is 60 mg/gr, whereas others might have 64 mg/gr or even 65 mg/gr. However, when performing calculations, the use of 60 mg/gr is customary.

BOX 4-1 APOTHECARY WEIGHTS

Dry Weight

1 gr	= 60 mg
15 gr	= 1 g
20 gr	= Ꙋ 1
1 dram	= Ꙋ 3
1 oz	= ʒ 8 or
	= Ꙋ 24
	= gr 480
	= 31.1 g
1 lb	= 16 oz
	= ʒ 96
	= Ꙋ 288
	= gr 5760
	= 454 g

Fluid Weight

1 dram	= ♏ 60
8 drams	= ♏ 480
3 scruples*	= ʒ 1

*Scruples (Ꙋ) and minims (♏) are not commonly used units.

TABLE 4-2 Conversion Table: Apothecary/Metric/Household

Apothecary volume	Apothecary weight	Metric volume	Metric weight	Common household
ʒ 1	ʒ 1	30 mL	30 g	2 tbsp
ʒ 4	ʒ 4	15 mL	15 g	1 tbsp
ʒ 2	ʒ 2	7.5 mL	7.5 g	½ tbsp
ʒ 1	gr 60	4 mL	4 g	1 tsp
ʒ ½	gr 30	2 mL	2 g	½ tsp

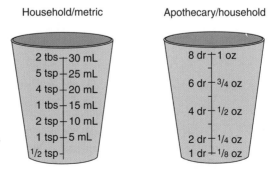

Household/metric   Apothecary/household

2 tbs	30 mL
5 tsp	25 mL
4 tsp	20 mL
1 tbs	15 mL
2 tsp	10 mL
1 tsp	5 mL
½ tsp	

8 dr	1 oz
6 dr	¾ oz
4 dr	½ oz
2 dr	¼ oz
1 dr	⅛ oz

One-ounce medicine cups (30 mL)

FIGURE 4-1 Oral cups show equivalent volumes between household to metric and household to apothecary.

TABLE 4-3 Standard Weights: Avoirdupois/Metric

Avoirdupois	Metric equivalent
Dry Weights	
1 lb	454 g
1 oz	30 g
1 gr	64.8 mg
Liquids	
1 fl oz	30 mL
1 pt	473 mL
1 gal	3785 mL

Avoirdupois System

The avoirdupois system is another type of measurement that originated in England. The avoirdupois system is similar to the apothecary system because it also uses grains, ounces, and pounds for weights. Table 4-3 shows the common avoirdupois weights.

Important Differences among Systems

You should know how metric system units vary from other units of measure such as ounces and grains. Most of the time they convert easily, but sometimes there are variances, making conversions between measurement systems approximate in these instances. Because the metric system is the most common system used in pharmacies, it is the measurement you use when preparing a compounded drug. However, you will see differences among manufacturers' products and their weights. For example, some manufacturers consider 473 mL to equal a pint, whereas others consider 480 mL or 500 mL to equal a pint.

As shown in the following, 1 lb is equal to 454 g in metric measurements, whereas it is only 373 g in the apothecary system. Although there is some difference between systems on the exact weight, the most accepted measurement is the metric system.

2.2 lb = 1 kg	Metric
1 lb = 454 g	Metric
1 lb ap = 373.2 g	Apothecary
1 oz = 28.35 g	Avoirdupois
1 oz = 31.1 g	Apothecary
1 oz = 30 g	Metric

Writing Units Using Each System

See the following for the most common units used for each of the systems discussed in this chapter. Although all four systems are used in writing prescriptions, the pharmacy primarily uses the metric system. However, regardless of which system is used in a prescription, it must be converted into household measurements for the patient. At the end of each section are quick check questions to answer. The answers to these problems are at the end of the chapter.

[handwritten in left margin: 5gr = 325mg]

METRIC MEASUREMENTS

1. You can use cc (cubic centimeter) and mL (milliliter) interchangeably, although mL is the preferred measurement.

1 mL = 1 cc

5 mL = 5 cc

100 mL = 100 cc

1000 mL = 1000 cc

2. Dry weights use microgram (mcg), milligram (mg), gram (g), and kilogram (kg).
3. Liquid volumes use milliliter (mL) and liter (L).

APOTHECARY MEASUREMENTS

1. Dry weights use pounds (lb), ounces (℥), drams (ʒ), scruples (℈), and grains (gr).
2. Liquid volume weights use fluidounces (f℥), fluidrams (fʒ), and minims (♏).

AVOIRDUPOIS MEASUREMENTS

1. Dry weights use pounds (lb), ounces (oz), and grains (gr).
2. Liquid volumes use fluid ounces (foz), pints (pt), and gallons (gal).

EXERCISE 4-1 QUICK CHECK

1 dram = _1_ tsp
8 oz = _1_ cup(s)
1 gal = _16_ cup(s)
5 cc = _1_ tsp
30 mL = _2_ tbsp
30 mL = _1 fl_ oz
1 gr = _60_ mg
1 pt = _2_ cup(s)
1 pt = _480_ mL
15 tbsp = _225_ mL
1 kg = _1000_ g

Conversions

When converting orders, you must know the basics. Once you have memorized the basic units of the preceding tables and figures, then continue.

METRIC SYSTEM SLIDE

When converting metric measurements from one unit to another, you need to move the decimal to the right or the left. All changes of the metric system involve dividing or multiplying by 10. The most common units used in pharmacy are kilogram, gram, milligram, and microgram. Each unit is a multiple of 1000. By moving the decimal by three spaces (to the right or left), you can change between these units. For example, changing units from 5000 mg to grams involves dividing the 5000 mg by 1000, or moving the decimal three places to the left. See the following scale. Remember, the difference between 1 kg, 1 g, 1 mg, and 1 mcg is

1000. Therefore, you always need to move three decimal places in one direction or another. One of the most frustrating problems is when you cannot remember which way the decimal must be moved when changing between large and small numbers or vice versa. Two ways are possible; choose the one that works for you and stick with it.

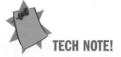

TECH NOTE!

Remember that there are 1000 g in 1 kg, 1000 mg in 1 g, and 1000 mcg in 1 mg.

Method A for Determining Metric Conversions

Left			Right
Largest			Smallest

— 1 _____ 1 _____ 1 _____ 1 _____

1000 kg	1000 g	1000 mg	1000 mcg
(3 decimals)	(3 decimals)	(3 decimals)	(3 decimals)
0.000000001 kg =	0.000001 g =	0.001 mg =	1 mcg
1 kg =	1000 g =	1,000,000 mg =	1,000,000,000 mcg

For the purpose of most pharmacy drug calculations, these are the only four units that you need to use. When going from a larger (1 kg) to a smaller amount (1 g), move the decimal to the right three spaces. In the following illustration the decimal is placed in this equation to show you how to count off the right number of spaces. Decimals are not placed at the end of a number *unless* there is a fraction, such as 1.1 kg. Decimals and periods have been a main source of mistakes in pharmacies because they can be mistaken for changing a number by a thousand: 0.10 and 01. for example. Do you know for sure what this number represents? This could have devastating effects if a medication were given to a patient and the doctor had intended 1 and not 0.1.

$$1 \text{ kg} = ? \text{ g} \rightarrow 1 \text{ kg} = 1000 \text{ g}$$

Count to the right three spaces and fill in your zeros.

$$1 \text{ g} = ? \text{ mg} \rightarrow 1 \text{ g} = 1\,000 \text{ mg}$$

$$1 \text{ kg} = ? \text{ mg} \rightarrow 1 \text{ kg} = 1\,000\,000 \text{ mg}$$

Move three spaces to the right twice.

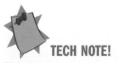

TECH NOTE!

This is an easy way using the calculator to get the number quickly, but sometimes it becomes confusing—divide or multiply? When going from a *Larger* to *Smaller* unit, do not *Divide (LSD)*; multiply to obtain the answer instead.

Method B for Converting Large Number to Small Number; Do Not Divide but Multiply

When converting from large to small, you multiply (use the previous ruler). When converting from small to large, you divide.

Try the following three questions using your calculator. All of these are larger units going to smaller units.

2 kg = ? g	2 kg × 1000 = 2000 g
2 g = ? mg	2 g × 1000 = 2000 mg
2 kg = ? mg	2 kg × 1000 × 1000 = 2,000,000 mg

Let's go in reverse, smaller to larger, using the calculator.

$$2 \text{ mcg} = ? \text{ mg}   \quad 0.002 \text{ mg}$$

$$2 \text{ mg} = ?g   \quad \frac{2}{1000} = 0.002\,g$$

EXERCISE 4-2 QUICK CHECK

Use both methods and see which one works best.
You receive a doctor's order for 0.88 mcg of levothyroxine.
What is the equivalent in milligrams?
How many grams?
How many kilograms?
Weight and volume are calculated the same way. Practice on small numbers until you become comfortable with this conversion.

Fractions

Rarely will you receive an order in fraction form that you need to convert; however, you should know how to do this in case the need ever arises. The conversion is a simple two-step process to convert simple fractions into percentages. For example, $^6/_9$ converted into a percentage requires dividing 6 by 9 and multiplying this by 100 to get the percentage. Remember that a percentage is always a portion of 100.

So, $^6/_9 = 0.66 \times 100 = 66.6\%$, or rounded up it would be 67%. To convert a decimal into a percentage, you simply multiply by 100 because decimals are just a different representation of a percentage or part of 100. For example, 1.5 is the same as 150%. If you are converting a fraction from grains into milligrams, however, you multiply by 60 rather than 100 because there are 60 mg per grain. For example, if you receive an order for $^1/_{150}$ gr of nitroglycerin SL (sublingual) tablets, you first divide 1 by 150 and then multiply by 60 to get the answer of 0.39999 . . . , which would be rounded up to 0.4 mg.

Percentages

Percentages represent a portion of a whole. The number 100 is used to represent the whole. 100% equals one whole. This whole could be anything—a pie, a cup of water, or a 1-L intravenous solution. If 100% is a whole, what is one half of a whole? Two tenths of a whole? Six thousandths of a whole? This is discussed, and how to make these conversions is explained.

First, let's convert fractions into percentages. In a fraction the numerator is the top number and the denominator is the bottom number. Let's start with an easy one, such as $^1/_2$. Simple division is used. Take the numerator and divide it by the denominator, that is, 1 divided by 2. Because 100 is used to represent a whole, carry out the division to a minimum of three spaces to the right of the decimal point.

$$\frac{1}{2} = 0.5$$

The next step to convert a fraction into a percentage is the easiest. See the decimal point? Move that decimal point two spaces to the *right* and add a percent sign (%), and you are done.

$$0.5 \times 100\% = 50\%$$

Let's try some conversions. Convert the following fractions into percentages:

1. $^1/_8 = \_\_\%$ Answers: 1. 12.5%
2. $^5/_2 = \_\_\%$ 2. 250%
3. $^3/_4 = \_\_\%$ 3. 75%
4. $^4/_{10} = \_\_\%$ 4. 40%
5. $^2/_3 = \_\_\%$ 5. 66.7%

Percentages are used in compounding, which is discussed later in this chapter. Percentages also are used in the pharmacy to calculate markup on

---

prices, payment discounts, net profits, and gross profits. You also will find problems on the Pharmacy Technician Certification Board exam dealing with percentages. Therefore, you must be able use percentages to determine what the price will be marked up for a drug or how much money the pharmacy can save by making payments quickly.

When working in a pharmacy, a technician may see an invoice or bill from a supplier. Usually underneath the total due of the invoice will be the terms for payment. It may read something similar to "1.5% 10 days/Net 30 days." What this means is that the supplier will give the pharmacy a 1.5% discount if the invoice is paid within 10 days, but the entire amount is due within 30 days. How is the discount figured out? To begin, convert the percentage into a decimal. Let's use the 1.5% as our example. Drop the percent sign. Next, move the decimal point two places to the *left*. You now have a decimal number. Easy, right? Let's now try some conversions from percentages to decimal numbers.

1. 50% = ___   Answers: 1. 0.50
2. 12% = ___   2. 0.120
3. 175% = ___   3. 1.750
4. 2.5% = ___   4. 0.025
5. 10.3% = ___   5. 0.103

Okay, you have gotten this far and you are asking yourself, "How will I use this information?" Let's say that you are responsible for figuring out how much the pharmacy can save on invoices if they are paid quickly. You have an invoice that says, "2.5% 10 days/Net 30 days." The total amount of the invoice is $3500.00. To figure the discount is really only two steps. First, convert the percentage to a decimal. Second, multiply the invoice total and the decimal number to obtain the discount. Using the foregoing example, convert the 2.5% to a decimal.

2.5% becomes 0.025

Now multiply the decimal and the invoice total.

$$\$3500.00 \times 0.025 = \$87.50$$

So the discount would be $87.50. It does not sound like a big discount, but remember that this is one invoice. A pharmacy could save thousands of dollars a year just by paying the invoices quickly.

Another use of percentages is to figure out the amount of markup for items so the pharmacy can make a profit. Remember, the pharmacy has to make a profit so that it can pay you, pay for rent and utilities, and give the owner enough to live off. Let's do a few practice exercises on how to figure markup.

The pharmacy must mark up all cold medicines by 56% in order to make a profit. The following is an example of three different products at different prices: Find the amount to mark them up, and then give the total cost of the product.

Daytime cold and cough liquid, $4.25	$4.25 × 0.56 = $2.38 (markup)
Total cost of this medication would be	$4.25 + $2.38 = $6.63
Tylenol cold and cough liquid, $5.50	$5.50 × 0.56 = $3.08
Total cost of this medication would be	$5.50 + $3.08 = $8.58
Pseudoephedrine tablets, $2.95	$2.95 × 0.56 = $1.65
Total cost of this medication would be	$2.95 + $1.65 = $4.60

Ratio/Proportion or Formula Method

When technicians compound certain products, they may be required to solve problems using ratios, which can be considered parts or fractions. For example, a concentration of 1:1000 means there is 1 part to 1000 parts, or 1 g of drug in

1000 mL of solution. If you receive an order for 5% hydrocortisone and you have 1:1000 concentration in stock, you can use a simple two-step ratio/proportion to solve the problem.

EXAMPLE 4-1 RATIO/PROPORTION

Step 1
5% is equivalent to 5 g per 100 mL or 5000 mg per 100 mL. This can be reduced to 50 mg/mL. Your stock solution is 1 g in 1000 mL, or 1000 mg in 1000 mL, which can be reduced to equal 1 mg/mL.

Step 2
Subtract what you have from what you need to find the final volume or strength. In this case it would be as follows:

> 5 g (needed) − 1 g (have) = 4 g needed to prepare the final product per 100 mL

About 90% of the orders you will encounter in the pharmacy will be ratio/proportion equations. This is a three-step process. One of the first rules to remember is to filter out the unnecessary information. Second, find what strength you have in stock and what strength you need (what the doctor is ordering). Finally, set up the equation and double check the calculations. You can use one of two methods: method A (ratio/proportion) (have = need) or method B (formula) using $\frac{D}{H} \times Q$ = medication to give, where D is the desired dose, H is what you have in stock, and Q is the quantity on hand.

For each of the following examples, both types of calculations are used. Try to solve the problems using both methods, and use what works best for you.

For other medication orders, finding the answer may not be as simple. For example, if a drug is ordered that does not easily convert, you can use these two methods. The most important point to remember is to place the correct units into the correct position. Try both methods, and choose the one that makes more sense to you.

EXAMPLE 4-2 RATIO/PROPORTION

Order: Prepare 240 mg of a drug using the pharmacy stock concentration of 80 mg/4 mL.

Method A: (Have = Need)
In this case, you need to determine how many milliliters of the stock solution are needed to fill the 240-mg order. Write your stock or given concentration on the left and your needed amount on the right. Make sure your milligrams and milliliters match across from one another. Then cross multiply by the quantity on the side of the *x,* and then divide by the numerator of your concentration, and you will have your necessary milliliters to draw from the vial.

$$\frac{80\,mg}{4\,mL} = \frac{240\,mg}{x}$$

$$960 = 80x$$

$$\frac{960\,mg}{80\,mL} = \frac{80\,mg}{x} \quad \text{Divide both sides by 80}$$

$$12\,mL = x$$

Answer: You will need to withdraw 12 mL of solution to equal 240 mg of drug.

Method B: D/H × Q = medication to give

Using a different method, you can set up the equation as the desired amount (240 mg) over the stock strength (80 mg) times the quantity of the stock volume (4 mL) as shown below:

$$\frac{240\,mg}{80\,mL} \times 4\,mL = 12\,mL$$

EXAMPLE 4-3 RATIO/PROPORTION

Method A: (Have = Need)

Order: You need to prepare 1 pt of 40 mcg medicated lotion. How many milliliters of the stock solution 5 mcg/mL will it take to prepare the final product? Write your stock or given concentration on the left and your volume needed on the right. Make sure your milligrams and milliliters match across from one another. Do not forget to cross multiply and divide by the quantity on the side of the *x*, and you will have your necessary volume to draw from the container.

$$\frac{5\,mcg}{1\,mL} = \frac{40\,mcg}{x}$$

$$40 = 5x$$

$$\frac{40\,mg}{5\,mg} = \frac{5\,mg}{x} \text{ Divide both sides by 5}$$

$$x = 8\,mL$$

Answer: You need a total volume of 8 mL of drug mixed into the lotion to equal 1 pt. To determine 1 pt (30 mL/oz; 8 oz/cup; 2 cups/pt; so, 30 mL × 16 oz = 480 mL). Therefore you subtract the amount of drug to be added from the total volume:

$$480\,mL - 8\,mL = 472\,mL$$

Answer: You will add 8 mL of drug to 472 mL of lotion to get a 40-mcg bottle of lotion.

Method B: D/H × Q = Medication to Give

Using a different method, you can set up the equation as the desired strength (40%) over the stock strength (5%) times the volume of the stock strength (1 mL). Remember that when setting up Method B, the units must match in the fraction as shown below:

$$\frac{40\%}{5\%} \times 1\,mL = 8\,mL$$

Answer: You will need to convert the pint the same way as indicated previously, and you will end up with the same answer.

EXAMPLE 4-4

You receive an order for clindamycin 450 mg q12h. To set up your equation, you need to know what you have on hand. Clindamycin is available in different sizes, but all of the sizes have the same concentration. The strength for clindamycin is 150 mg/mL. For each of the milliliters in the vial there is 150 mg of drug (clindamycin). We now have all the components we need to begin.

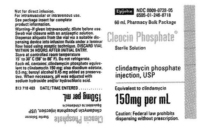

Method A (Have = Need)

What you have = What you need

$$\frac{150\,mg}{1\,mL} = \frac{450\,mg}{x\,mL}$$

You are solving for *x* because you do not know how much clindamycin to draw up into a syringe. To solve for *x*, you *cross multiply and divide.*

$$\frac{150\,mg}{1\,mL} = \frac{450\,mg}{x\,mL} \qquad \frac{1\,mL \times 450\,mg}{150\,mg} = x$$

$$x = 3\ mL$$

Method B (D/H × Q)

$$\frac{450\,mg}{150\,mg} \times 1\,mL = 3\,mL$$

In this case the desired amount of drug is 450 mg; the stock on hand is 150 mg/1 mL. When laid out in this linear fashion, the amount needed is 3 mL. You can confirm this by multiplying 3 mL by 150 mg to get 450 mg.

EXAMPLE 4-5

You receive an order for 0.5 mg of alprazolam (Xanax) 1 to 2 tabs qhs × 7 days prn insomnia.

 You only have 1-mg tablets in stock.
 How many tablets are needed to fill this order?

Method A (Have = Need)

What you have = What you need

$$\frac{1\,mg}{1\ tablet} = \frac{0.5\,mg}{x\ tablets}$$

$$\frac{1\,mg}{tablet} = \frac{0.5\,mg}{x\ tablets} = 0.5\ tablets$$

$$0.5\ tablets \times 2\ tablets = 1\text{-}mg\ tablets$$

In this case, multiply the answer by the maximum dosage ordered (1 mg), and then multiply it by 7 days.

$$1\ mg\ tablet \times 7\ days = 7\ tablets$$

Give seven tablets with the following instructions:

 Take one-half to one tablet at bedtime for 7 days as needed for insomnia.

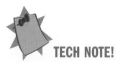

Method B (D/H × Q)

$$\frac{0.5\,mg}{1\,mg} \times 1\,tablet = 0.5\,tablets$$

$$0.5\ tablets \times 2\ tablets = 1\text{-}mg\ tablets$$

$$1\ mg \times 7\ days = 7\ tablets$$

Give seven tablets with the following instructions:
Take one-half to one tablet at bedtime for 7 days as needed for insomnia.

EXAMPLE 4-6

You receive an order for erythromycin 200 mg/5 mL suspension.
Give 150 mg every 6 hours per day for 10 days.

1. How many milliliters of suspension will be given per dose?
2. How many milliliters of suspension will be given per day?
3. How many milliliters of suspension will be given over the course of the treatment?
4. How much suspension will be discarded, if any?

To solve, do the following:

You have on hand a 200-mL container of 200 mg/5 mL. You need 150 mg/x mL (x mL = the volume).

Answer to question 1
Using Method A:

$$\frac{200\,mg}{5\,mL} = \frac{150\,mg}{x\,mL}$$

$$x = 3.75\ mL\ per\ dose$$

Using Method B:

$$\frac{150\,mg}{200\,mL} \times 5\,mL = 3.75\,mL\ per\ dose$$

Answer to question 2
Multiply the dose by times per day.

$$3.75\ per\ dose \times 4\ doses/day = 15\ mL/day$$

Answer to question 3
This requires a straight multiplication to get the answer.

$$15\ mL\ (per\ day) \times 10\ (amount\ of\ days) = 150\ mL\ over\ 10\ days$$

Answer to question 4
This requires subtraction of the total volume minus the used portion.

$$Erythromycin\ suspension\ 200\ mL - 150\ mL = 50\ mL\ that\ will\ be\ discarded$$

EXERCISE 4-3 QUICK CHECK

You receive an order for erythromycin 1.5-g dose stat to the hospital floor. You have 500-mg tablets in stock. How many 500-mg tablets will you need to fill this order? How many would you need for three doses?

EXERCISE 4-4 QUICK CHECK

Order 1: Metoprolol tartrate (Lopressor) 100-mg tablet twice a day for 30 days. You have 50-mg tablets. How many tablets will it take to fill this 30-day supply? — 60

Order 2: Ranitidine 75-mg syrup at bedtime. You have 1 pt of a 15-mg/mL bottle available. How many milliliters will it take to fill a 30-day supply? Do you have enough?

Try both methods for each of the problems listed previously.

Determine which method you find simpler to use, and then stick with that method.

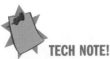

TECH NOTE!

Always pay attention to the dosage form. If you have a capsule, you cannot take one and a half capsules, but you can take a scored tablet. Also remember that not all tablets can be split, such as sustained-release tablets.

Filling Prescriptions

Following are more examples of basic calculations using ratio/proportion. When filling an oral tablet prescription using a different strength than what was ordered, use the following technique to determine the correct quantity.

EXAMPLE 4-7 DETERMINING QUANTITY

You need to fill cimetidine 600 mg tid (3 times a day) for 30 days.
     You have 400-mg tablets.

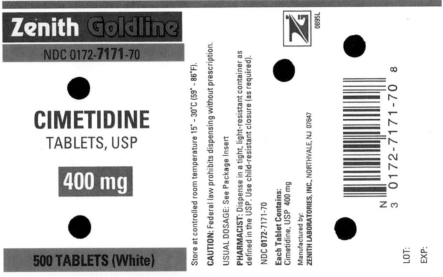

How many 400-mg tablets will you need to fill this order?
To solve, do the following:

$$600 \text{ mg} \times 3 \text{ doses} = 1800 \text{ mg per day}$$

$$\frac{1800 \text{ mg per day}}{400 \text{ mg}} = 4.5 \text{ tablets per day}$$

4.5 tablets (per day) × 30-day supply = 135 tablets to fill this order

Directions: The label would read as follows:

Take $1\frac{1}{2}$ tablets three times daily for 30 days

Pediatric Dosing

Many prescriptions are filled daily for children, and it is important that the parent understand how much medicine to give the child. When the strength needed cannot be measured with a teaspoon or is an odd amount, you must use droppers. Figure 4-2 shows various measuring devices that can be used to deliver suspensions. The pharmacist, not the technician, should show the parent of the patient how to measure the correct amount.

Household/metric   Medication Dropper   Syringe

oz/mL

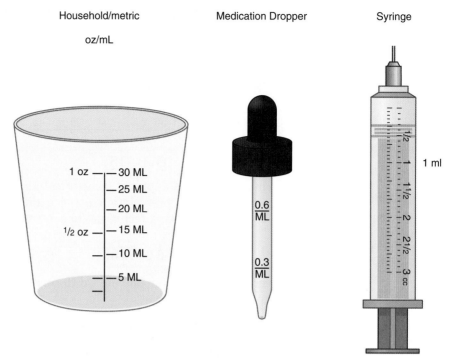

FIGURE 4-2 Common devices used for measuring liquid medications.

EXAMPLE 4-8 PEDIATRIC DOSAGE CALCULATION

You receive an order for carbamazepine suspension. The following is an example of what you have in stock.

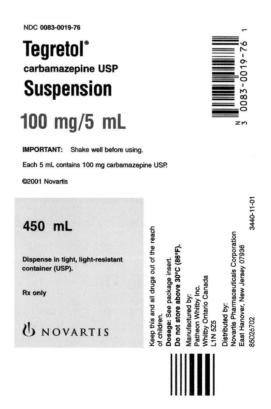

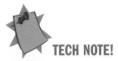

TECH NOTE!

This is how to remember kilogram conversion: Your weight is more than cut in half when put in kilograms (2.2 lb = 1 kg). If you weighed 200 lb, you would weigh 90.0 kg.

In stock: carbamazepine 100 mg/5 mL bottle of 450 mL.
Order: carbamazepine 250 mg tid (3 times a day) PO (by mouth)

1. How many milliliters are needed per dose?
2. How many milliliters are needed per day?
3. How many doses can be taken from the 450-mL bottle?

To solve, use method A or method B as explained previously:

Answer to question 1
Using method A:

$$\frac{100\,mg}{5\,mL} = \frac{250\,mg}{x\,mL}$$

$$1250 = 100\,x$$

$$\frac{1250}{100} = \frac{100}{100} \quad \text{Divide both sides by 100}$$

$$x = 12.5\,mL\ per\ dose$$

Using method B:

$$\frac{250\,mg}{100\,mg} \times 5\,mL = 12.5\,mL\ per\ dose$$

Answer to question 2
12.5 mL (per dose) × 3 (times per day) = 37.5 mL per day

Answer to question 3
If we have 450 mL of carbamazepine (Tegretol), divide by 12.5 mL to get 36 doses.

Determining Weight

Because all manufacturers provide proper dosing regimens based on kilograms, it is necessary to convert pounds into kilograms. Because most persons do not know their weight in kilograms, they will provide their weight in pounds. Therefore the pharmacy technician will need to convert the patient's weight. Although the steps are simple, it is important to remember that there are 2.2 lb per kilogram.

$$16\,oz = 1\,lb$$

$$2.2\,lb = 1\,kg$$

To determine how many kilograms there are in 1 lb, divide.
To determine how many pounds there are in 1 kg, multiply.

EXAMPLE 4-9 CONVERTING WEIGHT AND DETERMINING PEDIATRIC DOSAGE

The pharmacy receives an order for a baby girl weighing 7 lb.
The order calls for 20 mg/kg dose.
This means that for every kilogram the child weighs, she should receive 20 mg of medication.
To solve, do the following: find her weight in kg

$$\frac{2.2\,lb}{1\,kg} = \frac{7\,lb}{x\,kg}$$

$$\frac{7\,lb}{2.2\,lb} = 3.18\,kg$$

Now multiply the weight in kilograms by the recommended dosage.

$$20 \text{ mg} \times 3.18 \text{ kg} \times 1 \text{ dose} = 63.6 \text{ mg/dose}$$

EXAMPLE 4-10 CONVERTING WEIGHTS

Determine the total amount of drug to be given per day and then per dose.

For the same baby given in Example 4-9, we now have an order for 60 mg/kg per day to be given every 8 hours. To figure out the problem, first multiply the milligrams of medicine by the weight of the child in kilograms to obtain the daily amount. Then divide by the number of doses per day.

$$60 \text{ mg} \times 3.18 \text{ kg} = 190.8 \text{ mg/day}$$

EXERCISE 4.5 QUICK CHECK

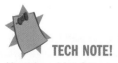

TECH NOTE!
When rounding off numbers, complete all of the calculations, and then round at the end if instructed to do so by the pharmacist. If you round off at each step, your answer will not be as accurate.

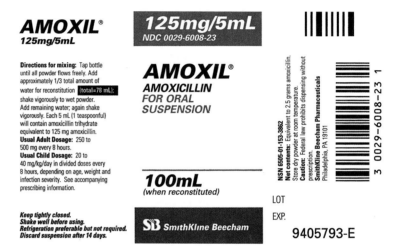

You receive an order for a pediatric patient.
Baby, male; weight 23 lb
Sig: Give amoxicillin suspension 30 mg/kg/day in divided doses q8h.
1. What is the weight of the baby in kilograms (rounded to the nearest tenth)?
2. What is the dose per day based on the baby's weight?
3. What is the strength of a single dose?
4. How many milliliters are to be given with each dose?

Drip Rates

Hospital pharmacy technicians deliver a 24-hour supply of intravenous solutions to the nursing stations daily, so the nurses can administer them to their patients. Most intravenous piggybacks are smaller intravenous solutions that are given over 30 to 60 minutes. Large-volume medications need to be given at a slow rate because veins can handle only a small volume. For large-volume drips, the pharmacy technician must be able to calculate the volume needed to last over a certain amount of time, or he or she may need to calculate how much longer a currently hanging intravenous solution will last. Depending on the order received, the technician must be able to manipulate the numbers to determine this information. This ultimately will determine the amount of intravenous solution to be prepared that will last for 24 hours (Figure 4-3).

TECH NOTE!
Here is a hint for determining drops. Remember drops are written as *gtt*. Amounts differ between dropper sizes. About 60 drops are in 5 mL (cc). Also, drops can be intended for drip rates. The number of drops per milliliter depends on the tubing.

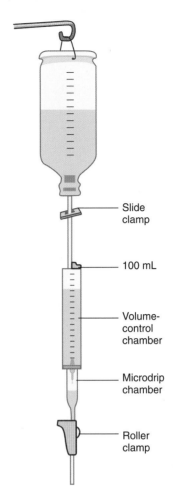

FIGURE 4-3 Intravenous (IV) drip system.

These calculations involve determining the following:

1. The right amount of drug that is to be given over time
2. The amount of time left until an IV runs out
3. The amount of drug needed to last a certain time

Basic conversions are as follows:

Time: 1 hour = 60 minutes, 24 hours = 1 day
Volume: 5 mL = 60 gtt

These calculations will be determined by the size of tubing used to deliver the medication. We will use a common drop factor to determine the volume. The drop factor is given on each set of tubing. If you have a tubing set that states 10 gtt/mL, this is the drop factor and will be used to determine the rate.

EXAMPLE 4-11 CALCULATING DRIP RATES

You receive an order for a 2-L bag to be given over 24 hours. Your tubing says it delivers 15 gtt/mL. What are the drops per minute? To find this out, prepare the problem.

Steps involved in determining drops per minute:

1. What is the drop factor? 15 gtt/mL
2. What will be the milliliters per hour?

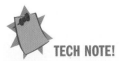

TECH NOTE!
Technicians and pharmacists do not determine the size of the tubing. This is predetermined by the doctor's orders to the nurse.

$$\frac{2000\,mL}{24\,hours} = \frac{83.3\,mL}{hour}$$

(24 hours/day)

3. What will be the milliliters per minute?

$$\frac{83.3\,mL}{60\,minutes} = \frac{1.38\,mL}{min}$$

(60 minutes/hour)

4. What will be the drops per minute?

$$\frac{1.38\,mL}{min\,mL} \times \frac{15\,gtt}{min} = \frac{20.7\,gtt}{min}$$

EXAMPLE 4-12 DETERMINING DROPS PER MINUTE

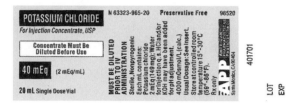

Order: 1500 mL of 20 mEq KCl for 12 hours. The tubing size is 20 gtt/mL. How many drops per minute will be delivered?

Answer

$$\frac{1500\,mL}{12\,hours} = \frac{125\,mL}{hr}$$

$$\frac{125\,mL}{60\,min} = \frac{2.08\,mL}{min}$$

$$\frac{2.08\,mL}{min} \times \frac{20\,gtt}{mL} = \frac{41.66\,gtt}{min}$$

EXAMPLE 4-13 DETERMINING VOLUME BASED ON DROPS PER MINUTE

Administer to patient a 3-L total parenteral nutrition bag over 24 hours. Tubing size delivers 15 gtt/mL.

How many mL/hr will be delivered?

How many milliliters per minute are being delivered to the patient?

How many drops per minute will be delivered?

Determine milliliters/hour:

$$\frac{3000\,mL}{24\,hr} = 125\,gtt/min$$

Determine mL/minute:

$$\frac{125\,mL/hr}{60\,min} = 2.08\,gtt/min$$

Determine gtt/minute:

$$2.08\,gtt/min \times 15\,gtt/min = 31.2\,gtt/min$$

EXAMPLE 4-14 DETERMINING DROPS PER MINUTE BASED ON VOLUME AND DROP FACTOR

How many drops/minute would an IV deliver to a patient receiving 40 mL/hr using a 20 gtt/mL set?

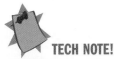

TECH NOTE!

A large-volume bag can hang for a maximum of 24 hours before it must be changed to prevent microbial growth.

Determine the milliliters/minute: 40 mL/hr ÷ 60 min = 0.666 mL/min

Determine the drops/minute: 0.666 gtt/min × 20 gtt/mL drop factor = 13.33 or 13 gtt/min

EXERCISE 4-6 QUICK CHECK

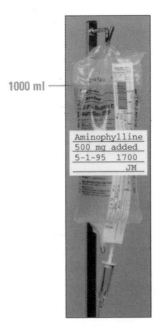

1000 ml —

Aminophylline
500 mg added
5-1-95   1700
        JM

Order: Patient to be given aminophylline 500 mg in 1000 mL over 24 hours. The drip rate is 25 gtt/mL. What is the flow rate in drops/minute? How many milliliters would be delivered per hour?

Alligation

Alligation is used when you need to prepare (compound) percent strength that you do not have in stock. To make this strength, you need to use two other strengths to attain the correct one. For example, if a doctor orders 20% KCl, but you only have 10% and 50% on hand, calculate the amount of each solution to attain a 20% solution. You can do this using any two strengths as long as only one is less concentrated than the final solution. This means that you cannot make a 20% solution from a 5% and a 10% solution because both are less than the needed amount. However, you can make a 10% solution from a 5% and a 70% solution. Also, water is another element you might use as one of the solutions. The percentage of water is considered 0%. Let's begin by working with these numbers.

Problem: You have in stock a 70% solution and a 20% solution. How much of each do you need in order to create 1 L of 40% solution?

This is as simple as tic-tac-toe; following these basic rules:

1. Draw a tic-tac-toe board.

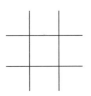

2. Place your desired strength in the middle square.

$$\begin{array}{c|c}\hline & \\\hline 40 & \\\hline & \\\end{array}$$

3. Put your higher-strength solution in the top left square.

$$\begin{array}{c|c}70 & \\\hline & 40 \\\hline & \\\end{array}$$

4. Put your lower-strength solution in the bottom left square. If you are using water, you will place a zero in this square.

$$\begin{array}{c|c}70 & \\\hline & 40 \\\hline 20 & \\\end{array}$$

5. Take the difference between top left square and middle square number, and place the new number in bottom right square. Do the same with the bottom left number, and place this result in the top right square.

$$\begin{array}{c|c}70 & 20 \\\hline & 40 \\\hline 20 & 30\end{array}$$ 40 – 20 = 20

    70 – 40 = 30

6. Create a fraction by adding the two new figures (top and bottom right squares) together for a common denominator. Place the top right number over the denominator and do the same for the bottom right number.

$$\begin{array}{c|c}70 & 20 \\\hline & 40 \\\hline 20 & 30\end{array}$$ $\dfrac{20}{20 + 30}$ $\dfrac{30}{20 + 30}$

7. Divide out each fraction, and then multiply by the total volume you need.

$$\begin{array}{c|c}70 & 20 \\\hline & 40 \\\hline 20 & 30\end{array}$$ $\dfrac{20}{50} \times 1000 \text{ mL} = 400 \text{ mL}$

    $\dfrac{30}{50} \times 1000 \text{ mL} = 600 \text{ mL}$

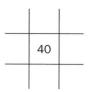

TECH NOTE!
Do not read your answer diagonally. Read your answer straight across!

8. Check your answer by adding the two parts. They should equal the total volume.

$$\begin{array}{c|c}70 & 20 \\\hline & 40 \\\hline 20 & 30\end{array}$$ 400 mL of 70% solution

    $\dfrac{600 \text{ mL}}{1000 \text{ mL of 20\% solution}}$

Answer: 400 mL of the 70% solution, and 600 mL of the 20% solution will prepare a 1-L solution of 40%.

EXERCISE 4-7 QUICK CHECK

> Prepare a 20% KCl 500 mL from your stock of 5% and 70% KCl.

Roman Numerals

The number system commonly used in the United States is the Arabic system, consisting of the numbers 1, 2, 3, and so forth. This system is not always used by physicians when ordering medications. Instead they may use Roman numerals indicating a quantity of tablets or capsules to be filled or to order the strength of medication. When adding Roman numerals, begin with I to III, then write IV (1 less than 5) to equal 4. Repeat the process at 9 by writing IX (1 less than 10) to equal 9. In the same way, if you were to write 49, you would write IL (1 less than 50) to equal 49. See the following for a comparison of Roman numerals and Arabic numbers.

Roman Numerals	Arabic Numerals	Roman Numerals	Arabic Numerals
I	1	XI	11
II	2	XIX	19
III	3	XX	20
IV	4	L	50
V	5	C	100
VI	6	D	500
VII	7	M	1000
VIII	8		
IX	9		
X	10		

RULES FOR DETERMINING ROMAN NUMERALS

1. When a numeral is repeated, its value is repeated.
   Example: II = 2
2. A numeral may not be repeated more than 3 times.
   Example: XL = 40, not XXXX
3. V, L, and D are never repeated. LL is incorrect.
4. When a smaller numeral is placed before a larger numeral, it is subtracted from the larger numeral.
   Example: XC = 100 − 10 = 90
5. When a smaller numeral is placed after a larger numeral, it is added to the larger numeral.
   Example: CL = 100 + 50 = 150
6. V, L, and D are never subtracted. LC is incorrect.
7. Never subtract more than one numeral.
   Example: 8 = VIII not IIX
8. When subtracting, only use a numeral before the next two higher-value numerals. For example, use I before V and X, X before L and C, and C before D and M.

EXAMPLE 4-15 WORKING WITH ROMAN NUMERALS

When working with Roman numerals, remember that if a larger number is placed in front of a smaller one, you must add both to determine the value.

XV   X(10) + V(5) = 15

However, if there is a smaller number placed before a larger number, then you must subtract.

IX X(10) − I(1) = 9

EXERCISE 4-8 **QUICK CHECK**

Determine the following:

a. XIV = _____
b. XC = _____
c. CIV = _____
d. XL = _____
e. VIII = _____
f. C = _____
g. IV = _____
h. LX = _____
i. IX = _____
j. III = _____
k. X = _____
l. XI = _____
m. XXXIX = _____
n. VII = _____

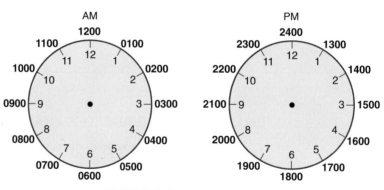

FIGURE 4-4 Military time clock.

International Time

In hospital settings, international time, also known as military time, is used exclusively. Because orders are written 24 hours a day, a system is needed to ensure that all medical-related caretakers understand exactly when the order was written and when the medication or treatment is to take place. The system is based on 100. Starting with the first hour of the day, the clock begins at 0100 (1 AM) through 2400 or midnight (Figure 4-4). This system is easy for most persons to use through 1200 (noon), but then it can get confusing. As the clock hands begin to make their second trip around the face of the clock, the numbers continue. For example, 1300 is 1 PM, and 1400 is 2 PM. When the pharmacy receives orders, the receiver needs to check date and time against previous orders to ensure that the most recent order is in effect. By using this system, one never has any question as to when an order was written or which order supersedes another.

EXERCISE 4-9 QUICK CHECK

Fill in the blanks:

From 0800 to 1500 hours is _____ hours.

A dose given at 0600, 1400, and 2200 hours is _____ hours apart.

A dose given at 0005, 1430, and 2045 would be given at _____, _____, and _____ on a 12-hour clock.

Write 4:20 PM, 7:15 PM, and 12:00 AM in international time: _____, _____, _____.

DO YOU REMEMBER THESE KEY POINTS?

- The basic measurements of the metric, apothecary, and avoirdupois systems
- That the primary system used in pharmacy is the metric system
- How to convert metric numbers from kilograms all the way to micrograms
- That all measurements must have units attached to keep them straight
- How to convert pounds into kilograms and vice versa
- That double-checking calculations is important before preparing medications
- How to determine how long an intravenous solution will last
- When to use ratio/proportion and the steps involved in both methods shown
- When to use alligation and how to set up the equation
- How to convert Roman numerals to Arabic numbers

REVIEW QUESTIONS

Convert the following units into percentages.

1. $^1/_5$ _____
2. 0.25 _____
3. $^{10}/_{25}$ _____
4. 2.275 _____

Convert the following fractions of grains into milligrams.

5. $^1/_{300}$ gr _____   .0033 × 65 = 0.2
6. $^1/_{150}$ gr _____   .0067 × 65 = 0.4

Write the Arabic numbers in Roman numerals and Roman numerals in Arabic numbers.

7. 20
8. 50
9. 100
10. 59
11. 2
12. CXL
13. XC
14. XXXIV
15. XIX
16. VIII

Convert the following metric units into the units indicated to the right.

17. 5 cc = ___ tsp
18. 15 cc = ___ tsp
19. 30 mL = ___ tsp
20. 1000 mL = ___ L
21. 2 kg = ___ lb
22. 1 mcg = ___ mg
23. 1000 mg = ___ g
24. 900 mL = ___ oz
25. 0.25 L = ___ mL
26. 0.25 mg = ___ mcg

Solve the following drug orders. Be sure to show your work. Use the following conversions.

qd = daily

bid = 2 times daily

tid = 3 times daily

qid = 4 times daily

PO = orally/by mouth

IV = intravenous

27. You receive the following order: Cimetidine 300 mg tab qid × 30 days. You have cimetidine 150 mg in stock. How many tablets will you need to fill this order?

28. Make a tobramycin IV 60 mg q8h in D_5W 50 mL. You have tobramycin 40 mg/mL in 2-mL vials. How much will you need in milliliters?

29. Make a vancomycin IV 750 mg q12h in D_5W 250 mL. You have vancomycin 1 g per 20-mL vial. How much will you take from the 1-g vial?

30. Make a 10% NS solution 1 L. You have 5% and 50% NS bags only. How much of each solution will it take to make a 10% NS 1-L bag?

31. Make amino acids 30% solution 0.5 L. You have 70% amino acids and sterile water in stock. How much of each solution is required to prepare a 30% solution?

32. Convert the following ratios into grams over milliliters.
A. 1:10   D. 100:100
B. 2:100   E. 100:100,000
C. 1:1000   F. 2:10,000

33. Prepare 5-mL of a 1:1000 epinephrine solution. You have 1:1000 1 mL stock solution. What will be the amount of epinephrine (in milligrams) in 5 mL?

34. Dispense ibuprofen liquid 40 mg/kg per day; give qid. You have ibuprofen liquid 100 mg/5 mL in stock. How much will this patient receive per dose if the patient's weight is 10 lb? How much liquid is needed to fill a 7-day supply?

35. Administer 500 mL heparin to be given over 20 hours. Tubing size delivers 10 gtt/mL. How many drops/minute are being delivered to the patient?

TECHNICIAN'S CORNER

A compounding order comes to the pharmacy with the following directions:

Gentamicin 15 mg/mL dispense 5 mL ii gtt os bid
You have a 5-mL bottle of gentamicin ophthalmic drops 40 mg/mL in stock. You must decrease the concentration from 40 mg/mL to 15 mg/mL using sterile water.

ANSWERS TO QUICK CHECK EXERCISES

Answers to quick check 4-1

1. 0.8 tsp or 1 tsp

2. 1 cup

3. 16 cups

4. 1 tsp

5. 2 tbsp

6. 1 oz

7. 60 mg

8. 2 cups

9. 480 mL

10. 225 mL

11. 1000 g

Answers to quick check 4-2

0.00088 mg

0.00000088 g

0.00000000088 kg

Answers to quick check 4-3

3 tablets = 1500 mg or 1.5 g

3 tablets × 3 doses = 9 tablets

Answers to quick check 4-4

Order 1: 120 tablets

Order 2: 150 mL; yes, because there are 480 mL in 1 pt

Answers to quick check 4-5

Baby weighs 10.5 kg

Dose per day: 315 mg/day

Single dose: 105 mg

Milliliters per dose: 4.25 mL

Answers to quick check 4-6

The flow rate is 17.36, or 17 gtt/min

41.66, or 42 mL/hr

Answers to quick check 4-7

115.38 mL, or (115 mL) of the 70% solution

384.61 mL, or (385 mL) of the 20% solution

Answers to quick check 4-8

a. 14

b. 90

c. 104

d. 40

e. 8

f. 100

g. 4

h. 60

i. 9

j. 3

k. 10

l. 11

m. 39

n. 7

Answers to quick check 4-9

a. 7 hours

b. 8 hours

c. 5 minutes after midnight; 2:30 PM; 8:45 PM

d. 1620; 1915; 2400

BIBLIOGRAPHY

Gray Morris D: *Calculate with confidence,* ed 4, St Louis, 2005, Elsevier.

Mizner JJ: *Mosby's review for the PTCB Certification Examination,* St Louis, 2005, Elsevier.

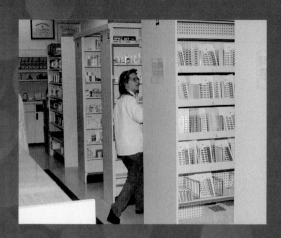

Dosage Forms, Abbreviations, and Routes of Administration

Objectives

UPON COMPLETING THIS CHAPTER, YOU SHOULD BE ABLE TO DO THE FOLLOWING:

- List at least three reasons why certain drugs need to be given by certain routes.

- Discuss the different components of medications and how that affects their bioavailability and pharmacological effectiveness.

- List the most common routes and dosage forms of drugs.

- List three different common drugs and their storage requirements.

- Describe why additives are necessary in the production of medications.

- Define the common abbreviations for extended-release agents.

- List both pros and cons for the various routes of administration outlined.

- Show the ability to translate abbreviations for dosage forms and routes of administration.

Dosage forms	Abbreviation	Main routes of administration	Abbreviation
Buccal tablet	buccal	Right ear	AD
Capsule	cap	Left ear	AS
Chewable tablet	chew tab	Both ears	AU
Cream	cr	Gastrostomy tube	GT
Elixir	elix	Inhalant	INH
Enema	enema	Intradermal	ID
Enteric-coated tablet	EC tab	Intramuscular	IM
Gel cap	cap	Intravenous	IV
Gelatin	gel	Intravenous piggyback	IVPB
Liquid	liq	Nasogastric	NG
Lotion	lot	Nasogastric tube	NGT
Lozenge	loz	Right eye	OD
Metered dose inhaler	MDI	Left eye	OS
Ointment	ung, oint	Both eyes	OU
Patch, transdermal	top	Orally or by mouth	PO
Powder	top	Rectal, per rectum	PR
Spray	spry	Subcutaneous	SQ/SC
Suppository	supp	Sublingual	SL
Suspension	susp	Topical	TOP
Syrup	syr		
Tablet	tab		
Tincture	tinc		
Troche	troches		
Vaginal cream	vag cr		
Vaginal tablet	vag tab		

Absorption *The taking in of nutrients from food and liquids*

Bioavailability *The amount of drug that reaches its intended destination by being absorbed into the bloodstream*

Bioequivalence *The difference between a drug that is manufactured in a different dosage form or by a different company; includes the rate of absorption, distribution, metabolism, and excretion*

Distribution *The ability of a drug to pass into the bloodstream*

Excretion *Elimination of waste products through stools and urine*

Half-life *1. The amount of time it takes a chemical to be decreased by one half. 2. The time required for half the amount of a substance such as a drug in a living system to be eliminated or disintegrated by natural processes. 3. The time required for a concentration of a substance in a body fluid (blood plasma) to decrease by half.*

Instill *To place into; instructions used for ophthalmic or otic drugs*

Metabolism *The physical and chemical changes that take place within an organism*

OTC *Over-the-counter*

Parenteral medication *Medication administered by injection, such as intravenously or intramuscularly*

Pharmacokinetics *The life of the drug, which includes absorption, metabolism, distribution, and excretion*

FOR A TECHNICIAN TO BECOME PROFICIENT, it is necessary to interpret orders correctly. Although it may be true that many doctors' handwriting is referred to as "chicken scratch," it is the responsibility of the pharmacy to interpret and clarify orders if necessary. Many of the abbreviations that are used in prescribing medication look very much alike. For instance, mg (milligram) can look much like mcg (microgram) when written quickly. In this chapter we explore the common abbreviations seen in pharmacy as they apply to dosage forms and routes of administration. In addition to learning the many different types of dosage forms that are available and the reasons why they are necessary, we will cover the pharmacokinetics related to the manufacturing of dosage forms.

Where Did Pharmacy Abbreviations Originate?

Much of the terminology in pharmacy and medicine comes from the Latin and Greek languages. Because pharmacy began in Europe, most of the abbreviations have their origins in a foreign language. The use of Latin and Greek has remained into the twenty-first century with little change. Although these abbreviations tend to be confusing at first, they serve an important function. For example, if each pharmacy used its own terminology, it would be virtually impossible for one pharmacy to fill another pharmacy's prescriptions. Therefore the medical community uses terms in Latin and Greek. These terms serve as a universal language that all medical doctors, nurses, pharmacists, technicians, and other medical personnel can understand. However, the ability to clarify doctors' orders is still a real dilemma in the United States. The number of errors caused by doctors' poor handwriting and by inaccurate transcribing of orders by pharmacists and technicians is of great concern. Correct interpretation of doctors' orders by pharmacy staff is obviously extremely important. This can be a time-consuming element of pharmacy that conflicts with the requirements of most pharmacies because patients want their medications quickly. This leaves the pharmacy staff little time to confer or call on all orders that seem unclear; however, this is what must happen if errors are to be avoided. When writing out the various abbreviations, be sure to write as neatly as possible because other technicians and pharmacists will be reading your writing. Scrolls, stylized, or fancy lettering easily can seem to represent the wrong meaning. The pharmacy technician must learn all of the dosage forms and their abbreviations to decipher doctors' orders (see Terms and Abbreviations at the beginning of the chapter).

Dosage Forms

A dosage form refers to the means by which a drug is available for use or the vehicle by which the drug is delivered. With individual packaging the dosage form is given on the package. For example, the form may be a tablet or capsule. However, more than one type of tablet and capsule exist. Tablets come in a wide variety of shapes and sizes. For example, they come scored or unscored and coated or uncoated (Figure 5-1). Much of what determines the dosage form of a medication is determined by the effectiveness of the drug. For instance, heparin (an anticoagulant) is available only in parenteral (intravenous [IV] or subcutaneous [SQ]) form because it becomes ineffective if taken by mouth due to the effect of stomach acids on the drug. Manufacturers prepare certain medications with the ability to release the active ingredient over an extended period. This allows the patient to take the medication less often, which increases compliance. Another consideration is given to the person taking the drug. This includes age and condition of the person. If the prescription of acetaminophen (Tylenol) is

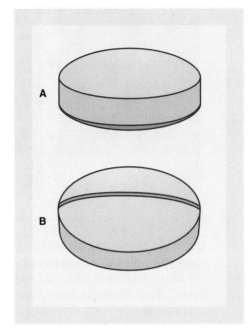

FIGURE 5-1 **A,** Unscored tablet. **B,** Scored tablet.

intended for a child, that dosage form should be available in liquid if at all possible for ease of administration. The following list of dosage forms gives a brief explanation of their differences. All the different forms can be broken down into three major categories that are composed of subcategories:

1. Solids: tablets, chewable tablets, enteric-coated tablets, extended-release agents, capsules, caplets, lozenges, troches, implant capsules, patches
2. Liquids: syrups, elixirs, sprays, inhalants, emulsions, suspensions, solutions, enemas
3. Semisolids: creams, lotions, ointments, powders, gelatins, suppositories

SOLIDS

Solid agents can be contained in various packages and administered by almost all routes except parenterally. The following brief descriptions explain the wide variety of solids available.

Tablets

Hundreds of types of tablets are available that range in size, shape, color, thickness, and composition. The most common type of tablet contains some type of filler. These fillers are composed of inert substances (no active ingredient) that serve to fill space or cover the tablet (sugar coatings). Sugar coatings improve taste and color or cover unpleasant odors. Finally, certain additives may be used to improve the absorption and/or distribution throughout the body. Some tablets are made to be administered sublingually (under the tongue) or vaginally. Also, some tablets come scored to allow the dosage to be cut in half if needed. Chewable tablets are convenient for persons who have difficulty swallowing tablets and for children who are unable to swallow large tablets. Other tablets are enteric-coated to help protect the drug through the acidic environment of the stomach until it reaches the more alkaline intestine. In other cases, the protective covering may delay the release of the drug while it travels through the stomach so that it will not irritate the stomach. Extended-release dosage forms

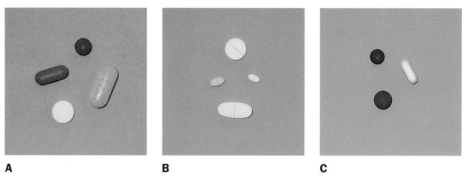

A   **B**   **C**

FIGURE 5-2 **A,** Plain tablets. **B,** Scored tablets. **C,** Enteric-coated tablets.

are made to control the amount of drug distributed over a set time. Figure 5-2 gives examples of plain, scored, and enteric-coated tablets.

Many medications have extended-release forms and regular forms. You must know which form the doctor has ordered. Abbreviations for agents that release medication over long periods are as follows:

CD	Controlled-diffusion
CR	Continuous/controlled-release
CRT	Controlled-release tablet
LA	Long-acting
SA	Sustained-action
SR	Sustained/slow-release
TD	Time-delay
TR	Time-release
XL	Extra-long
XR	Extended-release

Example: Aspirin tablets (over the counter [OTC]), aspirin tablets EC (OTC), nifedipine (prescription [Rx]), nifedipine XL (Rx)

Capsules and Caplets

Capsules are composed of a gelatin container. Caplet dosage forms are related closely to tablets, but they are smooth sided and are therefore easier to swallow. The word *caplet* refers to the shape of the tablet. Capsules can have a hard or a soft outer shell. The shells of hard capsules are composed of sugar, gelatin, and water. Their color is determined by the manufacturer and is used primarily for identification. Another type of capsule is the pulvule, which is shaped slightly different for identification purposes. Spansules are capsules that can be pulled apart to sprinkle the medication onto food for children, making it easier to administer. Because of the many sizes available in capsules and caplets, they can be produced to administer medication in many ways. For example, as seen in Figure 5-3, these capsules can even hold a small capsule or tablet inside. The reason behind this manufacturing decision is to determine the best absorption and distribution of the medication. The main difference between capsules and caplets is that capsules can be pulled apart. More medications are being prepared as caplets to ensure that they are tamper proof. Figure 5-4 shows more shapes and sizes of capsules.

Capsule sizes

Capsules come in different sizes, as seen in Figure 5-5. They vary in color, transparency, and identifying marks. The larger half of the capsule is known as the body, and the shorter half is known as the cap. Many companies produce a

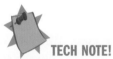

TECH NOTE!
Dosage forms that are especially made to release over time should not be crushed or broken into two. This would alter the delayed process. Some companies have their own unique names for extended-release agents. For example, Slo-Bid is a theophylline agent that is released over 12 hours, which is why the company has named it Slo-Bid (taken only twice daily).

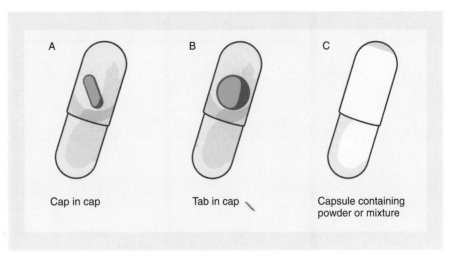

FIGURE 5-3 Different types of capsules.

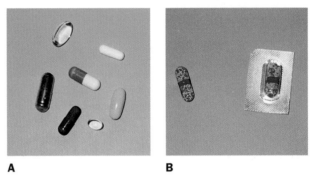

FIGURE 5-4 Types of capsules. **A,** Capsules. **B,** Extended-release capsules.

hard-shelled capsule that does not come apart to ensure that it is tamper resistant. Not all capsules are meant to be swallowed. Instead, specific dosages of medications are held inside the capsule. These medications can be sprinkled onto food or into liquid for administration. An example of this is Theo-Dur Sprinkles.

Example: Acetaminophen caplets (OTC), omeprazole capsules (Rx).

Lozenges/Troches
Lozenges and troches are other forms of tablets that are not meant to be swallowed but to dissolve in the mouth, which releases the medication more slowly. Many cough drops come in this type of package. Lozenges are similar to hard candy. Troches are larger than normal-size tablets and are flat; they usually have a chalky consistency in order to dissolve in the mouth.

Example: Lozenge—cetylpyridinium chloride (Cepacol; OTC); troche—clotrimazole (Rx)

Implants
A special type of capsule can be implanted under the skin and left in place for up to 5 years. This type of capsule comes in a set of six, each containing progestin, which acts as a contraceptive. The medication is released in a stair-step method starting with the highest amount of drug released in the first year and then tapering down from there to a minimum level that is maintained throughout the remaining time.

Number	Quantity	Example
000	1.37 ml	
00	0.95 ml	
0	0.68 ml	
1	0.5 ml	
2	0.37 ml	
3	0.3 ml	
4	0.2 ml	
5	0.13 ml	

FIGURE 5-5 Different sizes of capsules. Eight sizes are available; each holds a specific volume, and each holds a specific amount of medication. The size numbers are 5, 4, 3, 2, 1, 0, 00, 000—5 being the smallest and 000 being the largest.

TECH ALERT!
Never discard a medication patch after use. Because the medication is in a form that enables it to penetrate through the skin, a child might get hold of a potentially dangerous drug from the trash. The best approach is to wrap the patch in such a way that a child would not be able to grasp it.

Patches

Patches are solid pieces of material that hold a specific amount of medication to be released into the skin over time. Patches are convenient dosage forms because they are administered easily and eliminate possible upset stomach. Anginal medication such as transdermal patches can be placed on the chest once daily. Some motion sickness patches can be applied and left in place for up to 3 days. Fentanyl (Duragesic), a chronic pain medication, is a transdermal patch with a 3-day delivery time (Figure 5-6).

Example: Nitroglycerin patches (Rx), scopolamine transdermal patches (Rx), fentanyl patch (Duragesic; Rx)

LIQUIDS

Liquids are composed of various solutions. Their names relate to the types of liquid with which the medication is mixed. Depending on the type of taste, speed of action, or route of administration intended, a physician can choose the best agent for the job. Liquids can be administered by all routes, which makes them a popular choice. For example, enemas are liquid-filled bottles with a dispensing top that can be placed into the rectum to administer the solution into the lower intestine. This method works well for cleaning out impacted intestines. Other liquids are used in eye and ear products, which are used to treat a variety of conditions. Solutions also can be used topically to treat skin conditions. The following examples show the various types of liquids available.

Syrups

Syrups are sugar-based solutions that have medication dissolved into them. The sugar improves the taste of the drug. Syrups tend to be thicker than water.

Example: Vicks syrup (OTC), metaproterenol syrup (Rx)

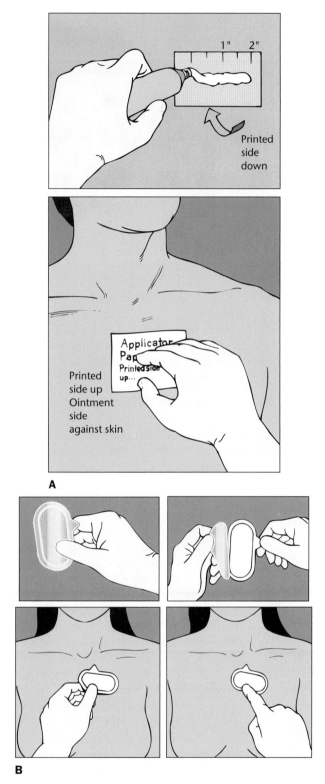

FIGURE 5-6 **A,** Example of nitroglycerin ointment patch. **B,** Example of a transdermal patch.

Elixirs

Elixirs contain dissolved medication in an alcohol base or water and alcohol (hydroalcoholic) base. The alcohol usually covers up the bad taste of the drug. Unlike syrups, elixirs have the same consistency as water.

Example: Dimetapp DM Elixir (OTC), theophylline elixir (Rx)

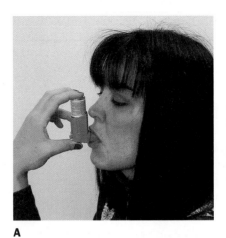

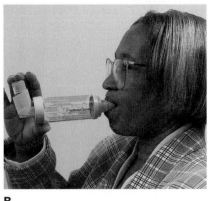

FIGURE 5-7 **A,** Inhaler. **B,** Inhaler attached to an aerochamber (also known as a spacer).

Sprays

Sprays are composed of various bases such as alcohol or water in a pump-type dispenser. Sprays are available for use in products such as nasal decongestants and sunscreens. A nitroglycerin translingual spray also is available for use under the tongue for relief of anginal pain.

> **Example:** Oxymetazoline (OTC), nitroglycerin (Nitrolingual; Rx)

Inhalants and Aerosols

Certain patients need to be able to get medication directly to the source of inflammation, such as the bronchial tree. Because these areas are so small, the particles must be extremely fine to reach these areas effectively. Inhaler agents come in a variety of forms, but all must be able to be inhaled easily into the lungs. Common devices of this type, available OTC, are vaporizers and humidifiers that distribute medications by adding agents to a container located on the device. In a hospital, respiratory therapists use nebulizers to give breathing treatments to patients, but patients also can use nebulizers at home if they are trained. Anesthetics come in solutions that are inhaled and are administered during surgery by an anesthesiologist. Many of the prescribed inhalants contain drugs that treat asthma and allergies. These agents are called metered dose inhalers and dispense a specific amount of drug with each puff or inhalation (Figure 5-7, *A*). Some aerosols are used to deliver medication into the nasal passages, whereas others are inhaled orally. For orally inhaled agents, although the sizes of the particles are extremely small, unless the patient uses this device correctly, much of the drug is swallowed rather than inhaled into the lungs where it is needed. Many physicians encourage the use of aerochambers or spacers (Figure 5-7, *B*). These allow the patient to take a breath of medication without worrying about poor timing, which would result in loss of medication. The chamber holds the medication until each puff can be inhaled.

> **Example:** Primatene Mist aerosol (OTC), albuterol metered dose inhaler (Rx)

Emulsions

A mixture of water and oil may be used with an emulsifier to bind the two together. Many different types of emulsifiers are used, depending on what the manufacturer is preparing.

> **Example:** Simethicone drops (OTC), milk of magnesia (OTC), Propofol (RX)

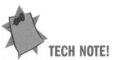

TECH NOTE!

Most inhalants are propelled out by the use of various gases. In the past, most propellants contained chlorofluorocarbons, which have been found to destroy the ozone. When ozone is decreased, ultraviolet light is allowed to enter the atmosphere at levels that are known to cause skin cancer. Because of this finding (years ago), new guidelines have been put into effect to switch over to another source of propellant. The replacements for chlorofluorocarbons must not harm the environment or alter or destroy the medication.

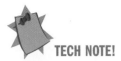

Suspensions

Suspensions are liquids that have very small, solid particles suspended in the base solution. Certain active ingredients are found to be unstable when dissolved in a solution but are stable in a suspension form. Also, these products can be used orally by children and seniors because the patients can take the medication more easily. In the case of dosing a child depending on age and weight, suspension dosages can be altered by adding more or less sterile water to the powder product. OTC products that are suspensions have a "Shake Well" ancillary label that is easily visible on the front of the bottle and in the directions. Proper mixing of suspensions before dispensing and attachment of auxiliary labels that instruct the patient to shake well before using and that include the date of expiration are important. Suspensions also are used in the eye and ear, rectally, and even parenterally.

>   **Example:** Prednisolone ophthalmic suspension (Rx), amoxicillin suspension (Rx), Ibuprofen suspension (OTC)

Enemas

Enemas may be administered for two different reasons—retention or evacuation. They can be used to deliver medication to the body, bypassing the stomach yet being absorbed. Conditions such as colitis (inflammation of the intestines) can be treated with agents in this manner to reduce the swelling. The most common reason for enemas, however, is to evacuate the lower intestine for a variety of reasons, such as preoperative care (for example, to prepare for surgeries involving the intestine) or for women about to give birth. These types of enemas can be administered from prefilled squeeze bottles. Some enemas are available OTC that are used strictly for the relief of constipation. However, because of the dramatic effects of enemas, physicians usually do not recommend these as the first line of treatment. Enemas come in a water base that is faster acting than an oil base. The typical amount of time it takes enemas to work is less than 10 minutes.

>   **Example:** Fleet enema (OTC)

SEMISOLIDS

Semisolid agents are different in their composition from liquids or solids. Although they contain solids and liquids, they normally are meant for topical application. Examples include creams, lotions, ointments, gels, pastes, and suppositories.

Creams

Creams usually have medications in a base that is part oil and part water and is meant for topical or local use. When an emulsifier is added, the water and oil will stay bound together. Creams are massaged easily into the skin and do not leave a heavy, oily residue. They also can be used vaginally or in the rectum.

>   **Example:** Hydrocortisone cream 1% (OTC), betamethasone (Diprolene) 0.05% (Rx)

Lotions

Lotions are thinner than creams because their base contains more water. They penetrate well into the skin and do not leave an oily residue after application.

>   **Example:** Jergens lotion (OTC), hydrocortisone lotion 2.5% (Rx)

Ointments

Ointments contain medication in a glycol or oil base, such as petrolatum. These work well on a skin surface to cover an area while keeping out moisture. Ointments can be used rectally, topically, and as an ophthalmic agent.

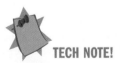

Example: Neosporin ointment (OTC), erythromycin ophthalmic ointment (Rx)

Gels

Gels contain medication in a viscous (thick) liquid that easily penetrates the skin and does not leave a residue. Many sunscreens come in this dosage form. Medications for various skin conditions are available in gels as well.

Example: Naftifine gel (Rx), bullfrog gel (OTC), Ora-Jel (OTC)

Pastes

Pastes contain a lesser amount of liquid base than solids. They are used for topical application and are able to absorb skin secretions, unlike other topical agents.

Example: Zinc oxide paste (Rx)

Suppositories

Suppositories can be used rectally and vaginally. They have several advantages over other dosage forms. Rectal suppositories bypass the stomach, which is important if the patient has nausea and vomiting. They can relieve these symptoms without requiring an injection, which is much more invasive. They also are good for relief of constipation. Vaginal suppositories are used mostly to treat infections of the vaginal area without having to involve other systems, such as the stomach.

Example: Bisacodyl suppositories (OTC), promethazine suppositories (Rx), miconazole vaginal suppositories (Rx)

Powders

Powders do not fit neatly into semisolids. Powders are solids, yet they are packaged in some forms that allow them to be sprayed similar to liquid dosage forms. Therefore, they have been included in the semisolids section. One of the main uses of powders involves decreasing the amount of wetness of an area. Most antifungal foot agents are available in powdered forms to keep the area as dry as possible, decreasing the ability of the fungus to thrive. Powders also can be spread over a wide area if needed.

Example: Tolnaftate powder (OTC), nystatin (Mycostatin) powder (Rx)

Injectables

Injectables normally are used for rapid response. The onset of an injectable drug only takes a few minutes as opposed to the up to 45 minutes that oral medications can take to work. Although diabetic persons are the most common users of injectable drugs outside the hospital, other treatments such as low-dose heparin and certain multiple sclerosis injectables are used by patients at home. Inside the hospital, many oral medications are available in injectable form, as well as those that are only available in injectable form. Technicians need to pay close attention to store injectables in the correct manner and environment. Storage temperatures range from room temperature to refrigerated. Some injectables, such as phytonadione (AquaMEPHYTON; vitamin K), must be kept in a light-protected ampule and should be stored at room temperature. Other injectables need to be stored in light-protected bags after being reconstituted into an IV bag, such as ciprofloxacin. Glass containers also are packaged more securely to protect them from breakage. Ampules are made of glass (Figure 5-8, *B*). Ampules can range in volume from 0.5 to 50 mL. When opening these various sizes of ampules, use the techniques outlined in Chapter 13 (Aseptic Technique). Many vials are in plastic and in glass containers (Figure 5-8, *A*) and range from 1 to 100 mL. Other medications that come in intraveneous form are

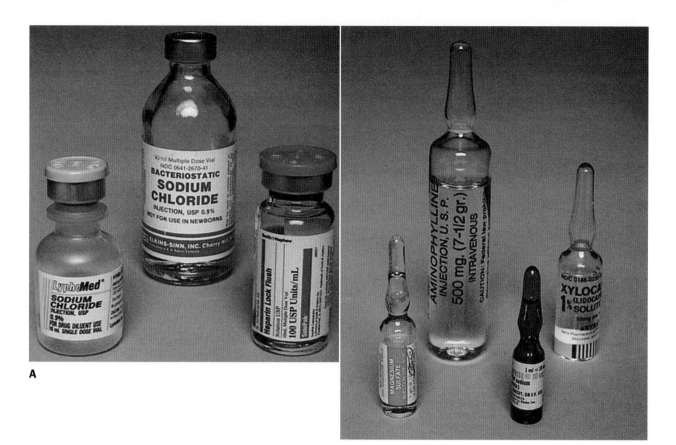

FIGURE 5-8 **A,** Medication in vials. **B,** Medication in ampules.

the premade IV bags and those prepared by a technician. Another form of vial is the Add-O-Vial that keeps the medication separate from the diluent until it is time to reconstitute. This saves waste when using an expensive drug that has a short shelf life after preparing the drug (Figure 5-9 gives instructions on mixing). Other types of containers include examples of premade, large-volume IV and an IV piggyback drug (Figure 5-10).

> **Example:** Furosemide (Lasix; Rx, light protected), sodium chloride 0.9% plastic vials (Rx)

Although many other types of dosage forms can be made by manufacturers or by compounding pharmacies, the various types covered in this chapter are the most commonly seen in the pharmacy. Because the types of dosage forms are kept in their respective areas in the pharmacy, it is important for the technician student to be familiar with the dosage forms to find them in the pharmacy. Table 5-1 lists the most common dosage forms and their routes of administration. The advantages and disadvantages of each type of route of administration determines the doctors' final decisions as to what type of agent the patients should receive. The following describes each route and its pros and cons.

Routes of Administration

BY MOUTH, OR ORAL (PO)

A positive aspect of taking tablets or capsules or any agent by mouth is the convenience of the drug to the patient. Most oral medications can be carried along

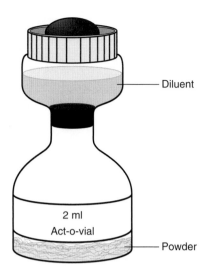

FIGURE 5-9 This type of vial is called Add-O-Vial or Mix-O-Vial. The advantage of this type of medication dosage form is its longer shelf life. **1,** First remove the sterile cap. **2,** The powder is below, and the sterile diluent is on top of the vial. The vial is divided by a rubber stopper in the middle. **3,** Push the plunger down, forcing the stopper to fall into the bottom of the vial. This allows the diluent to mix with the powder. Shake well. Once dissolved, the medication is ready to be used.

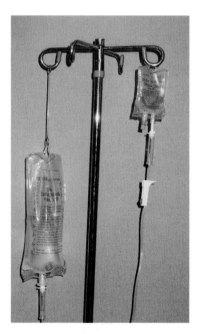

FIGURE 5-10 On the left is a large-volume IV. On the right is an IV piggyback.

throughout the day in a handy bottle. Tablets and capsules do not need to be measured, which increases their ease of use, and most oral forms are much less expensive than other alternatives. Oral medications are systemic, which means they are dispersed throughout the body. They are also one of the safer ways to take medication, because if too much is given, there is time to react before the drug begins to work. The downside of these drugs is that they do not work as quickly as parenteral medications; they take anywhere from 30 minutes to 1 hour to become active. This can be important, for instance, if the medication

TABLE 5-1   Common Abbreviations Used with Dosage Forms

Abbreviation	Route of administration	Specific site of action	Dosage forms
PO	Oral	Absorbed into bloodstream	Tablet Capsule Solution Syrup Suspension Powder Elixir Tincture Troche
SL	Sublingual	Under the tongue	Tablet Sprays
Buc	Buccal	In the cheek	Lozenge/troche
PR	Per rectum	Rectum	Suppository Solution Enema Ointment
IV	Intravenous	In the vein	Solution/suspension
IM	Intramuscular	In the muscle	Solution/suspension
SQ	Subcutaneous	Under the skin	Solution/suspension
IT	Intrathecal	In the spine	Solution
IA	Intraarterial	In the artery	Solution
TOP	Epicutaneous or percutaneous	On the skin surface	Ointment Cream Paste Powder Spray Solution Lotion
	Transdermal	On the skin surface	Patch Disk
OS, OD, OU	Ophthalmic	Eye	Suspension Ointment Solution Lens
AS, AD, AU	Otic	Ear	Suspension Solution
NAS	Intranasal	Nose	Solution Spray Inhalant
Inh	Inhalant	Mouth	Solution Aerosol
Va	Vaginal	Vagina	Solution Ointment Foam Gel Suppository Sponge
Urethral	Urethral	Urethra	Solution Suppository

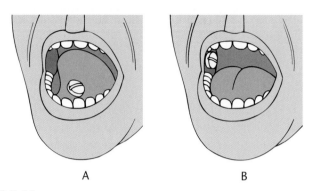

A   B

FIGURE 5-11 **A,** Sublingual tablet placement. **B,** Buccal tablet placement.

is intended for pain relief. Also, some drugs cannot be taken orally because they are not as effective. This complication is due to the acid pH of the stomach, which breaks down some substances and makes certain medications of little use.

SUBLINGUAL AND BUCCAL AGENTS (SL, BUCCAL)

Although not many medications are available at this time in the form of sublingual or buccal agents, the few that are used commonly are effective. Nitroglycerin is the most commonly used sublingual tablet that treats anginal attacks. Angina is a common heart ailment that affects millions of persons with symptoms that include shortness of breath and pain in and around the chest cavity. Nitroglycerin sublingual tablets (placed under the tongue) bypass the long trek through the gastrointestinal system and are absorbed readily into the bloodstream. This speeds up its action to a few minutes as opposed to the longer time requirement of oral agents (Figure 5-11, *A*). Many new prescription agents have been approved for sale. These include agents such as famotidine (Fluxid) for treatment of ulcers and gastrointestinal upset and carbidopa-levodopa (Parcopa), a medication for Parkinson's disease. Buccal agents are another type of dosage form. These oral tablets are placed between the gums and cheek where the medication penetrates the mouth lining and then enters the bloodstream (Figure 5-11, *B*).

RECTAL AGENTS (PR)

Rectal agents are used for many different reasons; an example is a person who is vomiting and cannot take oral medications. Suppositories or rectal creams can be used to treat the patient. Different preparations are available, depending on what result is desired. To reduce inflammation, ointments or creams can be used in addition to suppositories. These types of drugs work on a specific site rather than systemically. However, for treating nausea or motion sickness, a systemic-acting suppository can be used. Other agents include solutions that also are used locally for various reasons, usually to clear the intestines of fecal material. The downside is that most persons do not feel comfortable using suppositories. Also, the actual amount of drug absorbed is not as predictable as with those medications taken orally.

TOPICAL AGENTS (TOP)

Many different preparations of topical treatments are available. The effects of topical preparations range from systemic to localized for rashes. The skin is the largest organ of the body because of its large surface area. The skin has many portals through which drugs can pass into the body. Openings include sweat glands, hair follicles, and other small openings in the pores of the skin. Many topical agents fight skin infections, inflammation, and ultraviolet rays of the sun. Topical agents work at the site of action, which makes them effective. In addition, manufacturers have created topical treatments that work systemically, such as medications for the heart, blood pressure, hormonal replacement, motion sickness, and smoking cessation agents. These are prepared in a variety of dosage forms from ointments to patches or small disks that can be applied to the skin. The medication is absorbed through the pores into the bloodstream where it begins to work. An advantage of topical agents is the ease of application for the patient. Many topical medications act rapidly at the site of application to relieve itching or inflammation. Patches can be worn all day, which increases patient compliance because the patient does not have to remember to take the medication at various times during the day. In fact, some patches, such as those for motion sickness, can be applied and left in place for days. The downside of topical drugs is that they may cause a reaction; therefore, many agents cannot be given by this route of administration. Because patches are relatively new on the market, they tend to be a little more expensive than their counterpart, the oral medications.

PARENTERAL: INTRAVENOUS, INTRAVENOUS PIGGYBACK, INTRAMUSCULAR, AND SUBCUTANEOUS AGENTS (IV, IVPB, IM, SQ)

The word *parenteral* comes from Greek and means "side of intestine" or "outside the intestine," which is where oral medications travel. A wide range of parenteral dosages and sites are available where these agents can be given. The most common parenteral medications are given intravenously, into the veins; intramuscularly, into the muscles; or subcutaneously, under the skin. Very small–gauge needles are used, and the lengths depend on the sites being injected. This type of administration has clear benefits, such as the speed of action. Parenteral medications such as insulin have allowed millions of persons who suffer from diabetes to inject themselves daily, thus allowing them to function normally. In addition, parenteral drugs work faster than those given by the oral route. This is important for emergency situations, for those who are unconscious or combative, or for those who are unable to swallow. Also, smaller doses are needed because of the high bioavailability of the agents injected. The disadvantage of parenteral drugs as a group is the increased risk of infection. Any drug injection must be done using as sterile a technique as possible to avoid introducing any microbes into the body. Also, any injection is much more expensive than other routes of administration because of the required preparation and administration by trained personnel. Another downside is that, because injectable drugs work quickly, once the drug is injected, there is little time to alter its course if an allergic reaction should take place or too much drug is given.

EYE/EAR/NOSE (OU, AU, NASAL)

A wide variety of agents are used for treating a large assortment of conditions affecting the eyes, nose, and ears. A consideration one must remember when preparing and filling prescriptions for agents that treat the ear or eye is that doctors often use eye solutions to treat ear conditions; however, because the eye is sterile, ear solutions cannot be used to treat eye conditions. Therefore, all eye agents are sterile. Otic drugs (ear preparations) are not necessarily sterile because they treat the ear canal and do not penetrate a sterile environment. The pharmacy technician may prepare ophthalmic drugs in a laminar flow hood using aseptic technique (see Chapter 13). One must remember that all ophthalmic drugs need to be kept sterile. For the eye, ear, and nose there are different types of agents used, including ointments, solutions, and suspensions. Most treatments of the ear are for clearing up an infection or cleaning out ear wax buildup. Most nasal sprays are used to treat symptoms of colds and allergies, whereas eye treatments are for infections, inflammation, and conditions such as glaucoma (increased pressure of the eye). These types of dosage forms work on a specific site rather than involving the whole body. They can be administered with ease because of the small package size of the drug. Instructions for eye and ear preparations should say *instill* rather than *take* or *put.* The main disadvantage of these drugs is that solutions used for the eye, if not kept sterile, can introduce bacteria into the area being treated. Also, ophthalmic drugs do not last as long as other treatments because of the blinking of the eye and tearing, which washes away the medication. Therefore, dosing times may be more frequent. In addition, most ophthalmic ointments make it hard to see clearly.

INHALANTS (INH)

Many persons suffer from lung diseases and use inhalants to treat these conditions. Gases such as oxygen mixed with anesthetics are used to keep patients asleep during procedures as well. Dosage forms may be limited; however, they are effective if used properly. For patients suffering from conditions such as asthma, bronchitis, or emphysema, a metered dose inhaler often is used. Some agents open the passageways (bronchodilators) to the lungs, and some can be used afterward to prolong the effectiveness of the bronchodilators. For more chronic or severe conditions, corticosteroids are also available in metered dose inhalers.

A positive aspect of inhalants is that most aerosols come in handheld units, are convenient for carrying, and may be used when the need arises. The onset of action for these types of agents is quick and can make an extreme difference in a person's ability to breathe comfortably. The downside is that, if not used properly, little if any of the drug is able to get into the lungs. Breathing in as the inhaler is activated is important, and it is necessary always to shake inhalers before drug administration. Respiratory solutions that are packaged in unit dose ampules deliver a specific amount of drug per treatment.

MISCELLANEOUS ROUTES

Other routes include vaginal or urethral dosage forms. These forms are suppositories, ointments, foams, and gels. These types of delivery systems are used for treatment of infections and inflammation and, in the case of vaginal foams, for birth control. Although there are clear advantages in using these agents, such as bypassing a systemic effect and affecting the specific site, they are not necessarily applied easily and can be uncomfortable.

Other Considerations: Form and Function

Dosage forms are created based on the results from many clinical trials that delve into the pharmacokinetics of the medication or the function of the drug in experiments.

PHARMACOKINETICS

Pharmacokinetics is a (all inclusive) word that represents many different components concerning the actions of a drug. For example, from the time a person takes a tablet, various considerations are examined, such as levels of drug in the blood and tissues; the absorption or movement of the drug throughout the body; and the overall distribution, metabolism, and excretion of the drug. This includes the reaction of the drug with other drugs to see what may change in the course of its time in the body. As these components are tested and refined,

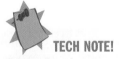

TECH NOTE!

To determine how much medicine is left in an inhaler, float the container in water. If it sinks, it is full; if it floats on top of the water, it is empty. If the container is half submerged, it is about half full.

TECH NOTE!

Remember that suspensions and inhalers always need to be shaken before use. Shaking evenly distributes the drug throughout the liquid to attain an even dosage of drug.

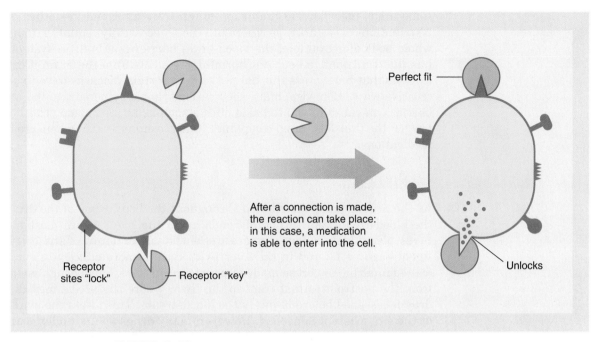

Receptor sites "lock"

Receptor "key"

After a connection is made, the reaction can take place: in this case, a medication is able to enter into the cell.

Perfect fit

Unlocks

FIGURE 5-12 Lock-and-key mechanism allowing absorption to take place in a cell. These common reactions take place naturally throughout the body. Only after the correct receptor makes a connection with the matching receptor site will the cell allow a reaction to take place. Medications often mimic this natural mechanism.

the eventual result is a dosage form that is tailor-made to work at its optimal level, while always keeping patient compliance in mind. Patient compliance is the level at which patients will or will not take their scheduled drugs (see Chapter 7). If a manufacturer can make a drug that can be taken once daily rather than several times a day, the odds increase that the patient will take the medication as directed.

Other areas in the overall pharmacokinetics or life of the drug includes the bioavailability (absorption, distribution, metabolism, and excretion), half-life and bioequivalence. Each of these areas is discussed briefly.

ABSORPTION

Medications are made specifically to get through natural body barriers such as the skin, stomach, intestines, blood-brain barrier (surrounding the brain), and other membranous tissues. How well the drug passes through these barriers is one factor that determines its ultimate effectiveness. Some considerations include whether the barrier is a lipid base (fatty) or not. Membranes surrounding organs, such as the intestine, have a variety of proteins and other structures implanted in a membranous protective structure that act as receptor sites. Important chemicals and drugs are able to pass a lock-and-key mechanism by latching onto receptive sites that allow the chemical or drug to pass into the organ to reach the final site of action intended for the drug. Figure 5-12 shows an example of this action.

DISTRIBUTION

After the absorption of a medication, the medication is distributed throughout the body from the bloodstream into tissues, membranes, and ultimately organs of the body. Not all systems are affected equally by the drugs administered, with some areas not allowing the drugs to infiltrate as rapidly as other areas. The distribution of a drug is therefore not necessarily equal throughout the whole body. For example, the blood-brain barrier is a built-in system the body has that functions to keep out harmful chemicals from the brain. Certain medications that must cross this barrier to help certain diseases have to be made in creative ways. Likewise, many medications that may penetrate the blood-brain barrier can cause unwanted side effects such as hypertension. These are just a few of the hurdles drug companies must contend with when creating new medications.

METABOLISM

As the drug is being distributed throughout the body, some of the drug reenters the bloodstream and ultimately ends up in the liver, where most metabolism takes place. Metabolism changes the chemical structure of the original drug. Agents can be altered in the liver to produce a more effective chemical agent (called prodrug) or can be made less toxic or effective. Some drugs can go directly from the gastrointestinal tract to the liver, where the active ingredient of the drug is lessened before it enters the bloodstream. This alters the available drug at the site where it is needed. However, many drugs do not undergo any change at all and are excreted from the body in the same form in which they started. Different influences can alter metabolism, such as age, gender, genetics, diet, and other chemicals ingested.

EXCRETION

Excretion is the last phase of the life of a drug in the body. Although excretion usually is associated with urination, it is important to know that there are many ways that a drug can be excreted from the body. In addition to excretion via the kidneys, drugs also may be expelled via the feces, exhalation, sweat glands, and even breast milk in women who are lactating. Urination and bowel movements are by far the most common methods of excretion. Less common methods such as through breast milk must be considered when a doctor prescribes a drug. For the doctor to give an appropriate drug, all drugs must be tested by the manufacturer for excretion into breast milk and the results reported in the package insert. All information concerning the proper dosing and pharmacokinetics are listed in several reference books (see Chapter 8) and drug package inserts.

BIOAVAILABILITY

Bioavailability is the proportion of the drug that makes it to its destination and is available to the site of action for which it was intended. Drugs that are intended for a certain organ or tissues in the body must pass many different obstacles such as stomach acids, which may break down any substance in the stomach. Many drugs travel into the liver before they have a chance to be absorbed into the whole system. This "first pass" therefore can metabolize the drugs and lower their bioavailability before the drug arrives at the site of action.

HALF-LIFE

Half-life refers to the time it takes the body to break down and excrete one half of the drug. For example, if a person takes a medication that has a half-life of 10 hours, this means that in 10 hours one half of the drug will be gone, and in another 10 hours another one half of the remaining drug will be gone. This is

an important factor in the creation of all drugs because this information tells the manufacturer how long it takes the body to rid itself of the drug. If a person takes too much medication or takes doses too close together, the liver or kidneys can have toxic buildup of the drug, which can be dangerous to the patient.

BIOEQUIVALENCE

Bioequivalence is the comparison between drugs from different manufacturers or in the same company but from different batches of drug. This is an important aspect of a drug because patients assume that every tablet they take is exactly the same as the one before and that all are the exact strength as listed on the label. Generic drug manufacturers strive to achieve the same equivalence as brand name manufacturers so that they can compete with the original manufacturer. Another reference to use in order to see whether the generic drug is rated as bioequivalent is the *Orange Book*. This book lists the approved drug products with therapeutic equivalence and evaluations.

Most of the final metabolism of a drug takes place in the liver. This is the final processing center of the body that extracts toxins and unwanted chemicals from the body and forwards them onto the excretion process (in the kidneys). The liver works hard but can process only so much within a given time. Persons suffering from any type of liver damage must be monitored closely when taking various medications to ensure that toxic levels are not present in the liver.

The Use of Additives

All medications are prepared with some sort of additive for many different reasons, as shown in Table 5-2. These additives include coloring for better appearance of the product and flavorings to cover taste and/or smell. Many times fillers are used to increase the size of the medication because there may be such a small amount of drug that it otherwise would be hard, if not impossible, to handle. Many different types of preservatives are available. Each prevents certain microbes from affecting the drug. These preservatives prolong the shelf life after the patient obtains the drug. Other types of additives include those that increase the dispersing of the drug once it reaches the intestines and others that release the medication much slower over a longer period. Again, many components that go into preparing dosage forms are done for the patients' convenience. Patients are more likely to take medication once or twice daily as opposed to multiple times per day.

TECH ALERT!

Not all generic drugs are bioequivalent to the trade/brand drugs. Even if a generic drug has the same active ingredient, it may vary in additional additives, making it different. An example is albuterol inhalant; although all generics contain the same main ingredients and propellants, they differ in types of additives. Also the size of the valve differs between trade/brand that may alter the amount of medicine being dispensed.

TABLE 5-2 Description of Additives

Type of additive	Example of chemical	Reason
Weak salt acid/base	Hydrochloric acid	Helps dissolve drug easier once it arrives in the gastrointestinal system
Preservative	Phenol	Increases shelf life
Sweetener	Sucrose	Improves taste
Flavoring	Cherry	Improves taste
Coloring	Yellow dye No. 5	Improves visual appeal
Buffer	Sodium acetate	Adjusts pH
Antifungal	Benzoic acid	Prevents fungal growth
Base	Petrolatum	Main component to which medication is added for ointments and creams
Filler	Starch, powdered cellulose	To increase size of dosage form

TABLE 5-3 Description of Dosage Forms

Dosage form	Types	Result
Oral tablet	Layered	Slow release
	Film coated	Protects against stomach acid
	Extended release	Releases medication slowly
	Compressed	Hard dissolves slower; soft dissolves faster
Coated tablet	Sugar and colored	Protects drug; covers taste
	Caplet	Hard, capsule-shaped tablet
	Colored	Appearance
	Gel	Smaller than a capsule, easier to swallow
	Enteric coated	Delayed release; easier to swallow
	Dissolving	Dissolve in the mouth on contact
Sublingual/buccal	Soft compressed	Dissolve in mouth
Chewable tablet		Chewed
Capsule	Gelatin cover	Allows for pharmacy-compounded agents; easy to swallow
	Spansule	Capsule holds small pellets or beads
	Pulvule	Manufacturer prepared (bullet shaped)
	Dry fill	Filled with powder
Hard gelatin		Filled with a tablet inside
		Filled with pellets
		Filled with another capsule
Soft gelatin	Wet fill	Filled with a liquid
		Filled with paste
Injectable vial	Multiple-dose vial	May be used more than once (see Figure 5-6)
	Single-dose vial	Must be discarded after one use (see Figure 5-6)
	Add-O-Vial	Rubber stopper is pushed, releasing diluent into powder product (see Figure 5-7)

Manufactured Products

After learning how many different routes of administration there are and the dosage forms used, you may think that is all there is. The ever-changing world of drug manufacturing has made available many different choices and has turned a simple compressed powder, known as a tablet, into an intricate, complicated, and highly structured format. A tablet is not just a tablet, nor a capsule merely a capsule. As seen in Table 5-3, there are many different types of dosage forms depending on the desired effect of the drug in question. All types of dosage forms must be approved by the Food and Drug Administration (see Chapter 2). This includes constant testing of the product from batch to batch to ensure continuity of the medication. Injectable dosage forms are discussed further in Chapter 13.

Miscellaneous Agents and Devices

OCULAR INSERTS (FOR THE EYE)

Ocular inserts are a new treatment for glaucoma. Lenses are inserted into the eye that release a continuous amount of drug over time.

TABLE 5-4 Examples of Storage Requirements

Medication	Location	Considerations
Suppository	Drug shelf or refrigerator	Meant to melt at body temperature
Latanoprost	Refrigerator	Stored in the refrigerator (2°-8°C) until opened; may be kept up to 6 weeks at room temperature after opening
Metronidazole IV	At room temperature	Most premade intravenous medications are stored in the freezer until thawed for use; store at 15°-30°C and protect from light
Vaccines	Refrigerator	Kept in the refrigerator (2°-8°C)
Insulin	Refrigerator	Although insulin is kept in the refrigerator, it may be kept at room temperature for up to 1 month
Penicillins (Wycillin, Bicillin)	Drug shelf or refrigerator	Must be stored in refrigerator after reconstitution
Mannitol	At room temperature	Mannitol crystallizes at room temperature; temperature of drug must be raised before using

INJECTABLE FORMS (LONG-ACTING)

An assortment of long-acting parenteral drugs are available that can be used in place of daily dosing, such as medroxyprogesterone acetate (Depo Provera) for birth control, which must be injected every 3 months. Other parenteral medications include haloperidol decanoate, which is used monthly for antipsychotic episodes, and the steroid dexamethasone, which is given intramuscularly every 1 to 3 weeks per doctor's orders.

Packaging and Storage Requirements

Medications are packaged according to manufacturers' specifications to ensure the effectiveness and shelf life of the drug. The various storage requirements of medications are important for the technician to learn. Medications that have specific storage requirements will be clearly marked on the container or box in which it arrives. Certain medications arrive in dry ice and must be unpacked and stored immediately at the proper temperature indicated. When the outside of a box is labeled "refrigerate or keep frozen," the contents should never be left lying around to thaw and become unusable. Listed in Table 5-4 are some examples of storage requirements for various drugs, along with special considerations. All medications have a package insert that describes the storage and stability of the drug. Technicians should become familiar with this type of information. In addition to manufacturer storage requirements, repackaging medications have their own guidelines, which have been set in place by the FDA and can be referenced in Chapter 12.

DO YOU REMEMBER THESE KEY POINTS?

- Various routes of administration
- Terms and definitions relating to pharmacokinetics
- Abbreviations for the routes of administration
- Reasons why different routes are used to administer drugs
- Form and function of medications
- Food and Drug Administration guidelines for proper manufacturing practices
- Types of additives used in manufacturing dosage forms and the reasons behind them
- How different dosage forms affect pharmacokinetics
- The importance of the half-life of a drug
- Storage requirements of medications

MULTIPLE CHOICE QUESTIONS

1. Why are sublingual tablets better for relieving anginal attacks than traditional tablets?
   A. They are smaller.
   B. They bypass the stomach, entering the bloodstream for quicker relief.
   C. They are cheaper.
   D. Both A and C.

2. Why do manufacturers make dosage forms that work over a longer time?
   A. To cut down on the cost of making the drug
   B. To save time preparing each dose
   C. To enable the patient to take the medication less often
   D. To meet Food and Drug Administration standards

3. Preservatives are often added to medications to _____.
   A. Increase their shelf life
   B. Decrease the possibility of contamination
   C. Cut down on the cost of having to make large amounts of the drug
   D. Both A and B

4. Often, parenteral medications are used because _____.
   A. They work fast
   B. They bypass the stomach acid secretions
   C. The patient is unable to take medication by mouth
   D. All of the above

5. The definition for pharmacokinetics can be best described as _____.
   A. The life of a drug within the body
   B. The absorption of a drug
   C. The pharmacy aspect of a drug
   D. The testing of a drug

6. An advantage of taking medications orally is/are _____.
   A. Lower cost
   B. Easier to take than other routes
   C. Less chance of infection with oral dosage forms
   D. All of the above

7. The organ that performs most of the metabolism of a drug is _____.
   A. The kidney
   B. The blood
   C. The stomach
   D. The liver

8. If a drug has a half-life of 20 hours, this would mean that _____.
   A. Half of the drug would be gone in the first 20 hours, followed by the second half in 20 more hours
   B. The drug will only last half as long as needed
   C. The drug will lose half its strength in half of 20 hours
   D. The drug will lose half its strength in 20 hours, followed by half of the remaining strength in the following 20 hours, and so forth

9. Of the body areas listed, which one is not a common route for excretion?
   A. Intestines
   B. Kidneys
   C. Mouth
   D. Skin

10. Dyes and sugars are used in preparing medications to _____.
   A. Improve looks and taste
   B. Improve taste and shelf life
   C. Improve sales
   D. All of the above

TRUE/FALSE If the statement is false, then change it to make it true.

_____ 1. Medications for the ear also can be used for the eye.

_____ 2. Depending on the type of rectal medication given, the medication can work systemically or locally.

_____ 3. Parenteral drugs are used only in emergency rooms.

_____ 4. A bioequivalent generic drug means it is equivalent to the brand name drug for effectiveness.

_____ 5. Phenol is used in making drugs because of its taste properties.

_____ 6. Fungal and bacterial contamination can occur if medications are not stored properly.

_____ 7. Some medications require tests to determine whether the liver is clearing medications appropriately.

_____ 8. Ophthalmic medications can be delivered in lenses.

_____ 9. Capsules can be manufactured to hold smaller capsules or tablets.

_____ 10. Pharmacy technicians are not responsible for making errors if the doctor's handwriting is illegible.

TECHNICIAN'S CORNER

The following examples list the proper way to transcribe orders along with an example of a prescription order for that route. Using these as a guideline, answer the question at the end of this Technician's Corner.

Remember that physicians may write in upper or lower case for these orders.

1. Oral routes, written PO
   PO = by mouth
2. Rectal routes, written PR
   PR = per rectal
3. Topically, written TOP
   TOP = to be applied to the surface of the skin
4. Ophthalmic, written OD, OS, OU
   D = right, S = left, U = both
5. Otic, written AD, AS, AU
   D = right, S = left, U = both
6. Parenteral drugs; written either IV, IM, SQ, or ID
   IV = intravenous
   IM = intramuscular
   SQ = subcutaneous (also written SC)
   ID = intradermal

Question

A patient brings in a prescription. Transcribe this order into lay person's terms, and list any auxiliary labels that should be adhered to the prescription. Finally, list any questions that you may have about the order and whom you would ask.

BIBLIOGRAPHY

Ansel HC, Allen LV, Popovich NG: *Ansel's Pharmaceutical dosage forms and drug delivery systems,* ed 8, Baltimore, 2004, Lippincott Williams & Wilkins.
Brown M, Mulholland J: *Drug calculations,* ed 7, St Louis, 2003, Elsevier.
Drug facts and comparisons, ed 53, St Louis, 1999, Wolters Kluwer.
Gray Morris D: *Calculate with confidence,* ed 4, St Louis, 2005, Elsevier.
Potter PA, Perry AG: *Fundamentals of nursing,* ed 6, St Louis, 2004, Elsevier.
www.drugtopics.com Wisniewski, RN, Carol Holquist, RPh. The absence of a trade name does not equal a generic drug. 10/10/2005.

WEBSITES

http.users.ahsc.arizona.edu/davis/bbb.htm (Blood brain barrier)
www.fda.gov/cder/ob (Orange book information)

6

Referencing

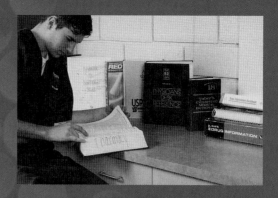

Objectives

UPON COMPLETING THIS CHAPTER, YOU SHOULD BE ABLE TO
DO THE FOLLOWING:

■ Demonstrate the appropriate way to reference drugs and other
information.

■ Describe the information contained in the following reference
books:
  ■ *American Hospital Formulary Service Drug Information*
  ■ *Drug Topics Red Book*
  ■ *Orange Book*
  ■ *Drug Facts and Comparisons*
  ■ *Goodman & Gilman's the Pharmacological Basis of
    Therapeutics*
  ■ *Handbook on Injectable Drugs*
  ■ *Ident-A-Drug Handbook*
  ■ *Physicians' Desk Reference*
  ■ *Remington's Pharmaceutical Sciences: The Science and Practice
    of Pharmacy*

■ Explain the specialized reference books necessary in hospital
pharmacy.

■ List other types of referencing materials in addition to books.

■ Explain the importance of journals and news magazines as they
pertain to pharmacy and continuing education.

Brand/trade name *Trademark of a drug or device created by the originating manufacturing company*

Chemical structure *The shape of molecules and their location to one another*

Drug classification *Categorization based on the action of a drug and its usage*

Formulary *A list of preferred drugs to be stocked by the pharmacy; also a list of drugs covered by an insurance company*

Generic name *Name assigned to a medication by the Food and Drug Administration; nonproprietary name of a drug*

Monograph *Medication information sheet provided by the manufacturer that includes side effects, dosage forms, indications, and other important information*

REFERENCE BOOKS ARE SOME of the most important tools that are used in pharmacy. Doctors, nurses, and other health care professionals call the pharmacy daily to ask questions concerning various medications. Pharmacists rely on good up-to-date reference books to help give the correct information to the caller. Although a few of the books in pharmacy are highly technical, most give basic information on drugs. Knowing which book to choose for referencing and how to access the information is an important skill for pharmacists and technicians. This chapter covers the popular books that most pharmacies stock. In addition, other types of referencing materials that can be of help specifically to the technician are listed.

Understanding the Correct Way to Reference

Before you begin to look for information, take these key points into consideration. First, what exactly are you looking for? Do you need to know the generic drug name only, interactions, classification, or maybe what the drug looks like? Let us begin with the making of a drug to learn the importance of each one of these components.

When a new drug is in the experimentation phase, the creators or the company give the drug a name based on its chemical attributes. Later, when the drug is approved through the Food and Drug Administration, a monograph is created to include the classification, indications, and important findings, such as side effects that were reported during the testing phase. The classification is important because it puts the drug into the proper category based on its chemical actions. Many times, drugs within the same class act the same way if they are taken with other drugs. This information can assist the pharmacist in knowing whether an adverse reaction might occur. The indication lists the main conditions for which this chemical is used. The founding company also gives the chemical a trade name. Many times names are closely related to the chemical name, but not always.

Most of the chemical names for beta-blockers end in *-olol*. Each drug company produces monographs, also known as package inserts, that list pertinent information.

Most reference books that pharmacists use list trade and generic names of drugs, indications, classifications, possible contraindications, and dosage

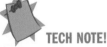

TECH NOTE!

Technically, all generic drug names are spelled in lower case as opposed to trade or brand names, which are capitalized, for example, atenolol (generic) and Tenormin (brand).

TABLE 6-1 **Sections in *Drug Facts and Comparisons***

Sections in order of reference	Contents of each section	Specific information
Section 1	Index	Generic and trade names
Section 2	Keeping up	Orphan, investigational, and temporary listings
Section 3	Drug monographs	14 chapters of drug descriptions
Section 4	Drug identification	More than 250 drugs are shown in color
Section 5	Appendix	Dosage calculations and list of manufacturers

strengths, and dosage forms. When studies are completed and all the data have been analyzed, the manufacturing companies make a list of contraindications. This list identifies types of persons who should not be given the medication. Reasons may range from certain serious drug-drug interactions to conditions that conflict with the action of the drug.

Technicians also must be at ease using reference books in the pharmacy. Good reference books have a section on how to use the text. This is an important step with which all users should become familiar. Knowing how to use books allows the technician to find the correct information in a timely manner. In this way the technician can assist the pharmacist in locating the correct information.

Main Reference Books Used in Pharmacy

Although many different types of reference books are available, this chapter covers only the most common types seen in a pharmacy setting. Many good reference books are available to technicians and pharmacists. Determining which book to use depends on what information you need and how easy it is to find in a book.

DRUG FACTS AND COMPARISONS

Drug Facts and Comparisons is the most often used book by pharmacists. This reference book was first published in 1946 and was created for quick and accurate reference and drug comparison. Because of its vital information and the ease of use, it is used in most pharmacies. *Drug Facts and Comparisons* has five sections, as shown in Table 6-1. *Drug Facts and Comparisons* may be purchased as a loose-leaf book that can be updated monthly. It is also available online and as a CD-ROM.

At the front of each classification section is extensive information on various aspects of the class of drugs. Included under each drug listing are indications for use. Also, a chart lists all of the dosage strengths, dosage forms, sizes, and manufacturers. Most pharmacies carry the unbound book to allow for monthly updates. *Drug Facts and Comparisons* answers most questions for the pharmacist.

PHYSICIANS' DESK REFERENCE

The *Physicians' Desk Reference (PDR)* is a popular book found in most doctors' offices and pharmacies. The *PDR* has been in publication for more than 50 years. The *PDR* has six sections, as shown in Table 6-2.

Each drug referenced in the *PDR* has a complete description of the drug, including its chemical structure and study results. This book is a compilation of

TABLE 6-2　Sections of *Physicians' Desk Reference*

Sections in order of reference	Contents of each section	Specific information
Section 1	Manufacturer indexing	Lists address and phone number
Section 2	Generic and trade names	Serves as an index for referencing manufacturers
Section 3	Product category index	Products are listed by classification or method of action
Section 4	Product identification guide	Drugs shown in color
Section 5	Product information	Most FDA-approved drugs
Section 6	Diagnostic product information	Information on drug products used as diagnostic agents
Miscellaneous section	Miscellaneous information	Drug information centers listed, key to controlled substances, key for FDA pregnancy ratings, U.S. FDA telephone directory, and poison control centers

FDA, Food and Drug Administration.

package inserts, which are small, printed information packets that are inserted with or attached to each drug as it leaves the manufacturer. Package inserts can be hard to read. Although most pharmacies have a *PDR,* physicians are the primary users, and again the *PDR* lists only Food and Drug Administration–approved drugs that the manufacturers choose. This book is not as important in a pharmacy setting as it is in a physician's office. The *PDR,* however, does contain useful drug manufacturer contact information such as addresses and phone numbers.

DRUG TOPICS RED BOOK

One of the longest published reference guides is *Drug Topics Red Book,* often known as *Red Book.* This book is a good source of information pertaining to drug costs. The newer *Red Book* has 10 sections, as outlined in Table 6-3. Community pharmacies, rather than hospital pharmacies, are more likely to use this book.

Red Book contains valuable information in the form of quick referencing charts that technicians can use, such as drugs that should not be crushed, sugar-free and alcohol-free drugs, and drugs excreted in breast milk. In addition, *Red Book* includes convenient tables showing pharmacy calculations and dosing instructions converted into Spanish. Although *Red Book* has an extraordinary amount of information, it is not an easy book to reference without knowing the abbreviations for the drug sections (Table 6-4). An added feature of *Red Book* is a listing of all nontraditional doctor of pharmacy (PharmD) programs, along with requirements and current enrollment numbers. This is information that few, if any other, books contain.

ORANGE BOOK

The *Orange Book* is a comprehensive listing of approved drug products with therapeutic equivalence evaluations. This is the book to use to determine whether a generic drug is the same as a brand drug. Other information includes discontinued drug product use list, orphan products designations, and approvals list. Information searches can be accessed by several different means: active ingre-

TABLE 6-3 Sections in *Drug Topics Red Book*

Sections in order of reference	Contents of each section	Specific information
Section 1	Emergency information	Lists address and phone number
Section 2	Clinical reference guide	Quick guide listings such as for sugar-free and alcohol-free products, sulfite-containing drugs, and drugs that cannot be crushed
Section 3	Practice management and professional development	Disease management programs, listed in alphabetical order with address and phone number
Section 4	Pharmacy and health care organizations	Lists 25 major organizations including ASHP, NABP, and American Association of Colleges of Pharmacy; no technician organizations are listed
Section 5	Drug reimbursement information	Lists State Aids Drug Assistance Programs for all states; lists Medicaid upper limit prices and rules on what units each type of drug must be billed
Section 6	Manufacturer/ wholesaler information	Address and phone number for manufacturers, wholesalers, OBRA '90 participating manufacturers (by identification number), and returned goods policies
Section 7	Product identification	Color photos of limited drugs; also includes look-alike, soundalike drug names list
Section 8	Prescription product listings	Contains *Orange Book,* which lists generic drug, manufacturer, National Drug Code, average wholesale price, direct price, and *Orange Book* code
Section 9	Over-the-counter/ nondrug products listing	This section lists drugs by generic name or trademark name and contains health-related item, universal product code, National Drug Code, average wholesale price, and suggested retail price
Section 10	Complementary/herbal product referencing	A short listing of popular herbal remedies along with a listing of those that may be contraindicated, those that require supervision by medical personnel, and interactions; followed by a list of both scientific and common herbal names

ASHP, American Society of Health-System Pharmacists; *NABP,* National Association of Boards of Pharmacy; *OBRA '90,* Omnibus Budget Reconciliation Act of 1990.

dient, patent, proprietary name, applicant holder, or application number. The *Orange Book* is updated annually and can be accessed online.

AMERICAN HOSPITAL FORMULARY SERVICE DRUG INFORMATION

Used mainly by hospitals, *American Hospital Formulary Service Drug Information* gives a comprehensive listing of approved formulary drugs, their uses, adverse reactions, and other pertinent information. This information is derived from experts in the fields of medicine, pharmacy, and management.

Formularies are lists of approved uses of medications. The criteria for a formulary include the best use of a drug based on effectiveness of the drug, cost,

TABLE 6-4 Abbreviations in *Drug Topics Red Book*

Abbreviations	Definitions	What information is given
AWP	Average wholesale price	Average price wholesalers charge the pharmacy
NDC	National Drug Code	Identifies each drug by number
OBC	*Orange Book* code	Gives therapeutic equivalence
DP	Direct price	The price for purchasing from manufacturer
NCPDP	National Council for Prescription Drug Programs	Standard billing units, such as milliliter and milligram
HRI	Health-related item	Nonmedication item required to treat patient (e.g., crutches, gauze, tape, or lancets)
UPC	Universal product code	Similar to the National Drug Code for drug items
SRP	Suggested retail price	Suggested price to charge patients

and other factors. A hospital pharmacist usually provides drug education for doctors, nurses, and other ancillary staff to identify the drugs that are on the hospital formulary. Doctors should stay within the formulary guidelines of their institution when ordering drugs.

UNITED STATES PHARMACOPOEIA DRUG INFORMATION

United States Pharmacopoeia Drug Information comes as a set of three volumes. Volume 1 gives drug information, including labeled and unlabeled uses for the drug. Volume 2 helps the pharmacist in advising patients about their medications. Volume 3 covers state and federal requirements, such as how the drug must be stored.

IDENT-A-DRUG

Ident-A-Drug lists tablet and capsule identifications. Most tablets and capsules have a code or number stamped onto them by the manufacturer for identification purposes. *Ident-A-Drug* is the most extensive reference book available, with more than 7000 listings. The drugs are not listed by pictures but by identifiable codes, colors, shapes, and whether the tablet is scored. Once these characteristics are identified, the book provides the manufacturer, generic and brand names, strength, and use of the drug. This type of referencing comes in handy when patients do not know what drug they are taking but have a capsule or tablet of the drug to show. Emergency departments often have a patient who has overdosed on a drug but who cannot identify it. If one tablet or capsule is brought in with the patient, the pharmacy probably can identify the drug using this book. Although some books such as *Drug Facts and Comparisons* do have some pictures of tablets and capsules, these are not extensive and are not the first choice to use in identifying a drug.

INJECTABLE DRUG HANDBOOK

Mostly used in the hospital setting, the *Injectable Drug Handbook* is a reference to the compatibility of various agents given parenterally. Although technicians cannot relay information from this book to doctors or nurses, they can find the information and have it ready for the pharmacist. In this way, they can facilitate a rapid response from the pharmacy to the necessary medical personnel.

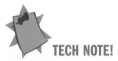

TECH NOTE!

Hospitals or pharmacies that work extensively with pediatric and/or geriatric patients may use these types of handbooks more often. Table 6-5 outlines specifics concerning each of the books listed previously or discussed in this chapter. This information includes how often the reference books are updated, along with which professionals most often use them.

TABLE 6-5 Main Attributes of Various Reference Books

Reference book	Who uses information	Updated
Drug Facts and Comparisons	Pharmacy	Yearly (hardbound) Monthly (unbound)
Physicians' Desk Reference	Physicians, pharmacy	Yearly
Drug Topics Red Book	Outpatient pharmacy	Yearly
Orange Book	Pharmacists	Yearly
Goodman & Gilman's The Pharmacological Basis of Therapeutics	Pharmacy students, practicing physicians, and registered pharmacists	Every 5 years
Remington's Pharmaceutical Sciences: The Science and Practice of Pharmacy	For registered pharmacists, physicians, and medical scientists	Every 5 years
United States Pharmacopoeia Drug Information	Pharmacy	Yearly
American Hospital Formulary Service Drug Information	Pharmacy	Yearly
Injectable Drug Handbook	Inpatient pharmacy	Yearly
Pediatric Handbook	Pharmacy	Yearly
Geriatric Handbook	Pharmacy	Yearly

ADDITIONAL PHARMACY REFERENCE BOOKS PHARMACISTS USE

Other reference books that pharmacists and technicians may use include the following:

American Drug Index
Goodman & Gilman's The Pharmacological Basis of Therapeutics
Handbook of Non-Prescription Drugs
Martindale's Extra Pharmacopoeia
Pediatric Drug Handbook
Remington's Pharmaceutical Sciences: The Science and Practice of Pharmacy

In addition to these well-known books, there are many specialty reference books such as those on lactating mothers, psychotropic medications, and antibiotics. Many pharmacies keep a wide range of these types of reference books (Table 6-5).

Learn What to Look for When Choosing a Reference Book

At times, technicians need to use reference books to find out more information on a drug or for billing purposes. Knowing the proper book to reference is important not only for the correct information but also for saving time and avoiding frustration.

The books listed previously are large reference books that are provided for the staff in the pharmacy. If you choose to buy your own reference books for home use or pocket versions for use at work, you should consider some basics. If your main use of the book will be to determine generic and trade names, indications, and side effects, then a book such as *Drug Facts and Comparisons* is a good choice. As pharmacies update their stock, you might be able to get a free copy of *Drug Facts and Comparisons*. Also, check bookstores on the internet for the previous year's edition. They can be sold at a decreased price and contain most of the information you require. You might check other book companies for

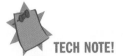

similar information. Many reference books contain the same type of information as *Drug Facts and Comparisons*. Another consideration may be the size of the reference book. For instance, although *Drug Facts and Comparisons* is a complete and up-to-date book, it is large and will not fit in your pocket for easy access; however, a pocket version is available. Other publishers also offer pocket versions of books.

Stay away from books that only reference drug names one way (only trade or generic names) because this can become time consuming. Most drugs have many names depending on the drug company that manufactures them. If you are going to keep the book at home or in your office, you might be looking for a larger book. If your space is limited, you may be more interested in a small book. Remember that smaller books will contain less information or will have harder-to-read print. If you are going to purchase a reference book at a bookstore, take a wide variety of drug names with you to reference in the store. If the book has all the drugs you are looking for and is easy to read, you will use the book more often.

Pocket-Sized Reference Books

Technicians traditionally have not carried pocket versions of drug books. As roles expand at work, the pharmacy technician needs to have his or her own reference books. Some manufacturers produce small pocket versions of trade/generic name drug books, but the drugs listed often are limited to their drug line only. For technicians to carry a good pocket guide not only of trade and generic names but also of the drug classifications, indications, and side effects is becoming more important. Thus it is important to check out as many pocket versions as you can to see what works for you. One of the best books to keep is one in which a drug can be looked up by trade or brand name without having to check the index. The cost of these pocket handbooks ranges between $20 and $40. The downside is that they are softbound and will need to be updated yearly to incorporate new drugs or discontinued ones. The upside is that most of the drugs remain the same year after year.

ELECTRONIC REFERENCE BOOKS

Handheld devices such as Palm Pilots are becoming more popular and economical. One can download an assortment of drug guides and other reference materials onto a handheld device for easy access. These devices are small enough to be carried in a coat pocket or purse. However, these devices are still one of the more expensive ways to obtain reference materials. As technology advances, the prices of these handheld devices will decrease, making them more affordable.

Journals and Newsmagazines

Nearly every pharmacy subscribes to journals and newsmagazines that pertain to pharmacy. These can be informative to the pharmacy technician. When a technician becomes nationally certified, he or she must complete continuing education units and may at some point use these journals for completing some if not all the necessary units. Journals offer continuing education at a reasonable cost; in addition, they allow the technician to keep up on the most recent drugs that are coming into pharmacy. Journals and newsletters may be published monthly, bimonthly, quarterly, or even weekly. They contain articles on new drugs, technicians, the future of pharmacy, and various legislative changes that may be taking place. The information they can give you on the field of pharmacy can be beneficial. Many different journals, newsletters, and magazines are available. Another source of journals that technicians may not see in the pharmacy setting are those written by pharmacy technician associations. These journals are geared specifically toward technician issues. Table 6-6 provides a sample of the types of journals and pharmacy magazines available.

TABLE 6-6 Types of Journals and Pharmacy Magazines Available

News magazine	Journal name	Published	Continuing education included	Website	Association
AAPT		6 times yearly	Yes	www.pharmacytechnician.com	Yes
Computertalk		6 times yearly	No	www.computertalk.com	No
Drug Topics		Monthly	Yes	www.drugtopics.com	No
Today's Technician		6 times yearly	Yes	www.pharmacytechnician.org	Yes
Pharmacy Times		Monthly	Yes	www.pharmacytimes.com	No
The Script		Monthly	No	www.pharmacy.ca.gov	No
U.S. Pharmacist		Monthly	Yes	www.uspharmacist.com	No
	AJHP	Twice monthly	Yes	www.ashp.org	Yes
	Journal of Pharmacy Technology	6 times yearly	Yes	www.jpharmtechnol.com	No

AAPT, American Association of Pharmacy Technicians; *AJHP*, *American Journal of Health-System Pharmacy.*

The Internet

Referencing should not be limited to books alone. The Internet has a lot of information; however, it is up to the reader to determine whether the information is reliable and accurate. Finding websites at universities and through publishing companies is a good way to look for information. Going to personal websites may give you a person's perspective but may not provide medically sound information. A list of reputable websites for news concerning medications is listed at the end of this chapter.

Pharmacy organizations have websites on the Internet, and many have weekly news boards that reference important information concerning pharmacy. Because so much is happening in pharmacy today, much of the information cannot be included in journals. The news links are listed on the website. This is a valuable tool used to keep members updated with accurate information. Also, these association sites have links to other pharmacy sites that may be of interest. Pharmacy associations also may offer Internet areas where the user can have questions answered by other members.

Additional Types of Information

In addition to large desktop books, pocket handbooks, journals, and the Internet, other sources of information can keep you current and on the cutting edge as a pharmacy technician. Joining an association can be rewarding and can serve as a good source of information and a way to network. Currently, the following associations provide continuing education and information for technicians:

> National Pharmacy Technicians Association
> American Association of Pharmacy Technicians
> American Society of Health-Systems Pharmacists
> American Pharmacists Association

All of these organizations offer a great way to stay up to date on new drugs, devices, and current and future pharmacy issues. In addition, they usually offer a vehicle to order pharmacy technician certification review books and other reference books, sometimes at a reduced membership rate. These reference books can be found on their websites or at their bookstores (this information may be

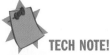

TECH NOTE!

Before you join an association, check out its website for information on how involved the association is with its technician members. Many associations do not have a technician division or offer continuing education classes specifically for technicians. Currently, only one association is run by technicians and allows only technicians as members; this is the National Pharmacy Technicians Association. They have yearly seminars and a bimonthly journal containing continuing education and other useful information pertaining specifically to technicians. Becoming familiar with the various conditions of patients and understanding the terminology is essential for a competent pharmacy technician. Table 6-7 lists good books that represent various aspects of health care. All health care workers never stop acquiring information.

TABLE 6-7 Additional Reference Books That Technicians May Find Helpful in Understanding Various Aspects of Health Care

Name	Useful information
Gray Morris D: *Calculate with confidence,* ed 4, St Louis, 2005, Elsevier. ISBN 0-323-02928-0	Math calculations for all types of dosage forms
Potter PA, Perry AG: *Fundamentals of nursing,* ed 6, St Louis, 2004, Elsevier. ISBN 0-323-02586-2	How nurses approach patients In-depth information on disease states
Mosby's medical, nursing, & allied health dictionary, revised reprint ed 6, St Louis, 2005, Elsevier. ISBN 0-323-03736-4	Fantastic diagrams along with definitions
Barkauskas VH, Baumann LC, Darling-Fisher CS: *Health & physical assesssment,* ed 3, St Louis, 2002, Mosby. ISBN 0-323-01214-0	Diagrams and treatment courses In-depth information on disease states
Gerdin J: *Health careers today,* ed 4, St Louis, 2007, Elsevier. ISBN 0-323-04474-3	Good description of more than 45 vocations in the medical field. Gives the technician a better understanding of health fields
Elkin MK, Perry AG, Potter PA: *Nursing interventions & clinical skills,* ed 3, St Louis, 2003, Elsevier. ISBN 0-323-02201-4	In-depth information on disease states

found at their seminars). The information and support they can provide is limited only by how much they are used. Also, many pharmacist associations such as the American Society of Health-Systems Pharmacists and American Pharmacists Association and their chapters have technician divisions that give technicians an avenue for learning new information. You must inquire about your local pharmacy associations to see what they have to offer. Some technician divisions are active in bringing continuing education courses to technicians and host various functions for networking and unifying pharmacy technicians from different types of pharmacies. As of today, only the National Pharmacy Technicians Association is completely run by and for technicians. For more information on all associations, refer to Chapter 1.

Seminars and continuing education dinners, provided by pharmacy associations, are sponsored mostly by drug companies and are another good source of information on drug topics, new drugs, and more. You do not need to be a member of an association to attend, but the cost usually is lower for members. Although seminars normally are held once or twice yearly depending on the association that is putting on the seminar, continuing education dinners may be hosted monthly by the local chapter of an association. At seminars, many of the technician classes include math, aseptic technique, the future of pharmacy technicians, law updates, and more. Monthly continuing education dinners or events usually have a limited amount of space available and, depending on the drug company sponsoring the event, there may be a speaker and a meal for a low cost or no cost. These costs usually are predetermined by the chapter of the association. All of these seminar classes and continuing education dinners can be used toward continuing education credit for pharmacy technicians.

DO YOU REMEMBER THESE KEY POINTS?
- The major sources of information that a technician most often uses in pharmacy
- The benefits of joining a pharmacy association
- Why continuing education is important for pharmacy technicians
- The key attributes of each of the books explained in this chapter
- Other sources available to technicians in addition to books, journals, and magazines
- Types of information on which a technician must keep up in pharmacy
- The difference between organizations and associations outlined in this chapter

MULTIPLE CHOICE QUESTIONS

1. Which of the books listed provides package inserts from manufacturers?
   A. *Drug Facts and Comparisons*
   B. *Goodman & Gilman's the Pharmacological Basis of Therapeutics*
   C. *Red Book*
   D. *Physician's Desk Reference*

2. Which book(s) listed below is(are) the best source for locating manufacturer addresses?
   A. *Red Book*
   B. *Physician's Desk Reference*
   C. *Goodman & Gilman's the Pharmacological Basis of Therapeutics*
   D. *Drug Facts and Comparisons*
   E. A, B, and D

3. If you need to look up the average wholesale price (AWP) of a drug, the best source to look in is _____.
   A. *American Drug Index*
   B. *Drug Facts and Comparisons*
   C. *Red Book*
   D. A journal

4. The book that comes hardbound and loose-leaf to allow for monthly updates is _____.
   A. *Drug Facts and Comparisons*
   B. *Red Book*
   C. *Goodman & Gilman's the Pharmacological Basis of Therapeutics*
   D. None of the above

5. The most widely used reference book in pharmacy is _____.
   A. *Goodman & Gilman's the Pharmacological Basis of Therapeutics*
   B. *Dictionary*
   C. *Remington's Pharmaceutical Sciences: The Science and Practice of Pharmacy*
   D. *Drug Facts and Comparisons*

6. A major pharmacy technician association run by technicians for technicians is _____.
   A. American Society of Health-System Professionals
   B. National Pharmacy Technician Association
   C. American Pharmacists Association
   D. All of the above

7. If you need to identify a specific tablet or capsule only by the markings and color, you will look in _____.
   A. *Drug Facts and Comparisons*
   B. *Ident-A-Drug*
   C. *American Drug Index*
   D. None of the above

8. The best way to choose a reference book is to _____.
   A. Ask a friend
   B. Choose the largest book because it will be the most comprehensive
   C. Choose the least expensive
   D. Choose one that you can use easily and covers the areas that you are interested in

9. One alternative to buying books is to _____.
   A. Wait until the pharmacy is going to throw out an old version
   B. Check for lower prices as a member of an association
   C. Use the Internet for information and read journals that your pharmacy provides for employees
   D. Both A and C

10. All of the following books are updated at least yearly except _____.
   A. *Drug Facts and Comparisons*
   B. *Red Book*
   C. *Goodman & Gilman's the Pharmacological Basis of Therapeutics*
   D. *Physician's Desk Reference*

TRUE/FALSE If a statement is false, then change it to make it true.

_____ **1.** Classification and indication mean the same thing.

_____ **2.** If a drug is contraindicated, it is not available in the United States.

_____ **3.** Monographs for a specific drug are produced after the experimentation phase and after approval from the Food and Drug Administration.

_____ **4.** A Palm Pilot is a device that allows referencing materials to be downloaded for individual use.

_____ **5.** Technicians can take continuing education only through pharmacists' journals.

_____ **6.** The Internet has information that is incorrect and should not be used as a source.

_____ **7.** Technicians do not need to use reference materials in a pharmacy.

_____ **8.** Many pharmacy associations have technician divisions for members.

_____ **9.** One of the best reasons to join an association and get involved is to network.

_____ **10.** Technicians are not expected to keep up with current medications or pharmacy trends.

TECHNICIAN'S CORNER

A patient comes into the pharmacy holding one capsule of medication that he or she needs to have refilled. The patient wants to know the price of the medication and whether it is available as a liquid. The capsule is white and has the markings "Watson 369" on one side and "5 mg" on the opposite. What is this drug, and what is it used for? Also list the average wholesale price, National Drug Code, and dosage forms.

BIBLIOGRAPHY

Billups NF, Billups SM: *American drug index* 2007, Philadelphia, 2006, Lippincott Williams & Wilkins.

Berardi RR, et al: *Handbook of non-prescription drugs,* ed 14, Washington, DC, 2004, American Pharmacists Association.

Drug facts and comparisons, ed 60, St Louis, 2005, Wolters-Kluwer.

Drug topics red book, ed 109, Montvale, NJ, 2005, Thomson.

Gennaro A: *Remington's pharmaceutical sciences: the science and practice of pharmacy,* ed 18, Easton, Pa, 1995, Mack.

Hardman JG, Limbird LE, editors: *Goodman & Gilman's the pharmaceutical basis of therapeutics,* ed 11, New York, 2005, McGraw-Hill Professional.

Jellin J, editor: *Ident-a-drug Reference 2006,* Stockton, Calif, 2006, Therapeutic Research Center.

Trissel, L: *Handbook on injectable drugs,* ed 14, Elk Grove Village, Ill, 2006, American Academy of Pediatrics.

US pharmacopoeia, ed 30, Rockville, Md, 2006, US Pharmacopeial Convention.

WEBSITES

www.fda.gov/cder/ob
www.dea.gov
www.drugtopics.com
www.webmd.com

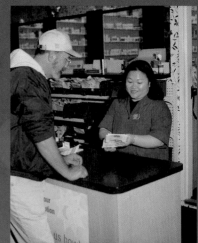

CHAPTER 7

Competency, Communication, and Ethics

Objectives

UPON COMPLETING THIS CHAPTER, YOU SHOULD BE ABLE TO DO THE FOLLOWING:

- List the primary responsibilities of a pharmacy technician.
- List the primary competencies of a pharmacy technician.
- Differentiate between morals and ethics.
- Describe the importance of good communication skills.
- List examples of ways pharmacy technicians can lessen errors in the workplace.
- Give an example of resolution techniques when dealing with irate patients.
- Explain the main psychological steps through which a terminally ill patient proceeds.
- Provide examples of situations in which pharmacy technicians must use their communication skills, ethics, and competencies.

Communication *The ability to express oneself in such a way that one is readily and clearly understood*

Competency *The capability or proficiency to perform a function*

Confidentiality *To keep privileged customer information from being disclosed without the customer's consent*

Ethics *The values and morals that are used within a profession*

Morals *Ethics; honorable beliefs*

Nationally Certified Technician *One who is proficient in minimum standards set by the Pharmacy Technician Certification Board*

Professionalism *Conforming to right principles of conduct (work ethics) as accepted by others in the profession*

A S THE NUMBER OF PHARMACY TECHNICIAN jobs increases in many different areas of pharmacy, so will the number of applicants for those positions. As the population grows older, use of prescription medications also continues to grow. Therefore, more technicians are needed to help fill those prescriptions. In addition, as pharmacists are becoming more involved in patient care (consulting with patients, conferring with physicians, and helping to make decisions in clinical aspects of patients' prescribing), pharmacy technicians are taking over the traditional role of a pharmacist. In addition to filling prescriptions, technicians also work in many other areas of pharmacy practice (see Chapter 3). The technician who can function in more areas of the pharmacy is more valuable as an employee; however, this alone does not guarantee a long-lasting career. Several factors must be considered before a person can be considered a competent employee, specifically whether he or she meets the state regulations (i.e., certification and/or registration) as a pharmacy technician. This chapter reveals the major competencies required of a pharmacy technician, which include job duties, communication skills, and ethics. In a growing industry that strives to deliver error-free medications to the patient, this aspect of the pharmacy job is one of the most critical. This chapter explores the types of common errors with which pharmacists and technicians are in a constant battle and ways to deflect such events from happening. In addition, this chapter covers the rights of a patient. Also, the five stages of a terminally ill patient are identified.

Responsibilities

Because of the varying types of settings in which technicians may work, technicians have many different duties as well. Box 7-1 references chapters that cover common responsibilities and competencies necessary to function in various settings. To fulfill the duties of a technician, one must become competent in those areas. The following competencies are outlined in this chapter. Although certain areas of pharmacy bring a technician close to the patient, others will not. Still, the technician converses with co-workers and other health care workers daily under various circumstances. Because of this, the technician must exercise competencies and communication skills daily.

BOX 7-1 COMMON RESPONSIBILITIES AND COMPETENCIES OF A PHARMACY TECHNICIAN REFERENCE

Conversions and calculations —*need to master.*	Chapter 4
Dosage forms, abbreviations, and routes of administration	Chapter 5
Referencing	Chapter 6
Prescriptions	Chapter 8
Inpatient pharmacy	Chapter 11
Repackaging and compounding	Chapter 12
Aseptic technique	Chapter 13
Pharmacy stock and billing practices	Chapter 14

BOX 7-2 EXAMPLES OF FEDERAL LAWS GOVERNING PHARMACY

- Required prescription label information: pharmacy name, address, and phone number; patient's name; prescription number; name of drug; strength; dosage form; quantity; date filled; doctor; refills; expiration date; and pharmacist's initials. If a technician fills the prescription, he or she also must initial label.
- Required prescription information: doctor's name, address, and phone number; patient's name; name of drug; strength; dosage form; quantity; date written; refills; doctor's Drug Enforcement Administration number; and signature.
- Verbal orders: Only a registered pharmacist within the pharmacy can take a doctor's verbal orders for prescriptions.
- Patient consultation: Only a registered pharmacist can give advice or consult a patient about his or her medications.
- Unit dosing: Proper documentation of a medication includes manufacturer, lot number, expiration date, dosage form, quantity prepared, date, technician's initials, and pharmacist initials. On each unit dose label, the following information must show drug, strength, dosage form, manufacturer facilities lot, and expiration date.
- Controlled substances: Only a registered pharmacist can sign controlled substances into the pharmacy inventory or send them back to the manufacturer. Within a hospital, only pharmacists, pharmacy technicians, nurses, and doctors may sign controlled substances into stock.

Competencies

TECH ALERT!

Remember that the strictest law (whether it's federal or state) is the one that you must follow. This is a guaranteed exam question on the National Certification Exam.

LAWS, REGULATIONS, AND PHARMACY COMPETENCIES

Knowledge of pharmacy law is essential before working in a pharmacy environment. The basics are listed in Box 7-2 (for more examples, see Chapter 2). Federal laws govern all 50 states. In addition each state also has specific laws, regulations, and guidelines that pertain to pharmacy practice and as governed by the boards of pharmacy. State laws may differ from Federal laws.

Each pharmacy has a binder of policies and procedures that are the protocol of the pharmacy. These standards pertain to medications, inventory, order of operations, work schedules, and specific skills and/or tasks required of pharmacy staff. Other information that can be found in this binder includes guidelines pertaining to job duties, employee benefits, job orientation, training, and evaluation methods. These policies are developed by management and are updated regularly. In addition to this information, procedures one must follow to report errors, discrepancies, or other areas of concern that may arise are outlined. This is an important tool with which every pharmacy technician should become acquainted as a component of professional behavior.

BASIC SKILLS

Typing

The speed required by most pharmacy employers does not exceed 35 words per minute, but a technician who has speed and a good knowledge of medication is cherished within the pharmacy setting. The number of prescriptions processed per day in a pharmacy directly relates to the speed of the typist. This makes a fast and accurate pharmacy technician typist a much-sought-after commodity.

Computers

One of the requirements imposed on pharmacies by the federal government is the reduction of pharmacy errors. This has influenced pharmacies to use computers for dispensing medications and keeping inventory. Dispensing medication systems accurately count and dispense medications and directly have led to a decrease in the rate of errors. Although these systems increase accurate dosing, human error still occurs. Nothing replaces the knowledge of a skilled pharmacy technician to decrease error rates.

Reports and Documentation

Many pharmacies expect technicians to prepare various reports. Knowledge of computers and programs such as Microsoft Word and Excel can make a technician a valuable asset to the pharmacy. Because all pharmacies have integrated computers into their ordering, filling, and documentation procedures, technicians must be computer savvy.

Ordering Supplies

The task of ordering stock usually falls on a specific person within the pharmacy, although everyone should know how to order stock when necessary. Learning how to order stock, return expired or damaged stock, and handle recalled items are among the duties in which pharmacy technicians should be competent. This skill is normally taught on-the-job as each pharmacy has its own way of handling stock inventory. An important aspect of an inventory technician is the storage requirements of the medications that arrive in pharmacy. For more information on this topic, refer to Chapter 5.

REGISTRATION AND CERTIFICATION

Meeting the specific guidelines of state regulations is the single most basic requirement of a pharmacy technician. Each state has a board of pharmacy that institutes regulations for pharmacy technicians. Regulations can be found on the respective website of each state. More states are requiring registration of technicians. Registration is an important tool for pharmacy management to ensure that each technician has a clean background to work in the pharmacy environment. By doing a simple fingerprint background check, the hiring pharmacy gains a measure of confidence in the pharmacy technician candidate; however, it is not a measurement of the competency of the technician. Thus certification is being used in more states and most likely will be used soon in some form or another throughout all 50 states (Chapter 3). This examination encompasses all types of pharmacy practice.

Registration and/or certification help pharmacy management more easily to choose the most competent technician to fill the position. The technician who is certified has a clear edge over a non-certified technician in the hiring process.

Of course, these qualifications alone do not necessarily cover all skills required of a competent technician. Thus a probationary period is imposed to assess the pharmacy technician daily. The following sections describe the areas of competency that, if met, increase the prospective pharmacy technician's chances of being chosen for a pharmacy position.

Professionalism

Pharmacy technicians are paraprofessionals and may be thought of as assistants to pharmacists. Because of the vast changes that have taken place during the last decade, pharmacy technicians are moving into an emerging field of pharmacy. As technicians assume more roles, such as clinical pharmacy technicians, inventory specialists, nuclear medication technicians, and other specialized roles, they must be knowledgeable in many areas of pharmacy. More technical colleges are offering associate's degrees for pharmacy technicians. The field of pharmacy technician is becoming a profession. According to the American Medical Association, pharmacy technician was the top new profession in 2001.

Although it is good that the job of a pharmacy technician is beginning to be thought of as a profession, there is a difference between a profession and professionalism. A profession is a job, occupation, or line of work that becomes a career. Professionalism is conforming to right principles of conduct (work ethics) as accepted by others in the profession. It takes time, hard work, and consistency to be respected as a professional. Because of the increasing depth of education and training that a pharmacy technician needs, pharmacy technicians of today are the first generation of pharmacy technician professionals. If they do not meet certain responsibilities, they will remain pharmacy assistants and not professionals in the eyes of other health care professionals. Measuring professionalism includes projecting the correct behavior. This includes your attitude and interpersonal skills, in addition to meeting the requirements of your state. Pharmacy technicians deal daily with patients, pharmacists, doctors, and nurses. How they handle themselves in various situations reveals their competencies in the pharmacy and their personal maturity. Probably one of the most prevalent concerns of pharmacy managers and pharmacists is the need for pharmacy technicians who are competent in the area of communication.

Communication

Pharmacy technicians communicate every day with family, friends, strangers, acquaintances, and customers that they help (Figure 7-1). Individuals depend on good communication skills to get a job; to buy products, and to have needs, wants, and concerns presented to others. Communication is defined as the ability to express oneself in such a way that one is understood readily and clearly; however, one of the major complaints from customers and managers is the lack of good communication skills. Most schools do not teach students to be good communicators; however, virtually all jobs require good communication skills. One of the most important areas in which effective communication is needed is in the pharmacy and other health care settings, because life and death issues are often faced there. Good communication skills include diplomacy, compassion, sensitivity, responsibility, tact, and patience. Communication skills, or interpersonal skills, also can be referred to as the ability to relate to another person, verbally or nonverbally.

Every person takes his or her health seriously. Going to the doctor is not enjoyable but is done out of necessity. Feeling sick or unable to perform does not put a person in a happy mood. After visiting the doctor, a person may have to start taking medication or add another medication to the many that the person already is taking. On arrival to the pharmacy, the first person with whom the

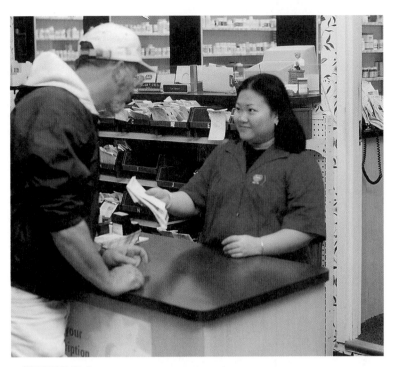

FIGURE 7-1 Technicians must be sensitive when helping patients.

customer may have to interact may be the pharmacy technician. This up-close-and-personal interaction reveals the best and worst communication skills of the pharmacy technician. One must consider several areas when assessing interpersonal skills, such as the different ways in which we communicate.

WAYS TO COMMUNICATE

Body Language

Have you ever heard the phrase "actions speak louder than words"? Many persons make an instant judgment of others within the first 30 seconds of meeting. This is true with respect to the pharmacy setting too. The primary goal of pharmacy personnel is to help others, which can be accomplished by being friendly and remaining calm. Facial expressions can show many different emotions, thoughts, and biases. As a professional, it is imperative that the only body language that should be conveyed is that of a helpful and concerned pharmacy staff member. A professional should not bring his or her outside personal problems to work. Stress manifests in various ways such as frowning, tensing the shoulders, biting one's lip, raising eyebrows, folding arms, placing hands on hips, or other idiosyncrasies. If and when stress begins to transform into this type of body language, it is time to take a step back and maybe a deep breath to bring oneself back into focus, as seen in an example in Box 7-3.

Listening Skills

Listen, listen, and listen. Sometimes just listening to a person is all that is required. If a customer is angry about the medication, regardless of the problem, just listening can ease the person's frustration. Rather than trying to beat the person to the next sentence and telling the person that he or she is wrong, try to listen until the person is finished and empathize with the dilemma. Most persons know a problem with medication is not the fault of the pharmacy technician, but they want to be heard. A professional does not allow himself or herself to be directed by another person's inappropriate behavior. Pharmacy technicians must remember the final outcome and behave professionally.

BOX 7-3 EXAMPLE OF NEGATIVE BODY LANGUAGE

Ms. Lehman walks up to the counter to have her prescription filled and asks whether it can be done within 5 minutes because her bus will be leaving. Pharmacy technician John rolls his eyes and shakes his head in disbelief that everyone thinks that he or she should not have to wait. He turns and walks away without saying a word.

Alternate response: John shows concern for Ms. Lehman and tells her they will fill her prescription as soon as possible. John can ask the pharmacist to please fill the prescription as quickly as possible.

BOX 7-4 EXAMPLE OF UNACCEPTABLE PHONE ETIQUETTE

Patient: Hello, I'm calling because my medication looks different than before and I need to know if it's the same drug or not.

Pharmacy technician: Would you please hold?

Patient: No, I need to know now because . . .

Pharmacy technician: [places the patient on hold and forgets to get back to the patient]

Alternate response: The technician waits to hear the patient's response to the question. When the patient says she cannot wait, the technician waits to hear why and then proceeds to help her.

Phone Skills

Pharmacies receive phone calls every few minutes. If there are multiple lines, the phone can ring almost constantly. This can lead to several problems. For example, most persons do not want to be placed on hold, but it is often necessary. For a customer to be placed on hold and then forgotten is not acceptable. When answering the phone, it is best to identify oneself, place the customer on hold, and check back every minute or so just to let the customer know that he or she is not forgotten. Customers are calling about medications, and often these are essential medications that are important. Patients must be treated with respect and courtesy (Box 7-4).

Appearance

Pharmacy technicians must interact daily with all types of customers or patients. In addition to customers, they must interact with nurses, doctors, and hospital staff. Knowledge, behavior, and good communication skills are essential to be considered a professional. But all of these attributes are inadequate if the pharmacy technician is not dressed professionally. A well-groomed person conveys self-confidence and professionalism. Of course, this should not be the only goal of the pharmacy technician; however, pharmacy protocol usually outlines what is acceptable and unacceptable regarding uniform, shoes, hair, jewelry, and other miscellaneous items. Consider the message conveyed to customers when the pharmacy technician who takes the prescription has messy hair, too much makeup, a nose ring, and tattoos. Does this convey professionalism? Probably not, prompting the management of most pharmacies to frown on facial jewelry, an unkempt appearance, and visible tattoos.

Good Writing Skills

One of the daily duties of a pharmacy technician is to answer the phones; talk to patients, nurses, and doctors; and take messages when the pharmacist is busy. It may seem simple just to write a question down quickly on a note pad, but if

BOX 7-5 EXAMPLE OF POOR WRITTEN COMMUNICATION SKILLS

Nurse Black calls and wants to know if the two drugs that she is about to administer are compatible. She's in a hurry. Joe North, CPhT, scribbles down the question but does not get the nurse's name or extension. By the time the nurse calls back to contact the pharmacist, the dose is late and the patient has been in pain while waiting.

Alternate response: The technician, Joe North, tells the nurse he will ask the pharmacist to call her back and then proceeds to ask her name, station, extension, and patient's name and medical record number.

done poorly, this task can lead to improper communication or possibly an error. For example, if a nurse calls the pharmacy with a question about a drug interaction, it is imperative that the technician write down all of the pertinent information. Make sure to spell the following information correctly:

- Nurse's name
- Floor location and extension in a hospital setting, or the physician's office in a community pharmacy
- The purpose of the call written in a concise question
- The time of the call
- The initials of the technician who took the call
- How soon is the information needed timewise

Only then can a pharmacist quickly and easily relay the correct information to the appropriate person. If your handwriting is illegible, it can cost time and possibly result in a preventable error. One has no excuse for poor handwriting. This is one of the reasons that doctors now are moving to electronic medication ordering. Thousands of preventable errors can be overcome through the use of computer ordering (Box 7-5).

Ethics

The morals with which children are raised stem from their family's beliefs in what is right and wrong. These morals and values extend throughout a lifetime and are passed to the next generation. Ethics are slightly different than morals, yet they are just as important. Ethics are the values and morals that are used within a profession. Each person has his or her own morals concerning issues such as abortion, and those morals can affect the ethics of a person in a professional situation. For example, if delivering medication used in performing abortions goes against a technician's morals, it may affect work ethics because the technician is required to deliver medications to the patient as prescribed, regardless of personal beliefs. The technician should not make a judgment about the patient. If a technician does not deliver the medication, he or she is not performing the assigned duties, which is a violation of professional duties. Most persons can separate their own morals from work ethics and are able to do their job without believing that they have betrayed their belief system. The bottom line is talk to your employer if any part of your job description is of concern to you.

CONFIDENTIALITY

Confidentiality is another aspect of working ethically. The definition of confidentiality is to keep privileged information about a customer from being disclosed without his or her consent. This includes information that may cause the patient embarrassment or harm. Patients have a right to privacy concerning their medications, treatment, or any aspect of their health care. The Health Insurance Portability and Accountability Act addresses patient confidentiality

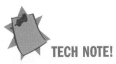

TECH NOTE!

Remember that working ethically is doing what is right for the patient, not what is right for you.

BOX 7-6 EXAMPLE OF BREACHING CONFIDENTIALITY

Ms. K has cancer. Two pharmacy technicians discuss her condition and the medications that she is taking. A co-worker of Ms. K overhears this information and tells her employer.

in the pharmacy (see Appendix E). These new laws affect all areas of medicine, including pharmacy, concerning issues of obtaining, transferring, and accessing patient information. Changes have been made throughout all medical facilities and medical information centers that limit access to patient information in charts and computer bases. A patient's approval is required for any information concerning the patient to be released to any third party, including insurance companies, doctors, and pharmacies. Because pharmacy technicians and other health care professionals have access to a patient's condition, medications, and other personal information, they are responsible to keep the patient's information confidential (Box 7-6).

Terminally Ill Patients

Special consideration should be given to those patients who are terminally ill. This can prove difficult. Although each person deals with his or her own mortality differently, there are "normal" progressive steps that persons experience. The five stages that terminally ill patients experience are as follows:

Stages	Example
Denial	"This can't be happening . . ."
Anger	"It isn't fair. I don't deserve this . . ."
Bargaining	"Please make me better, and I promise . . ."
Depression	"I will never be able to see you again . . ."
Acceptance	"I can do this, everyone does . . ."

Normally the first stage is denial. This is a defense mechanism in which the situation does not seem real. Perhaps the reality is too harsh for the person to accept. The next stage is anger. Sometimes one may have a feeling of unfairness. Bargaining usually follows anger. The person makes promises to himself or herself or to a higher power in the hope of a miracle. Depression may take over at this point when the realization sets in that nothing is going to change concerning the prognosis. The final phase is acceptance, in which the person concedes his or her own mortality and prepares for eventual death.

Each of these stages can manifest at any time and last for different lengths of time. Therefore, it is important that the technician be compassionate to the patient's situation. Most health care workers do not hesitate to help a dying patient; however, the problem is how to identify these patients. Unfortunately, unless the patient decides to share this information, the pharmacy staff does not necessarily know. Some medications indicate an advancing medical condition. These include pain medications, such as fentanyl patches or morphine; however, these drugs do not identify definitively a fatal condition. Therefore the pharmacy technician must be objective about each person who enters the pharmacy and realize that he or she does not know what each person is experiencing.

If the technician treats persons equally regardless of their disposition, then the pharmacy technician is behaving appropriately and professionally. The pharmacy technician can influence the development of a positive atmosphere within the pharmacy setting. Allowing customers to express frustration, being a good listener, and doing one's best to help others is what being a professional is all about.

BOX 7-7 AGENCIES THAT TRACK MEDICATION ERRORS

AHRQ	Agency for Healthcare Research and Quality
AMA	American Medical Association
ASHP	American Society of Health-System Pharmacists
CDER	Center for Drug Evaluation and Research
FDA	Food and Drug Administration
ISMP	Institute for Safe Medication Practices
JCAHO	Joint Commission on Accreditation of Healthcare Organizations
NCCMERP	National Coordinating Council for Medication Error Reporting and Prevention
USP	United States Pharmacopoeia

TABLE 7-1 Places Where Errors Can Occur

Location	Example of type of error that might occur
Hospitals/clinics	Dosing medications
Pharmacies	Wrong dosing information, drug interactions, wrong drug
Nursing homes	Dosing side effects, overdosing or underdosing
Doctors' offices	Poor doctor-patient communication, improper diagnosis
Patients' homes	Skipped dosing times, wrong dose taken, overdose

Medication Errors

One of the functions of the Food and Drug Administration (FDA) is to protect the consumer against harmful medications and devices. This includes medication errors that may originate within hospitals, clinics, doctors' offices, and pharmacies. According to current information provided by the FDA, medication error is the top cause of injury and death in the United States. A report issued in 1999 by the Institute of Medicine estimated that up to 98,000 persons die in hospitals yearly from medication errors. This statistic tops death rates linked to breast cancer, motor vehicle accidents, and acquired immunodeficiency syndrome. The cost of errors can reach the astounding amount of $75 billion annually. Because of these shocking statistics, decreasing medication errors has become a hot issue and has received the attention of all agencies and organizations that are linked to medicine and consumer information services. Box 7-7 lists some of these agencies. All of these agencies can be accessed on the Internet to keep one updated on new policies and practices that currently are being implemented across the United States.

The FDA and other agencies have proposed specific avenues and guidelines that ultimately will decrease drug errors to the consumer. The Institute for Safe Medication Practices is a nonprofit agency that works with the FDA and the United States Pharmacopoeia to analyze dangerous medication errors and what they refer to as "near misses." These agencies work together to try to prevent these errors from occurring again. The medical community and consumers have an avenue to report errors called MedWatch (Chapter 2, Figure 2-1). Information given is not meant to punish the person or place blame but to look into the reason behind the error in hopes that change may be implemented to prevent future errors.

Errors can occur almost anywhere and at any time (Table 7-1). Errors that occur in hospital pharmacies and pharmacies outside the hospital directly affect the performance of the pharmacy technician. Some common reasons why errors

TABLE 7-2 Types of Errors That Can Occur in the Pharmacy

Type of error	Example of errors made by technicians
Lack of or incorrect communication	Poor telephone message
Errors in repackaging medications	Wrong drug name or unit dose medication
Poor procedures or techniques	Poor aseptic technique used preparing drug
Poor training or knowledge	Improper calculations used in compounding
Poor doctor's handwriting	Assuming a drug name in error
Poor use of abbreviations	Transcribing an assumed drug abbreviation in error
Poor written directions for medication use	Typing a label based on assumption of doctor's poorly written prescription
Similar sounding drug name	Pulling wrong drug to be dispensed

occur are a stressful job environment resulting from understaffing, increased workload, and lack of training. Table 7-2 lists types of errors that can occur within the pharmacy.

Pharmacy technicians can prevent errors by taking certain steps. The misconception that pharmacists can and will catch every mistake that a pharmacy technician makes is incorrect and is thus a dangerous misconception.

The following sections outline necessary competencies in which every pharmacy technician must be proficient. All pharmacy personnel must strive continually to increase their knowledge in order to lessen the possibility of medication errors.

DOCTORS' ORDERS

You must know normal dosing of medications and those that are abnormal. A strong knowledge of generic and trade drug names and their strengths can enable the pharmacy technician to catch a possible prescribing mistake. All orders that are difficult to read should be brought to the pharmacist's attention before filling the prescription. Often the wrong medication is dispensed because of the physician's poor handwriting. Pharmacists and technicians may pull the wrong medication based on an assumption of what the order says. If the prescription is hard to read, the pharmacist must call the physician for clarification.

ASEPTIC TECHNIQUE

Daily preparation and compounding of various medications requires knowledge of aseptic technique. Although pharmacists are responsible for all medications dispensed from the pharmacy, they cannot watch every pharmacy technician every moment of the day to ensure that proper procedures are used. Competent pharmacy technicians have learned how to use aseptic technique and why it is important to cultivate their skills. Pharmacy supervisors periodically take samples of compounded intravenous drugs and send them to the laboratory to be tested for microbial growth. Because each sample has the name of the pharmacy technician who prepared it, this information may be used to assess his or her performance.

SOUNDALIKE, LOOK-ALIKE DRUGS

Drugs with names that are spelled similarly but are totally different classes of drugs have been the cause of many medication errors. For example, quinidine

TECH ALERT!

If anyone, including a pharmacist or technician, is caught taking any drug, especially a narcotic or controlled substance, or altering log sheets, there may be serious consequences. The penalties vary depending on the crime. Penalties may include suspension or a loss of your license and/or civil penalties. Also, the board of pharmacy has the right to list all persons by name along with their violations and actions taken in their monthly newsletter. No drug is worth the cost of your career and reputation. If you have a tendency to misuse any type of drug, you should seek counseling before working in a pharmacy or choose a different career that does not bring you into proximity of these types of medications. Also, know that most companies have mandatory drug screenings.

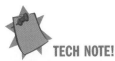

TECH NOTE!

One way to decrease errors is to read prescription labels three times. First, when pulling the drug from the shelf to fill an order, check the prescription against the drug label. Next, as you prepare the prescription, check the name of the drug, strength, and dosage form against the medication you have chosen. Finally, check the drug as you move it over to the pharmacist for final checking. It works!

and quinine have been mistaken for each other. Quinidine is for the heart, whereas quinine is for malaria. It can be even more confusing when the drugs are similar not only in name but also in the condition that they treat. For example, the drugs amrinone and amiodarone are used for various heart conditions, and their names sound and look very much alike.

Manufacturers that package several different drugs have been known to package all of their products in similarly colored packaging with similar print size and font for the cost savings. For example, unit dose packages of the generic version of promethazine 25 mg and promethazine 50 mg have the same packaging (font size, color, and package size) and can be confused easily if the technician is pulling a dose in a hurry. These types of errors have been documented over the years by the FDA. The FDA and others are encouraging drug companies to package their medications in packages that are considerably different (such as using various colors and different print) to distinguish each individual drug name and strength further for easy identification.

Because most drugs are kept on the pharmacy shelves in alphabetical order by generic name, a drug can be mistaken accidentally for another drug with a similar spelling. Each pharmacy must take steps to prevent this from happening by identifying these medications. For example, hydralazine and hydroxyzine are similar-sounding drugs and are close to one another on the shelf. The following provides several ways to decrease errors in the pharmacy:

✓ Verify any unclear orders (a technician must do this via the pharmacist)
✓ Ask what the condition being treated is; what is the drug's indication
✓ Ask for both trade and generic name to cross-reference the medication
✓ Keep similar drugs either away from one another on the pharmacy shelves or clearly mark them to avoid confusion

Pharmacist's Perspective
BY SUSAN WONG, PharmD

In recent years, there has been a national shortage of medical professionals, especially pharmacists and nurses. In some states, recent legislation has been approved to help pharmacies deliver better service in a timely manner. This allows pharmacists to spend more time counseling patients. As an example in California, more technician support for pharmacists is allowed (up to two technicians to work with each pharmacist in certain situations—the technician-to-pharmacist ratio.) Now the challenge will be to find enough qualified technicians to work in the pharmacies. More emphasis will be placed on competency, communication, and ethics/professional behavior as the growth and expansion of the pharmacy technician role continues.

As mentioned in a previous chapter, the technician role has evolved from a clerical role to a more technical one behind the scenes, helping pharmacists provide medicines to those who need it. The technician is part of the team, not an individual practitioner. The technician must be willing and competent to work anywhere from the front line helping customers to working behind the counter with the pharmacist answering phones, assist in filling prescriptions, preparing intravenous admixtures, and so on. Being competent in as many skills as possible is what sets the technician apart as a valued team member. Together, under the guidance and supervision of licensed pharmacists, this team functions as a well-oiled machine. This allows efficiency on the job, delivery of world-class pharmaceutical care, and personal job satisfaction. ■

DO YOU REMEMBER THESE KEY POINTS?

- The benefits of certification
- Information contained in the policies and procedures binder
- The major causes of medication errors
- The agencies that track errors
- Examples of how a pharmacy technician can decrease errors
- The difference between profession and professionalism
- The difference between morals and work ethics
- Five ways to communicate effectively to staff or patients
- The importance of patient confidentiality and the laws that cover them
- Examples of additional competencies of a pharmacy technician
- The five stages of a terminally ill patient

MULTIPLE CHOICE QUESTIONS

1. Of the skills listed, which one is not a competency required of a pharmacy technician?
   A. Providing prescription label information
   B. Transcribing doctors' orders
   C. Consulting a doctor to clarify orders
   D. Preparing unit dose medications, including documentation

2. Of the information listed, which one normally is not contained in the policies and procedures binder within the pharmacy?
   A. Work shifts
   B. Job duties
   C. Employee benefits
   D. Insurance forms

3. Which of these statements is not true pertaining to medication errors?
   A. As many as 98,000 persons die yearly because of medication errors.
   B. Costs resulting from drug errors can reach $75 billion annually.
   C. As of 2002, the Food and Drug Administration has just begun to gather information on drug errors.
   D. Deaths caused by drug errors surpass deaths caused by acquired immunodeficiency syndrome, auto accidents, and breast cancer.

4. Pharmacy technicians can decrease errors in all of the following ways except _____.
   A. Bringing prescriptions that are difficult to read to the pharmacist's attention
   B. Writing notes or messages clearly
   C. Using good communication techniques
   D. Relying on the pharmacist to catch mistakes

5. The best definition for communication is _____.
   A. Talking between two persons
   B. Telling information to another person
   C. Expressing oneself in a way that is understood by another
   D. Winning an argument

6. Communication skills involve all of the following except _____.
   A. Body language
   B. Listening
   C. Talking loudly
   D. Appearance

7. Concerning confidentially, which of the following statements is the most correct?
   A. Patients never have to worry about anyone talking about their personal health information.
   B. Patients give up their rights to confidentiality when they are admitted into a hospital.
   C. Pharmacy technicians do not have access to patient information other than their current drugs.
   D. All health care workers are responsible for keeping patient information confidential.

8. Of the skills listed, identify the important ones.
A. Computer skills
B. Inventory skills
C. Aseptic technique skills
D. All of the above

9. Which of the following stages of a terminally ill patient is not one of those outlined in this chapter?
A. Denial
B. Anger
C. Bargaining
D. Psychosis

10. Of the statements listed, which one is not true concerning technician-to-patient interaction?
A. Treating all patients equally is best.
B. Using compassion and patience is important.
C. Call security immediately when a patient becomes angry.
D. Call the pharmacist for assistance if a patient insists on speaking with one.

TRUE/FALSE If a statement is false, then change it to make it true.

_____ **1.** Registration and certification are done by the board of pharmacy of each state.

_____ **2.** Only the Food and Drug Administration keeps information pertaining to drug errors.

_____ **3.** Consumers and health care workers can report drug errors to MedWatch.

_____ **4.** Drug errors are likely to occur any time and any place.

_____ **5.** All persons who are in the profession of pharmacy technician are automatically professional.

_____ **6.** Facial jewelry, tattoos, and brightly colored hair on health care workers does not exhibit a professional appearance.

_____ **7.** *Morals* and *ethics* are exactly the same.

_____ **8.** Confidentiality is something that only doctors and nurses need to worry about.

_____ **9.** If pharmacy technicians are registered, this means they have had background checks done.

_____ **10.** Only pharmacists should talk to angry patients.

TECHNICIAN'S CORNER Go to the Food and Drug Administration website at *www.fda.gov* and find the area in which medication errors can be reported. Download the form used and attach it to one of the many incident reports that have come into the Food and Drug Administration from a consumer or health care professional.

BIBLIOGRAPHY

Koln LT, Corrigan JM, Donaldson MS: *To err is human: building a safer health system.* Retrieved March 2, 2003, from http://books.nap.edu/books/030906837/html/R1.html

Manual for pharmacy technicians, ed 3, Bethesda, Md, 2004, American Society of Health-System Pharmacists.

Nordenberg T: Make no mistake: medical errors can be deadly serious. *FDA Consumer* Sep-Oct 2000. Retrieved March 2, 2003, from www.fda.gov/fdac/features/2000/500_err.html

Western Career College curriculum, Sacramento, Calif, Western Career College.

Phillips J: Generic name confusion. FDA Safety Page, *Drug Topics* 10-6-2003; 147:90

WEBSITES

www.ama-assn.org—American Medical Association

www.ashpASHP.org—American Society of Healthcare Pharmacists

www.fda.gov—Food and Drug Administration

www.fda.gov/cder- Center for Drug Evaluation and Research

www.JACHOjointcommission.org—Joint Commission on Accreditation of Hospital Organizations

www.nccmerp.org—National Coordinating Council for Medication Error Reporting & Prevention

www.qualityindicators.ahrq.gov—Agency for Healthcare Research and Quality

8

Prescription Processing

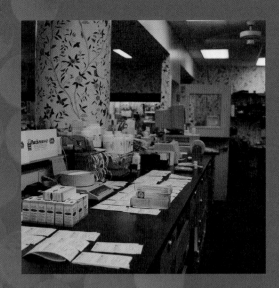

Objectives

UPON COMPLETING THIS CHAPTER, YOU SHOULD BE ABLE TO DO THE FOLLOWING:

- Describe the responsibilities of a technician filling prescriptions.
- List the necessary information required for prescriptions and labels.
- Demonstrate the ability to prioritize the filling of prescriptions.
- Differentiate filling methods between controlled substances and noncontrolled substances.
- Describe laws pertaining to the technician's responsibilities when filling prescriptions.
- List the 10 steps of carefully filling a medication order.
- Differentiate between inpatient and outpatient information requirements.
- List the types of automated machines used in filling prescriptions.
- Explain steps in reducing medication errors.
- List the 5 rights of a patient.

Auxiliary label *An adhesive label that is attached to a container with specific instructions or information pertaining to the medication inside*

Hard copy *The original prescription*

Rx *Latin abbreviation for "recipe," commonly used to mean "prescription"; legend drug; prescription drug*

Script *A prescription*

Sig *Medication directions written in pharmacy terms on a prescription*

FILLING A PRESCRIPTION is one of the most important and commonly performed duties of a technician, regardless of the setting. The art of transcribing doctors' writing into lay terms sometimes can be frustrating, if not impossible. However, with time and experience, a good technician can determine easily whether he or she can process a prescription quickly or if assistance from the pharmacist is needed. Often the pharmacist cannot decipher the doctor's writing either. In this case, the pharmacist is responsible for calling the physician and asking for clarification of the prescription, also known as the script. Whether a technician is working in a hospital or community pharmacy, the process of reading a doctor's orders and the documentation of that order is much the same.

This chapter first explores the various methods by which a prescription can arrive in a pharmacy and the fundamentals of reading a prescription. Inpatient and outpatient skills are covered under certain sections because they differ in methods. Then the chapter explores what to look for, how to fill, how to file, and finally, how to resolve discrepancies. In addition, the most common types of medication errors and how the technician can avoid some of the more common pitfalls are discussed. As with any skill, practice makes perfect.

Processing a Prescription: A Step-by-Step Approach

Five basic steps are required for filling a prescription. Four of these steps relate directly to the technician; the fifth relates directly to the pharmacist. Although these steps may seem simple, they require complete presence of mind and concentration. Within each step are several important points to remember that have been outlined in this chapter. The five steps include the following:

1. Taking in the prescription
2. Translating the prescription
3. Entering information into the computer system
4. Filling the prescription
5. Patient counseling*

Taking in the Prescription

A prescription can arrive in a pharmacy by various methods. A prescription can be in the form of a written order that is on a conventional prescription pad listing

---

*Counseling may be done by a registered pharmacist or pharmacist intern.

BOX 8-1 COMMONLY FOLLOWED RULES FOR TAKING IN PRESCRIPTIONS

Call-in

Calling in a prescription can be done by a doctor, nurse, physician's assistant, or a person designated by the doctor.

Taking a prescription over the phone must be done only by a registered pharmacist or pharmacist intern (in some states).

Fax

Faxed original copies mostly are used by hospitals but are becoming more common in community pharmacies. Schedule II medications, if faxed, must be followed by a written prescription received at the pharmacy in 72 hours.

Walk-in

Most prescriptions in a community pharmacy are taken into a pharmacy by the patient or the patient's relative. In hospitals, discharge orders usually are sent to the pharmacy via pneumatic tube system or are hand delivered by staff or volunteers. In an outpatient dispensing pharmacy of a hospital, prescriptions are handled in the same manner as a community pharmacy.

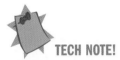

TECH NOTE!

Prescriptions may be faxed to a pharmacy. However, it is a good idea for the pharmacist to know the prescriber who will be faxing prescriptions, because forgery is more likely to occur otherwise.

the doctor's information (see Figure 2-5, *B*). A prescription can be carried into the pharmacy by hand or can be faxed from the doctor's office to the pharmacy. Computer-generated prescriptions are becoming more common. Prescriptions written in this way may be provided to the patient on discharge from the hospital or physician's office.

Prescriptions can be called into the pharmacy; the pharmacist transcribes the verbal order onto a blank prescription pad. Technicians should be aware of the specific rules of their state for taking in prescriptions. Box 8-1 shows the most commonly followed rules.

PRESCRIPTION INFORMATION

Outpatient Setting

If the order is written by a physician or other authorized person, it usually is hand carried to the pharmacy by the patient. Therefore the person at the take-in counter is the first one to handle the prescription. This is usually the clerk or technician who is on duty. This person must ensure that the correct information is listed on the prescription. Box 8-2 lists the information that needs to be on a prescription presented to the pharmacy for filling. Additional information, such as information regarding allergies, usually is needed for a new patient. This information is placed into the computer system for future reference.

The patient must know his or her medical record number if the patient is a member of a health maintenance organization or the specific medical coverage information. For a prescriber, the Drug Enforcement Administration number is necessary if a controlled drug is being dispensed. In addition, a controlled drug prescription must be written in ink or indelible pencil. See Chapter 2 for more information on Drug Enforcement Administration numbers.

Inpatient Setting

In a hospital setting the information required on a prescription is different. If the doctor works for the hospital, the license number and Drug Enforcement Administration number are on file. Therefore, it may not be necessary for the doctor to write out as much information. The same is true for the patient because that information is also more readily available. Box 8-3 shows the information that is required for in-house prescriptions.

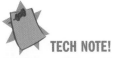

TECH NOTE!

An order written in the chart of a hospital patient is considered a legal prescription once signed by the prescriber.

BOX 8-2 REQUIRED PATIENT INFORMATION

Patient Information
Name
Phone number and address
Insurance information, if applicable
Age or date of birth

Provider's Information
Name
Phone number and address
Provider's license number
Provider's Drug Enforcement Administration number if applicable
Name of medication
Strength
Dosage form
Route
Quantity
Route of administration
Sig
Refill information
Provider's signature
Date written
"Brand necessary" if brand name drug is desired

BOX 8-3 REQUIRED PATIENT INFORMATION IN A HOSPITAL SETTING

Patient
Patient name
Medical record number
Room number

Other important information
Allergies
Height
Weight
Age

Prescriber
Name of medication
Strength
Route of administration
Dosage form
Sig (route and frequency)
Provider's signature
Date and time written

Other important information
Diagnosis
In pediatrics and geriatrics, the height and weight of the patient is needed for dosage
   calculations.

Because most dosing is set on a 24-hour period, the doctor writes only the actual dose to be given daily. For example, a multivitamin written as 1 qd (daily) will be loaded into the patient's medication tray every 24 hours and will continue until the doctor changes the order or writes D/C (discontinue). Exceptions to this are orders for antibiotics, which usually have an automatic stop date.

Translation of an Order

When reading an order that is difficult to decipher, make sure you look at the whole order. For instance, do you know from which clinic the order came? Can you make out the strength or dose? What is the route of administration? How often is the medication being ordered? What is the dosage form? Are there refills? If you are having a hard time reading the order, but you can see that the drug strength is 0.125 mg and it is to be taken daily, this limits the types of possible medications because of the strength and the dosing time. It may become clear to you what the order is for. Of course the bottom line is, if you are in doubt, ask another person such as the pharmacist.

WHEN TO ASK FOR HELP

When a job relies on reading another's handwriting and the handwriting is poor, it is common to need assistance in interpreting the writing. However, each person filling prescriptions is under intense pressure to fill them quickly, and this can lead to "guessing" at an order and then filling it. The following example is to help you feel comfortable in asking for help.

EXAMPLE 8-1 ASK FOR HELP

A patient's prescription is filled inappropriately with a strength of medication higher than ordered. The patient is admitted to the hospital suffering from a stroke. The probable cause is determined to be error in medication. Because the technician did not ask for help in deciphering the prescription and the pharmacist did not question the technician, the following occurred:

> The costs of the hospital stay for 3 days: $15,000
> Cost of litigation: $40,000
> Settlement amount: $100,000
> Overall stress and hardship on those involved in the case: [varies for each person]
> The pharmacist's license was revoked for 6 months and a fine was imposed

If the technician had asked the pharmacist for help, the pharmacist could have called the doctor who wrote the prescription and asked for clarification, and the order would have been filled correctly—time, 45 minutes. Was it a good idea to make an assumption when filling the prescription? The best way to deal with a questionable prescription is to inquire further rather than to make quick judgments and run the risk of errors.

Fact: Most court cases favor the patient and award him or her with cash settlements.

Fact: Most errors require a minimal amount of time to correct.

Fact: Most errors are caused by the technician and pharmacist trying to hurry.

Bottom line: Whenever in doubt, always ask for help.

Entering the Information into the Database

OUTPATIENT SETTING

Once you have read the doctor's order or prescription correctly, you then enter it into the computer terminal (Figure 8-1). In a community pharmacy setting, the technician usually does this. The computerized label is checked against the prescription after it is filled. Two labels are always discharged from the printer; one is placed on the vial for dispensing, and the other is placed on the back of

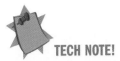

TECH NOTE!

When you ask someone to decipher a drug or instruction, do not first tell him or her your thought. This inadvertently can make that person see it the same way. Simply ask, "What does this look like to you?" If the answer matches yours, then you have an unbiased opinion. However, if you are not sure, ask the pharmacist to call the doctor to confirm the prescription.

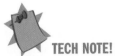

TECH NOTE!

As physicians begin to move into the paperless writing of prescriptions, the hope is that these difficult tasks will be a thing of the past. More and more hospitals are using preprinted order forms, and some have begun to use handheld computers capable of transferring a prescription to the pharmacy.

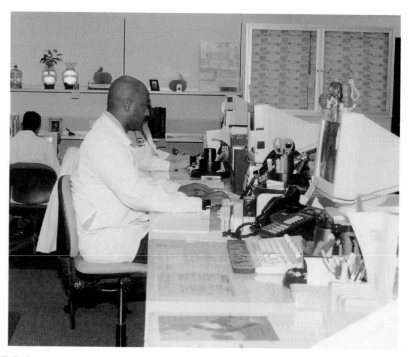

FIGURE 8-1 Technicians may enter information into the computer system in many pharmacy settings.

the original prescription. The pharmacist must initial both copies. Most pharmacies today copy prescriptions to the computer for verification. If a change must be made, the pharmacist can access the terminal easily and make the change to the order. At the time of consultation, the pharmacist also finds out which other medications the patient is taking.

INPATIENT SETTING

In a hospital, it is uncommon to have a technician enter new prescriptions into the computer. A pharmacist most likely has this responsibility. In a hospital, there are multiple orders sent on the admission of a patient and throughout the patient's hospital stay. Because all orders have to be verified by a pharmacist, it saves time if the pharmacist inputs the order and the technician fills the order. (Computer systems allow the technician to enter medications and flag them for the pharmacist to check. This must be done before a label is created.) Therefore, if the pharmacist enters the order, he or she only has to check the technician's work (pulled medications) once rather than twice—after the technician enters the order and after the technician fills it. In addition, most computers have a built-in system that alerts the person entering prescriptions that a drug interaction can occur. A technician cannot handle interaction problems; a pharmacist must initiate a phone call to the physician for an order change if necessary.

Filling the Prescription

INPATIENT AND OUTPATIENT SETTINGS

After the prescription label is prepared, it is matched with the original order and is sent to the counter for filling (Figure 8-2). This may be an automated dispensing system. Again, the technician (in most settings) receives the order. From the beginning, it is important that the technician pay close attention to the prescription he or she is filling because this is where many mistakes can be avoided.

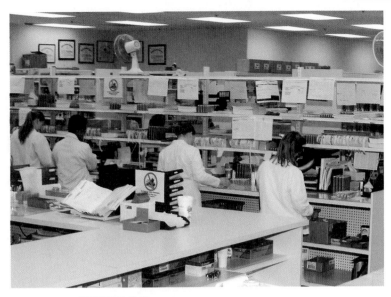

FIGURE 8-2 Technicians filling prescriptions.

Following these 10 simple yet important steps may prevent the technician from making a grievous error:

1. Check the label on the stock bottle and the National Drug Code in the computer against the original prescription for confirmation of the order.*
2. Pull the appropriate medication from the shelf.*
3. Measure or count out the necessary amount of the medication.
4. Fill the vial with the medication, taking care not to touch the medication.
5. Make sure that the lid is the appropriate type and is affixed properly onto the vial.
6. Apply the labels onto the vial and back of the prescription.*
7. Place the technician's initial on the bottom right hand side of all labels printed.
8. Apply any necessary auxiliary labels to the vial.
9. Put the medication on top of the original prescription.*
10. Pass the medication onto the pharmacist for final inspection. Usually the pharmacist on duty signs in to the computer with his or her initials that will appear on the prescription label.

CHECKING THE LABEL AGAINST THE PRESCRIPTION

When the label is passed along with the original prescription, it must be checked many times before it ever reaches the patient. The technician should hold the original prescription next to the label and check for any apparent errors or discrepancies. Look at the name of the drug, the strength or dose, dosage form, amount, and the sig (directions). Make sure all information matches. For direction abbreviations, see Chapter 5.

PULLING THE CORRECT MEDICATION

You will leave the counter to get the medication from the shelf. When doing this, make sure that you take the label with you for two reasons:

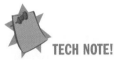

TECH NOTE!
If the order does not seem right, it probably is not. Ask for assistance if you cannot put your finger on what is wrong.

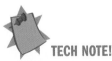

TECH NOTE!
When checking the dosage form, do not make assumptions. To assume that a spansule is the same as a capsule is easy (they look similar); however, they are different.

*The technician should check the medication against the prescription and/or against the label at these points.

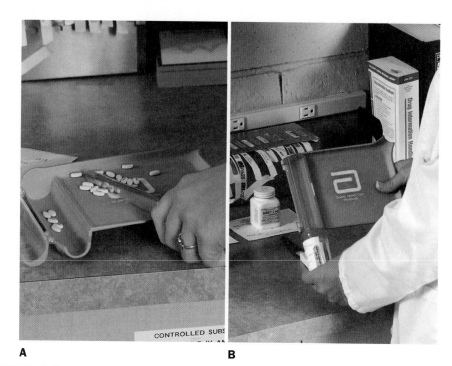

A   **B**

FIGURE 8-3 A, Technicians filling prescriptions using a pill counter and spatula. **B,** The remaining medication gets placed back into the original vial and the counted medications then are poured into a new vial with the patient's name and information.

1. You do not forget what you are looking for (which cuts down on time spent).
2. Once the bottle of medication is found, compare the label information to the bottle, checking the name, strength, and dosage form and the National Drug Code on refills.

COUNTING AND FILLING THE MEDICATION

After the technician locates the medication, removes it from the shelf, and returns to the counter, the prescription is filled.

Again, you should check your label and prescription against the medication bottle for accuracy. If the order calls for a bottle of 100, check to make sure that the manufacturer's package size matches your order. For example, many times bottles hold different amounts. Although there are various ways to count medications, many pharmacies still use counting trays, and then the medication is poured into the vial (Figure 8-3). Counting out more than 20 tablets is usually easiest, and it is quicker to count in multiples of five. Another way to count is with a device that uses a beam of light. As the light is broken, the digital counter adds another tablet or capsule on the monitor. High-technology filling is now done by semiautomated or automated machines. These range from Baker Cell systems to large hospital computer dispensing systems. Dispensing systems are discussed later in this chapter.

PRESCRIPTION LIDS

Once the vial is filled with the medication, the appropriate lid is applied to the vial. As the average human life expectancy increases, there is a growing segment of the population that is older than 70 years. Two of the problems that accompany aging are decreasing dexterity and strength. As most of us have experienced, there is a safety lid that even Godzilla cannot remove! Not surprisingly, many older patients do not wish to have safety lids on their medication. By law,

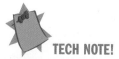

TECH NOTE!

Keep medications away from one another on the counter when filling to prevent grabbing the wrong bottle.

TABLE 8-1 Exceptions for Safety Caps*

Drug	Dispensed without safety lid	Reason
Nitroglycerin	Never has a safety lid	For emergencies
Isosorbide SL (sublingual)	May be dispensed without a safety lid	For emergencies
All other medications	If documented via doctor's request on prescription or patient's request documented in computer or in hard copy	Any conditions

*Refer to the Poison Control Act of 1970 for all exceptions.

the pharmacy must use safety lids in all cases except for a selected few. These cases are outlined in Table 8-1.

Most patients receive childproof caps; however, there are many older patients or those with disabilities who cannot manipulate prescription lids. If a waiver is signed by the patient or his or her physician has requested no child-proof caps, then the cap is replaced with a snap-on lid. This is listed on the patient information in the computer for future reference.

APPLYING THE LABEL

When labeling a bottle, you must remember professionalism. Do not place a torn label or place the label crookedly on a medication bottle. No one wants to believe that the prescription was put together in a rush, but rather with care and concern. When filling a prescription for a full bottle, such as cough syrup, you can place the label over the label of the existing bottle, making sure not to cover the lot number and expiration date. If the medication has to be counted, pour the medication into an appropriate-sized bottle.

Sometimes labels must be cut down in size because of lengthy directions. For example, a tapering dose of prednisone is a typical challenge, but it is possible to fit these labels onto a vial even if you must use a vial that is larger than normal to accommodate the label. Take care when cutting a label so that it will not be apparent to the patient. Also, the label must not cover any important print. In addition, auxiliary labels, when required, must be placed onto the bottle so that the patient can read the instructions easily. Many computer systems have a labeling system that allows the following information to be printed on one sheet:

- The prescription label
- A duplicate copy to be placed on the original hard copy
- Billing information
- Auxiliary labels

Once a prescription is entered into the computer system, the instructions and necessary information are printed out on labels (see Figure 2-5, *A*). Most labels contain preprinted information that is required by law, which consists of the following:

- Name, address, and phone number of pharmacy
- A prescription number, given automatically by the computer
- Patient name
- Drug, strength or dose, dosage form
- Manufacturer's name if not dispensed in manufacturer's bottle
- Instructions
- Date filled

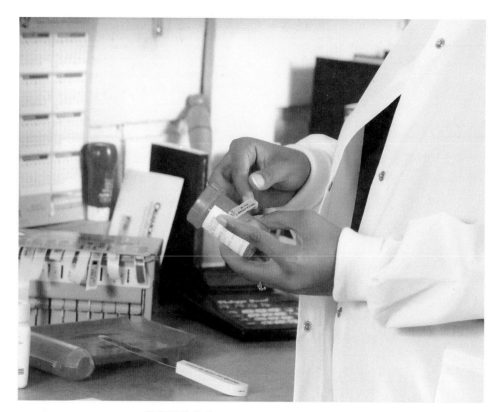

FIGURE 8-4 Applying an auxiliary label.

- Refill information
- Prescriber
- Expiration date if not dispensed in the manufacturer's bottle

TECHNICIAN'S INITIALS

All orders filled by a technician should be initialed by him or her as the prescriptions are filled per state law. This is important for several reasons. The pharmacist who will give the final approval now knows that the prescription is filled. If the pharmacist has any questions, he or she knows whom to ask. Finally, if there should be an error, the technician can be notified and learn from that error. In addition, the pharmacist must always sign off after completion. Some computer systems have the pharmacist's initials printed on the label, which is acceptable to most state boards of pharmacy.

AUXILIARY LABELS

All necessary auxiliary labels must adhere to the vial in a neat manner (Figure 8-4). These labels normally are printed out along with the label, making it easy for the technician. However, it is still important to know what medications need special auxiliary labels because not all pharmacies have this ability. If many auxiliary labels are printed out, it is necessary to choose the most important ones that can fit easily on the medication bottle. Care should be taken not to cover up any instructions, lot number, or expiration date.

For the technician to know which medications require an auxiliary label, he or she must know the classification of the drug, interactions, and side effects. Remembering a few common rules will help with the most general auxiliary labels (Table 8-2). For the most part, it takes time and experience to learn which

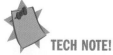

TECH NOTE!

Place auxiliary labels on top of the cap or lid of the medication to allow the pharmacist to select which one he or she deems necessary.

TABLE 8-2 Commonly Used Auxiliary Labels for Side Effects

Medication	Most common auxiliary label
Contraceptives	Take as directed
Nonsteroidal antiinflammatory drugs	May cause dizziness/drowsiness Take with food
Narcotics	Do not drink alcohol *and/or* Drinking may increase the effects of the drug
Macrolides	Take on an empty stomach Take with plenty of water
Antibiotics	Take until gone
Sulfa	May cause sensitivity to light Take on an empty stomach Take with plenty of water
Warfarin	Do not take aspirin

Suspension   shake well
diabetes   take w/food
high Blood pressure

auxiliary labels are the best. However, it is ultimately up to the pharmacist to choose which labels to place on the prescription bottle. Be sure to read auxiliary labels before adhering them to the bottle, because many different instructions are colored the same and may appear similar.

PHARMACIST'S FINAL INSPECTION

The last step in filling prescriptions is placing the filled vial, along with the medication container taken from the shelf, on top of the original prescription and passing it to the pharmacist for final inspection. Give the order one more inspection to ensure that the patient's name on the prescription matches the label and that all other information is correct. Only then should you pass the medication to the pharmacist and begin the next order.

It may seem as though all of these steps would take a long time; however, it takes only a few moments. Another important aspect of filling a prescription is to remember not to fill more than one prescription at a time; this is an invitation for error. You can pull several orders, giving each a double check for accuracy, but then place them back away from the prescription you are filling.

If a new stock bottle is opened to fill an order, mark it across the front with an *X* (in pen) to alert fellow employees that this is not a full bottle. Do not cover National Drug Code or expiration date with the mark. When the bottle finally is returned to stock, the next person pulling the bottle will know it is a partial. If a full bottle is needed, he or she will choose an unmarked one. The overall time that a prescription is in the hands of the pharmacy technician is not long, which is why it is so important to make each moment count when trying to fill a prescription flawlessly.

COMPUTER DISPENSING SYSTEMS

Another type of prescription filler besides the traditional pharmacist or technician is the emerging automated computer system. New and improved versions become available every year. Pharmacy personnel must become comfortable with manipulating these devices because they are here to stay. Several versions of dispensing systems are available: those made for filling outpatient prescriptions and those for hospitals, nursing care facilities, and large mail-order companies. Because of many differences between these types of pharmacy settings and

BOX 8-4 ADVANTAGES OF COMPUTER DISPENSING SYSTEMS

Speed up dispensing of medication	As the prescription is entered into the computer system, the information is transferred to the dispensing system.
Cut down on errors	The proper number of tablets or capsules then are dispensed into a container.
Inventory control	Medication can be scanned to keep accurate count of inventory.
	Daily printouts can be used by a technician or pharmacist to help the inventory technician keep the correct amount of drug on the shelf.

because each pharmacy has different requirements, the computer systems used in each one must be made specifically to handle their needs. Because of this, most manufacturers of automated systems offer various components to fit specific needs of each pharmacy.

Outpatient Dispensing Systems

Many chain pharmacies are using automated dispensing systems for three primary reasons: to cut down on errors, to increase productivity, and for inventory control (Box 8-4). Because of new laws that require pharmacies to decrease medication errors, pharmacies are converting rapidly to these types of systems.

Inpatient Dispensing Systems

Most hospitals use some type of computerized dispensing system because it is important that medication be available around the clock. Although many inpatient pharmacies are open 24 hours a day, 7 days a week, staffing is limited throughout the night, and computer dispensing systems can help reduce staffing needs. Medical personnel such as doctors or nurses should be able to access only stocked medications. Another major use of automation in hospital systems is to regulate controlled substances and track their movement.

An example of an automated medication dispensing system is the Pyxis MedStation 3000 system (Figure 8-5, *A*). This automated system uses a biometric user identification security system. This means the user's fingerprint is scanned and verified before the system grants the user access. Many automated systems similar to the Pyxis MedStation system rely on passwords or identification swipe cards to control access. This approach puts security at risk because the card could be given to or stolen by unauthorized personnel. The advantage of the Pyxis MedStation 3000 system is that it helps ensure the security of the system and ultimate control over access to medications. Once the fingerprint scanner verifies the user, the user has the ability to access the drawers in the station for filling or dispensing purposes according to the privileges the user is assigned.

After a nurse is granted access to the station, the nurse then selects the patient for whom the nurse wishes to remove medication by touching the name of the patient and the name of the medication on the display screen. The appropriate drawer with the medication will open. Once the drawer is closed, the amount of medication removed will be recorded for inventory tracking purposes. The pharmacy has the ability to run reports that identify who accessed the station, when the station was accessed, which medication was removed, and how much of each medication was supposed to have been removed. This information is valuable in solving discrepancies and managing inventory.

Other products offered by the Pyxis Products business of Cardinal Health include the Pyxis C^{II}Safe system (Figure 8-5, *B*) and the Pyxis Oral Solid Pack-

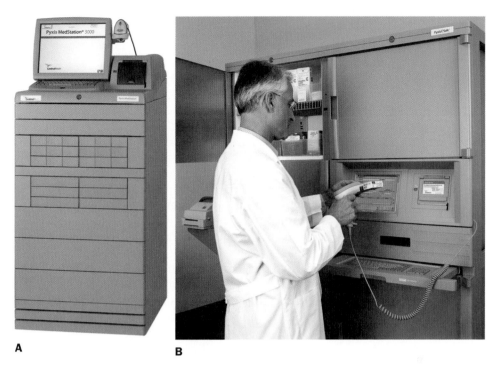

A   **B**

FIGURE 8-5 Pyxis Automated Systems. **A,** Pyxis MedStation 3000. **B,** Pyxis C^{II}Safe System.

ager. The Pyxis C^{II}Safe system is a controlled substance management system that creates detailed tracking and reporting for each transaction in order to improve inventory management. This system is separate from the Pyxis MedStation 3000 system, but the inventory management functions between the two systems can be integrated. The Pyxis Oral Solid Packager is an automated packager and bar code labeling system.

Another type of system being incorporated into hospital pharmacies is the robot-dispensing machine. This machine uses mechanical arms to scan bar codes on each unit dosed medication to identify the correct dose. (Dose information is fed into it by computer input from the pharmacist or technician.) The machine fills each patient's medication cassette with 99% accuracy as the cassette moves along a conveyer belt. Once the medication is filled, the cassette is delivered by the technician, who will bring back the previous day's cassette for the next day's filling. Examples of inpatient and outpatient dispensing systems follow:

Manufacturer	Type of System	Function
Amerisource	Med Select	Hospital
McKessonlosed	Loop Distribution	Outpatient
Omnicell	Medguard	Hospital
	Workflow Rx	Outpatient
Parata	RDS (robotic dispensing system)	Outpatient
Pyxis	ADS (automated dispensing system)	Hospital
Swisslog	PillPick System	Hosptial

The Rights of a Patient

When a technician takes on the role of filling a patient's prescription, it is very important that he or she always remember the basic rights of a patient. A good mindset is to think of you as the recipient of the medication that is being prepared. You would want extreme care taken in filling your medication; strive to do the same for others. Checking the prescription at least three times during the filling process helps to ensure accuracy. The rights of a patient are as follows:

1. The right medication
2. The right dose
3. The right route
4. The right time
5. The right price
6. The right dosage form
7. The right patient

Pharmacist Consultations: When and Who Needs Them

As the patient's medication is being entered into the computer system, one of the functions of pharmacy tracking is to determine whether it is a new prescription or a refill. First-time prescriptions usually are flagged in some manner so that they come to the attention of the pharmacist. If flagging is not automatic, it is up to the individual pharmacist to check the computer system for this information. If the prescription is a new one, a sticker is placed on the medication bag indicating to the technician or clerk that the patient needs a consultation. The federal law is that with all new prescriptions or changes in an existing prescription, a patient must be offered consultation. The patient can refuse consultation, but consultation must be offered per the Omnibus Reconciliation Act of 1990 (see Chapter 2). At this time, the pharmacist looks into the records of the patient to determine whether there are any possible "red flags," and explains the instructions to the patient and any side effects that he or she might encounter. At this time, the patient also can inquire about any questions or concerns specific to the medication.

Miscellaneous Orders

OUTPATIENT SETTING

Unlike first-time prescriptions, refills and transferring prescriptions can be done by technicians, clerks, and pharmacy interns over the phone as outlined in the following. Although these guidelines are enacted federally, they may be stricter depending on the protocol of each pharmacy.

Refills

A pharmacy technician may phone and receive authorization for a prescription refill. When a patient calls in a prescription refill or a request is faxed, the following information is necessary:

1. Patient's name
2. Home phone number
3. Prescription number
4. Name of the medication, strength, quantity, and prescription (abbreviated Rx) number
5. Prescription number

Zero Refill Reorders

Many pharmacies have an additional phone request line for prescriptions that have run out of refills. Typically, the patient should allow 2 days to get proper authorization from the prescriber, and technicians are able to perform this task under the pharmacist's direction.

Transfers

A pharmacist may transfer a previously filled prescription from one pharmacy to another. Most state boards of pharmacy prefer to allow transfers of a prescription to occur only one time; however, federal law stipulates that controlled substances may be transferred only one time. Always be aware of your board of pharmacy regulations. In general the following applies:

- A pharmacy technician may assist the pharmacist in the transfer of a prescription.
- Under the supervision of the pharmacist, the technician may fax a copy of the prescription to another pharmacy. The pharmacist directs the technician on what information may be needed from the receiving or transferring pharmacy.

Filing Prescriptions

Although times have changed with use of computers, it is still necessary to follow through on the manual filing of hard copy prescriptions. After the computer entry is made, the prescription makes its way down the filling counter, and all steps are completed, the hard copy must be filed for future reference. The law states that all prescriptions must be kept on file for a period of at least 3 years. This is done by using the prescription number. On the back of the prescription is a copy of the label used on the dispensed drug, along with the initials of the technician or pharmacist who filled the order. In addition, some states require that all controlled substances (schedules III and IV) that are filled together or with other prescriptions must be stamped with a red "C" 1 inch down on the right hand side of the prescription label to make it easier to find. The location of the stamp may differ depending on state law. All schedule II medications must be filed separately. Complete filing guidelines are discussed in Chapter 2. Usually, all prescriptions are filed at the end of the day. They are filed in small packets that are marked clearly on the outside with the date for easy reference. These are kept on the pharmacy premises. In addition to the hard copy, the computer copy indicates whether a drug is a controlled substance and lists all the other information required by the federal and state regulations. At the end of the workday, backup copies usually are made of all the orders in the system in case of a computer crash.

Medication Pickup

Patients can wait for their prescription, have it delivered, or pick it up another day. Occasionally, a patient has a relative pick up a prescription. For these cases, make a note in the computer listing the person or persons who are authorized to pick up another's prescription. Regardless of who picks up the prescription, it is important to ensure that the right person gets the right medication. Therefore, check all identification against the prescription before releasing the medication. In the case of a controlled substance, if the person picking up the medication is not the patient, that person must show identification to the clerk or technician and sign for it. All third-party prescriptions must have the signature of the receiver. Also, it is good professional practice to ask for identification on all schedule II controlled substance prescriptions.

Billing Patients

The billing portion of processing a prescription varies depending on what type of coverage the patient has, if any. If the patient does not have coverage, there is no additional paperwork to fill out because the patient simply has to pay full price for the prescription. Most persons have some type of coverage. Each type of insurance has its own limitations and conditions. Each pharmacy is responsible for contacting the coverage program. For more information on types of insurances and the new Medicare (Part D) medication plan, see Chapter 14.

Changing Trends

Interpreting, transcribing, producing labels, filling, and checking are the "meat and potatoes" of the pharmacy business. Laws such as the Omnibus Reconciliation Act of 1990 require that consultations be given to patients. The increasing age and population of Americans has moved the pharmacist away from the filling counter to interacting more with patients and prescribers. Because of this nationwide change, the technician has been placed on the front line. This responsibility requires the technician to fill prescriptions as quickly and with the same accuracy as a pharmacist. Technicians also must know their limitations at all times. In addition to these capabilities, many technicians are in charge of the billing process and must be well aware of the policies and procedures of their pharmacy and how to process various insurance claims. Patients expect perfection when it comes to their medications and proper billing practices. This weight clearly falls on the technician filling the orders and on the pharmacist in charge. This responsibility should never be taken lightly and requires continued education in all areas of pharmacy practice.

DO YOU REMEMBER THESE KEY POINTS?

- The various ways a prescription can be submitted to the pharmacy for processing
- The steps involved in filling a prescription
- Who can call in a prescription
- Who can transfer a prescription from one pharmacy to another
- The differences between information on inpatient and outpatient prescriptions
- What type of patient information is needed in different pharmacy settings
- The importance of knowing when and why to ask for help from a pharmacist
- The number of times a pharmacy technician should check a prescription while filling the order
- The necessary authorization to use snap-on caps rather than childproof caps
- The auxiliary labels needed for the medications outlined in this chapter
- Why computer dispensing systems are used
- The rights of a patient
- When patient consultations are done and who is authorized to do them
- How to process refills
- Requirements of filing prescriptions (hard copies)
- Requirements for patients or family members picking up medication from the pharmacy

MULTIPLE CHOICE QUESTIONS

1. Of the methods listed, which are the acceptable forms of receiving a prescription?
   A. By mail
   B. In person
   C. Called in
   D. Both A and B
   E. All of above

2. The best times to check for errors on a prescription while filling are _____.
   A. When the order is first received, during filling, and after filling
   B. While filling the order, after filling, and when handing to the patient
   C. When checking the original order against the label, against the stock bottle before filling, and before filling the vial and labeling
   D. Before applying the label, before applying the auxiliary labels, and before giving it to the pharmacist

3. Of the information listed, which is vital information needed from a patient before filling his or her prescription?
   A. Full name
   B. Address
   C. Insurance number or medical record number
   D. All of the above

4. When in doubt as to the directions on a prescription, it is best to _____.
   A. Call the doctor's office immediately
   B. Try your best to decipher the order
   C. Ask the pharmacist for help
   D. Ask a pharmacy clerk for help with interpretation

5. Of the reasons listed, which is(are) the main reason(s) for using automated dispensing systems in a community pharmacy?
   A. To increase the accuracy of filling prescriptions
   B. To help control inventory
   C. To decrease the time it takes to fill an order
   D. All of the above

6. What information is not needed from a prescriber on a prescription order?
   A. Directions
   B. Refills
   C. Manufacturer
   D. Date written

7. Which of the medications listed does not require a safety lid?
   A. All heart medication
   B. All diabetic medication
   C. Nitroglycerin sublingual tablets
   D. Acetaminophen (Tylenol)

8. Of the information listed, which is not necessary on a prescription label?
   A. Date filled
   B. Expiration date
   C. Prescriber
   D. Patient's home address

9. Which one of the rights listed is not considered a right of a patient?
   A. The right to the correct drug
   B. The right to the correct price
   C. The right to a lower price than listed
   D. The right to the correct strength

10. Of the following basic steps required in filling a prescription, which is not the responsibility of the technician?
    A. Filling the prescription
    B. Translation of a prescription
    C. Consulting the patient
    D. Entering the information into the database

TRUE/FALSE If a statement is false, then change it to make it true.

_____ 1. When a technician fills a prescription, only the pharmacist's initials should appear on the prescription bottle.

_____ 2. New prescriptions can be called in or taken into a pharmacy by the patient for filling.

_____ 3. When prescriptions are written by a physician for a patient in the hospital, it is not necessary for the order to be presented on a prescription pad.

_____ 4. Technicians regularly enter hospital orders and may call the doctor for additional information.

_____ 5. All prescriptions must have safety lids per federal law.

_____ 6. Most pharmacy labeling programs print out a second label to be placed on the back of the hard copy prescription.

_____ **7.** Technicians need to sign their initials or last name on all prescription labels before passing them on to the pharmacist for a final check.

_____ **8.** Antibiotics typically receive an auxiliary label "Take until gone" to ensure that the patient finishes the course of antibiotic treatment.

_____ **9.** The Omnibus Reconciliation Act of 1990 ensures that technicians can handle drugs.

_____ **10.** Technicians cannot take prescription orders over the phone.

TECHNICIAN'S CORNER   You fill a prescription with the wrong drug. The error is not caught until later that evening when the prescriptions are being filed. What do you do?

BIBLIOGRAPHY

Nielsen R, James JD: *Handbook of federal drug law,* ed 2, Philadelphia, 1992, Williams & Wilkins.

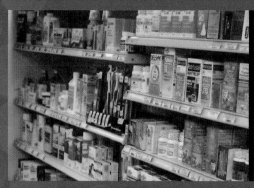

Over-the-Counter Medications and Skin Anatomy and Conditions

Objectives

UPON COMPLETING THIS CHAPTER, YOU SHOULD BE ABLE TO DO THE FOLLOWING:

- Describe why over-the-counter (OTC) medications are popular.

- List considerations concerning the use of OTC drugs.

- List the three categories used by the Food and Drug Administration for OTC drugs.

- Describe Food and Drug Administration regulations concerning the manufacturing of OTC drugs.

- Explain how legend drugs become OTC drugs.

- Describe the various types of conditions that OTC medicines treat.

- List major components of skin anatomy.

- List four types of noninfectious skin conditions and their treatments.

- List four types of infectious skin conditions and their treatments.

- Determine the right strength of sunscreen necessary to protect skin from ultraviolet rays.

- Define the various forms of acne.

- Describe psoriasis and the types of medications used to treat this skin condition.

Analgesic *A drug that relieves pain by reducing the perception of pain*

Antiinflammatory *A drug that reduces swelling, redness, and pain and that promotes healing*

Antiseptic *A substance that slows or stops growth of microorganisms on surfaces such as skin*

Antitussive *A drug that can decrease the coughing reflex of the central nervous system*

ASA *Acetylsalicylic acid (aspirin)*

Bulk forming *Fiber used as a stimulant to the intestines or to cause a feeling of fullness to decrease appetite*

Desquamation *A normal process of shedding the top layer of the skin, also known as exfoliation*

Expectorant *Chemical that causes the removal of mucous secretions from the respiratory system; loosens and thins sputum and bronchial secretions for ease of expectoration*

Keratolytic *A drug that causes shedding of the outer layer of the skin*

OTC *Over-the-counter*

Prophylaxis *Treatment given before an event to prevent the event from happening*

Protectant *A substance that acts as a barrier between the skin and an irritant*

Pruritus *Itching*

ROA *Route of administration*

Sunscreen *A substance that protects the skin from ultraviolet light, which causes sunburn; skin protection factor (SPF) rates effectiveness*

IF YOU WALK INTO A SHOPPING center or your corner drugstore, you will see the massive number of over-the-counter (OTC) medications that are available for personal use. No prescriptions are necessary, and no questions need answering to get these drugs. Most consumers give no thought to purchasing several different drugs to keep at home for themselves or their family. One almost could say that they are common staples of a home medicine cabinet just as staples are kept on hand in the kitchen. A basic shopping list may include items such as flour, sugar, eggs, acetaminophen (Tylenol), cough syrup, and ibuprofen (Motrin).

Since the mid-1980s, there has been a sharp increase of OTC drugs available to consumers. Many statistics can give useful information on the use and sales of OTC items that can affect drug interactions directly and give a sense of where the American consumer is heading. Here are some facts:

- 77% of Americans take OTC products to treat themselves (The Use of Over-the counter Medicines. Fact Sheet 9/2003)
- The U.S. retail sales of OTC drugs (excluding Wal-Mart) were $15.1 billion (ACNielsen, 2005)

TABLE 9-1 Common Over-the-Counter Brand Preparations

Brand name	Generic name	Classification
Fever/Pain Product		
Tylenol	Acetaminophen	Antipyretic/analgesic
Fever/Pain/Inflammation Products		
Bayer	Aspirin	NSAID, analgesic
Motrin, Advil	Ibuprofen	NSAID
Excedrin	Aspirin/caffeine/acetaminophen	NSAID (migraines)
Sleep Aid		
Benadryl	Diphenhydramine	Histamine blocker, sedative, antihistamine
Cold/Cough Products		
Robitussin	Guaifenesin	Expectorant
Benylin	Guaifenesin/dextromethorphan	Expectorant/antitussive
Benadryl	Diphenhydramine	Antihistamine
Sudafed	Pseudoephedrine	Decongestant
Nasal Products		
Neo-Synephrine	Phenylephrine	Vasoconstrictor
Privine	Naphazoline	Decongestant
Eye (Ophthalmic) Product		
VasoClear	Naphazoline	Decongestant
Sore Throat Products		
Sucrets	Dyclonine	Analgesic
Chloraseptic	Benzocaine	Topical anesthetic
Stomach Products		
Pepcid AC	Famotidine	H_2 antagonist
Zantac-75	Ranitidine	H_2 antagonist
Tagamet-HB	Cimetidine	H_2 antagonist
Milk of Magnesia	Magnesium hydroxide	Antacid, laxative
Tums	Calcium	Acid neutralizer/calcium carbonate supplement
Intestinal Products		
Metamucil	Psyllium	Fiber
Imodium A–D	Loperamide	Antidiarrheal
Anticonstipation Products		
Senokot	Senna extract	Laxative
Dulcolax	Bisacodyl	Laxative
Miscellaneous Products		
Compound W	Salicylic acid	Keratolytic (warts/corns)
Calamine	Calamine	Antipruritic
Tinactin	Tolnaftate	Antifungal
Lotrimin	Clotrimazole	Antifungal
Monostat	Miconazole	Antifungal
Anusol HC	Hydrocortisone	Antihemorrhoidal

NSAID, Nonsteroidal antiinflammatory drug.

- 73% of OTC medicines are used by women (ACNielsen Homescan Panel, 2005)
- Persons 65 years and older account for 33% of all OTC sales (American Pharmacists Association, 2001)
- Using OTC medications to treat upper respiratory problems saves the U.S. health care economy $4.75 billion each year (Northwest University, 2004)
- 61% of consumers are not concerned about experiencing side effects when taking an OTC medication

Obviously, OTC medications will continue to become available to consumers, and this means that it is increasingly important for consumers to learn about appropriate dosages and proper use of these medications. Although federal law requires that pharmacists counsel patients receiving new prescriptions, OTC medications do not fall into this category. However, when counseling a patient, the pharmacist should ask what OTC medications the patient is taking and should tell the patient what types of OTC drugs to avoid. The ability to buy drugs off the shelf can translate into substantial savings for consumers. This is only one of the many reasons why individuals want to buy their own medications. Drug companies know that customers want more drugs available to them. Following are three reasons why consumers use OTC products:

1. Consumers want to save money on OTC medication as opposed to using many expensive prescription drugs. They save money because they do not have to make doctors' appointments, which involves the cost of the office visit and missed time at work.
2. Consumers want to be involved in their own treatment; OTC medications give them this capability.
3. OTC medications are more easily obtainable than prescriptions because the many stores that carry OTC medications usually have longer hours than traditional pharmacies.

These are just three reasons that OTC medications are appealing to consumers. One should take some important considerations into account when purchasing OTC medications. See Table 9-1 for common brands of over-the-counter medications.

Over-the-Counter Drug Considerations

When patients decide to treat themselves, important factors should be taken into account. First, there are a wide variety of drugs from which to choose. Therefore, correctly identifying the cause of the problem is the first step. If the self-diagnosis is wrong, the OTC medication may mask the underlying condition from which the person is suffering. For example, if a person suffers from diarrhea and purchases an antidiarrheal medication, the diarrhea may cease for a short time, but the underlying cause could be something more serious that should be diagnosed by a physician. Ultimately, this can cost the person more money, or worse, in the long run. Many hospital stays have been attributed to patients' misuse of drugs, OTC and prescription. Most persons have not been trained to scrutinize OTC medications. This includes checking the drugs at home regularly for expiration dates. Another overlooked aspect of buying OTC drugs is tampering; these drugs are sitting out where anyone can tamper with them. Previously, several persons were the victims of someone who tampered with Tylenol. Since that time, manufacturers have taken steps to assure consumers that their medications are safe by adding tamper-proof wrapping. Consumers should check for any tampering before purchasing. Although there is only a slight risk, it is possible for someone to tamper with the product.

Most OTC medications do not recommend dosages for any child younger than 2 years of age. Thus parents should consult with their pediatrician before

TECH ALERT!

Because of the new laws governing the sales of OTC items that contain pseudoephedrine, ephedrine, and phenylpropanolamine, customers are limited on the amount they may purchase. This drug has been misused by illegal drug makers to produce dangerous street drugs. The Drug Enforcement Agency regulates these over-the-counter medications. The new laws governing the sale of these medications are covered under the Combat Meth Act 2005. For more information refer to Chapter 2.

giving children any OTC medication, especially any child younger than 2 years. In addition to these considerations, children with colds may develop ear infections and other conditions that warrant seeing a pediatrician for an appropriate prescription medication. Important considerations that consumers should think about before buying and using OTC medications follow:

- Various OTC medications have identical ingredients; however, consumers often purchase a more expensive name brand, not knowing that they are getting the same medication as the less expensive generic form.
- Manufacturers may swap "like ingredients" without notifying the consumer. The label will show the change. Many times a consumer overlooks this because the consumer does not read the labels carefully, if at all.
- The person who is on a special diet, has allergies, is a diabetic, or is taking other medications that may interact with OTC drugs should use caution.
- One should take extra care when purchasing medication for babies or young children; consumers should know and follow guidelines on the safety of agents based on the child's age. This includes topical agents.

When trying a new agent, one should watch carefully for any adverse reactions that may occur.

Many, if not most OTC and prescription medications cannot be taken if one is pregnant or nursing; always check with the physician before taking any medication.

Three FDA Categories Concerning Classification of Over-the-Counter Drugs

Although OTC medications may seem harmless, they can be deadly if taken inappropriately or if the person has a life-threatening allergic reaction. One may experience additional side effects from OTC medications, such as interactions with prescription medications. Before OTC medications are allowed to enter the market, the Food and Drug Administration (FDA) classifies them according to one of the following three categories. Obviously, only if the proposed medication falls under the first category would it eventually become available to the consumer.

1. Safe and effective for the claimed therapeutic indication
2. Not recognized as safe and effective
3. Additional data must be acquired to determine whether the drug is safe and effective

Food and Drug Administration Regulations

To determine into what category proposed OTC drugs fall, the FDA regulates five major areas concerning the safety of OTC medications. The following five areas are explored individually:

1. Purity
2. Potency
3. Bioavailability
4. Efficacy
5. Safety and toxicity

PURITY

The purity of a product represents the lack of contamination from environmental factors of the chemical (drug) contained in the product. Few agents are pure

BOX 9-1 TYPES OF PRODUCT ADDITIVES

Fillers	Enable manufacturers to make tablets or capsules large enough to ingest
Dyes	Used to color tablets and coatings for appearance
Solvents	Mixtures used along with chemical agents as a dissolvent
Buffers	Used to adjust the pH of a medication
Waxes	Used to mold various medications such as suppositories

BOX 9-2 MEDICATIONS MEASURED IN UNITS

Heparin	25,000 units/mL
Insulin	100 units/mL
Injectable penicillin	100,000 units/mL

because many medications are prepared on a large scale and dust particles are present in the mix. A certain amount of dust is allowed by government standards. Purity also is affected by other additives, such as those listed in Box 9-1. Various ingredients also are used in the preparation of medications to increase the size of the medication, to decrease absorption, and to make them taste better.

POTENCY

The potency of a medication refers to the strength of the drug. This measurement is done by chemical analysis and is measured in grams, milligrams, or micrograms. If the drug cannot be measured in a laboratory by the same methods, then it is tested on research animals, and the strength of the drug is measured in units. Examples of these medications are shown in Box 9-2.

BIOAVAILABILITY

Bioavailability is the percentage of a drug that is absorbed and transported to the site of action. Because of variances in absorption, the amount of drug that is able to enter the bloodstream can differ. The total bioavailability is measured by the concentration of the drug in the blood or tissue at a specific time of administration.

EFFICACY

Efficacy is the ability of the drug to produce the desired chemical change in the body. Clinical trials of the drug, which include the use of a placebo, are conducted to judge the effectiveness. Many variances may affect the end result. These variances are caused by other influences on a person, such as unknown health conditions, age, weight, lifestyle, gender, and genetic influences.

SAFETY AND TOXICITY

Safety and toxicity represent opposite effects of a drug being studied. After the drug is administered to test subjects, the number of adverse or undesirable effects is recorded. Laboratory animals often are used as test subjects in the beginning stages of trials, and it is sometimes impossible to know what effects might occur in human beings. In later years of the studies, published results include effects of drugs on pregnancy and other outside influences that cannot be replicated in a laboratory. All drugs can be toxic if not taken correctly. The

BOX 9-3 THREE FOOD AND DRUG ADMINISTRATION PHASES OF OVER-THE-COUNTER DRUG APPROVAL

Phase 1	Advisors evaluate the agent in question as to whether it is safe and effective when taken by the consumer/patient.
Phase 2	A final review is done on the ingredients of the agent in question. The public is able to give feedback. All data are taken into account, such as any new findings.
Phase 3	After sufficient evidence is presented and all aspects of the agent are exhausted, the final monograph is published.

difference between dosages that produce toxic effects and those that produce desirable effects is documented. This difference is referred to as the "margin of safety." If a dose of a drug falls into the margin of safety, it is considered a "therapeutic dose." Even so, before a drug is considered safe, the potential for adverse effects must be compared with the benefits.

How a Prescription Drug Becomes an Over-the-Counter Drug

The statistics on OTC sales are staggering. Sales were more than $15 billion in 2004 in the United States alone and continue to rise. Customers are estimated to have saved billions of dollars. Adults over the age of 65 are responsible for approximately a third of these OTC sales.

The amount of research that takes place before releasing a new OTC drug is extensive. The FDA must approve all new drugs entering the marketplace and has strict guidelines in place. The same standards of safety and effectiveness that are placed on legend drugs (those requiring a prescription) also are used to approve OTC drugs. The FDA uses three phases of testing as criteria for minimum standards of a new product or of a product that is going to be marketed as an OTC drug, as shown in Box 9-3.

A monograph is information about a drug that includes descriptive information about clinical trials, all side effects of the agent, appropriate dosing based on symptoms/disease state, and all types of reported interactions.

If the agent meets all the criteria, it is approved as an OTC medication. If the agent is approved already as a prescription drug and the manufacturer wants it to be changed to an OTC drug, it does not require further testing. However, the drug does need to be considered safe enough to self-administer before it is marketed as OTC. Many agents that have gone into the OTC section also continue to be marketed as legend drugs. The difference is the strength of the drug. For instance, ibuprofen is available OTC in 200-mg tablets; however, if 400 mg, 600 mg, or 800 mg are needed, a prescription (or Rx) is required. The same is true for many other agents, such as ranitidine (Zantac 75 mg and 150 mg is available OTC, whereas 300 mg requires a prescription).

The FDA is also in charge of all recalls. The FDA inspects manufacturing facilities to make sure they are adhering to good manufacturing practices. Manufacturers must show a consistency between batches of drugs daily. If they cannot, then the product cannot be distributed. In some cases, OTC medications have been taken off the market as well.

Although there are approximately 100,000 OTC products on the market today, only 1000 active ingredients are approved.[1] Although this list undoubtedly will continue to grow, it gives a sense of how OTC drugs are manufactured and combined to give the customer many more choices of products than ever before.

TABLE 9-2 Common Types of Over-the-Counter Products*

Type of drug	Symptom treated	Route of administration
Analgesics	Pain	Orally, topically, rectally
Antiinflammatories	Inflammation/arthritis pain	Orally
Antipyretics	Fever	Orally, rectally
Antiarthritics	Joint pain/inflammation	Orally, topically
Antihistamines	Congestion, sneezing	Orally, inhalation
Headache products	Pain	Orally
Sleep aids	Insomnia	Orally
Expectorants	Productive cough	Orally
Cough suppressants	Dry cough	Orally, inhalation
Colds/flu	Inflammatory	Orally, inhalation
Sore throat products	Pain	Orally
Sunscreens	Preventive sun barrier	Topically
Sunburn products	Pain/inflammation	Topically
Antacids	Indigestion	Orally
Antispasmodics	Spasms	Orally
Antidiarrheals	Diarrhea	Orally, rectally
Laxatives	Constipation	Orally, rectally
Antiacne products	Pimples	Topically
Antibiotics	Prevent infections	Topically
Antifungals	Dry, flaking skin and pain caused by fungus	Topically
Cold sore preparations	Painful canker sores	Topically
Wart removal products	Skin growth	Topically

*Other topical over-the-counter products are listed later in this chapter under skin care products.

Conditions Treated with Over-the-Counter Drugs

As stated before, thousands of OTC medications are available when you consider the brands, generic versions, combinations, various strengths, and dosage forms. Table 9-2 lists some of the most common OTC medications, the symptoms they treat, and the most popular routes of administration. As new medications enter the market as OTC drugs, the routes of administration from which consumers can choose will increase. For example, many analgesics are becoming available as topical patches, and many sore throat remedies are being produced as chewing gum.

Over-the-Counter Agents: Patient Information

This section contains a sample of common OTC agents such as those listed in Table 9-2. The following are common symptoms, indications, and generic and trade name drugs used in treatment. Some agents have added notes that commonly are seen on the product labels and that patients should read before taking the drug. Refer to your pharmacy drug handbooks for further information on these and other OTC drugs.

ANALGESICS AND ANTIPYRETICS

Analgesic and antipyretic agents help reduce or relieve pain (analgesic) and fever (antipyretic). Acetylsalicylic acid, abbreviated ASA and usually known by the more common generic name aspirin, has added effectiveness as an anti-inflammatory agent. Aspirin also decreases the clumping ability of platelets;

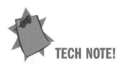

TECH NOTE!

Reye's syndrome is a rare condition that can affect children and teenagers who have an active case of chickenpox or influenza. The symptoms include vomiting, lethargy, delirium, and coma. Permanent brain damage can occur, and the infection can be fatal. Although the percentage of fatalities is less than 20%, it is safer to avoid the possibility of such adverse effects.

TABLE 9-3 Analgesics and Antipyretic Products

Condition	Product	Dosage forms
Fever/pain	Acetaminophen (Tylenol)	Tab, cap, liq supp
Fever/pain	Aspirin (Bayer, Alka-Seltzer)	Tab, cap, powder
Fever/pain	Ibuprofen (Motrin)	Tab, cap, liq
Pain/arthritis	Capsaicin (Zostrix)	Top

Tab, tablet; *cap,* capsule; *liq,* liquid; *top,* topical; *supp,* suppository.

TABLE 9-4 Common Interactions between Aspirin and Other Medications

Drug	Common use of drugs	Results of drug and aspirin
ACE inhibitors	Treat high blood pressure	Effects may be decreased
Alcohol	Lifestyle choice	May increase bleeding and risk of gastrointestinal ulcer
Antacids	Upset stomach	Decreases effectiveness of aspirin
Anticoagulants	To reduce the possibility of blood clots	May prolong or increase bleeding
β-blockers	To treat hypertension	Effects may be decreased
Carbonic anhydrase inhibitors (diuretics)	To decrease edema (fluid buildup)	Toxication of aspirin may occur
Corticosteroids	Antiinflammatory	Decreases effectiveness of aspirin
Loop diuretics	To reduce fluid retention	Effects may be decreased
Methotrexate	To treat certain skin conditions/cancer	Effects may be increased and excretion decreased
Nitroglycerin	To decrease angina (chest pain)	May result in hypotension
NSAIDs	To treat inflammation, pain, fever	Effects may be decreased
Spironolactone	To reduce edema	Effects may be decreased
Sulfonylureas/insulin	To lower glucose (diabetes)	May increase the effects of these agents
Valproic acid	To treat seizures	May decrease excretion, increasing potency of valproic acid

ACE, Angiotensin-converting enzyme; *NSAID,* nonsteroidal antiinflammatory drug.

therefore it also is used as prophylaxis to decrease the risk of blood clotting in heart disease and stroke. Examples are shown in Table 9-3.

Common Patient Information

Children and teenagers should avoid taking aspirin for chickenpox or flu symptoms without consulting a physician because aspirin has been associated with Reye's syndrome.

INTERACTIONS BETWEEN ASPIRIN AND OTHER AGENTS

Aspirin has many interactions that are important to note because they can result in an adverse effect to the patient. Table 9-4 provides a list of common interactions between various types of medications and aspirin. Interactions are not necessarily dangerous, but they can alter the absorption or metabolism of one of the two agents being taken concurrently. Many times, patients do not famil-

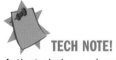

TECH NOTE!

Activated charcoal can be used to treat an overdose of aspirin or acetaminophen. It decreases the absorption of the drug.

TABLE 9-5 Decongestant Products

Condition	Product	Dosage forms
Common cold/allergies	Oxymetazoline (Afrin)	Spray
	Phenylephrine (Neo-Synephrine)	Spray
	Normal saline (Ocean)	Spray
Common cold	Pseudoephedrine* (Sudafed)	Tab, cap, liq
	Clemastine (Tavist)	Tab, liq

Tab, Tablet; *cap,* capsule; *liq,* liquid.
*Pseudoephedrine (Sudafed) is a decongestant and is less likely to cause drowsiness. Pseudoephedrine is used exclusively as a decongestant, not for allergies.

TABLE 9-6 Antihistamine Products*

Condition	Product	Dosage forms
Rhinitis, common cold	Chlorpheniramine (Chlor-Trimeton)	Tab, cap
Rhinitis, pruritus	Diphenhydramine (Benadryl)	Tab, cap, liq
Allergic rhinitis	Loratadine (Claritin)	Tab, cap

Tab, Tablet; *cap,* capsule; *liq,* liquid.
*These agents also come in many combinations with agents that treat cough, fever, and pain.

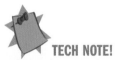

TECH NOTE!

Decongestants can interact with antidepressants. Patients using certain antidepressants and those with heart conditions should not use decongestant agents without the knowledge of their physician.

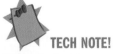

TECH NOTE!

Diphenhydramine (Benadryl) and chlorpheniramine (Chlor-Trimeton) are antihistamines that cause drowsiness. These agents should not be taken with alcohol because alcohol may intensify the effect. Patients suffering from glaucoma should not use these agents without their physician's knowledge.

iarize themselves with these types of interactions, which is why patient consultation is important and is a federal law. If a patient ever asks for advice from a technician or clerk, he or she must be referred to the pharmacist for advice. Technicians must know these interactions so that they can alert the pharmacist if they notice a possible interaction within the patient's prescriptions or medication orders.

ALLERGY AND COLD AGENTS

Decongestants (Table 9-5) and antihistamines (Table 9-6) are available for the relief of the common cold. These agents dry out mucous membranes and open airways. Persons suffering from severe allergies may require prescription medication. For mild allergies the antihistamines available are normally effective. Decongestants can be absorbed easily topically through nasal application. Because they cause vasoconstriction, they reduce congestion. Allergies require antihistamine agents.

ANTIHISTAMINES

Antihistamines are used with allergic symptoms which include pruritus, hives, sneezing, and runny eyes. The action is to block histamine (H_1) that causes allergic reactions. A common side effect of first-generation antihistamines is sleepiness. Many different types of these agents are available OTC. Loratadine (Claritin) is the first nondrowsy agent that has become an OTC drug. Second-generation agents are available as well that are more potent and do not cause drowsiness, but these are by prescription only.

DECONGESTANTS

Decongestants are indicated for stuffiness and congestion of the nasal passages and sinuses. Decongestants act to open these passages and allow the release of mucus. Decongestants used for chest congestion permit the coughing up of phlegm. Decongestants are available in prescription and OTC preparations.

TABLE 9-7 Antiinsomnia Products

Product	Dosage forms
Diphenhydramine (Benadryl)	Tab, caplet, liq
Diphenhydramine citrate/acetaminophen (Excedrin PM)	Tab, caplet
Doxylamine succinate (Unisom Nighttime Sleep Aid)	Tab

Tab, Tablet; *liq,* liquid.

TABLE 9-8 Cold and Cough Products

Condition	Product	Dosage forms
Congested cough	Guaifenesin/pseudoephedrine (Robitussin PE)	Tab, liq, syr
	Guaifenesin (Robitussin)	Tab, cap, syr
Dry cough	Guaifenesin/dextromethorphan (Robitussin DM)	Liq, syr

Tab, Tablet; *liq,* liquid; *syr,* syrup; *cap,* capsule.

Common Patient Information
Decongestants may cause drowsiness.

SLEEP AIDS

Many persons suffer from insomnia. Almost all OTC medications used to treat insomnia are a form of diphenhydramine or magnesium salicylate (Table 9-7). These agents can be used for transient insomnia, which is considered a short-term sleeping problem (nonchronic). Diphenhydramine is the most commonly prescribed agent ordered in hospitals to help patients sleep.

Common Patient Information
Sleep aids may cause drowsiness. Avoid alcoholic beverages while taking this medication. Do not take this product without consulting a physician if you are taking sedatives or tranquilizers. Do not use if you have asthma, glaucoma, emphysema, or an enlarged prostate. For chronic insomnia, consult a physician.

COUGH MEDICINES

The cold and flu section of the pharmacy is one of the largest; many manufacturers offer the same type of ingredients in different proportions (Table 9-8). For congested coughs, expectorants help one cough up phlegm. For dry, nonphlegm-producing coughs, an antitussive agent is commonly used.

Common Patient Information
Do not take this product without consulting a physician if you are taking sedatives or tranquilizers. Do not use if you have asthma, glaucoma, emphysema, heart problems, or an enlarged prostate.

SORE THROAT PRODUCTS

Sore, scratchy, and dry throats usually arise from a cold or flu. They can be treated with many different agents available as OTC medications (Table 9-9). If a sore throat continues without relief, one should see a physician to rule out an infection. A sore throat can be a symptom of a streptococcal bacterial infection, also known as strep throat. Strep throat should be treated with antibiotics.

TABLE 9-9 Sore Throat Products

Condition	Product	Dosage forms
Sore throat	Benzocaine (Chloraseptic)	Lozenges
	Dyclonine (Sucrets)	Lozenges

TABLE 9-10 Headache Products

Condition	Product	Dosage forms
Severe headache/ migraine	Aspirin/caffeine/acetaminophen combination (Excedrin)	Tablet
	Aspirin/calcium carbonate combination (Bayer Women's Aspirin Plus Calcium)	Caplet
	Acetaminophen/caffeine combination (Excedrin Tension Headache [aspirin free])	Caplet

TABLE 9-11 Stomach Products/Antacids

Condition	Product	Dosage forms
Heartburn	Cimetidine (Tagamet-HB)	Tab, liq
	Ranitidine (Zantac-75)	Tab
	Famotidine (Pepcid-AC)	Tab
	Nizatidine (Axid-AR)	Tab
Antacids	Calcium Carbonate (Tums)	Chewable tab
	Aluminum hydroxide/magnesium hydroxide/ simethicone (Mylanta)	Tab, liq, gel cap

Tab, Tablet; *liq,* liquid.

However, while the patient is taking antibiotics, he or she also may relieve throat pain with various syrups and sprays. The various agents used in these agents include menthol, alcohol, and benzocaine.

HEADACHE PRODUCTS

Depending on the severity of a headache, one can try many of the OTC medications. Those agents listed under analgesics are used mostly for pain. Some agents contain other additives such as caffeine that can help treat more severe headaches (Table 9-10). However, if a person suffers from severe migraines, usually a prescription drug is required.

STOMACH REMEDIES/ANTACIDS

Several classes of OTC medications are used to treat the common upset stomach (Table 9-11). Histamine$_2$ (H$_2$) antagonists are used to decrease acid secretion, which helps to decrease what is commonly known as heartburn. Proton pump inhibitors work differently than H$_2$ antagonists to relieve acid secretions. Although both work directly on the lining of the stomach, they each target different receptors. Antacid agents are used to balance the pH level in the stomach, which ultimately helps decrease heartburn. Each medication is effective in its own way.

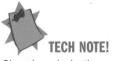

TECH NOTE!

Chronic pain in the stomach may be an ulcer caused by *Helicobacter pylori,* which is a bacterium that causes the symptoms of heartburn. If the problem persists for more than 2 weeks, it is better to seek advice for a possible underlying problem.

TABLE 9-12 Antiinflammatory Products

Condition	Product	Dosage forms
Inflammation/pain	Ibuprofen (Motrin, Advil)	Tab, liq
	Naproxen sodium (Aleve)	Tab, susp
	Ketoprofen (Orudis KT)	Tab, cap

Tab, Tablet; *liq*, liquid; *susp*, suspension; *cap*, capsule.

TABLE 9-13 Intestinal Products

Condition	Product	Dosage forms
Constipation	Combination stimulant (Ex-Lax)	Tab, chew tab
Stool softeners	Docusate sodium (Colace)	Gel cap
Diarrhea	Loperamide (Imodium A-D)	Tab, cap, liq
Flatulence	Simethicone (Mylicon)	Tab, chew tab, liq
Irregular bowels	Psyllium (Metamucil)	Powder

Tab, Tablet; *cap*, capsule or caplet; *liq*, liquid.

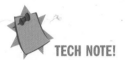

TECH NOTE!

Agents used to treat arthritis also are used to treat common inflammation and pain. Aspirin still is one of the best OTC treatments for arthritis.

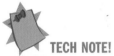

TECH NOTE!

Gas can be painful and embarrassing but is not life threatening, whereas diarrhea and constipation can have severe outcomes if they are not controlled. Babies can die of dehydration because of excess loss of electrolytes through watery stools. In extreme cases, constipation can cause a bowel rupture, which requires surgery to repair. Psyllium is the only agent that can be used for constipation and diarrhea because it works as a bulk-forming agent. Psyllium is also a natural agent and has been noted to reduce cholesterol.

Common Patient Information

Antacids are for short-term relief of heartburn. If problems persist, see your physician. Antacids may be taken without regard to meals.

ANTIINFLAMMATORIES

OTC agents that treat inflammation are referred to as nonsteroidal antiinflammatory drugs. They reduce pain by decreasing inflammation of soft tissue muscle strain. Nonsteroidal antiinflammatory drugs also are used as antipyretic and analgesics, as seen in Table 9-12.

Common Patient Information

Do not take this medication if you are allergic to aspirin. Antiinflammatory drugs may cause drowsiness and may upset the stomach. Take them with food or milk. Do not take these medications if you are in the last trimester of pregnancy.

INTESTINAL REMEDIES

Remedies for intestinal discomfort and pain resulting from constipation, diarrhea, or gas (flatulence) are listed in Table 9-13. Agents to stimulate the intestinal tract vary, but most contain an oil or saline solution that irritates the lining of the bowels and encourages the reflex action required to move the bowels. For diarrhea, an anticholinergic agent (one that dries out membranes) or a bulk-forming fiber such as psyllium powder works to dry out or absorb the excess water, creating bulk in the intestinal tract. Loperamide works well for immediate results. Psyllium (Metamucil) is a good natural choice that many doctors recommend. For the treatment of gas, simethicone (Gas-X) is the most commonly used agent, although there are other products available such as Beano, which contains the enzyme alpha-galactosidase. These agents neutralize the production of gas, which is created as a by-product from bacteria that reside in the intestines.

Common Patient Information

Do not use laxatives in the presence of abdominal pain, nausea, or vomiting. Do not use laxatives longer than 1 week. Loperamide may cause drowsiness or dizziness and may cause dry mouth.

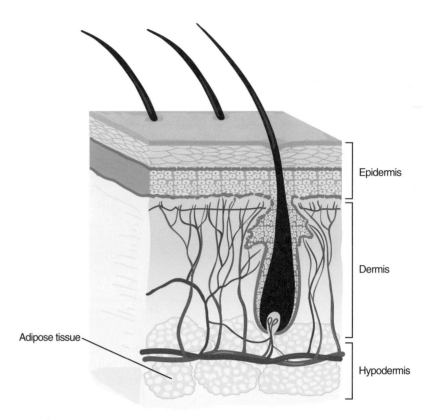

FIGURE 9-1 Anatomy of the skin. The three major layers of the skin.

SKIN ANATOMY

The skin, also known as the integumentary system, is the largest organ of the body. The integumentary system includes the skin, hair, and all tissues below the surface of the skin down to the muscle. Skin is one of the most abused organs of the body system. Skin holds up through weather, detergents, scratches, cuts, and bruises, and it repairs itself time and time again. Like other organs, it must be nourished, oxygenated, and taken care of. In return, it functions to protect the body, regulate temperature, and act as a sensor to stimuli.

On top of the skin are layers of keratin, which help protect the layers below. The two layers beneath the keratin are the epidermis and the dermis. Below the dermis lies the subcutaneous layers of fat that insulate the body, keeping it warm. Skin also protects the body from bumps and falls and is a food reserve in case of emergency. The epidermis does not have blood flow of its own; instead it receives nutrition from the tissues surrounding it. The dermis is much thicker than the epidermis and acts as a support system for the outer layer and holds the nerves, blood vessels, and other connective tissue (Figure 9-1). Also, the skin has the ability to absorb moisture and medications. Diabetics inject insulin subcutaneously under the skin, which means the needle penetrates through the subcutaneous layer. Another route of administration (or ROA) is the intradermal route, in which the needle penetrates between the dermal layer. An intramuscular dose requires penetrating through the subcutaneous layer and into the muscular layer.

Conditions Affecting the Skin

Many different types of agents can be used to treat skin conditions. The cause of the problem and what the physician wants the agent to do determines what

TABLE 9-14 Over-the-Counter Skin Products

Dosage forms*	Indications
Creams*	Dry, scaling, pruritic areas; thickened areas
Ointment*	Dry, scaling, pruritic areas; thickened areas
Lotions/gels	Hairy areas, lesions that ooze, wet areas
Sprays*	Acute weeping lesions

*Creams, lotions, and gels are absorbed through the skin; ointments and sprays remain on top of the skin to prevent moisture from evaporating.

TABLE 9-15 Antibiotic Products

Product	Trade names	Dosage forms
Bacitracin	Bacitracin	Ointment
Neomycin	Neomycin	Ointment
	Myciguent	Cream
Polymyxin B sulfate, neomycin, bacitracin	Neosporin	Ointment, cream

the physician prescribes. Table 9-14 lists common dosage forms and the type of conditions that the agents can treat. At some time everyone gets a cut or scrape to the skin; common skin problems involve minor infections that occur when bacteria get into a wound. There are several antibiotics available to treat these injuries. Popular antibiotic ointments and creams are listed in Table 9-15.

When unknown skin problems arise, a proper diagnosis may include a physical assessment, family history, drug history (including OTC and/or herbal medications used), laboratory tests, and possibly a biopsy. We begin with a short overview of the types of inflammatory skin conditions that can be treated with OTC agents. Other conditions require prescription agents. Following this is a discussion of more serious conditions, including psoriasis, melanomas, ulcers, herpes, and burns, along with some of the treatments given.

INFLAMMATORY SKIN CONDITIONS

Most skin conditions can be divided into the following two categories:

1. Noninfectious inflammatory conditions
2. Infectious inflammatory conditions

Many products are available that work well in treating noninfectious skin conditions, although if the symptoms continue, it is recommended that the patient visit a physician. Infectious inflammatory conditions are much more serious because they can be transferred from person to person; therefore, one should see a physician immediately for the proper treatment. Many of these conditions must be treated with prescription drugs. If a patient is unsure of what the skin condition is, it is best to visit a physician for the proper diagnosis (Box 9-4).

Sunburn, acne, and hives are common skin conditions that often are treated at home. These are noninfectious inflammatory conditions. Psoriasis, although noninfectious, normally is treated with prescription drugs.

SKIN PROTECTION FACTOR GUIDE

Skin protection factor (SPF) agents come in topical form and prevent sunburn. Ultraviolet A (UVA) rays and ultraviolet B (UVB) rays are the two main wave-

BOX 9-4 COMMON NONINFECTIOUS CONDITIONS AND THEIR DEFINITIONS

Condition	Defined
Urticaria (hives)	Usually caused by an allergic reaction
Eczema (red skin rash)	Allergic reaction
Psoriasis (plaques, scaly skin)	Genetic
Seborrheic dermatitis (rash)	Possible allergic reaction affecting the scalp area; color usually ranges from red to brown
Atopic dermatitis (rash)	Associated with allergic reaction; may be genetic

BOX 9-5 SUNSCREEN PRODUCTS

Action	Block or absorb ultraviolet A and B sun rays
Products	Hawaiian Tropic
	Bullfrog
	Sundown
Indications	See Table 9-16

lengths of solar rays that are of concern. Both affect the healthiness of the skin. UVA and UVB rays given off by the sun penetrate the earth's atmosphere and the skin layers. UVA rays can enter into the dermal layer. Although UVA rays do not cause the skin to redden, these rays cause premature aging of the skin and possible changes in DNA in the cells where it is absorbed. If the skin is left unprotected, the UVB rays cause erythema and even blistering of the skin. This is what normally is seen as sunburn.

Constant overexposure to the sun over time raises the likelihood of mutations within the structure of the DNA from UVA and UVB rays. When this happens, cancer can occur, as well as discoloration of the prematurely aged skin. To protect oneself from both of these harmful ultraviolet rays, one must wear the proper amount of SPF. The two types of protectants are sunscreens and sunblocks. Sunscreens protect the skin from UVA and UVB rays by allowing the skin protectant to absorb the ultraviolet rays, rendering them harmless. Sunblocks work by reflecting the ultraviolet rays. Ultimately, the best protection one can provide the skin is a sunblock/sunscreen combination. To judge how much protection is needed, divide the amount of time it takes you to burn. If you wear a sunscreen with an SPF of 20, then it will take you 20 times longer to burn. For example, say it takes you only 10 minutes to burn in the sun. If you apply a sun block of SPF 20, multiply that by the time you take to burn (10 minutes) and your coverage would last about 200 minutes, or about 3.2 hours. Reapplication is necessary based on the type of activity in which you are participating. For swimmers, there are water-resistant and waterproof agents that increase longevity of the product from 40 to 80 minutes, respectively, before it must be applied again. Because ultraviolet rays are always present, even on cloudy days, it is possible to choose the best coverage for specific skin types, as shown in Box 9-5. See Table 9-16 for sunscreen indications.

ACNE DEVELOPMENT AND TREATMENT

Acne affects not only teenagers but adults as well. In most cases, acne is caused by hormonal changes, which is why it is so prevalent in teenagers. However, genetics can influence acne too. The old belief that eating too much candy or greasy foods such as fries causes acne is incorrect. These foods do not cause acne, although they can worsen existing acne.

TABLE 9-16 Skin Protection Factor Guide for Application of Sunscreen

Skin type	Skin characteristics after 10 minutes of sun exposure	Suggested minimum coverage
I	Burns easily/rarely tans	20 to 30 SPF
II	Burns easily/tans minimally	12 to 20 SPF
III	Burns moderately/tans gradually	8 to 12 SPF
IV	Burns minimally/tans well	4 to 8 SPF
V	Rarely burns/always tans	2 to 4 SPF
VI	Never burns/deeply pigmented	None

SPF, Skin protection factor.

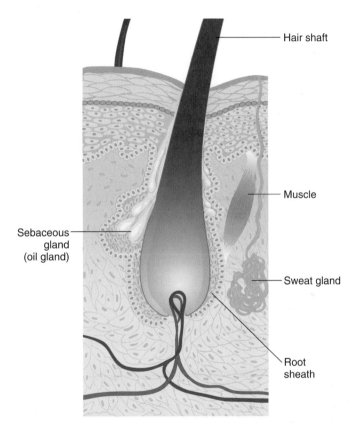

FIGURE 9-2 Diagram of sebum skin pore. Location of hair follicles and surrounding region.

Hormones have an ability to enlarge the glands of the skin. Two of the most productive glands are the sweat glands and sebaceous glands. Sweat glands are regulators of temperature. As a person sweats, the water evaporates and cools the body. The sebaceous glands are responsible for the production of skin oil called sebum. The oily layer it produces protects and lubricates the skin. When sebum production increases and traps bacteria at the base of the hair follicle, the likelihood of acne increases (Figure 9-2). The only treatment for acne is to keep the skin clean and free from bacteria, decrease the sebum production, and finally remove dead skin (Table 9-17).

Acne can be classified into the following two groups:

1. Noninflammatory
2. Inflammatory

TABLE 9-17   Acne Treatments

Product	Trade name	Dosage forms
Benzoyl peroxide	Clearasil Max Strength	Cream
	Oxy 10 Cover	Cream
	Oxy 5	Lotion
	Dry and Clear	Lotion

TABLE 9-18   Topical Antiinflammatory Products

Product	Trade names	Dosage forms
Calamine/diphenhydramine	Caladryl	Lotion, cream
Hydrocortisone		Cream, ointment

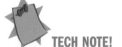

TECH NOTE!

Soap and water have always been a good way to remove bacteria from our skin. However, they do not necessarily kill all bacteria. Antiseptics are necessary for the healthcare worker because they do kill and/or inhibit the growth of germs. Unfortunately, both good and bad germs are killed when these agents are used. It is wise not to overuse antiseptics because bacteria have the capability to mutate into strains that are not necessarily inhibited or destroyed. Using gloves eliminates constantly washing one's hands, which also dries out the skin. See proper techniques for washing hands and gloving them in Chapter 13. Learn more about microbial growth in Chapter 29.

In treating noninflammatory acne, a mild medication can be used, such as keratolytics. These agents dry oily skin, remove dead skin, and fight bacteria. Examples include salicylic acid and benzoyl peroxide.

Painful, swollen pustules are usually present on the face in inflammatory acne. Benzoyl peroxide is the most common OTC product recommended to help dry out the sores, called pimples. More severe inflammatory acne may require the use of antibiotics in addition to keratolytics. Prescription antibiotics such as tetracycline, erythromycin, and clindamycin (also in topical form) may be prescribed. Topical agents include retinoic acid medications such as isotretinoin (Accutane) and tretinoin (Retin-A). These agents increase the growth of skin around the acne areas, which allows the infected cells to fall away as new cells replace them. With this type of treatment, the acne may seem to worsen initially but usually improves over several weeks.

Urticarias, commonly known as hives, are bumps that are extremely itchy. They are believed to be caused by a hypersensitivity to food or drugs. Topical agents can be used for hives and other skin rashes that cause inflammation of the skin resulting from severe itching yet are not infectious (Table 9-18).

INFECTIOUS INFLAMMATORY SKIN CONDITIONS

Although infectious skin conditions treated with prescription drugs are common, certain conditions such as warts, tinea infections (such as athlete's foot), cold sores, and lice can be treated with OTC medications. Other infections such as herpes and impetigo must be treated with prescription medications.

Warts
Skin irritation can arise from viral warts. Warts are contagious, although most disappear on their own within 6 months. Verruca plana commonly are seen in children and may appear in areas such as the hands, face, and neck area. These warts are caused by a papovavirus (Figure 9-3, *A*). Table 9-19 lists various treatments. Genital warts are caused by the human papillomavirus, which is a sexually transmitted disease. A physician should be seen for appropriate treatment, which may include liquid nitrogen or surgical removal. This type of wart can be linked to cancer and must be treated immediately (Figure 9-3, *B*).

Athlete's Foot
Tinea infections can appear anywhere on the body The name of the tinea infection depends on where it is located. A commonly known condition, tinea pedis

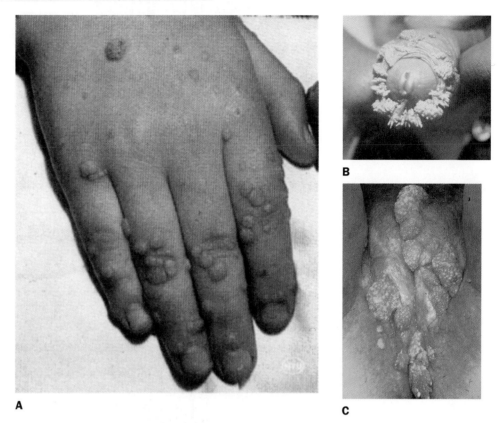

FIGURE 9-3 Warts. **A,** Verruca vulgaris (viral skin wart). Genital warts (male, **B**; female, **C**), which are caused by a sexually transmitted disease, human papillomavirus.

TABLE 9-19 Products to Treat Warts

Product	Trade names	Dosage forms
Salicylic acid	Wart Off	Liquid
	Compound W	Liquid

TABLE 9-20 Products to Treat Athlete's Foot

Product	Trade names	Dosage forms
Tolnaftate	Tinactin, Aftate	Cream, solution, spray, ointment, powder
Undecylenic acid	Desenex	Ointment, cream, powder, spray powder
Clotrimazole	Lotrimin	Solution, lotion, cream

(athlete's foot) causes dry, cracked skin, pain, and irritation. It can be spread by contact from shower floor surfaces and sharing socks. Antifungals that kill the fungus are used to treat athlete's foot; they are usually in powder or spray form. Keeping the feet dry and in comfortable shoes helps prevent athlete's foot. Other types of tinea infections include tinea capitis (head) and tinea corpus (nonhairy skin). Many tinea infections are caused by a fungal infection of the species of *Trichophyton* and are treated with various OTC agents as listed in Table 9-20 (Figure 9-4). Depending on the species and severity of the infection, one may need to see a physician for a prescription.

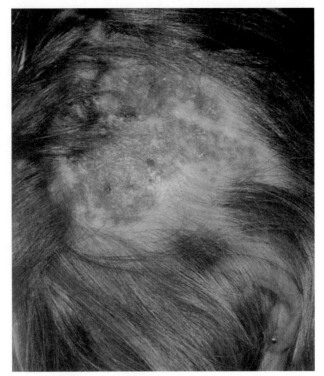

A

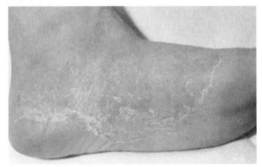

B

FIGURE 9-4 Two types of tinea infections. **A,** Tinea capitis (head). **B,** Tinea pedis (foot).

TABLE 9-21 Canker Sore Products

Product (ingredients)	Trade name	Dosage form
Benzocaine 20%	Orajel	Swab
Phenol, camphor, and miscellaneous additives	Campho-Phenique	Gel
	Neosporin Lip	
Vitamin E, cocoa butter, and miscellaneous additives	Treatment LT	Ointment

Canker Sores

Canker sores are located in the soft tissue of the mouth, usually inside the cheek or on the tongue, causing stomatitis. They are small topical ulcers that tend to disappear within 2 weeks but can be painful (Table 9-21).

Lice

Many children come home from school with head lice. Lice can be transferred easily when children use the same brush. Other ways include sleeping next to

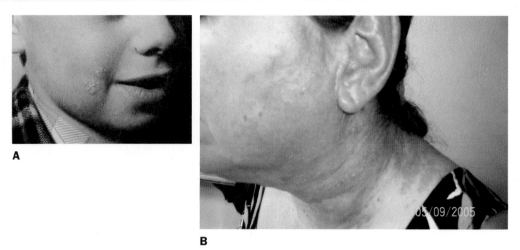

FIGURE 9-5 **A,** Herpes simplex. **B,** Herpes zoster.

someone with lice and sharing clothes. Lice also have been known to jump from one host to another. Therefore, there is a high risk of catching lice even without body contact. Several products on the market treat this infestation. Treatment of the whole family is important even though the infestation affects only one child. All brushes, combs, and hats must be cleaned in hot, soapy water or alcohol and should not be shared.

Herpes
The two different types of herpes are called herpes simplex and herpes zoster, and both can be painful. Herpes simplex is a form of virus that usually causes welts and sores around the mouth (cold sores) or vaginal area (herpes genitalis). This type of herpes is a sexually transmitted disease and commonly is treated with a prescription antiviral. Both types of herpes affect the nervous system, and persons are prone to repeated outbreak (Figure 9-5, *A*) when the immune system becomes weakened.

Herpes zoster causes lesions on the head, neck, arms, and legs. Antiviral medications are used to lessen the side effects along with pain medication. This condition is caused by varicella-zoster virus and affects adults more often (Figure 9-5, *B*).

Impetigo
Impetigo can affect the face, limbs, and abdomen. Impetigo is a contagious condition caused by streptococcal organisms or *Staphylococcus aureus* (see Chapter 29). A thick yellow crust is formed. The infection is contagious from the discharge from the lesions. Treatment includes antibiotics and Burow's solution (Figure 9-6).

SERIOUS SKIN CONDITIONS

Serious skin conditions require a visit to the hospital or doctor and may require hospitalization. These include skin melanomas, psoriasis, and burns. Although psoriasis is not infectious, it may become debilitating. Many types of lesions, burns, and damage to the skin usually are treated with prescription drugs. The following figures show samples of various serious skin conditions that include cancerous tumors, ulcers, and third-degree burns.

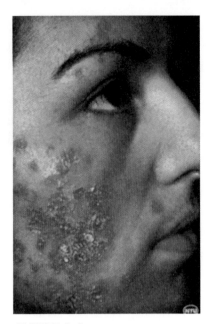

FIGURE 9-6 Impetigo contagiosa.

Malignant Melanoma

Melanomas are cancerous skin growths emanating from moles and areas of the skin that may have been sunburned. One must take several risk factors into consideration. Typically the appearance of melanomas is marked by irregular shape, elevation off the skin, discoloring, and change in size and shape. The normal course of treatment is removal of the melanoma and, if necessary, a skin graft. Figure 9-7 shows two types of skin cancers.

Ulcers

Many external ulcers are caused by bed sores and affect the elderly. They are slow to heal and may harbor methicillin-resistant *Staphylococcus aureus*. This is a highly contagious infection that must be treated with a strong antibiotic and must be reported to the county health department. In the case of ulcers, the wound must be kept moist and sterile. In addition, antibiotics are given. The patient usually has a lab sample taken after treatment to make sure there is no evidence of methicillin-resistant *Staphylococcus aureus*. Ulcers can be caused by sexually transmitted disease (Figure 9-8).

Psoriasis

Psoriasis is a genetic skin condition that cannot be cured and may last a lifetime. The onset of this painful disorder is usually during the teen years but can occur later in life. Persons can suffer from mild to severe cases of this disease. This condition is not contagious, although the lesions appear inflamed. Most affected areas are around the joints, limbs, neck, and even scalp. More potent drugs are used on psoriasis such as corticosteroids (Table 9-22). These drugs relieve inflammation and pruritic dermatosis and act as a vasoconstrictor. Agents used to treat psoriasis require several topical prescriptions as listed in Figure 9-9.

In addition to these medications, sometimes the patient is given sunlight treatments to cause mild sunburn of the skin and subsequent peeling. The mechanism of action of potent corticosteroids is the suppression of T cells and other constituents that cause inflammation and an increase in cell growth. Thus these agents must be used carefully because they impede the immune system.

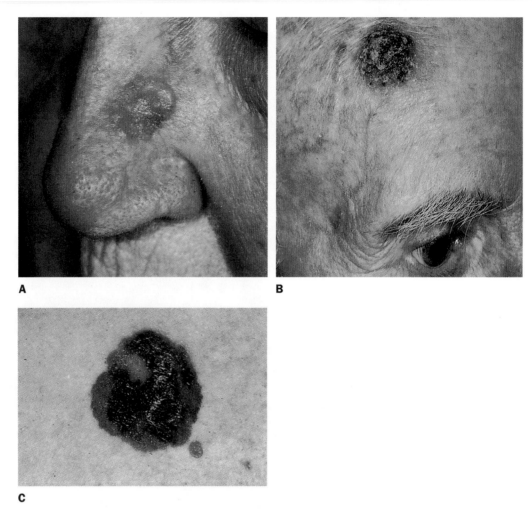

FIGURE 9-7 **A**, Squamous cell. **B**, Basal cell. **C**, Malignant melanoma.

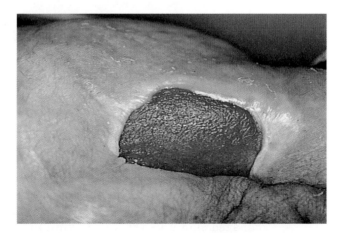

FIGURE 9-8 Pressure ulcer, which is common among bedridden patients. This picture is an example of the last stage, in which necrosis (death) and even damage to the patients underlying tissues and bone have occurred.

TABLE 9-22 Agents Used to Treat Psoriasis

Product	Trade name	Dosage	Potency
Dexamethasone (Rx)	Decaderm	Cream, ointment	Low
Betamethasone benzoate/ betamethasone valerate (Rx)	Uticort/ Valisone	Cream, ointment	Medium
Fluocinonide (Rx)	Lidex	Cream, ointment	High
Betamethasone/desoximetasone (Rx)	Diprosone/ Topicort	Cream, ointment	High
Bethamethasone dipropionate (Rx)	Diprolene	Cream, ointment	High

Rx, Prescription.

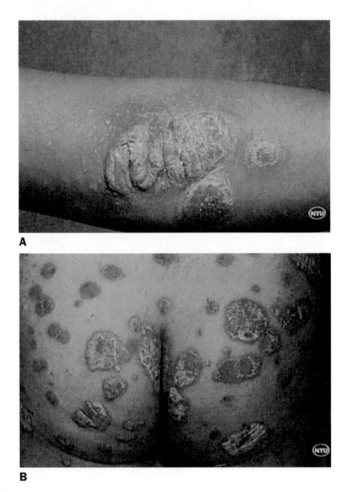

A

B

FIGURE 9-9 Psoriasis, which is commonly found on joints such as elbows and knees, although breakouts may occur anywhere.

Burns

Burns range in severely from first-degree, being the least severe, to third-degree, the most severe. Depending on the size of the third-degree burn, the patient must undergo surgery to replace the burned layers of skin. This is done by removing healthy skin from another part of the body. The new skin then is thinned out through a rolling process and then adhered by staples to the damaged skin area. This is a painful process. Medications used include silver sulfadiazine (Silvadene) cream. Burn hospitals require specialized solutions and medications from the pharmacy in order to treat patients who stay in the burn unit (Figure 9-10).

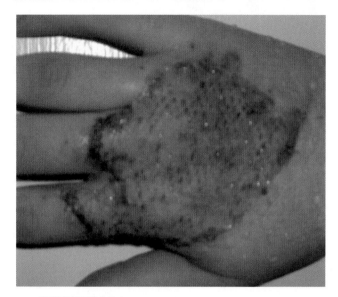

FIGURE 9-10 A third-degree burn prior to grafting.

DO YOU REMEMBER THESE KEY POINTS?

- The responsibility of the patient to know what type of OTC product that he or she is taking
- The problems associated with more drugs becoming OTC
- Guidelines regulated by the FDA for a legend drug to become an OTC product
- Guidelines regulated by the FDA for the manufacturing practices of OTC products
- Terms and definitions associated with OTC products
- Why consumers desire to diagnose and treat themselves
- The difference between generic and trade drugs
- The three categories of OTC products
- Main interactions between aspirin products and other medications
- The importance of skin protection against UVA and UVB rays
- The differences between infectious inflammatory and noninfectious inflammatory conditions
- The common interactions between aspirin and other medications

MULTIPLE CHOICE QUESTIONS

1. All of the medications listed are H_2 antagonists except _____C_____.
   A. Cimetidine (Tagamet)
   C. Loperamide (Imodium)
   B. Famotidine (Pepcid)
   D. Ranitidine (Zantac)

2. Which of the areas listed are not regulated by the Food and Drug Administration?
   A. Purity
   C. Color and texture
   B. Bioavailability
   D. Potency

3. Children under the age of _____ do not have recommended dosages listed on over-the-counter products.
   A. 1 year
   C. 5 years
   B. 2 years
   D. 8 years

4. What does MRSA stand for?
   A. Medication resistant staff A
   B. Methicillin-resistant *Staphylococcus aureus*
   C. Medical recommendation for surgical approval
   D. None of the above

5. Fillers are used to _____.
A. Make the drug taste better
B. Change the pH
C. Change the shape
D. Make the tablet larger

6. The best definition for the word *efficacy* is _____.
A. The ethical use of drugs
B. The ability of a drug to produce the desired chemical change in a person
C. The laboratory testing phase of a drug to determine its effectiveness
D. The results seen in a person's illness

7. Two major over-the-counter agents for use as nasal decongestants are _____.
A. Oxymetazoline and acetaminophen
B. Oxymetazoline and phenylephrine
C. Phenylephrine and dyclonine
D. Dyclonine and pseudoephedrine

8. The skin has many functions. Which one of the following is not one of its main functions?
A. Regulates temperature of the body
B. Acts as a sensor to stimulus
C. Protects the internal organs from the elements
D. All of above are main functions

9. Which of the following drugs cannot be used as an antiinflammatory?
A. Aspirin
B. Ibuprofen (Advil)
C. Acetaminophen (Tylenol)
D. Naproxen sodium (Anaprox)

10. The over-the-counter product most commonly used for insomnia is _____.
A. Aspirin
B. Ibuprofen
C. Diphenhydramine
D. Chlorpheniramine

11. The terms *UVA* and *UVB* relate to the _____.
A. Amount of sun that a person can withstand
B. Ultraviolet rays of the sun
C. Wavelength of rays emitted from the sun
D. Both B and C

12. If you burn easily and rarely tan when out in the sun and you decide to use an SPF of 10, how long can you be out in the sun before you would need to reapply the lotion?
A. 10 minutes
B. 100 minutes
C. 1 hour
D. 10 hours

TRUE/FALSE If a statement is false, then change it to make it true.

_____ **1.** Drug manufacturers can swap or replace "like ingredients" without notifying the public.

_____ **2.** Betamethasone (Diprolene) is a high-level corticosteroid that can be used for skin conditions such as psoriasis.

_____ **3.** The skin is the largest organ of the body.

_____ **4.** Herpes simplex and herpes zoster are caused by the same bacterial infection.

_____ **5.** Athlete's foot is caused by bacteria.

_____ **6.** Acne is caused by hormone levels, not eating habits.

_____ **7.** The epidermis contains the blood vessels and nerves that nourish the skin.

_____ **8.** Waterproof sun lotion increases the longevity of effectiveness by 40 minutes.

_____ **9.** Psoriasis is an infectious, inflammatory condition of the skin.

_____ **10.** The most used over-the-counter agent for acne is tetracycline.

TECHNICIAN'S CORNER

1. A patient comes into the pharmacy asking for a drug that is sold over the counter and can remember only the name of the ingredient benzoyl.
   How do you answer this question?
   Where is this product found?

2. A patient comes in with a toddler and asks what type of stool softener to use for her baby because she has not had any bowel movements and is cranky.
   How do you answer this question?
   What will you tell the patient?

3. A patient comes up to the counter with two bottles of cough syrup, guaifenesin/pseudoephedrine (Robitussin PE) and guaifenesin/dextromethorphan (Robitussin DM), in hand. She wants to know the difference between them.
   How do you answer this question?
   At what point would you call in the pharmacist?

REFERENCE

1. Sorial S: California Society of Health-System Pharmacists seminar, Oct 22, 2005.

BIBLIOGRAPHY

American Association of Retired Persons: *Using meds wisely: over-the-counter drug fact labels.* Retrieved 10/20/2005, from www.aarp.org/health/usingmeds/health/usingmeds//l

Barkauskas VH, Baumann LC, Darling-Fisher CS: *Health & physical assessment,* ed 3, St Louis, 2002, Mosby.

Consumer Healthcare Products Association: *OTC facts and figures.* Retrieved 2005, from http://www.chpa-info.org/ChpaPortal/ForConsumers/Drug_Facts_Label/

Consumers Health Education Center: *OTC fast facts.* Retrieved 10/20/05, from http://www.chpa-info.org/ChpaPortal/ForConsumers/CHEC/

Drug facts and comparisons, ed 60, St Louis, 2005, Wolters Kluwer.

Gerdin J: *Health careers today,* ed 4, St Louis, 2007, Elsevier.

McCuistion L, Gutierrez K: *Real world nursing survival guide: pharmacology,* Philadelphia, 2002, Elsevier.

Mosby's medical, nursing, & allied health dictionary, revised reprint, ed 6, St Louis, 2005, Mosby.

WEBSITES

www.bemedwise.org
www.aarp.org
www.chpa-info.org
www.heall.com
www.medic8.com/healthguide/search.htm

10

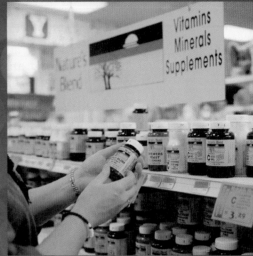

Complementary
Alternative Medicine

Objectives

UPON COMPLETING THIS CHAPTER, YOU SHOULD BE ABLE TO
DO THE FOLLOWING:

- Define the term alternative medicine.

- Differentiate between Eastern and Western medicine.

- Describe why alternative medicine has become popular.

- Explain what is meant by the placebo effect.

- Describe the following treatments and the belief systems of each:
  - Acupressure/acupuncture
  - Ancient Chinese medicine
  - Aromatherapy
  - Art therapy
  - Ayurveda
  - Biofeedback
  - Chiropractic manipulation
  - Herbal remedies
  - Homeopathy

- Identify common herbal preparations and their common uses.

AGENTS COVERED IN THIS CHAPTER

Common Name	Species
Aloe vera	*Aloe vera* (family Liliaceae)
Black cohosh	*Cimicifuga racemosa*
Chamomile	*Matricaria recutita*
Feverfew	*Tanacetum parthenium*
Garlic	*Allium sativum*
Ginger	*Zingiber officinale*
Ginkgo	*Ginkgo biloba*
Ginseng	*Panax quinquefolius*
Goldenseal	*Hydrastis canadensis*
Hawthorn	*Crataegus laevigata*
Purple coneflower	*Echinacea purpurea*
Milk thistle	*Silybum marianum*
St. John's wort	*Hypericum perforatum*
Valerian	*Valeriana officinalis*

THIS CHAPTER COVERS THE CURRENT VIEWS on complementary alternative medicine in the United States, including the origins of various nontraditional therapies from Eastern and Western cultures. This chapter also explores the reasons why nontraditional therapies have become popular and how they are being integrated into traditional medicine. An in-depth review of herbal remedies is presented using examples of top-selling herbs such as ginkgo, feverfew, and ginseng. Common uses and known interactions of these herbs are covered. In addition, the placebo effect is discussed.

Physicians are prescribing herbal medications for conditions such as sleeplessness and forgetfulness. For doctors and pharmacists to ask patients what herbal medications they are taking is common practice in order to determine any drug-drug interactions that may occur with traditional medications. Although various treatments outlined in this chapter are not necessarily effective or appropriate for treatment, nevertheless they are here to stay. Because of this, it is important that the technician have a working knowledge of these types of alternative treatments. This chapter outlines considerations concerning traditional medicine and its herbal counterparts. Ten popular alternative treatments also are discussed.

What Is Alternative Medicine?

To find out the meaning and scope of alternative medicine, one first must define traditional medicine. Traditional medical treatment includes medication prescribed by physicians, consisting of common agents or treatments for medical conditions. This includes doctor visits, possibly followed by radiographic examinations, laboratory tests, or other tests to enable the physician to make a correct diagnosis. Traditional medicine includes the use of legend (prescription) and over-the-counter (OTC) medications. Follow-up visits ensure the success of the treatment and regular visits to monitor the patient's condition.

The alternative approach might consist of visits to a chiropractor, homeopathic doctor, or other practitioner, followed by treatments used within those specific areas of study. These treatments might include herbs, acupuncture, acupressure, or yoga. Many alternative approaches have been in existence for thousands of years, whereas traditional medicine has existed for only a few hundred years. Nevertheless, traditional medicine is the standard for the Western world today.

Alternative medicine has been viewed as ineffective, ancient, and more closely related to superstition than "real" medicine. Many alternative treatments were thought of as extreme measures taken only by those who have lost all hope of recovery using traditional methods. The more controversial types of nontraditional medicine and therapies became labeled "alternative medicine" and were grouped with ancient remedies such as Ayurveda and Chinese medicine. Other controversial therapies include treatments such as hydrotherapy and crystal, spiritual, and magnetic healing. However, alternative medicine now is making a comeback. Why? This chapter answers this question and explains the considerations one must give to traditional medicine and complementary alternative medicine.

Overview of Eastern versus Western Medicine

Eastern medicine includes treatments originating from eastern Asia, parts of Arabia, India, Japan, and other Far East countries. Over the centuries, advancements made from each of these cultures have helped lay the foundation for Western medicine. As medicinal knowledge was gathered over the ages, it was transcribed and translated into other languages and was subjected to further experimentation. European scientists added their own herbal remedies to the growing list of herbal treatments made from varieties of plants indigenous to their terrain.

With the invention of the first microscope in the 1600s, scientists had new pathways to explore. This was the beginning of the golden age of microbiology (Chapter 29). Illnesses that were once thought of as caused by evil spirits now were identified as microbial diseases and treated. As science advanced through the age of antimicrobial therapy, it was possible to produce chemical agents that could produce a predetermined specific action within the body. The term *magic bullet* identifies specific medications that target only specific organs or cells within the body. This science is the cornerstone of Western medicine today and will continue to be in the future. One must not forget that Western medicine has been influenced by thousands of years of experimentation gathered from many different cultures.

Western medicine has omitted all cultural superstition and has relied on scientific methods to prove effective treatments. Yet some of the most powerful drugs have come from ancient herbal remedies or are derived from the plants used in those remedies. For example, digoxin, one of the most prescribed heart drugs in the geriatric community, has its origins in the 1700s. Digoxin is made from the plant foxglove and cannot be manufactured synthetically. Digoxin helps the heart beat in slow yet strong beats and is used to treat many persons who have congestive heart failure. Another example, homeopathy (discussed later in chapter) was practiced first in the late 1700s when diseases were treated with herbal medications that caused symptoms of illness when given to healthy persons. Homeopathy is based on "like treating like" in disease versus medication. Plant derivatives used in Western medicine include quinine for malaria, psyllium for high cholesterol and bowel regularity, and reserpine for high blood pressure.

Trends toward Alternatives

For thousands of years, practitioners of Eastern philosophy took the whole person into consideration in making a proper diagnosis and plan of treatment. This holistic approach included the person's diet, dreams, and even smell. According to the World Health Organization, alternative medicine now is estimated to be used by more than 70% of the world's population. Most of the countries that use alternative medicines are developing countries. These cultures use herbs as their main form of treatment because they cannot afford or obtain traditional medicine. Also there is a strong belief system in place that continues from generation to generation.

Starting in the 1980s, Eastern medicine, specifically herbal remedies, became popular in the Western world. Because herbs are not considered a form of traditional medical treatment, they became grouped with all types of nontraditional remedies that were considered ineffective, including crystals and aromatherapy, hydrotherapy, and sound therapy. However, during the past 2 decades, many of these nontraditional methods of treatment have become commonplace in the Western world. Consumers spend millions of dollars annually on alternative treatments. Until recently, most traditional practitioners have discounted all types of nontraditional or alternative medicine. However, if there were no truth to any of these alternative medicines, then why is interest still growing within the American people?

Because of current lifestyles, stresses, and emerging diseases, persons are becoming aware that traditional medicine has its limitations. As one ages, one's body experiences more age-related problems, such as diabetes, dementia, and strokes. As new medicines are produced by drug manufacturers, the risk of side effects and the rising cost of drugs can lead a person to try alternative medicine. Also, many manufacturers of herbal remedies and other therapies claim they can increase the life span in good health. This claim is sometimes enough for consumers to give these therapies a try. Another reason alternatives to traditional medicine are becoming more popular is that many times they claim to treat extreme illnesses. A person diagnosed with a cancer for which there is no current medication or therapy available may seek alternatives as a last resort for treatment.

Using Traditional and Alternative Medicine

In the 1990s alternative therapies were a topic of discussion within the traditional medical community. As medical practitioners researched the types of treatments used by their patients, it was necessary to put together a list of all types of known alternative treatments. The National Center for Complementary and Alternative Medicine (NCCAM) was formed in the early 1990s to deal with these issues. The three main goals of the NCCAM are to do research on alternative treatments, train individuals who are interested in learning techniques, and provide the consumer with information on the various types of therapies available. NCCAM has identified and classified various therapies and continues to receive funding from the U.S. government for more research. More than half of the medical schools in the United States currently are offering classes on alternative medicine. Areas of study include supplement therapy, such as vitamins and minerals; herbal medicine; acupuncture; and homeopathy.

The term *complementary* is used concurrently with *alternative* because nontraditional therapies have found a place alongside traditional medicine. Therefore the term *complementary alternative medicine* is an accurate description of how these two forms of treatment are being used together. More doctors, nurse practitioners, and other health care providers are suggesting herbal treatments and nondrug alternatives in place of, or concurrently with, traditional treatments. Nondrug alternatives may include remedies such as biofeedback, massage, and meditation. Self-hypnosis has been found clinically to reduce surgical pain in patients. Acupuncture has been used in hospitals to treat adolescent patients. Table 10-1 lists types of complementary therapies.

The Placebo Effect

One must consider the effectiveness of placebo drugs when discussing nontraditional medication. A placebo is an inert drug, meaning it contains no active ingredients. Therefore its ability to help a patient recover from illness or to decrease pain is based on the power of the patient's belief that the medication worked. Many persons believe so strongly in certain remedies or therapies that it is hard to determine whether the therapy or the belief of the patient is the likely cure. Through extensive double-blind tests, more information is becoming available as to whether various treatments and herbal medications are truly effective. Double-blind tests are conducted in which the patient and the treating physician are not told whether the patient is receiving the investigational drug or a placebo (inert drug). In this way the patient's bias cannot influence the findings and should give a clearer picture as to whether the drug is working or whether positive results are caused by the placebo effect.

Acupuncture

Acupuncture has been used for thousands of years with extensive studies in the Eastern and Western world. Acupuncture is used for conditions such as chronic pain, depression, addiction, and other ailments. Acupuncture is based on the Chinese belief that the body is made of energy channels. When these channels become blocked, sickness may result. The use of needles at specific points throughout the body is thought to release these channels, bringing the body into harmony once again (Figure 10-1).

Acupressure

Acupressure is closely related to acupuncture because it also uses specific energy points across the body. Instead of using needles, pressure is applied by hand to the specific point to unblock the channels. Insurance companies are beginning to pay for acupuncture and acupressure treatment if recommended by a physician for the treatment of pain. Classes are available on acupressure so that one can perform the technique on oneself (Figure 10-2).

TABLE 10-1 Twelve Alternative Treatments

Type of treatment	Description of alternative treatment
Acupressure	Acupressure is based on the same principles as acupuncture. Instead of using needles to unblock the pathways carrying energy, the practitioner uses his or her hands to apply pressure to specific points on the body.
Acupuncture	Acupuncture is based on the meridians in the body. These lines are believed to carry energy to specific parts of the body. When they become blocked, illness or pain can occur. The practitioner relieves blocked pathways with the use of needles.
Aromatherapy	Using the nasal senses, various blends of fragrances bring about relief of certain ailments. Herbs and perfumes are used. Mostly oils are used because they are considered more healing than the whole plant or portions of plants.
Art therapy	Art therapy is based on psychoanalysis and how the mind can manifest specific images. These images then can be expressed in drawings or paintings, hopefully stimulating enlightenment. Then the patient can work on the problem through feedback.
Ayurveda	Ayurveda is based on the spiritual side of the body and all that affects the body, including the environment, emotional stability, and physical health. Practitioners find ways to change what is necessary to enable the patient to be more in tune with the world. This includes various postures, meditation, and massage. Changing habits is a large part of this treatment.
Biofeedback	Biofeedback is a learned technique that enables self-control of various physiological responses of the body. This includes voluntary systems and involuntary systems of the body. A practitioner teaches it only until the patient is proficient in using the technique.
Chinese medicine	Chinese medicine is based on the body spirits of the yin (meaning man) and yang (meaning woman) that are acknowledged as having similar elements yet that are different in order. Therefore, each is treated differently. Diagnosis is based on the person's dreams, tastes, sensations, smell, and other senses. Various types of treatments are used, including herbal remedies and acupuncture.
Chiropractic	Chiropractic treatment is based on the belief that the realignment of the body, specifically the spine, can remedy certain conditions. Periodic adjustments usually are required to align the spine and various joints throughout the body. In this way, pressure or pain is relieved.
Crystal healing	Continual use of various stones and gems are required to produce healing. Practitioners of crystal healing place specific stones on parts of the body for certain lengths of time to draw out disease. Patients are taught which types of stone can be used for their healing abilities.
Herbal remedies	Medicinal purposes of herbs have been learned through historical literature and by word of mouth. Trial and error are the main guidelines of herbal treatments if used without consultation from an authority, such as a practitioner who has a legitimate degree in herbal use. Currently, many herbal agents are being tested, and testimonials of side effects and interactions are being compiled for reference.
Homeopathy	Homeopathy is the traditional belief that "like cures like." Various types of toxins are mixed in extreme dilutions to the point at which they are often undetectable by scientific means. This minute amount of the same disease from which the patient is suffering allows the patient's body to fight the illness.
Spiritual healing	In the belief system of spiritual healing, the patient's treatment is attained through prayer of the practitioner and patient. The practitioner claims to be a pathway for divine intervention. Recovery is instantaneous, and no follow-up visits are necessary.

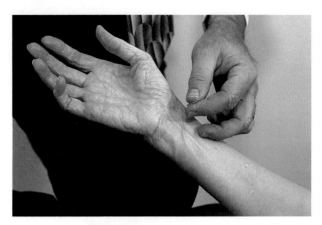

FIGURE 10-1 Acupuncture.

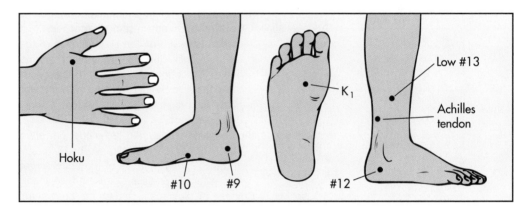

FIGURE 10-2 Acupressure points.

Ancient Chinese Medicine

For more than 4000 years, Chinese medicine has been a well-known art based on years of trial and error. Although herbal remedies might come to mind readily when the topic of Chinese medicine is discussed, it involves much more than the use of herbaceous plant parts. The heart of Chinese practice is the yin and yang, which represents male and female entities, respectively. The ancient Chinese belief contends that although men and women are made of the same substances, their spirits are different, and therefore appropriate treatment is different. Female spirits are thought of as a darker color, which coincides with the earth, whereas male spirits are lighter color, like the color of the sky.

Practitioners conduct an examination by asking the patient about dreams, strange tastes, or smells experienced. Also, a visual examination of the skin and voice tone is performed. Once the diagnosis is completed, the practitioner may prescribe the necessary treatment that could include a variety of herbs, minerals, and/or vegetables. Herbs are used extensively in Chinese medicine and can treat more than one ailment at a time. For example, goldenseal may be used for headaches, allergies, and infections concurrently. Also, various herbal plants have the ability to work for or against a specific physiological condition, such as raising or lowering blood pressure levels, depending on the person's condition. Herbs and other remedies are used in Chinese medicine to cure the body of the original illness as well as a prophylaxis. Chinese medicine is still in use today; many health care providers, including pharmacists, take classes based on Chinese knowledge of herbs and their medicinal uses.

Art Therapy

Art therapy became popular in psychology in the late 1960s. Psychiatrists had patients who were mentally disturbed or traumatized draw their feelings on paper if they were unable to discuss problems verbally. Such therapy was a way for patients to express themselves, relieve anxiety, and begin the road to recovery. Art therapy can be used for simple stress relief therapy or as therapeutic treatment for persons suffering from life-threatening illnesses, such as cancer. Patients may gather in groups or individually with a practitioner who guides them through the techniques of mental and visual awareness concerning their disease state or condition. This type of therapy is meant to supplement counseling.

Art therapy is used extensively in children with autism or other psychological conditions and now is used for many types of treatment in adults as well. Various forms of expression include painting, working with clay, making facial masks, and making batik. A master's degree is offered in this area of study through various colleges. Other art therapies include music, poetry, drama, and dance. The National Coalition of Creative Arts Therapies Association offers information on these types of therapies and schools for training.

Ayurveda

Ayurveda is an ancient Indian approach to medicine still practiced today. Dating back thousands of years, Ayurveda is based on the person knowing the spiritual self. This knowledge encompasses the body and all that affects it. With an insight into the various effects of outside influences on the body's spirit, it is possible to make assumptions. One can predict whether something will have a positive effect or negative effect on the body. For example, certain colors, sounds, clothing, and other environmental stimuli are taken into consideration. The types of food and herbs that are consumed also play a role in the overall health of the person. These assumptions then are applied to physical and spiritual activities of the ill person. Based on the type of personality of the subject, the practitioners suggest ways to alter food and/or lifestyle to cure and prevent illnesses. This form of treatment exists today in many parts of the world. Medical schools teaching this approach are located in India. Courses in Indian medicine also are offered in various medical schools in the United States.

Biofeedback

Biofeedback has been around for approximately 50 years and has been proved to be effective for treatment of stress, hypertension, and other conditions. Biofeedback uses the patient's mental ability to alter vital signs such as blood pressure, heart rate, and even gastrointestinal activity. The body is divided into two types of movement, voluntary and involuntary. Voluntary movements include the musculoskeletal system and involve purposeful actions such as walking, sitting, standing, and bending over. Persons have control over these functions daily; therefore, adjusting behavior does not take much conscious effort. However, with biofeedback one also is taught the ability to tap mentally into and alter involuntary bodily functions, such as heart beat, breathing, and digestion. These functions do not normally require conscious thought.

Biofeedback usually is taught by an instructor who uses electrical leads that provide a readout of data. Patients are hooked up to monitors that allow them to see what their bodies are experiencing. A monitor can show the activity of a specific organ. For example, the instructor might have the patient alter the heart

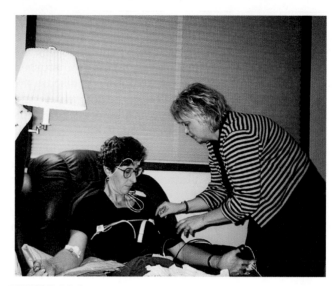

FIGURE 10-3 Biofeedback. Example of electrode placement.

rate to a certain level through concentration. When that level is reached, a new level is set. Gradually, the person is able to adjust body functions as needed without the use of a monitor. Biofeedback is a way of connecting the mind to the body. Patients are supposed to practice these techniques often for full effects. Biofeedback is used as an alternative for medication for anxiety, low back pain, neuromuscular dysfunction, tension headaches, and other conditions. Biofeedback is covered partially by many insurance companies with a doctor's approval. Once the technique of biofeedback is perfected, it can be done at any time without supervision (Figure 10-3).

Chiropractic

Chiropractic therapy is an orthopedic approach to treating pain resulting from misalignment of the bones. Chiropractic began in the late 1800s when it was believed to have cured deafness in a man after his back popped into correct alignment. Certain changes in the skeletal structure are believed to interfere with the nervous system and other organ systems. The treatment given to a patient by a chiropractic doctor is referred to as *manipulation*. Treatment can include hands-on adjustments of the spine or joints and application of massage and heat therapy. Research has proved that some forms of manipulation can be helpful, specifically manipulation of the lower back. Although use of chiropractic therapy is on the rise, various forms of treatment are controversial. Some doctors promote the use of manipulation of certain parts of the skeletal structure, whereas other physicians believe it may be harmful. This is especially true when chiropractors have been used to manipulate skeletal structures to cure infections or treat conditions such as hearing loss or diabetes.

Skepticism about the ability of manipulation to treat many common illnesses abounds, and studies are being done to find out exactly what therapy works and why. Practitioners must attend an accredited school to become a doctor of chiropractic. Many insurance companies cover chiropractic treatment based on scientific evidence and referrals from a physician such as an orthopedic doctor. Chiropractic therapy usually takes many sessions of treatment.

Pharmacist's Perspective
BY SUSAN WONG, PharmD

Educate Yourself When It Comes to Complementary and Alternative Medicine and Health

Many questions arise when it comes to a person's health. What is health? Some may believe that it is not getting sick, in other words, staying well. Others may think it is fixing something that has gone wrong or broken. Still others believe it is maintaining overall happiness and balance. All of these play an important role in being healthy. How to do this is another story. The four important steps follow:

1. A patient or customer must become a good self-observer.
2. A patient or customer must learn to recognize that he or she has control of lifestyle and choices.
3. A patient or customer must make lifestyle changes or other changes as necessary.
4. A patient or customer must follow the results of changes, as well as document and communicate them with the health care provider.

Your role as a pharmacy technician may be as a bridge of information between the pharmacist and the patient to help the patient become or stay healthy.

To do any and all of these things, one first must understand what makes a person tick. Over many centuries, different philosophies have developed that address health. Native Americans chewed on willow leaves for relief from pain or swelling. In Europe, this eventually led to the discovery and concentration of the active component, salicin, and with a little chemistry, acetylsalicylic acid (aspirin). In Chinese medicine, a practitioner prescribes a tailored mixture or formula to cure pain and restore balance, or one can use one of the patent medicines (ready-made formulas for a general condition). Many Eastern philosophies incorporate emotional, mental, and spiritual balance into the equation. Unfortunately, how these remedies and philosophies interact may not always be clear. That is why it is important to educate oneself and communicate to others; especially important is the communication between a patient and the health care provider.

In the world of drugs, herbs, and nutritional supplements, it is important to distinguish clearly what types there are. Learn how each of these single or multiple agents can affect a particular situation before its use. Sometimes one therapy may counteract another or actually may augment the effects of another. This may be good or bad depending on the person's situation and overall health. Patients should keep a diary of what has been used, what they are currently using (if anything), and any questions they may have. Patients should keep track of how they feel and what may have caused it, including any prescription drugs, OTC drugs, herbs, or supplements, and let the health care provider know exactly what they are using. The patient must let the medical doctor, pharmacist, chiropractor, herbalist, nutritionist, or anyone who is involved in the patient's health and well-being know what he or she is taking. Health care providers may not know exactly how some things interact, but they will find out for the patient before they recommend its use.

In Western medicine, drugs are highly refined chemicals (of plant and synthetic origin) that are taken for a specific purpose or endpoint. They have been studied extensively and documented in the scientific literature. These drugs are available mostly as single-agent pills or capsules. Multiple-agent compounds are designed to work together on one symptom or take care of many symptoms. New ways exist of getting those medicines into the body, such as injections or shots; skin patches; creams, lotions, and ointments; inhalers; suppositories when the patient cannot swallow or keep things down; drops for eyes, ears, and nose; and drops or liquid to swallow. All of these dosage forms have developed in the last 10 to 50 years and are designed to get the medicine to exactly where it is needed. This allows a smaller effective dose with fewer side effects.

Just because a drug can be bought OTC does not mean that it is the best thing to use. For example, the asthma inhalers that can be bought OTC certainly work but can cause some serious side effects in persons with a heart condition or anxiety. The patient should always consult the pharmacist if the patient is not sure. Also important is that the patient gets the right kind of drug in the right form and that the patient knows why, when, and how to use it.

For herbs, a similar situation exists in which there are single-agent herbs and multiple-agent formulas that work for different ailments. Fortunately, most are available in an oral form that can be swallowed or taken as a tea or infusion. Unfortunately, herbal medications are not regulated as closely in the United States as drugs are. Drugs are tested much more rigorously and take longer to reach the market. However, herbs have been used for centuries, even millennia, to heal and cure patients when used correctly. The patient must be aware of the exact genus and species of herb to ensure the right effect. Similarly named herbs can have different effects. Be aware of where the active agents are derived from—roots, leaves, berries, and tree bark. Also of importance for some herbs is when they are harvested: spring and fall harvests may have different chemical characteristics. Always be aware of the labels. Read and learn about exactly what

Pharmacist's Perspective—cont'd

the patient needs and how to take herbs. Use reputable sources and standardized extracts (standardized to known active ingredients) when buying herbs.

Food and dietary supplements are similar to herbs in that they are much less regulated than the drugs. We know we need certain foods, vitamins, and minerals to survive—too much or too little can affect health adversely. Different diets can rob patients of certain essential nutrients, so it is best for the patient to check with the physician/consultant before starting a diet. Most persons who follow a well-balanced diet do not need additional supplements. Others who may have chosen certain vegetarian diets or weight loss diets may be missing some nutrients and need supplements. Remember that different types or amounts of exercise can affect one's diet and nutrient needs.

For example, osteoporosis can occur in men but most commonly occurs in women. A well-balanced diet with plenty of exercise can help prevent long-term detrimental effects. Some persons take calcium supplements to augment their bone and mineral stores. The normal recommended daily allowance for calcium in adults is about 1200 mg. By taking calcium supplements of 1000 to 1500 mg per day, a healthy adult can avoid detrimental bone loss. Recently, a new and innovative supplement hit the market that is not a pill but a chocolate-flavored chew. It provides 500 mg of calcium just like old-fashioned oyster shell calcium but in a candylike form. Sounds good, doesn't it? In the fine print, there is also a tiny amount of vitamin K added. For those folks on a closely monitored blood-thinning agent to prevent strokes, this could be really bad news. Even this tiny amount of vitamin K can counteract the good effects of a blood-thinning agent and put a patient at risk for developing a stroke.

Green tea also has high amounts of vitamin K that can counteract blood-thinning agents. As persons get older and try to take better care of themselves, they could be doing harm if they do not pay attention to what they take and how.

In today's medicine, we really do not know how the Western philosophy of treating illness and promoting health interacts with the Eastern philosophy. A few terms to think about follow:

- Allopathy—a system of medical practice making use of all measures that have proved value in the treatment of disease
- Homeopathy—a system of medical practice that treats a disease especially by the administration of minute doses of a remedy that would in healthy persons produce symptoms similar to those of the disease
- Vegetarianism—the theory or practice of living on a diet made up of vegetables, fruits, grains, nuts, and sometimes animal products (e.g., milk, cheese, and eggs)
- Nutriceuticals/nutritional supplementation—whole foods, vitamins, minerals, enzymes, amino acids, phytochemicals, and other natural resources that are designed for use in the immune system, the inner healing force
- Herbal or botanical medicine—plants or plant substances that are used for medicinal purposes or crude drugs of vegetable origin used for the treatment of disease states, often of chronic nature, or to attain or maintain a condition of improved health
- Phytotherapy—the use of vegetable drugs in medicine
- Aromatherapy—the treatment of medical conditions with the aromatic essential oils of fragrant herbs
- Ayurveda—a holistic medical system that covers all aspects of heath and well-being (physical, emotional, mental, and spiritual). Ayurveda includes methods of healing from diet, herbs, exercise, and lifestyle regimens such as yoga and meditation and is based on a person's dominant *dosha,* one of three body/personality types
- Traditional Chinese medicine—a system of acupuncture, herbs, and diet based on the parallelism and synchronicity of events in the inner and outer world of the human organism; based on a person's Tao (one of five archetypes that symbolize human character or personality types); the five organ networks and their climates; and finally the balance (yin/yang) between qi (the life force), blood (governing the tissue), and moisture (governing the internal environment)

Lastly, age, gender, and body type can affect how a body responds to what is put in it. Well known in Western medicine is that pediatric (birth to 18 years old) and older patients (60 to 65 years and older) tolerate medications differently because of natural metabolic changes. Lifestyle issues such as smoking and alcohol use also affect responses to medicines. Medication doses are adjusted according to these factors and to the desired endpoints. It might be safe to infer that these changes may have similar effects when using Eastern medicines and therapies as well. Patients must be careful before starting any new therapies and must consult experts if necessary.

All patients must keep track of any and all agents they put into their bodies. They need to educate themselves on health and how they choose to maintain it. Patients should always inform their health care providers of any herbal remedies they are taking. This decreases the probability of a drug-drug or drug-food interaction. ■

Herbal Medicine

Although herbal remedies have been in existence for thousands of years (see Chapter 1), this basic therapy has gained renewed popularity during the past decade. The herbal remedy market is expected to grow even more in the coming years because of many factors, such as the increasing age of the population and the increasing costs associated with traditional health care and medications. The technician must know various interactions between legend drugs, OTC drugs, and herbal remedies. Most persons believe that it is not important to notify their physician or pharmacist that they are taking herbal medications because they believe them to be natural and therefore not harmful. However, there are many documented reports of harmful interactions between natural products, legend drugs, and OTC medications.

Many of the drugs used in traditional medicine today are medications derived from herbs. The main difference is that extensive testing and documentation has preceded their use. Through testing, specific chemicals have been isolated in many herbal plants. Those chemicals that have proven effectiveness against certain conditions then are made synthetically in a laboratory if possible. Therefore, most American medicine discovered from plants does not incorporate the whole plant or even parts of them. Also, over time, if literature has proved the effectiveness of herbs, the herbs are subjected to the regulations enforced by the Food and Drug Administration. However, the Food and Drug Administration does not regulate herbs because they are considered a nutritional supplement.

This section discusses some of the more popular herbs and the caution to take before self-administration. Because many herbs have been used in different cultures for thousands of years, they often have many different names. For example, *Echinacea* is also known as black sampson, sampson root, narrow-leafed purple coneflower, and red sunflower.

HERBAL TREATMENTS

Aloe vera is one of the most popular herbal agents is a succulent plant called *aloe*. Many different species are used to produce agents to treat minor burns, acne, and various skin irritations. If taken internally, aloe works as a laxative and also is used for bleeding ulcers. Dosage forms are gels, powder, capsules, tonic, and juice. Pregnant women should not take aloe internally.

Black cohosh *(Cimicifuga racemosa),* from the family Ranunculaceae, is used primarily for hormone replacement. Other indications are rheumatism and cough; black cohosh also can be used as an insect repellent (called bugbane). Short-term studies have concluded that black cohosh is safe if used for short periods. No extensive scientific studies have been done on this agent. One must not confuse black cohosh with similar sounding herbs, such as blue or white cohosh. These are not used for the same purpose and have different interactions with other medications.

Chamomile is from the family Asteraceae (Compositae) and has more than 20,000 known species. The species of *Matricaria recutita* is used for motion sickness, flatulence, and gastrointestinal disturbances. In the topical form, chamomile is used for open ulcers, hemorrhoids, and other inflammation of the skin. When taken orally, chamomile has been documented to cause emesis, and if used topically, one should keep the medication away from the eyes because it can cause irritation. Oral chamomile is contraindicated in pregnancy and (because of lack of testing) during lactation. Chamomile also has been reported to worsen asthma attacks. Chamomile has several interactions with anticoagulants, benzodiazepines, and central nervous system depressants. Most of these interactions can cause an additive effect of the medication if taken with chamomile.

Feverfew also is derived from the family of Asteraceae. The species *Tanacetum parthenium* is used for many different ailments including fever, headaches, gastrointestinal upset, arthritis, and asthma. Feverfew can be used in topical and oral forms. In the oral form, feverfew is known to cause irritation of the mouth and tongue and a variety of gastrointestinal upsets such as nausea, vomiting, and diarrhea. Side effects, such as increased bleeding, have been reported when feverfew is taken with anticoagulants. Nonsteroidal antiinflammatory drugs may decrease the effects of feverfew.

Garlic is from the family Amaryllidaceae (Liliaceae) and is most well known as a common herb used in most kitchens in America. Although it is known for its wonderful flavor, it has medicinal uses as well. The species *Allium sativum* has several uses that range from stress relief to an anticancer agent. Some persons use garlic to treat high blood pressure, colds, and flu and for overall wellness. Although garlic is safe most of the time, it is important not to overmedicate because it has been reported to cause adverse side effects such as heartburn, gastrointestinal burning, and even a kill-off of normal intestinal flora. (This normal flora of the gut is necessary for breakdown of food and some vitamin absorption.) Garlic should not be used medicinally when one is taking anticoagulants because it may increase bleeding. Garlic should not be taken by diabetic persons because it may interact with ongoing medication therapy, such as insulin or hypoglycemic agents. Persons suffering from gastrointestinal disorders should beware of possible interactions with garlic use.

Ginger is from the family Zingiberaceae, known as the ginger family, and has 1000 species. The species *Zingiber officinale* is known for its antiemetic and antivertigo properties and is used in gastrointestinal upset and other gastrointestinal conditions, including bleeding, flatulence, stomachache, diarrhea, and more severe conditions such as malaria and cholera. Like garlic, ginger has been shown to have interactions with anticoagulants, producing possible increased bleeding. Ginger also may interact with gastrointestinal medication such as H_2 antagonists (ranitidine) and proton pump inhibitors (omeprazole). Use of barbiturates with ginger may increase the effects of such agents. Ginger also may affect blood pressure medication, cardiac drugs, and diabetic agents.

Ginkgo biloba is the only remaining species of the family Ginkgoaceae and sometimes is referred to as a living fossil. Its most popular use is to treat poor circulation, but it also is used for asthma and other less documented uses, such as regulating blood pressure, improving liver function, increasing memory, and treating heart disease. Some drug interactions include increased bleeding when taken with anticoagulants and increased blood pressure when taken with antihypertensive medications. Persons suffering from bleeding disorders, epilepsy, or infertility should avoid ginkgo. Many medicinal herbs are made from different parts of a plant; therefore, it is important to know what part of the plant is used for which type of condition. Primarily, the ginkgo leaf is used as the medicinal agent, but seeds are also available. Studies have not shown their effectiveness, but raw seeds are known to be dangerous if taken orally.

Ginseng is from the family Araliaceae. Ginseng species *Panax quinquefolius* is used widely for overall wellness, including boosting the immune system. Ginseng also is used for other ailments such as inflammation and depression and as a diuretic. Drug interactions of ginseng include decreasing the effectiveness of anticoagulants and altering the effectiveness of some cardiac agents, diuretics, diabetic agents, and antidepressants.

Goldenseal is from the family Ranunculaceae, known as the buttercup family. The species *Hydrastis canadensis,* when taken orally, is used for gastrointestinal conditions, inflammatory conditions, and painful menstruation. Topically, goldenseal has been used for dandruff, eczema, and itching rashes. Goldenseal has been reported to have interactions with H_2 antagonists (ranitidine), blood pressure medication, anticoagulants, and central nervous system sedating drugs.

Hawthorn is available in many different preparations depending on the part of the plant used; however, all are members of the family Rosaceae (the rose family). The species *Crataegus laevigata* is used mostly to increase blood circulation and improve heart conditions, although studies have not proved its effectiveness conclusively. However, hawthorn has been reported to have possible interactions with various cardiac agents such as vasodilators, antiarrhythmics, antianginal agents, and antihypertensive drugs. Hawthorn also may interact with central nervous system depressants.

Purple coneflower is in the family Asteraceae or Compositae, depending on the species used. The species *Echinacea purpurea* has common uses that include treating colds and infections and use as a general immune booster. Therefore, persons on any type of immunosuppressive agents should be aware that *Echinacea* might alter the effects of such agents. In addition, diabetic persons and any persons who have a condition that involves the immune system should not take *Echinacea* because this herb may worsen the problem.

Milk thistle is from the family of Asteraceae or Compositae. The species *Silybum marianum* is used primarily for liver conditions. Like several other herbs, various parts of the plant are used. The effect varies depending on what part is used. Unlike many other herbs, milk thistle does not have any reported major contraindications and is one of the few herbs that is used intravenously for mushroom poisoning.

St. John's wort comes from the Clusiaceae family. *Wort* means "flower" in Old English, not to be confused with *wart,* which is a viral growth on the skin. More literature has been written on the effectiveness of this herb than on many others. Some of its uses include improvement of sleep disorders, anxiety, agitation, depression, and fatigue. One should take care if using St. John's wort with other herbs that increase sedation, such as valerian. St. John's wort has many documented interactions with medications such as antianginal agents, antidepressants, and anticoagulants.

Valerian is from the family Valerianaceae. The species *Valeriana officinalis* is used mostly for sleeplessness and depression. Because of its strong ability to induce sleepiness, it should not be taken with alcohol, barbiturates, benzodiazepines, or any other sedative type of medication. Valerian may increase the effects of such drugs and/or their side effects.

Knowledge of the family name of the herb is important in case of possible unwanted interactions or reactions. For instance, if someone is allergic to corn, then any herbal drug from the same family may cause an allergic response. Therefore, that person should avoid all herbs from this family. Several herbal books can be referenced to determine the family of an herb. Knowing the species of the herb is also important because species can vary even if they are closely related (Table 10-2). Some studies have been completed on only one of many species of herbs used to prepare herbal supplements.

Use of correct or safe dosages is difficult because the ingredients of each batch of herbs can vary widely. Therefore the strength of each tablet or capsule may vary from one production lot to another. The time of harvesting, which parts of the plants used, concentrations, and consistency in the method of preparation can alter their effectiveness.

HERBAL PREPARATIONS

How herbs are prepared can determine the strength of the active chemicals. Herbs that are brewed for teas are usually more potent than those prepared in capsule form. Teas can be prepared by various methods. Infusions consist of pouring hot water onto the herbs and letting them brew (steep) for a few

TABLE 10-2 Common Uses and Cautionary Notes for Herbals

Herb	Species	Various uses	Caution
Black cohosh	*Cimicifuga racemosa	Menopause, premenstrual syndrome	Should not be used if pregnant Studies not complete
Chamomile	*Matricaria recutita	Gastrointestinal upsets, skin conditions	Should not be used if pregnant Safe if used in small quantities and short term
Feverfew	Tanacetum parthenium	Migraine	Should not be used if pregnant
Garlic	Allium sativum	Antiinfective, antibiotic	Safe if used in small quantities
Ginger	Zingiber officinale	Motion sickness	Safe if used in small quantities
Ginkgo	Ginkgo biloba	Increases circulation	Should not be used if pregnant
Ginseng	Panax quinquefolius	Stress relief	Safe if used in small quantities
Goldenseal	Hydrastis canadensis	Urinary tract infections	Should not be used if pregnant or if hypertensive problems exist
Hawthorn	Crataegus laevigata	Chest pain, increases blood flow	Studies not complete
Purple coneflower	Echinacea purpurea	Antiinfective, antibiotic	Studies not complete because of the many different species and parts of herbaceous plant used
Milk thistle	Silybum marianum	Liver and spleen	Safe if used in small quantities
St. John's wort	Hypericum perforatum	Antidepressant	Safe if used in small quantities
Valerian	Valeriana officinalis	Sleep aid	Safe if used in small quantities

*Various species are used; some side effects may differ depending on species.

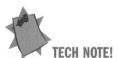

TECH NOTE!

As the popularity of alternative therapies increases, the medical community must meet the responsibilities of keeping up on information about such therapies. Increased use of herbal remedies may have a great impact on medication interactions because herbal remedies have a direct effect on other drugs being prescribed or bought over the counter by the patient. The technician must know the most common interactions between common herbal remedies and legend drugs. In this way the technician is able to assist the pharmacist in identifying persons who may want or need counseling.

minutes. Decoctions are herbs that are simmered over heat in water for 15 to 20 minutes, and cold infusions are left to soak in cold water over many hours. Various methods are suggested depending on the type of herb being prepared (Table 10-3). Medical schools are including studies of herbal remedies because of their prevalence and possible benefits when used correctly along with traditional medicine.

Homeopathy

Homeopathy, translated from Greek, simply means "like suffering." The premise of homeopathy is the belief that "like cures like." Homeopathy also is referred to as the law of similars. The belief is that if a small amount of the substance that caused a person's disease or condition is consumed, it will enable the body to fight off the disease. In the late 1700s, homeopathy was made well known by Samuel Hahnemann, a German physician. After ingesting a small amount of quinine, he showed symptoms of having malaria, the disease that quinine cured. Over time he perfected the necessary minute amount of agent that was needed

TABLE 10-3 Herbal Preparations

Dosage form	Route of administration	Ingredients	Use, strength, onset of action
Syrups, diluted; tinctures	Internal	Alcohol, glycerin	Usually this is a potent form
Tablets, capsules	Internal	Powdered	Slower to act; these are broken down in the stomach
Teas	Internal	Syrups, sweeteners	Better tasting when sweeteners added; teas are stronger than tablets, capsules
Aromatic solutions, baths	External	Scented water	Used to treat skin conditions and burns
Oils	External	Extracted oil from herbs	Used for sore muscles and skin conditions
Compresses, salves	External	Made from teas, salves from herbal oils	A cloth soaked in herbal tea is applied to skin site; used for conditions such as bruises and cramps

If a patient asks about herbal medications, the best advice is to tell the patient to talk to the pharmacist or to his or her physician. A technician should never comment on any specifics even if he/she has in-depth information. Keeping current on new scientific findings is important in case any major side effects or contraindications are found.

to bring about cure rather than disease. Homeopathy made its way to the United States in the 1800s and was a popular treatment. Although homeopathy has remained a popular form of treatment in parts of Europe, it became an alternative treatment in the United States. Homeopathy, however, has regained some popularity over the last decade along with all other forms of alternative medicine.

Thousands of homeopathic remedies are available, but only one right one for each illness; therefore, homeopathic doctors must know what will work for the patient. Unlike herbs and other alternative treatments, the FDA oversees the manufacturing of homeopathic drugs. They are in the same category as OTC medications. Although more medical schools are offering classes on homeopathic medicine, it is still somewhat controversial in the traditional medical community.

All drugs are prepared following guidelines in the *Homeopathic Pharmacopoeia of the United States.* Many of the remedies include herbal treatments. The process of preparing homeopathic agents involves blending and condensing the main ingredients, followed by diluting the active ingredients, and finally preparing the dosage form. The dilution of these active ingredients renders a trace amount of the agent that can equal as little as one part per million. Many times this minute amount is so small that it cannot be detected by chemical analysis.

More information on homeopathic medicine can be obtained from the National Center for Homeopathy. Although most homeopathic agents are available OTC, there are homeopathic practitioners who can oversee treatments. Various credentials are available, such as diplomate of the Homeopathic Academy of Naturopathic Physicians (DHANP), diplomate in homeotherapeutics (DHt), and certified in classical homeopathy (CCH).

DO YOU REMEMBER THESE KEY POINTS?

- The difference between Eastern and Western beliefs concerning medicine and healing
- Why alternative medicine is becoming more popular
- What the function of the National Center for Complementary and Alternative Medicine is concerning alternative medicine
- How the placebo effect fits into the healing process
- What the major alternative therapies are and how they work
- The current regulations pertaining to herbal remedies
- How individuals feel about informing their physicians about taking herbal medicines
- The main uses for the herbal medications covered
- How different dosage forms of herbal medications are used when prepared in different forms
- How homeopathy originated and the belief systems behind it

MULTIPLE CHOICE QUESTIONS

1. Of the following statements regarding biofeedback, which is *not* true?
   A. It is used to treat low back pain.
   B. Treatment may be covered partially by insurance companies.
   C. The patient is able to adjust his or her body functions to a degree.
   D. It must be used with supervision from a biofeedback therapist.

2. Chamomile most likely would be used to _____.
   A. Treat an upset stomach
   B. Relieve stress
   C. Increase circulation
   D. All of the above

3. Art therapy often is used for all of the following conditions or patients *except* _____.
   A. Severe illnesses
   B. Children with autism
   C. Persons who have a difficult time communicating
   D. For persons with an artistic ability

4. Homeopathy is known as the law of similars, which can be best described as _____.
   A. Taking a similar drug that works but at a much reduced cost
   B. Taking a drug that is similar to legend drugs but does not require a prescription
   C. Taking a drug that causes the same illness as the one you are trying to cure
   D. Taking a drug that causes a similar reaction to traditional agents

5. The herb that is known to increase circulation and memory is _____.
   A. Garlic
   B. Goldenseal
   C. Ginger
   D. *Ginkgo biloba*

6. Which of the remedies listed is regulated by the Food and Drug Administration?
   A. Herbal agents
   B. Homeopathic agents
   C. Healing gemstones
   D. Acupuncture

7. The most common use of *Echinacea purpurea* is _____.
   A. As an immune builder
   B. To treat gastrointestinal conditions
   C. To treat skin conditions
   D. As an antioxidant

8. *Silybum marianum* is known commonly as _____ and is used most commonly as _____.
   A. Ginger, motion sickness
   B. St. John's wort, depression
   C. Milk thistle, liver and spleen conditions
   D. Garlic, antiinfective

9. Garlic has been shown to _____.
   A. Interact with anticoagulants
   B. Increase flatulence
   C. Affect blood pressure medication
   D. Both A and C

10. The one drug classification that has unwanted interactions with many herbal drugs is

_____.

A. Antiulcer agents
B. Anticoagulants

C. Vitamins
D. Heart medications

TRUE/FALSE

If a statement is false, then change it to make it true.

_____ **1.** Acupuncture is used in hospitals within the United States to help relieve pain.

_____ **2.** *Ginkgo biloba* is the last remaining species of the Ginkgoaceae family.

_____ **3.** Ayurveda is an old Chinese form of medicine no longer in use.

_____ **4.** Chinese philosophy relies on the belief of spiritual healing.

_____ **5.** Herbal drugs are safe because they are natural.

_____ **6.** Ingesting herbal tea is less potent than taking tablets or capsules.

_____ **7.** Acupressure uses the same techniques as acupuncture.

_____ **8.** The main purpose of the National Center for Complementary and Alternative Medicine is to inform the public about herbal remedies.

_____ **9.** The terms *alternative* and *nontraditional* medicine describe all forms of treatments other than the commonly used methods of Western physicians.

_____ **10.** When taking any herbal agent, it is important to know the species name in case of possible allergic reactions to the specific species.

TECHNICIAN'S CORNER

1. A customer walks into your pharmacy and inquires about which herbal remedies are good for colds. What should you tell the customer?
2. An elderly customer suffering from the flu asks you if it is okay to take garlic tablets with her warfarin? What do you know about drug interactions (if any) between these two agents, and what should you tell the customer?

BIBLIOGRAPHY

Freeman LW: *Mosby's complementary & alternative medicine,* ed 2, St Louis, 2004, Elsevier.

Loecher B, Altshul O'Donnell S: *Women's choices in natural healing,* Emmaus, Pa, 1998, Rodale Press.

Potter PA, Perry AG: *Fundamentals of nursing,* ed 6, St Louis, 2004, Elsevier.

Skidmore-Roth L: *Mosby's handbook of herbs & natural supplements,* ed 3, St Louis, 2005, Elsevier.

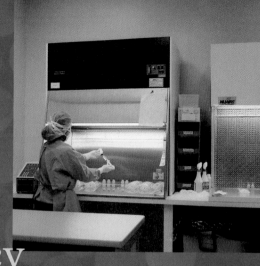

Hospital Pharmacy

Objectives

UPON COMPLETING THIS CHAPTER, YOU SHOULD BE ABLE TO
DO THE FOLLOWING:

- Define the most common tasks performed by hospital pharmacy technicians.

- Identify hospital units according to their specialty.

- Explain the functions of various hospital pharmacies.

- List the patient information required for processing orders.

- Describe the functions of satellite pharmacies.

- Recognize the differences in floor stock depending on the area of the hospital.

- List special unit services and the type of stock they require.

- Explain the reasons for stock rotation, PAR levels, and ordering practices.

- Describe the differences between horizontal and vertical laminar flow hoods.

- List the types of medications used on crash carts and the areas they are stocked in.

Aseptic technique *The procedures used to eliminate the possibility of a drug becoming contaminated with microbes or particles*

Code blue *A coded message to indicate an emergency in a hospital situation*

Floor stock *Supplies kept on hand in different units of a hospital*

Inpatient *A hospitalized patient*

Inpatient or in-house pharmacy *Hospital pharmacy*

NKDA *No known drug allergy*

On-call *A medication to be administered when directed, usually for preanesthesia*

PAR *Periodic automatic replacement*

Post-op *After surgery*

Pre-op *Before surgery*

PRN *Latin term (pro ra nata) meaning "as needed"*

Protocol *A set of standards and guidelines within which a facility works*

Stat order *A medication order that must be filled as soon as possible, usually within 5 to 15 minutes*

PROBABLY ONE OF THE MOST CHALLENGING areas to work in as a technician is a hospital pharmacy, also known as the inpatient pharmacy. The dynamics of this environment can be exhilarating and exhausting, depending on the circumstances. Because hospitals are not as abundant as community pharmacies, there are fewer job openings for pharmacy technicians in hospitals. However, because of the changes in the pharmacist's role within the hospital setting, more highly skilled technicians are required. Pharmacists once made all intravenous antibiotics, chemotherapy drugs, and large-volume parenteral medications in addition to other inpatient tasks. Because of the increase in patient census and the need for pharmacy interventions and evaluations as they pertain to patient profiles, pharmacists do not have time to perform many important tasks they once performed. Technicians have taken over these tasks, which include preparing intravenous medications, loading patient medication drawers, and entering patient data into the computer systematically. As the health care industry continues to change and improve, so will the vital roles that pharmacy technicians play in providing health care services.

Types of Hospitals

Depending on the function of the hospital (facility), patient populations vary. The size of a hospital may be thought of as the number of beds available for patient use. Many small cities or towns may have small facilities with a bed capacity of 50 or less. Larger urban areas have facilities that can range from 50 beds to more than 250 beds. Other factors that differentiate hospitals from one another are their capabilities for diagnosis, surgery, and outpatient services. For instance, many hospitals do not have computed tomography scanners, which are large and expensive; patients needing computer tomography scans are sent to another hospital to have procedures performed or diagnostic examinations done.

Another important difference between hospitals is the layout of their pharmacies. Many older hospitals may have one central inpatient pharmacy (or in-house pharmacy) that is responsible for supplying the entire hospital and all clinics. Larger hospitals or those with specialized areas may have a central pharmacy and smaller satellites located at various points throughout the facility. For instance, a large teaching facility may have specialized areas of treatment such as pediatrics, burn units, intensive care units, and cancer units. Because of the large volume and specialty of the medications needed for these areas, these units may have small pharmacies that stock specific medications to speed up the turn-around time of a medical order. Listed in Table 11-1 are hospital facilities and types of pharmacy layouts.

Policies and Procedures

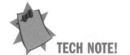

TECH NOTE!

Ask for the policies and procedures binder on your internship to familiarize yourself with specific rules and regulations of the pharmacy.

All pharmacies have a policies and procedures handbook that outlines the rules of the facility. These rules apply to all pharmacy employees. The information contained in the policies and procedures binder concerns daily work routines, benefits, emergency situations, mandatory training, and other important and useful information. Technicians should be familiar with the policies and procedures handbook of their facility.

Hospital Protocol

Protocol is another term used to define the guidelines within the hospital setting, such as the type of medications that are available for dispensing. These rules must be enforced and updated constantly. A committee composed of pharmacists, doctors, nurses, other health care workers, and administrators meets to discuss appropriate changes to the protocol. The purpose of the committee is to choose the best medicine for patients at the best cost. A drug education coordinator is a pharmacist who helps educate the health care providers about the changes in protocol concerning drug coverage and also helps the hospital pharmacy implement these changes. Not all hospitals have the extra help needed to perform these duties; therefore, the tasks of the drug education coordinator may fall onto the staff pharmacists or pharmacy manager.

Hospital Standards

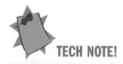

TECH NOTE!

All pharmacists and technicians must have their license, registration, and/or certification visible within the workplace for inspection by the board of pharmacy at all times.

All hospitals must meet federal and state guidelines if they are to be reimbursed for patients who have Medicare or Medicaid insurance coverage. Various agencies such as the U.S. Department of Health and Human Services ensure that hospitals meet all standards of safe operation. The board of pharmacy may inspect all pharmacies to ensure that all personnel are working within legal guidelines. The board has the authority to impose fines on any pharmacy not in compliance with current laws and can close noncompliant pharmacies.

The following are some of the agencies that govern the operations of hospitals:

- Joint Commission on Accreditation of Healthcare Organizations (JCAHO). Hospitals pay a fee for JCAHO accreditation. This inspection is done every 3 years and is conducted over a 2-day period. JCAHO inspects only hospital pharmacies, not community pharmacies, as well as the entire hospital.
- Health Care Financing Administration. Programs include Medicare, Medicaid, and the Health Insurance Portability and Accountability Act (see Chapter 14).
- Department of Health and Human Services. This department is the primary agency that protects the health of the American people and also provides services. This agency includes more than 300 programs and is linked to the

TABLE 11-1 Example of Various Sizes and Types of Hospitals

Types of hospitals	Bed capacity	Usually one pharmacy	Central pharmacy and satellites	Each pharmacy independent from one another	Type of care given
Small	25-50	X			Limited, minor surgeries; critical care is temporary
Medium-sized	50-100	X			Most surgeries, a coronary care unit and an intensive care unit
Large	100	X	X	X	Treats most conditions; physical therapy, intensive care unit, coronary care unit; may have specialty areas such as burn or pediatric units
Teaching	100	X	X	X	Covers all conditions and has specialty areas for teaching purposes; trains medical doctors and other health care providers
Institution	10-100	X		X	Care ranges from treating severe emergencies to continuing treatment but also may include triage to a larger facility that specializes in a particular area; found in institutions such as prisons and mental facilities
Convalescent or long-term care	100	X			Depending on the type of convalescent home, the level of care given may vary; some patients are sent to a hospital for surgery and recovery, and then are sent back to their main resident home

Health Care Financing Administration and Medicare and Medicaid Standards.

- Board of pharmacy. The board develops, implements, and enforces standards for the purpose of protecting the public.

Flow of Orders

When a doctor visits a patient in the hospital and writes medication orders for the patient, the orders are equivalent to a prescription. Figure 11-1 gives a visual

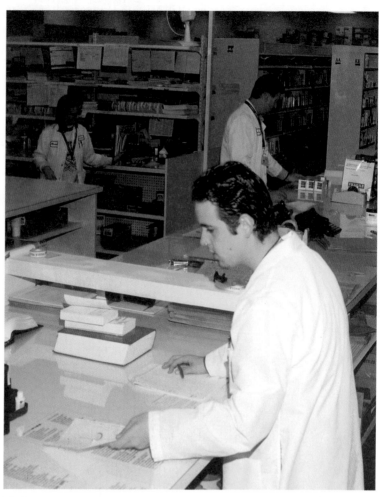

FIGURE 11-1 The flow of orders. As orders arrive, they are entered into the computer. If an order is unclear or if there is a question, the pharmacist calls the doctor.

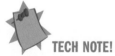

TECH NOTE!

The abbreviation NKA means no known allergies, while the abbreviation NKDA means no known drug allergy. Both of these abbreviations are used in pharmacy.

representation of the flow of orders. The order is written on a doctor's order sheet and is placed in the patient's record (Figure 11-2). This record contains all of the medical records written by medical staff and remains in the patient care area where the patient is admitted. The unit clerk or nurse periodically checks all records for new orders that need to be sent to various areas of the hospital. These include dietary restrictions to be sent to the dietary department, laboratory test requests to be sent to the laboratory, and orders for medications to be sent to the pharmacy. The doctor, nurse, or unit clerk must include all the necessary information on the patient's admitting record and subsequent medication orders to ensure that the orders are filled correctly. This includes the patient's full name, date of birth, medical record number, room number, diagnosis, weight, and, of course, drug allergies.

Although many hospital pharmacies are not open to the public 24 hours a day, orders arrive at the pharmacy around the clock, 365 days a year. Various methods are used to send orders. One is a pneumatic tube system that allows a person to send orders and other small items by way of an air-propelled system. In another system, cylindrical canisters carry intravenous bags and other medications to the hospital floor (Figure 11-3).

The downside of this system is that the tube can get jammed easily or by accident can end up in another department. Also, fragile items, like those

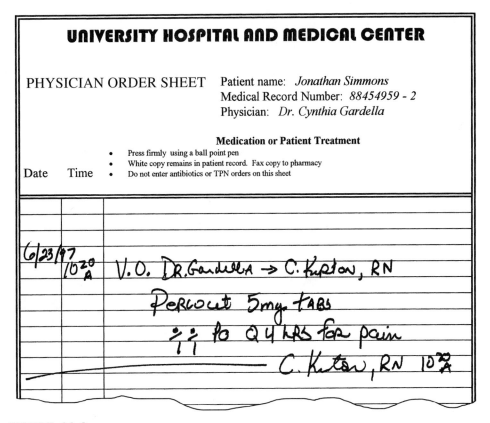

FIGURE 11-2 Example of a physician's order. Note the medical record number in place of a prescription number. Also the patient's room number and allergies should be listed (*not shown*).

encased in glass; controlled substances; expensive medications; or protein-derived medications should not be sent via the pneumatic tube system because they can break during the rough ride or become lost in the system. A growing method of receiving orders is via a fax machine. Although the fax machine is an effective way to get orders to the pharmacy quickly, often the quality of the fax can cause a delay in filling the order. Pharmacists need to verify all unreadable orders over the phone or have the order faxed again. Other methods of obtaining doctors' orders include the use of volunteers or paid staff to deliver the orders to the pharmacy.

Once the orders are received in the pharmacy, they need to be processed in the same way that a regular prescription is processed. However, instead of using the name, address, and phone number for identification, the pharmacy uses the patient's medical record number. Even though this method is the primary way patients are identified, all information, including name and room number, should always be verified against the order. In this way, errors are decreased, especially when two patients with the same last name are on the same floor. The pharmacy uses name alert stickers that are placed on the patient's drawer and medication when two patients have the same last name and are on the same floor. Many computer systems also have name alert functions to help distinguish between patients with similar identifying characteristics.

Most computer systems allow pharmacy technicians to enter the patient's medical record number and drug orders, although it is more common for the pharmacist to enter the order because the information, if entered by the technician, has to be checked by the pharmacist to ensure accuracy. Many pharma-

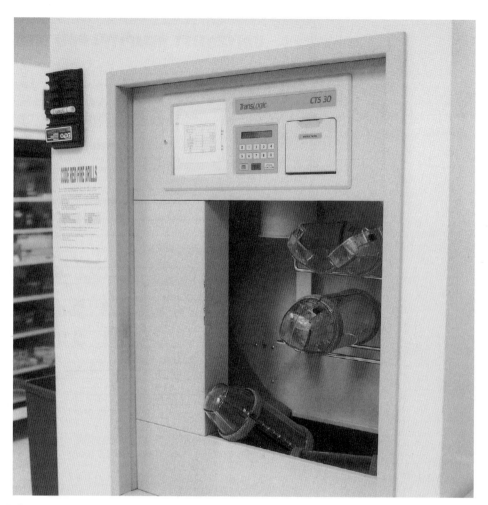

FIGURE 11-3 Pneumatic tube system. A pneumatic tube system is used to transport orders to the pharmacy and medications to hospital floors.

cists feel that it is double work if the technician enters the order but the pharmacist has to reread the order. As the orders are entered, labels are produced from a printer that has the patient's name, medical record number, and room number along with the medication information. The name of the drug, strength, dosage form, route of administration, dose, and the dosing time are included on printed labels.

Because the labels are being produced continually, the technician usually pulls them off the printer and fills the order. Labels are placed on small ziplock baggies so that the medication can be checked visibly against the label by the pharmacist before they are placed in a tube or are taken to the patient's floor. Some orders that are sent to pharmacy have "at once" (stat) or "as soon as possible" (ASAP) stamped on the order. These orders need to be filled immediately because they are ordered in this manner only when an emergency situation exists.

Responsibilities of an Inpatient Technician

Pharmacy technicians must have many skills in today's pharmacy; because the roles of the pharmacists are ever expanding, so must the roles of the pharmacy technicians. Because pharmacists have more interaction with the proper dosing of medications and implementation of formulary, the pharmacy technician completes many of the daily tasks that otherwise would require a pharmacist. The inpatient pharmacy has many different functions that depend mostly on the size of the hospital and number of pharmacies in operation. Many hospitals have 24-hour pharmacies and are open 7 days a week. Technicians need to be flexible to work all shifts, including holidays. They also need to be multifunctional because there are usually half as many technicians and pharmacists working on night and weekend shifts in most hospital pharmacies. However, the patient load may remain the same or even increase during these times. Therefore, it is essential that the technician be able to perform all of the functions necessary for all shifts.

Table 11-2 outlines some of the more common pharmacy job descriptions. Because hospital pharmacies need to be staffed year-round, it is important to have employees who can function in all areas. As a technician learns more skills throughout the pharmacy, he or she becomes more valuable.

Aseptic Technique

Aseptic technique is a method to prevent contamination of an object by microorganisms. The use of this technique is important in preparing all intravenous medications, chemotherapy, and compounded ophthalmic medications. All technicians must be tested periodically on the proper guidelines of aseptic technique, which usually is done by management at the yearly evaluation. Samples normally are taken from a newly prepared parenteral medication and are sent to the laboratory for testing. This is done to make sure that microbial contamination is not present in the patient's medication. To learn more about bacteria and harmful microbes, see Chapter 28. Aseptic technique is discussed in more detail in Chapter 13.

Intravenous Technician

DESCRIPTION

Most intravenous technicians are responsible for labeling and preparing all parenteral antibiotics; large-volume drips such as heparin, aminophylline, and an assortment of potassium drips; and lactated Ringer's solution. Some hospital pharmacies are responsible only for the large volumes of intravenous medications that need to be prepared; the nurses on the floor maintain a floor stock of premade, large-volume bags that can be supplied by central supply or by the pharmacy. This varies from hospital to hospital.

DUTIES

The daily routine usually includes printing all intravenous labels that are currently in the computer system. This intravenous medication information is added or deleted as patients are admitted or discharged and as order changes occur. All changes in intravenous medication information are kept updated by the technician and the pharmacist who work in the intravenous room. Normally, while the technician labels all premade intravenous antibiotics and other intravenous medications, the pharmacist answers the phones and enters new and changed orders. Pharmacists are also responsible for contacting the nurse or doctor if there is a problem with the order. For example, if an order is sent to the pharmacy for ampicillin/sulbactam (Unasyn) and the patient has an allergy to penicillin, the pharmacist calls the doctor and asks the doctor to substitute this antibiotic with one that will not cause an allergic reaction in the patient. The technician then begins to reconstitute and prepare all intravenous medications that must be compounded in a horizontal laminar flow hood.

TABLE 11-2 Common Job Descriptions

Technician responsibilities	Description
IV room	Prepares all parenteral intravenous preparations, including large-volume drips and parenteral nutrition; prepares drugs that are under investigational trial and logs these special medications in the appropriate manner as required by law
Chemotherapy	Prepares chemotherapy and other medications that may accompany these agents
Controlled substances	Gathers all controlled substance inventory sheets from all areas of the hospital; technician also may fill and deliver all controlled substances; the pharmacist is required to verify pharmacy inventory daily
Patient medication filling	Fills medication drawers on a pharmacy cart that will deliver medications to all hospital patients; also may deliver carts to all patient areas and restock any floor stock medications; if the hospital uses an automated medication dispensing system instead, the technician will need to fill this unit on all floors; fills prescriptions for patients who will be discharged on an as-needed basis
Preparation of medication	Fills unit dosing bulk medications; compounds drugs such as for ointments, creams, and solutions
Filling requisitions	Fills all requisitions sent to the pharmacy; stocks inventory; orders pharmacy stock; controls narcotics inventory, and audits narcotics if required; transports medications throughout the hospital facility
Inventory	Orders all medications and supplies for the pharmacy; also may order specialty items for other areas of the hospital; handles all returns and recalled items that need to be sent back to the manufacturer; responsible for handling all invoices and for putting all stock away in the appropriate bins; rotates stock, performs nursing floor inspections and inspects other pharmacy supply areas for outdated drugs and inventory levels; restocks these areas if necessary; this may include the operating room, postoperative area, preoperative area, and other sterile areas
Discharge pharmacy	Fills prescription orders as patients are discharged from the hospital; medications are sent to the floor for the patients, or patients may come to the pharmacy window to pick up the medications
Satellite pharmacy	May be responsible for all tasks related to a small, isolated pharmacy such as answering phones, ordering and putting away stock, preparing parenteral medications, transcribing, pulling all medication orders, and making deliveries to nursing stations
Miscellaneous duties	Ability to work in all areas of the pharmacy as needed; answers phones, trains new technicians and pharmacist interns; works on a team with other technicians, clerks, and pharmacists

Intravenous Therapy and Chemotherapy Preparation

DESCRIPTION

The hospital technician may be responsible for preparing intravenous therapies and chemotherapies. However, some hospitals have separate chemotherapy centers where a technician works side by side with a pharmacist in preparing these medications for patients. The same aseptic techniques are used in preventing contamination when preparing any parenteral medication. However, a few differences between the intravenous and the chemotherapy settings should be noted. One major difference involves the types of hoods used when preparing the medications. A horizontal flow hood is used for preparing intravenous medications. The air of a horizontal hood flows outward, away from the back of the hood, toward the technician. In this way, the environment stays bacteria free inside the hood (Figure 11-4, *A*). Chemotherapy hoods have cycled air that is sent in a vertical flow. The air is pulled down toward the tabletop filter, away from the ceiling of the hood. The chemotherapy hood does not allow the air to leave the container compartment, but the air gets recycled through a special filter that removes any particulate matter (Figure 11-4, *B*). The size of a chemotherapy hood is normally smaller than a horizontal laminar flow hood. In addition, technicians must wear a gown and double gloves or special chemical-safe gloves within chemotherapy hoods; it is not necessary to wear a gown or a second pair of gloves within a horizontal flow hood.

When working inside the horizontal flow hood, the orientation of the hands must not block the airflow. This means that hands cannot be moved behind the vial, needle, or intravenous bag. In a vertical flow hood, hands must not move over the top of any vial, needle, or intravenous bag. If the hands do move into these areas, then aseptic technique has been broken. Regardless of which hood is in use, it is most important that aseptic technique is always practiced. (See Chapter 13.)

DUTIES

Each morning at the beginning of the day shift, all intravenous labels representing all current orders are printed from the computer system. Throughout the day, intravenous medication information is deleted or intravenous medications are ordered as new medication orders arrive to the pharmacy. Orders differ depending upon the time of day within an inpatient pharmacy. In the morning, there may be several pre-op medications ordered and later in the morning post-op medications ordered for patients who have had surgery. Also, more diagnostic exams are done in the morning or afternoon hours than in the evening. Medications that are required for these diagnostics must be sent by pharmacy. The pharmacy technician is responsible for stocking the intravenous room with all of the supplies needed for the day; the supplies also must be restocked at the end of the day for the next shift. The technician also must make sure that the work area stays clean. Usually the same technician prepares all intravenous medications, and then at the end of the shift, he or she delivers them to the nursing floors. When the intravenous medications are delivered, the unused intravenous medications are returned to the pharmacy. If they have not expired, they are placed in the refrigerator or back into stock for future use; otherwise, they are wasted. Because each intravenous preparation must be accounted for, most pharmacies keep a binder or book in which information about all wasted intravenous preparations is written. The technician must remember that it is important to complete all tasks before the end of the shift and to replace all stock items as much as possible.

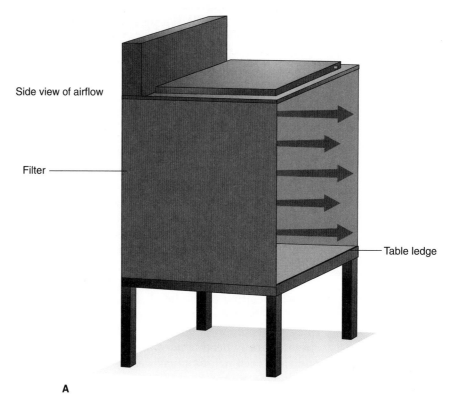

Side view of airflow

Filter

Table ledge

A

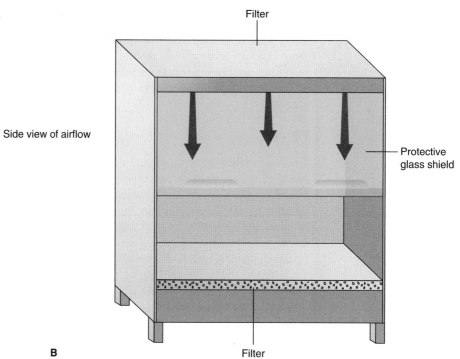

Filter

Side view of airflow

Protective glass shield

Filter

B

FIGURE 11-4 A, Horizontal flow hood. **B,** Vertical flow hood.

Labeling

DESCRIPTION

The proper placement of labels is important to ensure visibility of the solution and contents (Figure 11-5). The technician must initial all medications even if

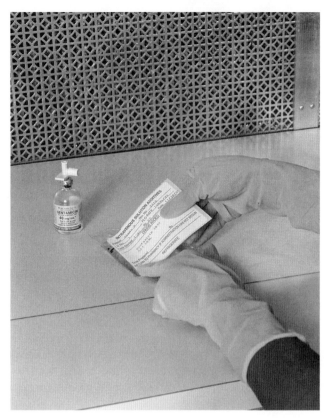

FIGURE 11-5 Placement of intravenous piggyback label onto intravenous bag. The name of the solution (D₅W or NS) inside the bag should not be covered up. This allows the pharmacist to check the type of solution against the order and label.

he or she only places a label on a premade bag. Before the intravenous piggybacks and drips are delivered to the appropriate floors, the pharmacist must check each one and countersign his or her initials. Labels usually contain the same type of information regardless of the facility. In addition to labeling parenteral medications, the technician must know additional information such as medications that need to be placed in light-protected bags and those requiring refrigeration. The technician must know the storage requirements and the stability of the medications he or she prepares.

DUTIES

All drugs must be labeled before they leave the pharmacy. The required parts of a label include the patient's name, patient's medical record number, room number, name of the drug, strength of the medication, the name of the solution with which the medication was mixed, and the rate of infusion. The pharmacy technician must check this information several times before he or she applies the label to the medication. Additional information contained on a label includes the time the dose should be given, the date, and the expiration date. Expiration dates are important because all intravenous preparations are returned to stock if not expired. Many pharmacies use the Julian date. This is the day of the year that does not take into account the month. For instance, if the day is February 1, the Julian date is 32 because it is the 32nd day of the year (January has 31 days plus February 1 equals 32). Determination of the expiration date from the Julian date is much easier because it is not necessary to remember how many days are in a particular month.

All labels must be placed squarely onto the medication and should be clear and easy to read. The pharmacist must check and initial every drug label that is applied and initialed by the pharmacy technician before the medication leaves the pharmacy.

Controlled Substances

DESCRIPTION

The task of counting, dispensing, and tracking controlled substances is a critical job that requires perfection. Within each hospital unit that stocks controlled substances, two nurses must conduct an actual count at the change of every shift. Therefore, all controlled substances are counted 3 times daily. One nurse counts the controlled substances while the other nurse confirms the count on the controlled substance sheet. At the beginning of the new day the count is moved over to a new sheet, and the last day's sheet is sent to the pharmacy. Periodic automatic replenishment (PAR) levels are written at the top of the controlled substance sheets that list the amounts of medications that should be kept on the floor at all times. Often the technician is responsible for retrieving these sheets daily from all units and beginning assessment of how many controlled substances of various sizes and strengths must be provided to keep the unit at or close to its PAR level. In the pharmacy, controlled substances normally are kept in a locked room, which may be under surveillance. All written records must be written in pen, and all inventories must be completed by a registered pharmacist.

DUTIES

After the technician has confirmed the pharmacy-controlled substances count for the day, he or she must sign out each drug onto a dispensing sheet that is used to deliver the controlled substances, which is confirmed by the pharmacist. A pharmacist must do all counts and monthly inventories. Many hospitals still require pharmacists to perform the task of preparing the controlled substances for delivery; technicians are allowed to deliver them.

Each hospital has its own system of delivering controlled substances, but one of the most important aspects is to keep the controlled substances non-identifiable. For instance, many pharmacies put controlled substances in brown paper bags that are stapled shut; most persons would never know that controlled substances are being delivered in this type of container. Even so, the pharmacy technician should never let these controlled substances out of sight when delivering them throughout the hospital. All controlled substances are signed into the department by adding them onto the controlled substances sheet. This can be done by the pharmacy technician or the nurse. All controlled substances then must be countersigned off of the pharmacy inventory sheet. The actual counting of the current levels of controlled substances should be done by the nurse and pharmacy technician to verify all existing controlled substances before adding additional ones into stock. The narcotic sheet must be signed by the RN and the technician. In addition to delivering controlled substances, the technician may be asked by the nurse to return certain ones to the pharmacy. The same validation system is used to enter onto the pharmacy inventory sheet those drugs that are to be returned to the pharmacy. Only registered nurses, not licensed practical nurses, can sign in controlled substances.

On return to the pharmacy, all controlled substances must be signed back into the pharmacy stock. This normally is done by a pharmacist. One of the most important parts of this job is to make sure that all numbers are correct. The pharmacist must never sign in controlled substances without first visually counting the existing stock.

Additional Areas of Pharmacy

Aside from the typical inpatient pharmacy there are additional types of pharmacies that are more specialized. For instance, more hospitals are incorporating satellite pharmacies to expedite order preparation and delivery. Within these pharmacies, specialty medications can be stocked, as is the case for units such as oncology, pediatrics, and intensive care. Certain hospitals connect both inpatient and discharge pharmacies together; this is an area where a technician may work both inpatients and outpatients concurrently. Additional information on specialty areas within the pharmacy field is discussed below.

SATELLITE PHARMACIES

Description

Satellites are small specialty pharmacies that supply a clinic such as the emergency department or an entire floor of a hospital. Most are small and minimally staffed. The satellites fill most of the daily medications for patients on their floors. Most of the floor stock used by the satellites is supplied by the large central pharmacy of the hospital.

Duties

Technicians who work in the satellites are responsible for filling all medication orders and delivering them to the nurses' stations. Other duties include answering phones, keeping satellites stocked, filling stat orders, and stock replenishment.

DISCHARGE PHARMACY

Description

Many hospitals have a discharge pharmacy that fills prescriptions in the same manner as a community pharmacy except that it is located in the inpatient pharmacy. Doctor's orders are written on special discharge order forms that are sent down to the pharmacy with other orders via the fax machine, pneumatic tube, or by volunteers.

Duties

Pharmacy technicians normally process the prescription in the same fashion as in an outpatient pharmacy. After the patient information is input into the computer system, the order is filled. All auxiliary labels are attached if required, and the medications must have a final check by the pharmacist. Once these orders are completed, the medication can be sent back to the floor for the nurse to give to the patient or, if the drug is a controlled substance or a new medication for the patient, the nurse can bring the patient down to receive the medications and be consulted by the pharmacist if necessary.

INVENTORY CONTROL TECHNICIAN

Description

Most hospitals have a technician who is in charge of maintaining stock levels and completing the special ordering of medications. The technician who orders the stock is responsible for the actual ordering, billing, and restocking of the pharmacy shelves; however, it takes a group effort in the pharmacy not to let stock levels drop to the point at which the stock person has to borrow items from another hospital or special-order them at a higher cost. Many methods of keeping stock at necessary levels are available. For instance, a hospital pharmacy may have ordering cards that are used to reorder stock when it is low.

Each person is responsible for pulling the card (normally kept with the medications) and placing it in a designated area where the inventory technician can place the order. When the order arrives, the card is put back into the box along with the new stock. Another method uses bar codes that are read by a handheld device for electronic ordering. In this case, the inventory technician must check visually to see what needs to be ordered. A third alternative requires each item to be tagged with a manufacturer's sticker as it arrives in the pharmacy. Stickers are provided by the manufacturer and must be adhered to each item before it is placed on the shelf. This sticker lists the stock number of the medication along with the price. When an item needs to be reordered, the sticker is taken off the container and placed on an ordering sheet. Medications may come from a warehouse or directly from the manufacturer. Either way, some medications must be ordered on an as-needed basis. This is due to the short expiration dates and expense of medications. This includes ordering large-volume solutions kept in central supply.

Duties

The pharmacy runs out of drugs and supplies daily. Although pharmacies have different systems of ordering the medications, most orders normally are placed using a computer. Depending on where the warehouse or manufacturer is located, the turnaround time for the shipment may vary. For example, if a medication comes from across the country, then it must be ordered earlier than the drug that simply is sent over from the pharmacy warehouse (which usually takes less than 24 hours). Knowing the right time to order medications is a skill that pharmacy technicians must acquire; it is crucial to keep the pharmacy completely stocked with necessary medications.

When the shipment arrives, all included medications and supplies must be verified against the inventory list. Initialing and writing *received* on each invoice is important. Some medications are back-ordered; these items are currently not in stock from the manufacturer but will be sent as soon as they are available. If the medication is one that cannot be left out of stock for any amount of time, it may be necessary to borrow from another pharmacy. This can be done by calling a pharmacist at a neighboring hospital and asking whether that pharmacy has enough to share. A loan/borrow sheet is filled out, and either a taxi or hospital courier normally is sent to carry the medication from one location to the other. After the original ordered stock arrives, replacements for the borrowed items are then returned to the lending pharmacy.

Placing stock onto the shelves is another important duty; it is the point at which the stock is rotated. Making sure that the later expiration dates are placed farthest back on the shelf ensures that the medications with the earliest expiration dates will be used first. The inventory technician is also responsible for returning damaged items and expired agents and handling recall items following the manufacturer's guidelines. Timing is probably one of the most important aspects of keeping inventory at a constant level. The technician can order appropriately if he or she learns the pharmacy protocol for ordering and compensating for items that take longer to arrive, upcoming holidays, and patient load. In the winter and spring, typically more patients are in the hospital. This directly relates to the types of heavily used agents and the overall increase in the use of medications.

Supplying Specialty Areas

In several areas of a hospital the pharmacy must maintain a PAR level of medications. Technicians must recognize each of the abbreviations representing the units and clinics that require medication from the pharmacy. Box 11-1 gives a breakdown of each major area of a hospital. The supplies kept on hand in these

BOX 11-1 PRIMARY UNITS AND CLINICS THAT REQUIRE MEDICATION FROM PHARMACY

CCU	Coronary care unit
CLINICS	Patients may visit a clinic to be seen by a physician or nurse practitioner
ED	Emergency department; area of hospital where patients can receive emergency care with doctors and nurses on staff 24 hours a day
ICU	Intensive care unit
L&D	Labor and delivery; unit where mother goes through labor and delivers a baby
MED	Medical unit for patients who have had surgery or who may be under observation
NICU	Neonatal intensive care unit
NSY	Nursery; unit where babies are taken for care and observation by nurses
OB/GYN	Obstetrics/gynecology; unit that takes care of expectant mothers or those who have just had a baby
ONCOLOGY	Unit that takes care of patients with cancer
OR	Operating room
ORTHO	Orthopedics unit that takes care of patients who may need treatment or surgery on bones or joints
PACU	Postanesthesia care unit
PED	Pediatrics; unit for children younger than age 14 years
POST-OP	Unit where patient is kept after an operation or procedure
PRE-OP	Unit where patient is kept before an operation or procedure
UROLOGY	Unit that takes care of patients who may need treatment, surgery, or procedures on the urinary system

units are referred to as *floor stock*. The technician must be fully aware of the types of medications used in each of the following areas because each unit, ward, or clinic has its own special stock. Because of the specialty of each of the following areas, many pharmacies have special forms that are preprinted with complete descriptions of commonly used drugs. This helps to decrease the incidence of stock being sent to the wrong areas within the hospital. The pharmacy normally receives the supply ordering forms from the specialty areas daily. Although they are not a high priority task, these orders should be filled before the end of the day. In addition, the technician may need to deliver the medications and check various areas of the hospital for any outdated medications. This task should be done monthly, preferably before the end of the month. Outdated medications normally can be returned to the pharmacy if they will expire within 3 months. Expired medications may be sent back to the manufacturer for credit (most manufacturers accept returned expired medications in batches of 100) or they may be taken away by an independent company and destroyed in a proper manner. This depends on the contract between the hospital and the manufacturer. Also, some hospitals contract an outside company that specializes in drug inventory to come into the pharmacy periodically to document all expired medications before they are sent off to be destroyed.

Each department—such as the operating room, post-anesthesia care unit, wards, and clinics—is stocked with its own types of medications depending on what type of services it provides. Because of the many different areas throughout a hospital, the pharmacy must stock a wide variety of medications in different dosage forms. Therefore the pharmacy technician must have a good understanding of which medications are appropriate for each department. Departments such as the emergency department, operating room, and intensive care unit stock many drugs in injectable form and a wide variety of oral and injectable controlled substances. Pediatrics uses many of the same medications

TABLE 11-3 Commonly Used Crash Cart Medications and Their Classification

Medications	Classification	Dosage forms
Adenosine	Antiarrhythmic	Vial
Amiodarone	Antiarrhythmic	Ampule
Atenolol	Beta-blocker	Ampule
Atropine sulfate	Anticholinergic	PFS, vial, ampule
Bretylium	Antiarrhythmic	PFS, vial, ampule
Calcium chloride	Electrolytes	PFS, vial, ampule
Dextrose 50%	Carbohydrates	PFS, IV bag, vial, ampule
Diazepam (Valium)	Benzodiazepine	Vial, ampule
Digoxin	Cardiac glycoside	Tubex, ampule
Diltiazem	Calcium channel blocker	Vial
Dobutamine	Vasopressor	Vial
Dopamine	Vasopressor	PFS, vial, ampule
Enalapril	ACE inhibitor	Vial
Epinephrine	Vasopressor	PFS, vial, ampule
Furosemide	Loop diuretic	Vial
Glucagon	Glucose-elevating agent	Vial
Heparin	Anticoagulant	IV bag, vial
Isoproterenol	Vasopressor	PFS, vial, ampule
Labetalol	Alpha-blocker/beta-blocker	Vial
Lidocaine	Antiarrhythmic	PFS, vial, ampule
Magnesium sulfate	Anticonvulsive	PFS, vial, ampule
Mannitol	Osmotic diuretic	Vial
Naloxone	Narcotic antagonist	PFS, vial, ampule
Nitroglycerin	Antianginal	Vial, ampule
Nitroprusside	Antihypertensive	Vial
Norepinephrine	Vasopressor	Ampule
Procainamide	Antiarrhythmic	PFS, vial
Propranolol	Beta-blocker	Vial, ampule
Sodium bicarbonate	Electrolyte	PFS, vial
Sodium chloride	Electrolyte	Vial
Verapamil	Calcium channel blocker	PFS, vial, ampule

PFS, Prefilled syringe; *IV,* intravenous.

TECH ALERT!

When refilling a crash cart, NEVER assume that the unused drugs left inside the tray are correct. A prime example is the common error between pediatric and adult strengths of lidocaine. Epinephrine is always stocked on a crash cart. Both strengths are packaged in prefilled syringes and appear similar in appearance. *Note the dosages of pediatric (1:100,000, [0.01 mg/mL]) and adult strength (1:10,000 [0.1 mg/mL]). Placement of adult-dose epinephrine in pediatric trays is a common error.* If an adult dose of lidocaine or another adult dose medication were filled into a pediatric tray, this could cause death rather than save a life. Always remove all medications and start anew. Following the prepared list, check all the strengths of the medications and the expiration dates.

that are used in the other departments, except in lower doses, as well as medications that are in suspension form. Labor and delivery departments stock injectables and other drugs meant for labor, contractions, and cesarean births. The tasks of collecting and filling all floor stock medications are part of the daily routine of a technician. As always, it is necessary that all orders be verified and initialed by a pharmacist before they can be delivered to the correct departments.

Another important pharmacy task is the refilling of crash carts. These are trays used by all areas of the hospital. They contain the injectable medications used for a code blue (respiratory distress) situation. Table 11-3 lists examples of the types of commonly used injectable drugs. Pharmacy stocks extra trays in case of a stat call for another tray. The three types of trays are adult, pediatric, and neonatal. Each type of tray contains a different strength of drug. When a tray has been used, the pharmacy technician will take a new tray, retrieve the used tray, and refill the missing contents. Also at this time the technician checks expiration dates on all medications. These dates are listed on a preprinted form. All crash cart medications should always be placed in the tray in the same order.

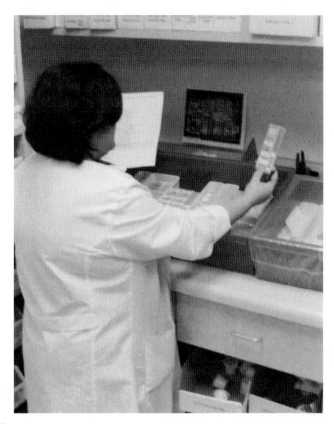

FIGURE 11-6 Refilling a crash cart is done by technicians and is checked by a pharmacist.

BOX 11-2 SPECIAL DEPARTMENTS STOCKED BY THE PHARMACY

Anesthesia	Doctors or nurse anesthesiologists who administer medications used before and throughout surgery
Respiratory	Therapists who administer breathing treatments to hospitalized patients
Injection clinic	Nurses administer adult and pediatric immunizations and also may perform allergy skin tests
Radiology or imaging department	Technicians and physicians may administer dyes for imaging and may need to use a medication cart (known as crash cart) for adverse reactions or incidents

(Figure 11-6) The reasoning behind this is the ability of the nurses quickly to grab a medication. If all crash carts were in a different order, the nurse would have to search for the lifesaving medication. As always, it is necessary that all orders be verified and initialed by a pharmacist before they can be delivered to the correct departments.

Nonclinical Areas the Pharmacy Stocks

Nonclinical areas of a hospital can include areas that a patient never sees or those areas that are used as an in-and-out clinic. Some examples of these special areas of the hospital, along with the types of medications that the pharmacy may be responsible for ordering and stocking, are included in Box 11-2.

Patient Medication Filling

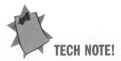

DESCRIPTION

One of the traditional roles of the pharmacy technician is filling the medication orders for hospitalized patients. In the past, the most common way to provide a 24-hour supply of medications for the floors was manually to fill the patient medication drawer for each patient. Once the drawers were filled, the pharmacist verified them against the doctor's orders. The drawers then were taken to the floors where the patients were admitted. Nurses then could get their patients the necessary medication from this drawer. Medications were divided between routine medications, located in the front of the drawer, and as-needed (abbreviated *prn*) medications, which were placed in the back of the drawer. Although some hospitals still use this system, more facilities are implementing automated dispensing systems. Not only do these systems speed up delivery of medication to the patient but also help to ensure accuracy. Some of the automated systems used in hospital settings include PYXIS, SUREMED, and Robot RX. Whereas the robot mechanically fills the drawers quickly and accurately located in the pharmacy, PYXIS and SUREMED are machines that are preloaded with a variety of commonly used medications located on the nursing floor. (Refer to Chapter 8.) The pharmacist needs only to type in the order, and the nurse then can retrieve the medication on the patient's floor by using an access code. Although these systems seem to replace the technician, they require constant filling and updating of new medications daily. Technicians now are trained properly to use these sophisticated computer systems to fill patient prescriptions and to complete many other pharmacy duties.

DUTIES

All medications are delivered to the patient floors using two carts that are rotated daily. Before loading the patients' drawers with the next 24-hour supply, all previous medications should be emptied from the drawer. This is to decrease the possibility of errors. The front of the drawer contains the routine medications and the back contains the as-needed medications. Routine medications are those that have to be taken on a schedule everyday, whereas as-needed medications are those medications that can be taken if needed. For example, most acetaminophen (Tylenol) is ordered as needed for headache or fever; therefore, many as-needed medications are not used for more than one 24-hour period. All bulk items normally are sent to the floor labeled with the patient's name and room number; these items may be left in the drawer. Per pharmacy protocol, certain medications can be sent to the floor as a bulk item. These are medications that contain more than a single dose. Many patients may be taking medications such as Mylanta or Pepto-Bismol. These medications can be sent once to the floor to last for the patient's stay in the hospital. Some medications that are not available in unit dose may be sent as well. For example, a bottle of medicated shampoo is a bulk item. Other pharmacies may make their own unit dose cups from their bulk stock; this would be done by a technician following repackaging guidelines outlined in Chapter 12.

If the hospital uses an automated medication dispensing system, a cart exchange is not necessary. However, these systems do require regular and frequent fillings with new medications; the dispensers throughout the hospital also must be refilled. When a new medication is ordered, it can be entered into the dispensing system computer, which is located within the hospital. This automatically is prompted as the pharmacist or technician enters the order into the terminal.

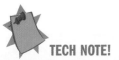

A multiple-day supply is entered and delivered to the unit on the next scheduled round. For example, if a medication given once daily is ordered, a total of five or more doses may be stocked in the dispensing machine. This allows the nurses to access the medications they need without having to wait for the medication cart to arrive each day. All transactions made on a medication dispensing system are recorded, and a receipt is generated. Only receipts for controlled medications are kept as records in the controlled substances room.

Controlled substances also are stocked in the dispensing machines each day. Counting of the controlled substances stocked in the machine is necessary before adding additional doses. The machine generates a receipt after each entry, and is transmitted electronically to the pharmacy computer system.

Pharmacy and Nursing Staff Relationship

The pharmacy staff probably works more with nurses than with anyone else in the hospital. Nurses depend on the pharmacy for all of their medications; they generally make more than 80% of the total calls that come into the inpatient pharmacy. The subjects of these phone calls include inquiries about the status of their patients' medications, as well as requests for information about drug interactions, dosing ranges, and pharmacy calculations. By far the most common question asked of the pharmacy is, "Where are the medications that I ordered?" Any pharmacy technician can answer this question by simply checking the computer system to see whether the medication was sent or checking the orders that have not yet been entered. However, for all other questions, the technician turns the phone over to the pharmacist. Good communication between the pharmacy and the nursing staff can alleviate a lot of anxiety.

Stat and ASAP Orders

Medication orders that need to be filled within minutes are referred to as stat orders. When the pharmacy receives a stat order, it should take precedence over all other orders. Normally, a stat order can be filled in 15 minutes, depending on the preparation time required for the medication. Some stat orders can be filled quickly using stock off the shelf, whereas others may require special preparations, such as the mixing of an intravenous preparation. When this happens, the medication must be made as quickly as possible while using proper aseptic technique. Stat orders are those that literally can mean the difference between life and death; they must be taken seriously. If possible, a stat order should be hand-delivered to ensure that it gets to the correct destination safely and quickly.

An ASAP order is not normally as urgent as a stat order. However, these orders should be put in front of the new orders to ensure fast processing by the pharmacist.

Specialty Tasks

In addition to the previously outlined tasks that technicians commonly perform, there are additional duties that require the skills of a technician. These duties include assisting with clinical duties and anticoagulant therapy tasks. Some hospitals that have nuclear medication pharmacies are using technicians to prepare these medications. These agents may be used in diagnostic procedures. As the role of the pharmacy continues to change, so will the tasks of the pharmacy technician. (For other types of jobs pertaining to technicians, refer to Chapter 3.)

DO YOU REMEMBER THESE KEY POINTS?

■ Duties of a pharmacy technician, including the areas described in this chapter
■ How often medications are supplied to nursing units using a cart-filling method
■ Steps in and frequency of filling automated medication dispensing systems
■ The difference between a centralized pharmacy and a satellite pharmacy
■ Duties involved in ordering and maintaining the stock levels of the pharmacy
■ Hospital areas that the pharmacy stocks
■ Specialty areas of the hospital for which the pharmacy stocks or orders medication
■ Abbreviations of units located within a hospital and the types of service they provide
■ What PAR levels are and who is responsible for maintaining them
■ Different types of hospitals, what differentiates them from one another, and how that affects the overall service that they may provide
■ Which agencies monitor hospitals, including pharmacies within the hospital
■ The various ways that orders are processed by the pharmacy

MULTIPLE CHOICE QUESTIONS

1. Policies and procedures binders contain information pertaining to all of the following except _____.
   A. Employees' weekly schedule
   B. Emergency situations
   C. Training
   D. Daily work routines

2. The JCAHO is an agency that inspects and accredits _____.
   A. Hospitals
   B. Hospital pharmacies
   C. Pharmacists
   D. Both A and B

3. Hospital orders contain which of the following information?
   A. Laboratory orders
   B. Dietary restrictions
   C. Medications
   D. All of the above

4. All of the following information is necessary on a doctor's order except _____.
   A. Patient's name
   B. Patient's room
   C. Patient's next of kin
   D. Patient's medical record number

5. Hospital technicians must be available to _____.
   A. Work various shifts
   B. Work weekends
   C. Fill different jobs per operational needs
   D. All of the above

6. Technicians have all of the following responsibilities except _____.
   A. Printing intravenous labels before filling them
   B. Preparing antibiotics
   C. Discontinuing intravenous medications per doctor's orders
   D. Calling the doctor for order clarification

7. By law, which of the following tasks cannot be done by a technician?
   A. Ordering pharmacy stock
   B. Filling chemotherapy orders
   C. Filling controlled substance orders for schedule III to V medications
   D. Final checking and signing off of orders

8. The following areas are stocked by the pharmacy except _____.
   A. Respiratory therapy
   B. Emergency department
   C. Central supply
   D. Injection clinic

9. Technicians can answer which of the following questions over the phone?
   A. Generic or trade name of drug
   B. Whether or not the drug is in stock
   C. If the drug order has been filled and sent to the floor
   D. All of the above

10. The differences between intravenous therapy and chemotherapy parenteral preparation include all of the following except _____.
    A. The type of flow hood used
    B. Hand placement
    C. Size of the hood
    D. Aseptic technique

TRUE/FALSE If the statement is false, then change it to make it true.

_____ 1. Protocol is policy that is set by the pharmacist on duty.

_____ 2. Hospitals must meet state and federal guidelines if they are to be reimbursed.

_____ 3. Orders written by doctors in a hospital setting are not the same as prescriptions.

_____ 4. Medications normally are placed in see-through ziplock containers for security reasons only.

_____ 5. Only pharmacists can fill orders that are received from the hospital floors.

_____ 6. Technicians need to use aseptic technique only in the chemotherapy hood.

_____ 7. A PAR level refers to the location and capabilities of the pharmacy within the hospital.

_____ 8. All units within a hospital have the same floor stock to treat patients.

_____ 9. Technicians cannot answer any questions that nurses direct to the pharmacy.

_____ 10. It is best to identify yourself as a technician when first answering the phone.

TECHNICIAN'S CORNER

While in the pharmacy, you get an order for Ms. Jen Baranowski. Only her name and her room number are written on the order. The order is for ceftriaxone 1g q6h. This is not the appropriate dosing regimen for this medication.

What information must you have before you can process this order?

What do you do concerning the wrong dosing times for this medication?

BIBLIOGRAPHY

Ansel HC, Allen LV, Popovich NG: *Pharmaceutical dosage forms and drug delivery systems,* ed 8, Baltimore, 2004, Lippincott Williams & Wilkins.

Elkin MK, Perry AG, Potter PA: *Nursing interventions & clinical skills,* ed 3, St Louis, 2003, Elsevier.

WEBSITES

www.hhs.gov
www.redcross.org/
www.vchca.org/mc/medstaff/formularies/HIGHRiskMeds2005.pdf

Repackaging and Compounding

Objectives

UPON COMPLETING THIS CHAPTER, YOU SHOULD BE ABLE TO
DO THE FOLLOWING:

- List the steps in the repackaging of medications.

- List five reasons pharmacies often repackage bulk medications
into unit dose packages

- Describe the proper handling of medications during repackaging.

- Describe the way in which ointments or creams should be packed
into jars.

- List the requirements for assigning expiration dates for unit dose
medication.

- Explain the calculations used to determine expiration dates when
repackaging.

- List the common reasons behind using unit dose medications.

- Define terms used in compounding procedures.

- Describe the equipment used in compounding drugs.

- Differentiate between types of scales used to weigh compounds.

- Explain the correct methods in the preparation and cleanup of
compounding areas.

TERMS AND DEFINITIONS

Blister pack *Container usually made of plastic that holds a single-dose tablet or capsule*

Calibration *The markings on a measuring device*

Compounding *The act of mixing, reconstituting, and packaging a drug*

Cream *A hydrophilic base*

Elixir *A base solution that is a mixture of alcohol and water*

Emulsification *To make into an emulsion, or bind together*

FDA *Food and Drug Administration*

Flocculation *The process by which a solute comes out of a solution in the form of flakes or precipitation; the solute then can be filtered out of the solution*

Hydrophilic *Water loving; any substance that easily goes into water*

Hydrophobic *Water hating; any substance that does not go into or mix in water*

Levigate *To make into a smooth paste or into a fine powder depending on the agent used*

Mortar and pestle *A bowl and rounded knob used to grind substances into fine powder*

Ointment *A hydrophobic product such as petroleum jelly*

Punch method *Filling of capsules by hand with powdered medication premeasured*

Reconstitution *To mix a liquid and a powder to form a suspension or solution*

Repackaging *The act of reducing the amount of medication taken from a bulk bottle; unit dosing is a form of repackaging*

Solute *The ingredient that is dissolved into a solution*

Solution *A water base in which the ingredient or ingredients dissolve completely*

Solvent *The greater part of a solution*

Suspension *A solution in which the powder does not dissolve into the base and which must be shaken before using*

Syrup *A sugar-based liquid*

Tincture *A base solution of alcohol*

Triturate *To grind or crush powder such as a tablet into fine particles*

Unit dose *A single dose of a drug*

REPACKAGING BULK DRUGS INTO UNIT DOSE containers more often is done for hospitals and long-term care facilities. In addition, many patients who have their medications ordered by mail may receive unit dose containers. A hospital usually will prepare unit dose blister packs each of which contains one medication, whereas nursing and home health care facilities may use a bubble pack, which may contain one to several medications for each timed dose. Medication compounding is common in hospital and community pharmacies. Although the types of products compounded may differ, many of the same rules apply for both. This chapter covers both of these skills required by

TABLE 12-1 Example of Good Manufacturing Practice Guidelines

Item	Guidelines
Drugs and labels	All medications must be checked by a registered pharmacist
Equipment	In good condition and clean
Expiration date	6 months or one fourth of the time of the drug's manufacturing date, whichever is less (recently updated to a maximum of 1 year of the manufacturer's expiration date or, if manufacturer's date is less than 1 year, then that date may be given). The bulk container may not have been previously opened.
Package	Appropriate for the drug
Preparation	Not more than one item prepared at a time
Records	All items repackaged are logged for referencing

technicians. Unit dose packaging is discussed first; compounding is discussed in the second half of the chapter.

Repackaging (Unit Dose)

The U.S. Food and Drug Administration (FDA) is responsible for providing guidelines for all manufacturers that package medications. Expiration dates are determined based on tests run by manufacturers and the FDA; however, these rules do not apply to medications repackaged in a hospital setting for individual patient use. The expiration date for repackaging products is set by each state. Items repackaged for use within a hospital or for a specific patient's use cannot be mass-produced. Manufacturing drug companies following FDA guidelines are in the business of mass production. Following are five reasons that a pharmacy repackages a bulk drug into unit dose medications:

1. Certain drugs cannot be bought from a manufacturer prepackaged in unit dose strips. The pharmacy must make its own.
2. The cost of unit dosing certain medications may be cheaper when done by the hospital than if purchased from a manufacturer.
3. Because of the packaging, speed and efficiency is increased.
4. Because of the label on each dose of drug, the chance of errors is decreased.
5. If unit dose medication is not used, it can be put back into stock and used for another patient at a later time.

Whatever the reason, unit dosing makes sense. By using unit dose medications, a hospital saves a substantial amount of money per patient. Although packaging guidelines are not exactly the same between pharmacies and manufacturers, both entities use good manufacturing practices. Good manufacturing practices are FDA guidelines designed to guarantee safe and effective products for the consumer. Table 12-1 lists some of the guidelines that the technician and pharmacist should follow.

DRUGS AND LABELS

Common dosage forms of drugs that normally are repackaged in a pharmacy include oral medications such as tablets, capsules, and liquids. Tablets may be cut in half and repackaged per protocol.

Many different types of computer labeling programs are used to generate unit dose labels in the pharmacy. Usually the pharmacy technician is responsible not only for determining which drugs are needed to replenish the pharmacy

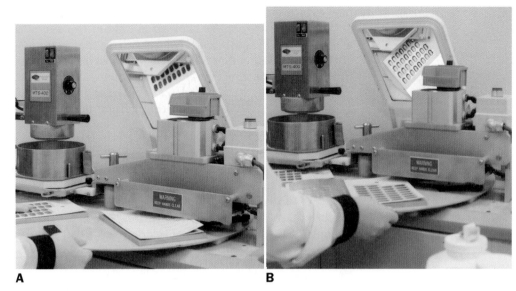

A   **B**

FIGURE 12-1 A technician is responsible for the proper preparation and labeling of all repackaged medications. **A,** The empty medication card is rotated under the hopper where the medication is placed into the card and then rotated to the heating element where the seal is made to enclose each tablet. **B,** The technician uses a mirror to verify that each sheet is filled completely.

stock but also calculating the correct expiration date, documenting the essential components of the drug, generating the labels, and loading the medication. Finally, the pharmacist checks the completed work to ensure that the label, drug, and logging of the medication are correct.

EQUIPMENT

Types of unit dosing equipment vary. Some packaging machines not only fill the unit dose containers but also may generate labels for the drugs and adhere them to the containers as they pass through (Figure 12-1). Other equipment is much less high-tech, and the technician manually places each tablet or capsule into the individual blister pack and adheres the labels. Although this type of repackaging is considered nonsterile, one should take care to keep the process of preparing medications as clean as possible. The process of repackaging should take place in a designated area of the pharmacy, away from high-use areas. This cuts down on air flow over the medication that may cause contamination. All equipment should be kept clean and in good condition. If the technician is using manual methods to load medications into blister packs, it is important that the technician wears gloves after washing his or her hands. If pill counters are used to guide tablets or capsules into their containers, the tray should be washed after each use.

In addition to pill counters, all equipment should be cleaned after use following manufacturer's guidelines. Keeping the area clean and well-organized not only helps avoid contamination of drugs but also reduces the chance of error during repacking.

EXPIRATION DATE

Assigning the expiration date of a repackaged medication is a simple yet important process. Once a bulk bottle is opened, the manufacturer's expiration date is no longer valid. The correct length of time is determined by calculating the

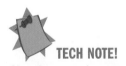

TECH NOTE!

Cleaning counting trays after each use is for protection for the next patient. If residue is left behind on the pill counter and the next patient is allergic to the previously counted medication, it is possible for that patient to have an allergic reaction. When chemotherapy medication is counted, a tray marked for counting chemotherapy should be used to avoid cross-contamination.

new expiration date from the bulk medication. One common and simple way of dating drugs is to set the expiration date at the end of the month. For example, when you are preparing a label for a drug that you have determined will expire at the end of September 2009, you would write 9/09. This means the drug is good through the month of September. Because laws change concerning appropriate expiration dating, two methods are outlined in this chapter; the specific requirements of your state determine the method to use.

Method 1

The life of a repackaged drug is 6 months or one fourth of the manufacturer's expiration date, whichever is less. The best way to determine this number is by determining the number of months that the drug is good for and divide by 4. This gives the exact amount of time the drug is in date. However, if that answer is more than 6 months, the expiration date is set at the least amount of time—6 months. The two examples provided show the calculations for proper dating.

EXAMPLE 12-1 EXPIRATION DATING (6-MONTH VERSION)

Acetaminophen 500-mg tablets Today's date: August 2010
Expires in December 2013 Calculation: 8/10 to 12/13 = 3 years × 12 months
  = 36 months ÷ 4
  = 9 months

You may give this drug only 6 months, or until 2/11.

Method 2

The medication is given a maximum of 1 year as long as it does not exceed the safety margin given by the drug company. If the medication expires in 6 months, then 6 months is the maximum allowable expiration date. For example, a drug that expires in 5 years can be given only 1 year if the drug company's data supports its safety. The bottom line is to remember that the most important aspect of determining the proper expiration date is documentation.

EXAMPLE 12-2 EXPIRATION DATING (1 YEAR VERSION)

Cimetidine 300-mg tablet Today's date: August 2009
Expires in August 2014 Calculation: 8/09 to 8/14 = 5 years × 12 months
  = 60 months ÷ 4
  = 15 months

You may give this drug a 1 year expiration date maximun, it would expire in 8/10.

UNIT DOSE PACKAGING

The types of packages used in pharmacy include liquid cups, vials, blister packs, ziplock bags, and light-resistant bags (Figure 12-2). Each type of container holds specific amounts and types of medications. Liquids normally are placed in bottles, cups, or vials. Tablets and capsules usually are placed in blister packs (Figure 12-3) or vials.

PREPARATION TECHNIQUES

The preparation required to repackage medications is simple. If tablets or capsules are to be unit dosed, the main task is to have enough packages and labels ready for use. In addition to these supplies, keeping medications separate from one another is important. Only one item at a time should be made because leaving multiple drugs on a countertop leads to errors. Part of the preparation of repackaging is accurate calculations for expiration dates and logging the med-

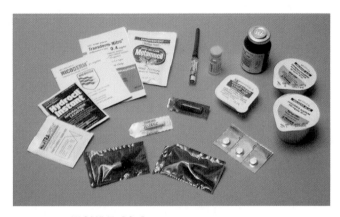

FIGURE 12-2 A sample of containers.

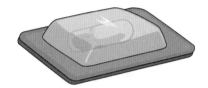

FIGURE 12-3 A sample of a blister pack container.

ications to be prepared in a logbook. Two common types of repackaged medications are the following:

1. Unit dose: one medication per container
2. Monthly supply: typically a 30-day supply; packaged for long-term care facilities or in standard prescription processing.

RECORDS

Keeping track of the products that you are repackaging is one of the major steps that should not be overlooked. Just as manufacturers must know how to find drugs they have packaged, so must the hospital pharmacy. For instance, if a manufacturer recalled a drug that had been repackaged, it is important to have an accurate count of how many unit doses were made and an identifying mark on each of them. Therefore, documentation for repackaged drugs must have the information shown in Table 12-2. Table 12-3 gives a few examples of how the drug manufacturers' names normally are abbreviated. It is important to fit as much information onto the records form and on the medication container. Usually a separate binder is used for record keeping. Figure 12-4 shows a sample of the type of unit dosing log record.

Compounding

Nonsterile compounding consists of compounding medications on a countertop in a pharmacy setting. Figure 12-5 shows a typical work area using a class A balance for weighing powder. Sterile compounding is discussed in Chapter 13. The most common items made in pharmacies are creams, ointments, and oral suspensions. Less common drugs that can be made include capsules, suppositories, and syringes. Only the most common compounding techniques are discussed in this chapter. Table 12-4 lists common compounding guidelines followed in pharmacies.

TABLE 12-2 Example of a Unit Dose Record Log Sheet Information

Item	Description
Date	The date that the drug is made, which includes day, month, and year
Drug	Drug name, usually by generic name then brand name if indicated on log sheet
Dosage form	Tablet, capsule, spansule, troche, liquid
Manufacturer	Manufacturer of the drug, usually abbreviated
Manufacturer's lot number	Control number located on the side of the label or on the bottom of the bottle
Manufacturer's expiration date	Located with the lot number; remember that if the date indicates only month and year, the drug is good through the end of the month
Pharmacy lot number	Each item repackaged in the pharmacy is given a number consecutive to the previously made batch
Pharmacy expiration date	Calculate the new expiration date, which is 6 months or one fourth of the time of the manufacturer's expiration date, whichever is less
Technician	Must initial the logbook entry
Pharmacist	Each item made must be checked off by a pharmacist

The information on the label of the unit dose item is much less than what is required in the logbook, but it is just as important. The following sample lists the components necessary on a typical unit dose label:

Name of drug
Generic name
Trade name (trade name commonly given for the easy identification of the proper medication)
Strength
Dosage form
Pharmacy lot number
Pharmacy expiration date

DRUGS AND LABELS

The types of drugs that can be mixed to produce a customized medication include elixirs, suspensions, ointments, creams, lotions, capsules, tablets, and suppositories. Most pharmacies do not have the staff, supplies, or time to prepare specialized doses of medications. For this type of task there are compounding pharmacies that specialize in this area. However, there is still a fair amount of compounding that the average technician will be exposed to. These are the areas that will be discussed further.

Solutions

There is a wide range of solutions that can be easily prepared for the patient. These include elixirs, syrups, and tinctures. In the preparation of these types of solutions there is no need to place a shake-well label on the container as they easily mix once added together. Flavoring is commonly used to improve the taste. When reconstituting drugs such as an amoxicillin suspension, the label already is attached to the product. All the technician must do is read the side panel and follow the directions for the proper amount of sterile water to be mixed with the powder. The expiration date is marked clearly on the side of the medication and is effective as soon as the suspension is mixed. Therefore, after mixing the drug, you must mark down the expiration date on the front of the label for the patient. In addition to this information, any necessary auxiliary labels must be attached. Table 12-5 lists common auxiliary labels.

TABLE 12-3 Manufacturer Abbreviation Codes

Manufacturer	Code	Manufacturer	Code
3M Pharmaceuticals	3MP	Knoll Laboratories	KNO
Abbott	ABB	Lederle	LED
A H Robins	ROB	Marion Merrill Dow	MMD
Astra	AST	Mead Johnson	M/J
Barr Laboratories	BRR	Merck & Co	MSD
Bausch & Lomb	B-L	Novartis	NVR
Bayer Corp	BYR	Novo Nordisk Pharmaceuticals	NNP
Boehringer Ingelheim	B-I	NovoPharm	NOV
Burroughs Wellcome	BW	Parke-Davis	P-D
Ciba Pharmaceuticals	CIB	Pfizer Pharm	FD
Colgate Oral Pharmaceuticals	COP	Pharmacia & Upjohn	UPJ
Dey LP	DEY	Procter Gamble	P + G
Dupont Pharma	DUP	Purdue Pharma	PUR
Econo Med Pharmaceuticals	ECO	Roche Pharmaceuticals	ORC
Eli Lilly & Co	LY	Roxane Laboratories	ROX
Endo Laboratories	END	Rugby Lab	RUG
Eon Laboratories	EON	Sandoz	SAN
Fujiswawa Pharmaceutical	FUJ	SmithKline Beecham Pharmaceuticals	SKF
G and W Laboratories	G&W		
Geigy Pharmaceuticals	GEI	Taro Pharmaceuticals	TRO
Geneva Pharmaceuticals	GG	Teva Pharmaceuticals	TEV
		Upsher Smith Laboratories	UPS
Glaxo Wellcome	GLX	Wyeth Ayerst	WY
Hoechst Marion Roussel	HMR	Zenith Goldline Pharmaceuticals	Z/G
ICN Pharmaceuticals	ICN		
Johnson & Johnson	J + J		

When reconstituting a suspension, if the manufacturer calls for 110 mL of sterile water to be mixed with the powder in the bottle, you should add only one half of the water at first. This allows the powder to mix with the water, which brings down the volume within the bottle and makes it easier to mix in the remaining amount.

EQUIPMENT

Graduated cylinders (Figure 12-6) come in conical and cylindrical shapes to measure liquids. In addition to proper balances and cylinders, other pieces of equipment commonly used are a mortar and pestle, which are needed to crush tablets and other solid substances into a fine powder to be mixed with other ingredients (Figure 12-7). Mortars and pestles are made of two different substances, glass and porcelain.

If the items that need to be compounded require specialized equipment, often the pharmacy orders the product from another pharmacy that specializes in compounding products.

Compounding in the pharmacy requires many different pieces of equipment. Table 12-6 lists common types of equipment. One of the most expensive pieces is the balance or scale used to weigh powders. Scales differ in their range of

	Date	Drug (generic)	Strength	Dosage form	Amount	MFG	MFG lot#	MFG exp date	Pharmacy expiration date	Pharmacy lot #	Tech	RPH
1	2/11/2007	aspirin	81mg	tab	100	Bayer	JGH405	7/15/2011	Aug-07	A1001	LP	TG
2	2/12/2007	perphenazine	2mg	tab	100	Schering	XYZ124	12/1/2007	Apr-07	A1002	TK	DS
3												
4												
5												
6												
7												
8												
9												

FIGURE 12-4 A unit dose log record.

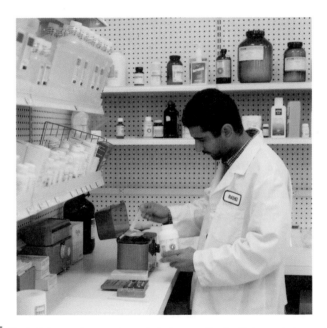

FIGURE 12-5 Technician using a class A balance. Each dial must be set accurately for precise measurement.

TABLE 12-4 **Example of Common Compounding Guidelines**

Item	Appropriateness
Equipment	In good condition and clean
Preparation	Not more than one item to be prepared at a time
Drugs and labels	All medications checked by a registered pharmacist
Package	All containers appropriate for each drug compounded
Expiration date	Cannot be longer than the expiration date of any of the ingredients used to prepare agent
Weighing	All ingredients must be weighed on a pharmacy balance
Meniscus	The concave upper surface of a liquid in a container. Measurement must be read at the bottom of the meniscus (see Figure 12-11)

TABLE 12-5 Common Auxiliary Labels Placed on Medication Containers

Dosage form	Type of auxiliary label
Suspensions	Shake well
Ophthalmic preparations	For the eye
Otic preparations	For the ear
Ointments, creams, lotions	For topical use; for external use
Suppositories	For rectal use; for vaginal use
Patches	Apply to skin

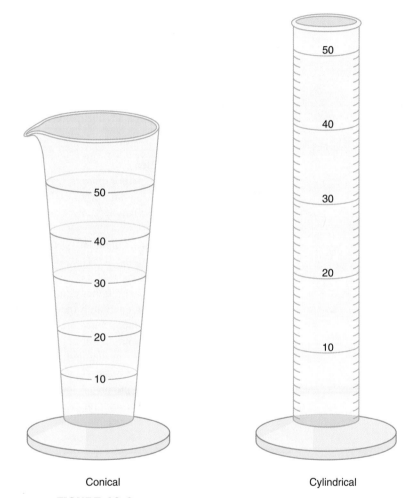

Conical   Cylindrical

FIGURE 12-6 Graduated cylinders for liquid measurement.

weight and style. A class A balance (Figure 12-8, *A*) is required by law and weighs lighter substances between 120 mg and 120 g, whereas a class B balance (optional) weighs heavier substances more than 650 mg. Each scale has special weights that are labeled in milligrams or grams (Figure 12-8, *B*). Class A and B balances are mechanical, using independent weights for reference. Another style of balance is the electronic balance that has a digital readout of the weight. No weights are used with this balance; instead the calibrations are electronic. In either case, appropriate care and cleaning of these sensitive instruments is a must.

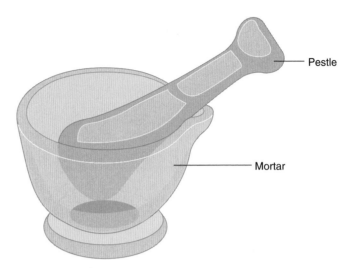

FIGURE 12-7 Mortar and pestle used to crush solids.

TABLE 12-6 Common Types of Equipment Used in Compounding

Equipment	Use
Types of Mortar and Pestles	
Glass	Mixing porous liquids, suspensions, or substances that may stain other containers
Porcelain	Blending powders
Other Compounding Station Equipment	
Filter paper	Used under compounding product to be weighed or as a filter in a funnel
Glycine paper	Used under compounding product to be weighed
Beakers/graduate	A calibrated measuring container used for liquids
Glass stir sticks	Used to stir products such as suspensions
Glass compounding slab	Smooth surface on which to mix ointments and creams
Spatulas	For mixing and filling jars
Blender	For mixing larger products or those that require high-speed or prolonged low-speed blending
Funnel	For filtering or pouring liquids into smaller bottles
Sink	For washing hands, equipment, and countertop
Solvents	For cleaning

EXPIRATION DATES

Several factors affect the stability of a drug. The amount of light, air, temperature, and even pH alters the longevity of a drug. Legally, the date given to a pharmacy-prepared product cannot be longer than any of the ingredients in the product. The pharmacist or the pharmacy technician must find the appropriate expiration date from the manufacturer's literature. In addition to this reference, many compounding books contain calculations that determine appropriate expiration dates.

PACKAGING

The types of containers used for compounded products must be appropriate. The container must protect the contents, have a child-resistant cap (if applicable),

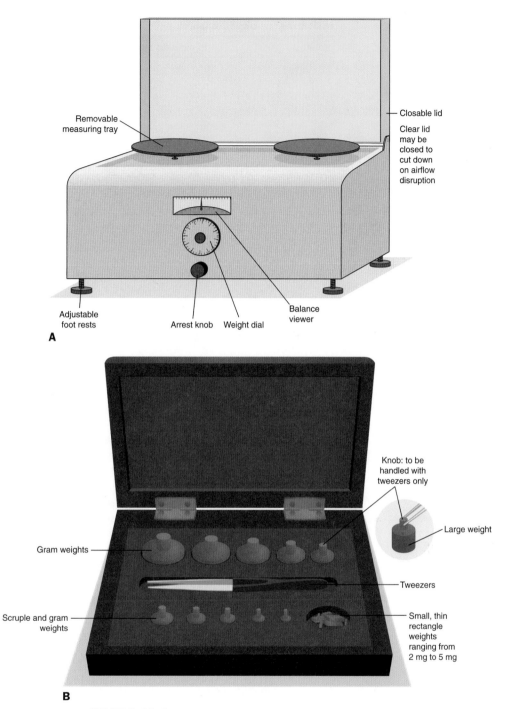

FIGURE 12-8 **A,** Class A balance. **B,** Pharmaceutical weights.

and have the appropriate label(s). Once mixed to the proper concentration, all products are filled into the appropriately sized container. This should be done neatly to avoid waste. Containers vary in size and in manufactured materials, depending on the use of the drug. In addition to the more traditional containers (such as bottles and jars), capsules, suppositories, and syringes also are used, although capsules normally are acquired from the manufacturer. If a physician writes an order for a compound not available by a manufacturer, the pharmacy may have to make the capsules. Eight sizes of capsules are available; each

TABLE 12-7 Capsule Sizes

Number	Approximate amount contained	Example
000	1000 mg	
00	750 mg	
0	500 mg	
1	400 mg	
2	300 mg	
3	200 mg	
4	150 mg	
5	100 mg	

holds a different amount of drug that is measured in milligrams, as shown in Table 12-7.

Syringes sometimes are used to prepare vaginal compounds. Once the drug is loaded into the barrel of the syringe, a cap is placed over the top to keep the contents inside. Suppositories rarely are made in most pharmacies because of the time required. When they are prepared, plastic or metal molds are used to shape the suppositories. The base ingredient of a suppository is usually a combination of cocoa butter, wax, and mineral oil that holds its shape until it reaches body temperature, at which point the drug can be released. Once the suppositories harden in the mold, they can be wrapped, packaged, and labeled for dispensing. Other containers used to package compounded products include glass and plastic bottles, dropper bottles, and jars of various sizes. Jars and syringes are the only two packages that do not have childproof caps or lids.

PREPARATION TECHNIQUES

Most pharmacies have a countertop station set aside for compounding products. At this station all necessary equipment for compounding is kept so that it is readily available. The technician who will be preparing the compounds is responsible to make sure that all items are clean and in good working order. Before compounding, be sure your state allows compounding by a pharmacy technician. The technician should tie back long hair and wear a lab coat and gloves to reduce contamination of the product. In addition to these personal considerations, a technician who is sick or has any open wounds should not make any compounding products. Only one compounding product should be made at a time to decrease the possibility of errors. For commonly compounded items, a recipe book or formula cards listing compounds, their weights, and step-by-step instructions may be used to guide the technician (Figure 12-9).

Additional ingredients that many pharmacies have in stock help reduce the bad taste of a drug and make them look more palatable. Sweeteners for taste, flavorings for smell, and colorings are among the main ingredients of a compounding area. Table 12-8 gives a list of the common additives.

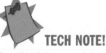

TECH NOTE!

Read all instructions before beginning to compound materials. Make sure that all the ingredients are available to avoid a delay in the product preparation. Also important is to reorder stock after ingredients are depleted so that the ingredients are available for the next time.

Ranitidine suspension		
Formulation ingredients	15 mg/ml	
Ingredients	150 mg tablets	#6
Simple syrup		30 ml
Distilled water		qs to 60 ml
Compounding procedure	1. Pulverize tabs in mortar	
	2. Levigate with a small amount of distilled water to disintegrate the film-coating fragments	
	3. Add, by geometric proportion, the syrup and levigate until a uniform mixture is obtained	
	4. Transfer the contents of the mortar to a conical graduate	
	5. Qs ad to 60 ml with distilled water	
	6. Pour into an amber bottle and shake vigorously	
Auxillary labels	**Shake well**	
	Protect from light	
Stability	1 week at 20 to 30 degrees Celsius	

FIGURE 12-9 A recipe book or formula cards.

TABLE 12-8 Common Additives for Taste and Appearance

Ingredient	Used in
Vanilla, berry	Antibiotics, antihistamines, barbiturates
Lemon	Decongestants
Grape	Electrolytes, antihistamines

If you have any questions on how to prepare a product, ask the pharmacist at the beginning of the compounding process, not in the middle. The only type of compounding that may be done away from the compounding area is the reconstitution of oral suspensions. These products are simple to prepare and do not need to be logged or labeled in the same manner as compounded products.

RECORDS

Just as in repackaging, documentation of compounded medications is important. By keeping accurate records, the integrity of the product dispensed is ensured and falls within FDA guidelines under quality assurance. Although protocol varies between hospital settings, most compounding ingredients and steps are put into a recipe format for the person preparing the medication. Along with the recipe, document the information shown in Box 12-1. Figure 12-10 shows a sample compounding record sheet.

BOX 12-1 INFORMATION NECESSARY ON COMPOUNDING LOG SHEET AND MEDICATION LABEL

Log Sheet Information
Date prepared
Name of ingredients
Manufacturer of each ingredient
Lot number and expiration date of each ingredient (this includes sterile water container, if used)
Amount or weight of each ingredient
Dosage form of each ingredient
Pharmacy lot number assigned
Pharmacy expiration date assigned
Technician's initials
Pharmacist's initials
Date dispensed
Patient's name and medical record number
Documents are kept on the pharmacy premises for no less than 3 years from the time the medication was prepared.

Medication Label Information
Name of patient and medical record number
Date
Drug
Doctor
Sig: Directions
Pharmacy lot and expiration date
Initials of technician and pharmacist

Once the label is affixed to the container, all necessary auxiliary labels are then chosen. Many auxiliary labels not only tell the patient what the intended use for the product is but also indicate the appropriate storage requirements. In addition, some labels allow for expiration dates to be written in.

Techniques for Compounding

WEIGHING TECHNIQUES

TECH NOTE!

Always place the weights on the right side of the balance. This is done to ensure continuity of measurement.

The components of a typical balance in a pharmacy include paper and weights. In the container that holds the weights is a pair of tweezers for grasping the metal weights. This is to prevent the oils from the hands getting onto the metal. Oils corrode the metal, altering the exact weight of the metal. Each balance also has an arrest knob that is used to lock the scale in place, reducing the chance of damage to the balance. The proper setup of a balance requires six steps; each one is critical to obtain the proper weight of a substance. The balance instrument guides are shown in Box 12-2.

MEASURING TECHNIQUES

Pharmacy balances are very sensitive. Regardless of the substance that you are measuring, it is important to keep the air flow around the balance to a minimum.

Product prepared: Ranitidine suspension

Quantity: 60 ml

Pharmacy lot # 100215

	MFG	MFG Lot number	Ingredients	Amount needed	Weighed or measured by	Checked by (RPH)
1	ACH	A08EA	Karo syrup	30 ml	RT	TG
2	AB Inc.	943555	Distilled water	60 ml	RT	TG
3	Glaxo	5ZPT220	Ranitidine	6 tablets		
4						
5						

Explanation of preparation technique: *Crushed 6 tablets of ranitidine 150mg. Added small amount of distilled water, added syrup and mixed well. Then transferred into amber bottle from mortar, then shook bottle well to mix suspension. Applied label and auxillary labels to bottle.*

Date prepared: 6-15-2008

Expiration date: 6-22-2008

Prepared by: *CH*

Approved by (RPH): *LC*

FIGURE 12-10 A sample compounding record sheet.

BOX 12-2 INSTRUCTIONS FOR USING A CLASS A BALANCE

The balance must be steadied on the counter. Every balance has adjustable legs.

Lightweight papers then are added to both sides of the balance to protect the weighing plates and to hold the substance being weighed.

The balance must be "zeroed out" to prevent the paper from being included in the weight of the drug.

At this point the counterweight can be placed on the right side of the balance.

Once the weight is in place, the balance must be set to the proper weight.

The substance to be measured then can be placed on the opposite plate until the two plates balance.

Even the motion of a person walking by can set the balance into a rocking motion, making calibration difficult. Pharmacy balances have a glass lid that can be used to cut off air currents, but it cannot be used easily while weighing compounds. As the balance begins to come into balance, it is important to add less and less substance to the balance. One way of doing this is to use a spatula and pick up a small amount of substance, then lightly tap the side of the spatula (from behind the substance) to flick on a few granules at a time. This technique is easier with powders than with other substances. Compounding is time consuming. It is important to keep the goal of accuracy in mind at all times. Thus you must take your time. Rushing to prepare a compound is a recipe for disaster.

Measuring liquids requires a few simple steps to ensure the proper volume. Because of the water molecules clinging to the sides of a container (called

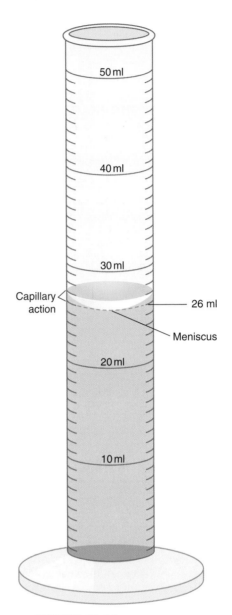

FIGURE 12-11 The meniscus.

capillary action), the amount of liquid appears to be more than the actual amount. When reading the calibrations of a beaker or graduate you must have the liquid at eye level. You must read the graduated cylinder at the bottom of the liquid line, also known as the meniscus as shown in Figure 12-11.

When choosing a vehicle in which to measure your liquids, remember that it is best to choose the container size closest to the volume required because the calibrations are more accurate than in larger containers.

COMPOUNDING TECHNIQUES

Depending on the type of product being prepared, different techniques are required. For each type of compounded product, there are specific steps that must be carefully followed as well as appropriate labeling. Pharmacy technicians often prepare compounded products and should be familiar with the behavior of each type of additive as well as the final product.

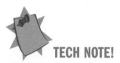

TECH NOTE!

When orders indicate a solution to be a specific strength then to "qs" the solution to a final volume, this means that after the proper strength is prepared, the solution is to be topped off with the additive liquid (such as sterile water) to yield a final volume as ordered by the physician.

Suspensions are different from solutions because they mix a hydrophobic (not water-soluble) ingredient into a hydrophilic (water-soluble) solution. For example, in the case of an amoxicillin suspension, the powdered ingredient is suspended in sterile water after mixing. Therefore, all suspensions must be shaken well to mix the powder evenly, which then can deliver the proper amount of medication. Most suspensions should be mixed by adding one half of the additive solution to the powder, mixing well, and then adding the remaining solution. This ensures thorough mixing. Remember to add the "SHAKE WELL" auxiliary label to the bottle.

Semi-solids

If an ointment is prepared, a hydrophobic base such as petroleum jelly is mixed with the drug. For preparing creams, hydrophilic bases such as Eucerin or Aquaphor creams are used. To prepare a simple mixture of 2.5% hydrocortisone cream in a 50-g Dermabase, follow these steps:

1. Use a mortar and pestle for trituration of tablets or coarse granules for mixture.
2. After properly weighing the base and drug, place the base on the center of a glass compounding slab. Add a small amount of glycerin to the powder (levigate it) to help it mix with the base more easily.
3. Slowly add the powdered drug to the base using a spatula to mix the two components well.
4. Once mixed thoroughly, use the spatula again to fill the medication jar. As the jar is being filled, periodically tap the jar on the counter to compact the contents.
5. When the jar is filled, place the spatula flat across the top of the contents and slowly turn the jar to level off the top and give the final product a professional look.

Solids

For preparation of capsules, the punch method commonly is used. This involves keeping the thickness of the powder in the middle of the compounding slab about one third of the length of the capsule. Then push the opened capsule into the powder, fill the entire capsule with powder, and then attach the other half of the capsule. As you can imagine, this technique is slow and arduous; therefore, most pharmacies order capsules to be prepared by a compounding pharmacy. Some machines load capsules quickly and accurately, saving the pharmacy staff hours of compounding the more difficult drugs.

Solutions

When preparing solutions, you must understand the major parts of the liquid: the solvent is the larger part of the overall solution, the solute is the ingredient or agent used within the solvent, and the solution is the final dosage form that results from these two types. Most solutions are simply mixed by adding the solute to the solvent in portions for proper mixing or by adding two solutions together. One of the most important techniques of mixing solutions is to measure carefully and mix thoroughly. Always check the final solution for any possible precipitation or discoloration that indicates a bad ingredient.

Other types of mixtures

Gels are made by the method of flocculation. These mixtures often include a water or alcohol base along with a solid that is dissolved or suspended into the mixture using a method that enables the solid to evenly mix into the base. These types of medications can be made in the pharmacy but are not as common as the previous ones discussed. In addition, capsules, tablets, and suppositories can be made to deliver medications for both fast-acting or sustained effects.

DO YOU REMEMBER THESE KEY POINTS?

- The proper steps to follow when repackaging medication
- The documentation necessary for repackaged and compounded products
- The proper steps to follow when compounding a product
- The various types of scales that are used in compounding
- How expiration dates are determined when repackaging
- Why pharmacies repackage products
- The various types of equipment used in packaging medications
- The sizes of capsules used in compounding
- Common auxiliary labels used on compounded products
- The various types of containers used in compounding products

MULTIPLE CHOICE QUESTIONS

1. Of the reasons listed, which is not a common reason for repackaging medication?
   A. Cost effectiveness
   B. More competitive against other hospitals
   C. Reusable
   D. Reduction of errors

2. The best description of the guidelines for assigning an expiration date of a repackaged drug is _____.
   A. Half of the manufacturer's expiration date
   B. Less than the manufacturer's date
   C. One sixth of the manufacturer's expiration date or 6 months, whichever is less
   D. One fourth of the manufacturer's expiration date or 6 months, whichever is less

3. Keeping a compounding area clean ensures _____.
   A. Avoidance of contamination of the products
   B. Less chance of errors
   C. Ability to mix several medications at the same time
   D. Both A and B

4. Using the 6-month expiration dating method, determine the expiration date of a drug to be unit dosed that has a manufacturer's expiration date of 3/10. If today's date is 2/09, the drug will expire in _____.
   A. 6/09   C. 3/10
   B. 8/10   D. 3/09

5. Of the information listed, which is not required to be logged into a repack logbook?
   A. The date the drug was made
   B. The patient's name
   C. The initials of the pharmacist
   D. The pharmacy lot number

6. The type of balance(s) that can weigh 10 g of powder accurately is(are) _____.
   A. Class A   C. Both A and B
   B. Class B   D. None of the above

7. The type of mortar and pestle that is best used for grinding coarse granules into a fine powder is(are) _____.
   A. Glass   C. China
   B. Porcelain   D. All of the above

8. A meniscus is best described as _____.
   A. A beaker filled with a small amount of water
   B. Water molecules attaching to the sides of a container
   C. A container used to measure very small amounts of liquid
   D. The lowest level of liquid, which is the point that should be used to measure

9. The arrest knob on a balance is used to _____.
   A. Measure the weight of a compound
   B. Balance the feet of the balance
   C. Adjust the balance's weights
   D. Lock the balance

10. Emulsification is a process that binds_____additives into solutes.
   A. Alcohol
   B. Hydrophilic
   C. Hydrophobic
   D. None of the above

TRUE/FALSE If the statement is false, then change it to make it true.

_____ **1.** Good manufacturing practices are a set of hospital standards on the practices of compounding medications.

_____ **2.** If gloves are worn for repackaging, washing hands is not necessary.

_____ **3.** A unit dose medication delivers only one dose of a drug.

_____ **4.** When compounding, it is better always to place the weights on the same side of the scale.

_____ **5.** Spatulas commonly are used for mixing and for loading compounds into jars.

_____ **6.** Most pharmacies have recipe books for compounded products.

_____ **7.** When compounding, it is not necessary to document the expiration date of all ingredients.

_____ **8.** All mortar and pestles are used for the same purpose.

_____ **9.** Tapping a jar of cream or ointment eliminates smoothing out the top of the compounded product.

_____ **10.** A bulk bottle refers to a compounded or repackaged product made in a pharmacy.

TECHNICIAN'S CORNER

You receive an order for 2.5% hydrocortisone cream in 50 g. You have 2.5% hydrocortisone powder and Dermabase in stock.

What is the strength of the hydrocortisone used (in grams)?
How much Dermabase do you need to equal a total volume of 50 g?
What documentation is required for these items?
What would you place on the label (include auxiliary labels needed)?

BIBLIOGRAPHY

Allen L: *The art, science, and technology of pharmaceutical compounding,* Washington, DC, 2002, American Pharmaceutical Association.
Ansel HC, Allen LV, Popovich NG: *Pharmaceutical dosage forms and drug delivery systems,* ed 8, Baltimore, 2004, Lippincott Williams & Wilkins.
Shargel L, Mutnick A, Souney P et al: *Comprehensive pharmacy review,* ed 5, Baltimore, 2003, Lippincott Williams & Wilkins.

WEBSITES

www.fda.gov/cder/pharmcomp/
www.fda.gov/cder/pharmcomp/survey.htm

CHAPTER

13

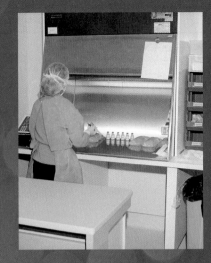

Aseptic Technique

Objectives

UPON COMPLETING THIS CHAPTER, YOU SHOULD BE ABLE TO
DO THE FOLLOWING:

- List the sizes of syringes and needles used in the pharmacy setting.

- Describe how often hoods must be inspected.

- Describe how to care properly for laminar flow hoods.

- Explain the use of aseptic technique within a horizontal flow hood.

- List the types of stock used within an intravenous room.

- Explain the differences between total parenteral nutrition and peripheral parenteral nutrition.

- Describe how properly to dispose of needles, vials, and cytotoxic supplies.

- Describe how to prepare and transport medications in syringes.

- List the medications that must be placed in glass containers.

- Describe aseptic technique within a vertical flow hood.

- List various containers used in the laminar flow hood.

- Explain the anatomy of a syringe and needle.

- Describe five medication delivery systems.

- Demonstrate the seven steps of preparing medications from ampules.

ONE OF THE MOST CRUCIAL RESPONSIBILITIES a hospital pharmacy technician has is the proper preparation of parenteral medications. Preparation of all parenteral medications in a manner that reduces the possibility of contamination is important. This is possible only through the proper manipulation of materials used within the hood. All parenteral and ophthalmic medications should be prepared within a laminar flow hood. Various sizes and types of hoods are available; all are capable of keeping out bacteria and other unwanted particulates if the technician uses proper aseptic technique.

The pharmacy technician may prepare sterile products in settings such as a pharmacy as part of a home health service and pharmacies in long-term care facilities. This chapter predominantly focuses on the technician working in a hospital pharmacy. A wider variety of parenteral medications are used in the hospital than in any other setting. Within the hospital the pharmacy technician is responsible for many daily tasks. Just as pharmacists are required to do everything from processing doctors' orders to performing clinical duties, a pharmacy technician must be versatile to complete the many tasks that will be asked of him or her. Each skill has its own set of guidelines. This chapter explores all types of parenteral medications—the terminology and the equipment commonly associated with them—and the various methods used in their preparation. Parenteral medications are prepared by pharmacies in or associated with hospitals, in long-term care facilities, and in home health clinics. Although these pharmacies may differ somewhat in their overall patient responsibilities, all still use the same techniques, which are outlined in this chapter. One must understand many important aspects of parenteral medications before an order can be filled, including information about inventory processes, the technician's responsibilities, and the variety of abbreviations that are used in medication orders.

Terminology

When doctor's orders are written, it is important to understand the symbols and abbreviations used in filling the prescription. Box 13-1 lists some of the most common abbreviations used for intravenous supplies. Also important is to pay attention to the strength, form, and timing of the dosage, as well as to the route of administration.

Supplies

Before discussing the actual techniques required to prepare intravenous drips, chemotherapy, and other sterile products, one first must learn about the types of supplies necessary for these processes. Many different tools are available, but cost can be the determining factor when pharmacies are choosing the equipment that is best suited for their purposes. For instance, many different types of automated pumps automatically fill intravenous bags and other sterile containers (Figure 13-1). These pumps range in complexity and cost. Usually pharmacies rent the machine and purchase the tubing that is required for that specific pump. Table 13-1 lists common supplies stocked by pharmacy intravenous rooms.

SYRINGES

Syringes used in the pharmacy are available in seven basic sizes: 1-, 3-, 5-, 10-, 20-, 30-, and 60-mL. As the size of the syringe increases, the accuracy decreases (Figure 13-2 gives the anatomy of a syringe). This is important to remember because it is necessary to obtain the exact amount of drug ordered. Syringe tips come in two types. A tension-type syringe comes in a 1-mL volume. In this case the needle is held on by friction only, as seen in Figure 13-3, *A,* and can be used for withdrawing insulin and other medications that require volumes equal to or less than 1 mL. However, tension-type tips cannot be used when preparing chemotherapy doses because of the risk of the needle coming off the syringe and causing a spill or a possible needle stick to the technician. All other sizes of syringes hold their needles in place by a lock mechanism referred to as a Luer-Lok (Figure 13-3, *B*). This ensures a safe seal for the withdrawal of medication.

Most syringes are made of plastic and should be disposed of after one use. Glass syringes may be available in some facilities. Glass syringes rarely are used in the pharmacy, although they can be used when a patient has an allergy to plastics. Glass syringes, unlike plastic syringes, can be sterilized and reused.

Another type of syringe is a Tubex, as seen in Figure 13-4. Tubex syringes can hold a variety of medications and are available in 0.5-mL to 3-mL volumes. The bottom of the syringe is screwed into the Tubex holder. Tubex holders are reusable and normally are dispensed to the nursing units by the pharmacy upon request. The Tubex or Carpujet is disposed of after use.

NEEDLES

Needles are made of aluminum or stainless steel. Needles come in many different gauges (sizes) and lengths, and most are used by nurses to administer injections. The nurse determines which gauge of needle to use depending on the

BOX 13-1   ABBREVIATIONS AND DESCRIPTIONS OF PHARMACY STOCK

Types of Containers Used for Preparing Parenteral Medications	Description of Container and/or Contents
Amp	Ampule; 1- to 50-mL glass container
Vial	0.5- to 100-mL glass or plastic container with a rubber stopper
MDV	Multidose vial; holds multiple doses of medication
SDV	Single-dose vial; holds one dose of medication
Flexible bag	Plastic container (empty or filled with various fluids ranging from 50 to 3000 mL)

Types of Solutions Used/Ordered for Parenteral Agents	
Diluent	Solution used to place medications in solution. Can be sterile water, normal saline (NS), or others
D_5NS	5% dextrose in normal saline
$D_{10}NS$	10% dextrose in normal saline
NS	0.9% normal saline, 0.9% sodium chloride
$\frac{1}{2}NaCl$	One-half normal saline (0.45% sodium chloride)
LR	Lactated Ringer's solution; isotonic solution containing sodium, potassium, calcium, and chloride
$\frac{1}{4}NS$	One-fourth normal saline (0.225% sodium chloride)
$D_5\frac{1}{2}NS$	5% dextrose and 0.45% normal saline contained in the same bag of solution*
SW	Sterile water, usually used to reconstitute
D_5W	5% dextrose in water
$D_{10}W$	10% dextrose in water

Routes of Administration for Parenteral Agents	
IV	Intravenous; into the vein
IV push	Into the vein quickly and forcefully
IM	Intramuscular; into the muscle
ID	Intradermal; upper layers of the skin (up to 1 mL)
SQ, SC	Subcutaneous; under the skin
IT	Intrathecal; into a sheath, such as the lumbar sheath located at the base of the spine

Miscellaneous Terms Used Concerning Parenteral Medications	
On call	Doctor wants dose to be ready when he or she decides to give the medication; most anesthesiologists order preoperative medications as on call
NPO	Nothing by mouth
Pre-op	Medication ordered is to be given before surgery; usually sedative/antiemetic
Post-op	Medication to be given after surgery
PRN	Medication is to be given as needed
QS	Quantity sufficient; adding enough diluent or medication to attain the correct amount needed
Drip or infusion	Usually an intravenous bag greater than 500 mL that runs over a specified amount of hours

*Normal saline comes in many different combinations of dextrose to saline.

injection site. In the pharmacy, needles are used to draw solutions into a syringe, not to administer medications to patients. A limited number of needle gauges are available in the pharmacy, and the larger-gauge needles make drawing medications easier. Choosing an appropriately sized syringe is more important for the pharmacist or technician than determining the correct needle gauge. The rule to remember in sizing needles is that the gauge (size) number of a needle

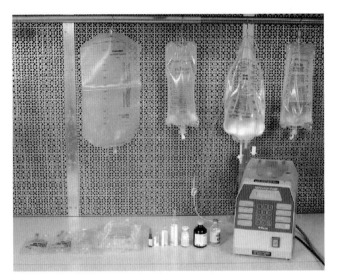

FIGURE 13-1 Supplies used with parenteral medications. These are sterile containers ranging from large-volume intravenous bags *(top)* to small intravenous piggyback bags, ampules, and vials *(bottom)*. The automated system shown pumps preset volumes from large-volume bags into vials *(bottom right)*.

TABLE 13-1 Commonly Used Intravenous Room Supplies

Supplies	Common description
70% isopropyl alcohol	Antiseptic for cleaning hood
Alcohol pads	Alcohol on pads for convenience
Ampule breaker	Plastic device; one end smaller for small ampules, other end for larger ampules; helps to prevent crushing the glass or cutting oneself when opening ampules
Filter needles	A needle that includes a filter that eliminates glass from entering the final solution when drawing from an ampule
Filter straws	For pulling medication from ampules
Filters	Used for specific medications to trap particles 5 to 0.22 μm from entering intravenous fluids
Male/female adapter	Universal size; fits a syringe on each end for mixing the two contents
Syringe needles	The most common bore sizes used in pharmacy are 16 to 20 gauge
Syringe caps	A sterile cap used to prevent contamination of syringes during transportation out of pharmacy
Syringes	Instrument that holds between 0.3 to 60 mL for administration of medications
Transfer needles	A needle on both ends used to transfer a vial to a bottle
Tubing for pumps	Tubing is specific for manufacturer's machine
Tubing transfer sets	Blood transfer sets; used to transfer large containers into empty containers
Mini spike	Large spike that is pushed into vial with a syringe attachment at the other end
Forceps	Instruments that lock; used to close off tubing while transferring medications

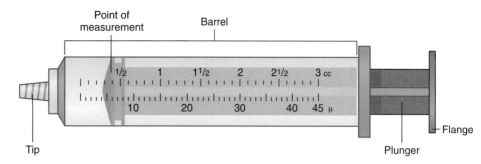

FIGURE 13-2 Anatomy of a syringe. As the syringe decreases in size, the calibrations (volume markers) become larger, allowing a more accurate dosage.

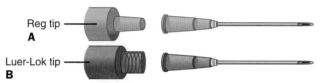

FIGURE 13-3 Two types of syringes. **A,** Reg tip syringe. The regular tip is held in place by pressure as seen in the 1-mL syringe. **B,** The Luer-Lok syringe has spirals to secure the needle as seen on a larger 3-mL syringe.

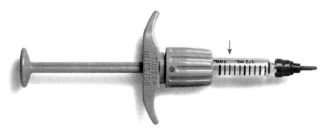

FIGURE 13-4 Tubex holders are meant to be reused. They hold the disposable Tubex or Carpujet cartridges. Each cartridge is prelabeled with the medication name, strength, volume, and concentration. The pharmacy stocks holders and cartridges.

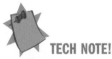

TECH NOTE!
You should not wipe needles with alcohol. If you touch the needle with alcohol or something unintended (such as the outside of a vial), the needle must be discarded and replaced with a new one.

is inversely proportional to the bore (opening) size of the needle. This means that as the bore size increases, the gauge decreases. For example, a 25-gauge needle has a much smaller opening than a 19-gauge needle. In the pharmacy setting the most common sizes used for preparing intravenous medications are 19 gauge, 18 gauge, and 16 gauge, which are used to draw medications from vials or other containers (Figure 13-5). The length of these needles is normally 1 to $1\frac{1}{2}$ inches. One must remember that as the bore size increases, the risk of coring the vial rubber stopper increases. When a vial is cored, a chunk of rubber is dislodged and may fall into the vial. To avoid coring, the bevel edge should face upward. If coring does occur, a filter needle must be used to prevent the piece of cored rubber from entering the intravenous solution.

The anatomy of a needle can be seen in Figure 13-6 and should be memorized because it is necessary to know which areas cannot be touched when assembling needles to syringes within a laminar flow hood. No part of a needle below the hub should be touched. The point and shaft must remain sterile.

FILTERS

Different types and sizes of filters can be used when preparing parenteral medications. The smallest filter is the 0.22-μm filter, which removes all unwanted

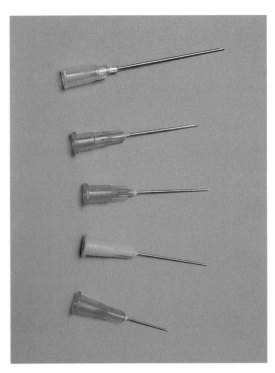

FIGURE 13-5 Needle sizes shown range from *(top to bottom)* 19 gauge, 20 gauge, 21 gauge, 23 gauge, and 25 gauge. Technicians may use a 19-gauge needle for small volumes such as 1 mL or less. Larger gauges *(not shown)* include 18 gauge and 16 gauge for larger volumes.

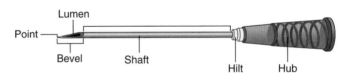

FIGURE 13-6 Anatomy of a needle.

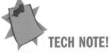

TECH NOTE!

To use a filter needle, first pull the solution into the syringe using a regular needle, replace the needle with a filter needle, and then push the solution through the filter into the intravenous container. When using a filter straw, withdraw the solution, and then place a regular needle on the syringe before pushing the solution out.

particles larger than 0.22 μm (thousandths of a millimeter) from the solution. Another type of filter is the filter straw. This strawlike needle can take a large amount of solution quickly, sifting it through a filter located in the hub of the needle. The filter straw often is used to remove any fine particles of glass from an ampule.

STOCK LEVELS

All of the items stored in the intravenous room of the pharmacy must be kept in stock and at their minimum levels at all times. Before and after each shift, the intravenous technician is responsible for reordering and restocking the intravenous room for the next shift. Many intravenous supplies can be ordered from the central supply area of the hospital and will arrive by the next shift. However, in cases in which the manufacturer or a centralized distribution center is located off site, delivery can take from 2 days to 1 week. Therefore the technician ordering stock must know how long the shipment normally takes to arrive so that the pharmacy will not run out.

Many intravenous antibiotics are available in premade bulk packs; 12 or 24 come frozen in boxes. Although they are convenient, they are more expensive than having technicians make intravenous stock. Most of the time, technicians make extra IVs to be used throughout the week. Intravenous medications can be frozen, but each box must be marked with the date of reconstitution as well as the expiration date, which is determined by using the manufacturer's information. Once intravenous medications are thawed, they must be marked with the new expiration date, also determined by the manufacturer. Large, temperature-controlled refrigerators may be used to store thawed intravenous medications and to recycle medications. Antibiotics and other medications that are in multiple-dose vials can be stored in the refrigerator, sometimes for days, and used day to day.

Medication Delivery Systems

Many different types of containers are used to deliver medications. Such containers are developed to be stable and easy to use. Also, because many of the medications are not premade by the manufacturer and must be made in the pharmacy, it is important to determine whether the medication will be wasted if the treatment is not given to the patient. Once the medication is reconstituted, it must be used within a certain time or it expires and money is lost. Sometimes, the drug may not be given to the patient for whom it was prepared; the doctor may have decided to use a medication of a different dose, type, volume, or solution. This type of waste only adds to the high costs of health care. Therefore, if methods can be devised that can decrease this waste, pharmacies will adopt these methods. Of course, sometimes methods of reducing waste are costly. However, as new innovative methods are created and adopted, the cost will decrease. The following examples show the types of delivery systems used in pharmacy.

PIGGYBACK CONTAINERS

Flexible bags and bottles are the two main types of piggyback containers. Containers can be purchased prefilled with solutions or empty for use in preparing a custom intravenous solution. The sizes and types of piggyback containers and solutions vary from 50 to 500 mL. Some medications, such as insulin, cannot be placed in viaflex bags and must be put into glass containers. Examples of specialized containers used for medication dispensing include large- and small-volume drips, syringe pumps, and miscellaneous dispensing systems.

Large- and Small-Volume Drips

Large-volume drips include viaflex bags in three sizes: 1, 2, and 3 L. Bottles are available in various sizes up to 1 L. These can deliver a variety of fluids, including parenteral nutrition. Parenteral nutrition is a combination of essential nutrients that is administered through a drip system over several hours or up to 24 hours. These will be discussed later in the chapter. The sizes of small-volume piggyback containers and solutions are available in 50, 100, 150, 250, and 500 mL. Small-volume drips can be piggybacked onto large-volume drips as seen in Figure 13-7.

SYRINGE PUMPS

Technicians also may prepare syringes that are placed into a pump that dispenses medications over time. These pumps can be set for short or long durations, not to exceed a 24-hour period. These pumps often are used to dispense controlled substances at a specific rate of infusion. Another type of syringe dispensing system relies on gravity for delivering the solution.

VOLUTROL SYSTEMS

Another type of administration system holds a specific volume within a chamber. This system allows the nurse to administer small amounts of medication over a

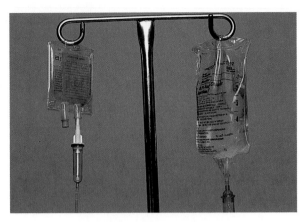

FIGURE 13-7 This gravity pump system intravenous piggyback setup shows a 100-mL viaflex container *(left)* piggybacked to a large-volume 1-L IV *(right)*.

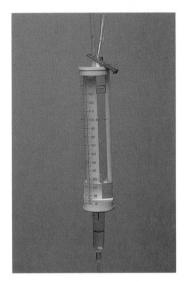

FIGURE 13-8 Volutrol drip systems are used mostly for pediatric patients. Nurses prepare these.

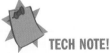

TECH NOTE!

All dosage forms of controlled substances that are delivered to nursing floors must be signed out of the pharmacy stock and into the floor stock of the receiving station. These documents are maintained, and all controlled substances should be counted at the end of every shift to account for all narcotic use or waste.

predetermined period. Macrodrip and microdrip chambers are available; the microdrip chambers are used most often for pediatric patients. An example is given in Figure 13-8. Patients who require analgesics after major surgery or those persons who are in hospice normally have their medications prepared in the pharmacy. Within the hospital setting, nursing stations stock various strengths of controlled substances aimed at relieving extreme pain. Depending on the doctor's order, the nurse can prepare intramuscular or IV push doses from the controlled-substances cabinet. For those patients who require large volumes of morphine sulfate or patients who are sent home with strong analgesics, the pharmacy technician prepares the medications. As mentioned previously in the section on containers, syringe pumps and controlled analgesic devices are two common types of devices that can be used to load controlled substances. Many controlled substances also are prepared in viaflex bags and are dispensed to the nursing floor after being documented on the controlled substances board.

CONTROLLED ANALGESIA DEVICE AND PATIENT-CONTROLLED ANALGESIA PUMPS

Another type of device that can be used to administer controlled substances is a controlled analgesia device. Moreover, patient-controlled analgesia is a method

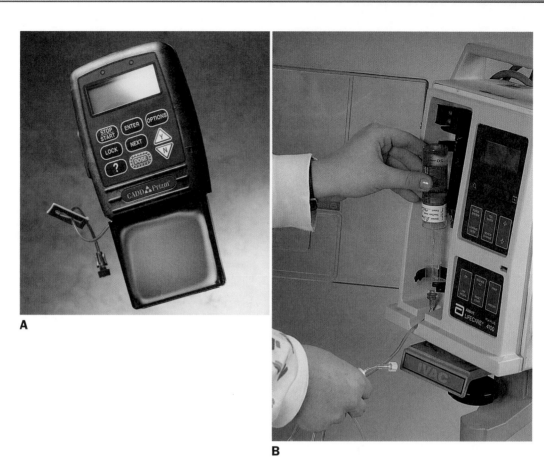

FIGURE 13-9 A, Controlled analgesia device pump. **B,** Patient-controlled analgesia pump.

of supplying analgesics that allows the patient to control the rate at which the drug is delivered for the relief of pain, usually using an infusion pump. These devices can be used within a hospital setting, or the patient may wear the cassette home, which is one of the biggest advantages of the device. Figure 13-9 shows examples of both. Tubing is connected to a catheter plug that automatically dispenses medication. An additional bolus may be programmed into the pump. A bolus is a preset amount of drug that can be administered by the patient when his or her pain intensifies. The patient has access to a button located at the end of a cord attached to the controlled analgesia device; when depressed, the button triggers the administration of additional medication. Because the boluses are preset for amount and frequency, even if the patient presses the button many times, he or she will receive only the predetermined amount of drug. This safeguards the patient from overdosing.

VIALS

Many types of vials, such as the ADD-Vantage system (Figure 13-10), can be placed onto a small piggyback solution via an adapter; these are not mixed with the solution until right before it is administered. The pharmacy technician is responsible for the proper attachment of the vial to the proper solution, but the nurse is the person responsible for breaking the adapter seal between the vial and the piggyback and mixing the drug with the solution. The advantage of this system is the avoidance of wasted medication.

Controlled-release infusion system is another type of delivery system in which the vial is reconstituted (mixed) but is not added to the piggyback. At the time of administration, the vial is attached to a special port on the side of the

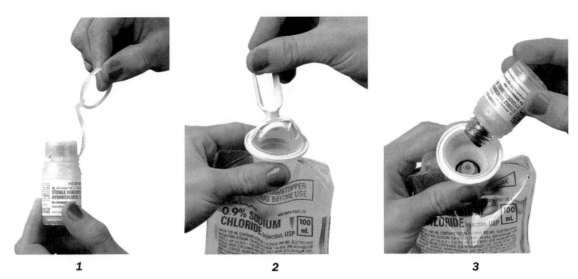

FIGURE 13-10 ADD-Vantage system: To prepare IV, follow the three steps listed. *1,* Take off the vial top. *2,* Pull up flange, removing the seal on the intravenous bag. *3,* Screw the vial into the port. Do not break the seal between vial and bag.

tubing set that allows the medication to enter the piggyback, where it then is delivered into the patient's bloodstream.

Aseptic Technique

All parenteral medications must be prepared using aseptic technique. Normally, nurses do not have the advantage of using a laminar flow hood; however, they too need to use strict aseptic technique. Aseptic technique goes hand in hand with universal precautions. Universal precautions are guidelines followed by all health care workers when dealing with body fluids or blood products. These precautions are used to keep contamination from occurring by a product or to a product. Aseptic technique is a set of guidelines used by nurses when they prepare intravenous treatments outside a laminar flow hood; technicians who use a laminar flow hood for preparing certain agents also must use aseptic technique. For technicians, the importance of using aseptic technique cannot be stressed enough. A medication that contains any microbes or unwanted debris can cause a dangerous infection, or even death, when it is administered into a patient's vein. Steps used in aseptic technique begin with washing hands as shown in Figure 13-11; follows with proper donning of gloves (Figure 13-12), gowning, hood cleaning, then preparation of the parenteral medication. These aseptic techniques are outlined in Box 13-2.

HOOD CLEANING AND MAINTENANCE

Depending on the type of sterile product being prepared, there are two main types of hoods used, a horizontal or a vertical flow hood. A horizontal flow hood is used for many types of parenteral medication preparations or sterile product mixtures. For all chemotherapeutic agents, only a vertical flow hood should be used because of the direction of the airflow and the specifications of the hood. A vertical flow hood can be used to mix nonchemotherapeutic agents if needed; however, chemotherapeutic agents should never be mixed in a horizontal flow hood. All hoods used in the pharmacy for preparing sterile products should be inspected yearly by an authorized inspector to ensure the effectiveness of the filtering system. The direction of airflow in each type of hood is shown in Chapter 11 (Figure 11-4).

In a horizontal flow hood, the outside air flows into the back of the hood, through a special filter, and out toward the opening. This special filter is a high-

TECH ALERT!

Did you know that all rooms are highly contaminated with microscopic debris such as dust? Droplets from sneezing can attach themselves to dust particles and remain in the air for weeks. If these contaminants get into a medication that is intended for intravenous use, they can cause infections, or worse. The intravenous route is the most dangerous to a patient because it bypasses our most protective barriers and directly enters the bloodstream.

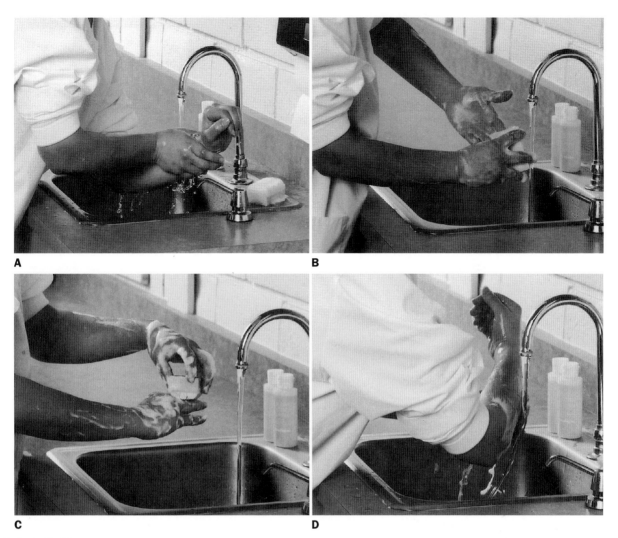

FIGURE 13-11 **A,** Wet hands and arms with warm water. **B,** Scrub top and bottom of hands. **C,** Scrub between fingers and up to the elbow. **D,** Rinse arms and hands thoroughly. Foot pedals may be used rather than handles.

efficiency particulate air (HEPA) filter that traps all particles larger than 0.2 μm. The sides of the hood and items within the hood create a disruption of airflow. For this reason, the technician must work 6 inches in from the sides and front of the hood. Also, movement within the hood should be kept to a minimum to decrease disruption of airflow. Box 13-3 gives an example of cleaning a horizontal flow hood.

In a vertical flow hood, the concept is similar, although air cannot be released back into the room. For this reason, vertical hoods have a Plexiglas shield that separates the technician from the inside work surface. The air comes into the HEPA filter and then into the workspace area. A grid at the front of the tabletop draws in the air and filters it once again through a HEPA filter before it is released out into the open or is vented to the outside, depending on the type of venting system used. The vertical flow hood should be cleaned as follows:

1. Wet a 4 × 4-inch gauze pad or other disposable cloth with 70% isopropyl alcohol and wipe down the inside of the hood. This includes the back, sides, and tabletop. Do not spray the ceiling inside the vertical hood because this is where the filtering system is located.
2. Start on the (inside) back of the hood and wipe from the top right across to the left-hand side, drop down a few inches, and then back across the wall to the other side. Continue this until the back wall is wiped completely.

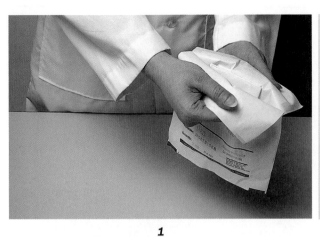

1

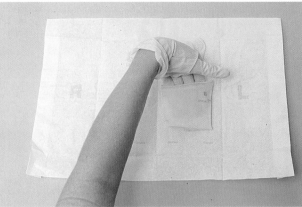

4

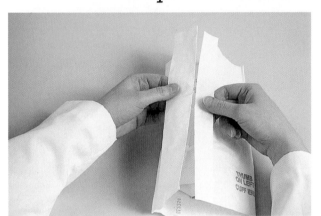

2

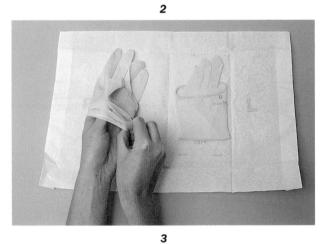

3

FIGURE 13-12 Steps for proper sterile gloving. *1,* Open glove packet. *2,* Open glove cover without touching gloves. *3,* Holding cuff of glove, pull glove over hand. *4,* Slide gloved hand under the cuff of the second glove. Carefully pull on glove.

3. Then repeat the cleaning procedures, working from the top right-hand side, across the tabletop, and up the other side until the whole hood is done.

4. In addition to the sides, tabletop, and back of the vertical flow hood, you also should wash down the inside of the Plexiglas protective shield.

BOX 13-2 TWELVE ASEPTIC TECHNIQUES FOR TECHNICIANS*

1. Do not wear jewelry in the hood. This includes artificial nails because of microbial growth around or underneath the nails.
2. Tie back long hair away from the face.
3. Wash hands after entering the intravenous area and before entering the laminar flow hood (Figure 13-11).
4. Wash hands, wrists, and arms to the elbow with antimicrobial soap and hot water for at least 30 seconds; no more than 90 seconds.
5. Gloves can be worn but should be washed down with 70% isopropyl alcohol after being put on.
6. Wash down the surface of the hood with 70% isopropyl alcohol using proper method (explained earlier in this chapter).
7. The hood must run at least 30 minutes before placing medications inside.
8. Wipe down all vials and ports with alcohol. They should not be sprayed because the alcohol can make contact with the filter in the back of the hood, which breaks down the filter.
9. Hands or any object within the hood cannot block the airflow at any time.
10. Work at least 6 inches into the horizontal hood; keep pens and other objects out of the hood.
11. Dispose of all needles, syringes, vials, and other by-products in proper receptacles.
12. No sneezing, talking, or coughing can be directed toward the airflow in a laminar flow hood.

*Sanitation of hands is found in Appendix F.

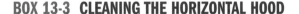

BOX 13-3 CLEANING THE HORIZONTAL HOOD

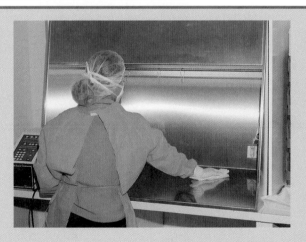

- Before cleaning the laminar flow hood, properly don an appropriate gown. Remove all items from the hood before cleaning.
- Moisten a 4 × 4-inch gauze or other disposable cloth or gauze with 70% isopropyl alcohol and wet down the inside of the hood. This includes the sides and tabletop. Make sure you do not spray the high-efficiency particulate air filter at the back or the ceiling inside the hood.
- Then, starting from the top right-hand side of the hood, wipe down, across the surface, and up to the top of the left-hand side of the hood.
- Moving forward a few inches, repeat the motion in the opposite direction.
- The side-to-side, back-to-front motion is essential for cleaning before use of the hood each day. In addition, clean the hood periodically throughout the course of the day to ensure a sterile environment.

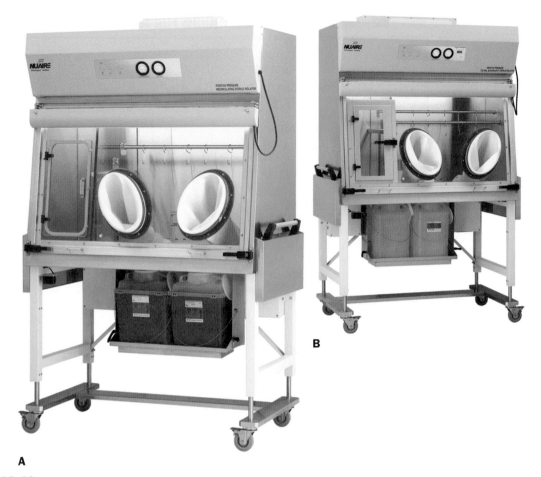

A

B

FIGURE 13-13 NuAire PharmaGard Systems. The technician never comes into contact with the contents within the hood. This minimizes the possibility of cross-contamination more than a traditional high-efficiency particulate air filter flow hoods. **A,** PharmaGard PR (positive pressure) hood is made specifically for the handling of nonhazardous drugs. **B,** PharmaGard NR/NTE (negative pressure) is made especially for the handling of hazardous drugs. This automated compounding system can be installed into the PharmaGard PR hood for larger tasks.

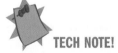

TECH NOTE!

To find out more about special glove box hoods, visit these websites: *www.NuAire.comb, www.Isotechdesign.com, www.pharmacy.com, www.isolators.com,* and *www.gloveboxes.com.*

BARRIER HOODS

Another type of hood for preparing intravenous medications is totally enclosed (Figure 13-13, *A*) and is referred to as a glove box or barrier isolator. This type of hood reduces the risks of contamination caused by accidental mishandling of drugs while compounding and environmental microbial contaminants, thus increasing the sterility of the product being prepared. This ultimately protects the patients from possible harmful medications. The air is redirected through a HEPA filter and uses an additional airflow system to help decontaminate the medication preparation. This type of hood has no horizontal flow.

After the technician washes his or her hands in the appropriate method outlined and after cleaning the hood, the technician can place all of the necessary materials and medications needed inside a holding chamber. After a disinfecting period, the technician may take the materials from the sterile chamber and transfer them into the main hood. At this point the technician may prepare the medication using the attached gloves. Almost any medication can be prepared in this type of hood except chemotherapeutic agents, which require specialized filtering. This type of totally enclosed hood is discussed in the chemotherapeutics section. Although these types of hoods are relatively new to pharmacies, they most likely will be incorporated into more locations that prepare a large volume of medications. For preparation of large quantities or volumes of intravenous medications, the NuAire Barrier has an automated compounding system (Figure 13-13, *B*).

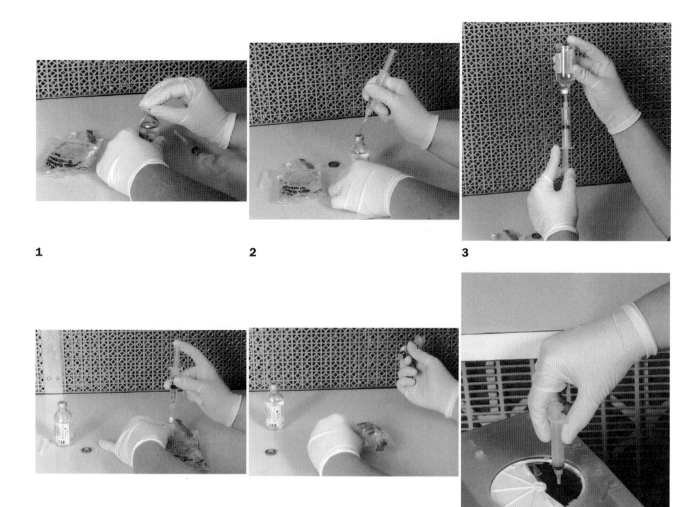

1 2 3

4 5 6

FIGURE 13-14 The six-step process of aseptic technique in the hood is as follows:

1. Using alcohol, swipe the top of the vials and the ports on the intravenous bags from back to front (move around the vial and bag rather than over or behind).
2. Place the needle bevel side up and push it into the rubber stopper of the vial. Preload the syringe with the necessary amount of air to replace solution.
3. Invert the vial and syringe 180 degrees. Push in the air from the syringe and pull out the solution.
4. After removing the syringe from the vial, insert the needle into the intravenous bag and inject the medication using a steady hand.
5. After injecting the intravenous bag with the medication, immediately flip the bag over. This decreases the possibility of forgetting which bags have been injected and which ones have not.
6. Never recap the used needles; instead, throw away each syringe in a sharps container along with the uncapped needle after use. Syringes cannot be reused when changing from one drug to another. This decreases the chance of drug-to-drug contamination.

HAND PLACEMENT

Regardless of which type of hood is used, the placement of the hands is one of the most important aspects to consider when preparing sterile medications. One should practice some simple yet important techniques. These techniques decrease the possibility of contamination and errors when preparing sterile products. Figure 13-14 outlines the necessary steps to take when working in the hood.

TABLE 13-2 Example of Suggested Dosing Times, Solutions, and Appropriate Volumes for Antibiotics

Generic name	Trade name	Common dosing regimens (in hours)	Common solutions	Common volumes
Ampicillin	Omnipen	q8-q6	NS	Less than 1.5 g (50 mL), more than 1.5 g (100 mL)
Cefazolin	Ancef, Kefzol	q8-q6	D$_5$W or NS	Less than 2 g (50 mL), more than 2 g (100 mL)
Cefotaxime	Claforan	q6-q12	D$_5$W or NS	Less than 2 g (50 mL), more than 2 g (100 mL)
Ceftazidime	Fortaz	q8-q6	D$_5$W or NS	Less than 2 g (50 mL), more than 2 g (100 mL)
Ceftriaxone	Rocephin	q8-q24	D$_5$W or NS	Less than 2 g (50 mL), more than 2 g (100 mL)
Doxycycline	Vibramycin	q12	D$_5$W or NS	250 mL
Erythromycin	E-Mycin	q6-q24	NS	250 mL* 10 mg/20 mg lidocaine
Gentamicin	Garamycin	q8-q18[†] based on glycosidic levels	D$_5$W or NS	Less than 100 mg (50 mL), more than 100 mg (100 mL)
Imipenem-cilastin	Primaxin	q6-q12	NS	Less than 500 mg (100 mL), more than 500 mg (250 mL)

D$_5$W, 5% dextrose in water; *NS,* normal saline.
*Erythromycin stings when given intravenously; therefore, it commonly is mixed with lidocaine to kill the pain.
[†]See Chapter 23 for more on antibiotics.

CLEANUP

Once the technician has finished using the hood area, he or she should clean up all unused materials and discard any empty or used products. Wiping down the hood countertop should be the final step in the cleanup, preparing it for the next product to be processed. In a vertical flow hood there are several steps that must be taken to maintain a sterile environment. These steps are detailed under Chemotherapeutic Agents later in this chapter.

PARENTERAL ANTIBIOTICS

Manufacturers have suggested guidelines for dosing regimens that most doctors follow. As shown in Table 13-2, the manufacturer's guidelines are determined by which microbe is being attacked. Pharmacies have a chart that instructs the person preparing the medication as to the type and amount of diluent needed, the normal dosing times, and expiration dates. Antibiotics also differ in how they should be prepared and how long it takes for the powder to dissolve in the diluent. Once the drug is reconstituted, the solution should be checked for color and clarity.

Use of Ampules to Prepare Medications

Intravenous push or intramuscular medications can be prepared by the nurse at the nursing station or at the patient's bedside; however, the pharmacy does prepare some IV push and intramuscular medications. These agents are placed in a syringe and sealed with a syringe cap until it is time to administer the medication. One must follow seven procedures when preparing these syringes from

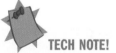

TECH NOTE!

Each type of medication has its own unique properties. For example, ceftazidime produces gas when reconstituted. Therefore, to prevent the solution from shooting out of the vial, the gas must be released first. This can be done by puncturing a needle into the vial. Erythromycin is difficult to get into solution form; therefore, it is important to allow additional time when reconstituting erythromycin. Let the vial sit in the hood (shaking it every so often) until the powder turns into a solution. These are the types of details that one learns over time in the pharmacy.

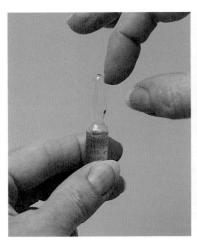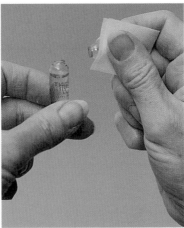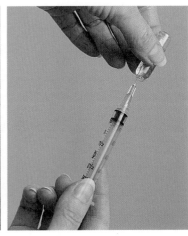

FIGURE 13-15 Ampule sizes range in from 1- to 50-mL glass containers. For larger ampules, an ampule breaker is suggested. For smaller ampules, follow these steps: (1) Tap top of ampule to empty top of container. (2) Using an alcohol swab, wipe the neck of the ampule and snap open (away from you). (3) Tilt the ampule at an angle (the solution will not come out) and withdraw needed amount of drug.

ampules, procedures that differ from using a vial. These steps are outlined next and in Figure 13-15:

1. The liquid inside the ampule must be untrapped from the tip of the ampule by snapping, tapping, or whipping the ampule around in a half circle to force the liquid from the tip. Only then can you proceed.
2. When breaking an ampule, you can use an ampule breaker or wrap an alcohol pad around the neck of the ampule and snap at the narrowest point. This decreases the possibility of crushing the ampule or cutting your fingers.
3. If the drug is taken from an ampule, you must use a filter needle to remove all microscopic pieces of glass that can remain at the bottom of a broken ampule.
4. Syringes cannot be transported from the pharmacy with needles attached; therefore a sterile syringe cap must be adhered to the tip of the syringe.
5. Syringes must be flagged with a label. This may involve cutting the label down so that it fits the length of the barrel of the syringe.
6. When flagging a syringe, do not cover the calibrations on the side of the syringe; the nurse must be able to see how many milliliters are in the syringe.
7. Never fill a syringe to the maximum when preparing an intramuscular or IV push syringe. The nurse must have some room to pull back the syringe before injecting the medication.

Other injectables are available premade from the manufacturer, including Tubex ampules. These are stocked in the pharmacy and are dispensed by request by the nursing station or area.

HYPERALIMENTATION

Hyperalimentation (also known as hyperals) are large volumes of parenteral medications normally made for persons who cannot take in nutrition orally (they cannot eat). Reasons for this inability to eat can range from recent stomach or intestinal surgery to various conditions that affect the gastrointestinal system. Two main types of hyperalimentation are prepared in the pharmacy: total parenteral nutrition (TPN) and peripheral parenteral nutrition. In a hospital setting, after the initial hyperalimentation is prepared and hung, daily laboratory tests of electrolyte levels are drawn from the patient to determine necessary changes. For example, if a patient's potassium levels begin to drop, then

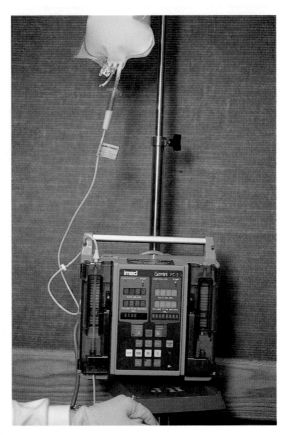

FIGURE 13-16 A total parenteral nutrition preparation hooked up to an infusion set.

the next hyperalimentation will be altered to compensate for the decrease. In this way, the patient gets exactly the nutrients needed each day. Home health clinics and some hospitals prepare a week's worth of hyperalimentation preparations; electrolyte levels are tested weekly instead of daily. Some patients may remain on this type of nutrition for many months. Figure 13-16 shows TPN hooked up to an automatic infusion pump system.

Many different protocols are used to prepare parenteral nutrition; following is an example of the solutions of a hospital pharmacy. These large volumes are premixed and ordered in cases from the manufacturer. Added to these solutions are the various electrolytes and other medications requested by the patient's attending physician:

- TPN normally contains 50% dextrose, 10% amino acids, and 20% fat
- Peripheral parenteral nutrition normally contains 25% dextrose, 10% amino acids, and 10% fat

These two preparations are administered differently because of their different concentrations. TPN is given intravenously via the subclavian vein and superior vena cava because of the higher concentration of nutrients. Patients must have a surgically inserted catheter. Peripheral parenteral nutrition is given via a large peripheral vein located in the back of the hand or in another peripheral area located in the upper extremity and therefore is less complicated. Most facilities have a standard order to start a patient on hyperalimentation. The volume of hyperalimentation typically ranges from 2 to 3 L. The doctor determines the rate of infusion over the course of 24 hours. Regardless of how many milliliters run per hour, the hyperalimentation must be changed at least every 24 hours to ensure the sterility of the solution. A standard rate of infusion is 100 mL/hr; therefore, 2400 mL may be used over the course of a day. If 3 L of TPN is hung at 1700 hours, then the following day at 1700 hours a new bag is hung and the remaining 600 mL of

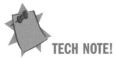

TECH NOTE!

Some chemicals can precipitate other chemicals, creating solid flakes in the intravenous solution. Always check your intravenous bag for clarity after you finish preparing the solution.

TPN ORDER SHEET

HOME HEALTH	DATE

PATIENT	ADDRESS

TPN FORMULA:

AMINO ACIDS: ☐ 5.5% ☐ 8.5% ☑ 10% ☐ WITH STANDARD ELECTROLYTES	425 ml
DEXTROSE: ☐ 10% ☐ 20% ☐ 40% ☐ 50% ☑ 70% (check one)	357 ml
LIPIDS: ☐ 10% ☑ 20% FOR ALL-IN-ONE FORMULA	125 ml

FINAL VOLUME qsad STERILE WATER FOR INJECTION 400mL	1307 ml

Calcium Gluconate	0.465m Eq/ml	5	mEq
Magnesium Sulfate	4m Eq/ml	5	mEq
Potassium Acetate	2m Eq/ml		mEq
Potassium Chloride	2m Eq/ml		mEq
Potassium Phosphate	3m M/ml	22	mM
Sodium Acetate	2m Eq/ml		mEq
Sodium Chloride	4m Eq/ml	35	mEq
Sodium Phosphate	3m M/ml		mM
TRACE ELEMENTS CONCENTRATE	☐ 4 ☐ 5 ☐ 6		ml

Patient Additives:

☐ MVC 9 + 3 10 ml Daily

☐ HUMULIN-R __10__ u Daily

☐ FOLIC ACID _____ mg
 _____ times weekly

☐ VITAMIN K _____ mg
 _____ times weekly

☐ OTHER: __MVI 12 1.5mL/daily__

☐ OTHER: _____

Directions:

INFUSE: ☑ DAILY

☐ _____ TIMES WEEKLY

OTHER DIRECTIONS:

_____

_____

_____

_____

Rate:	☐ CYCLIC INFUSION: OVER _____ HOURS (TAPER UP AND DOWN)	" " "	☐ CONTINUOUS INFUSION: AT _____ ml PER HOUR	" "	☑ STANDARD RATE: AT __110__ ml PER HOUR FOR __12__ HOURS

LAB ORDERS:

☐ STANDARD LAB ORDERS
 SMAC-20, CO2, Mg+2 TWICE WEEKLY
 CBC WITH AUTO DIFF WEEKLY
 UNTIL STABLE, THEN:
 SMAC-20, CO2, Mg+2 WEEKLY
 CBC WITH AUTO DIFF MONTHLY

☐ OTHER: _____

_____

_____

VALIDATION:

_____
DOCTOR'S SIGNATURE

Print Name: _____

Office Address: _____

_____

Phone: _____

WHITE: Home Health   CANARY: Physician

FIGURE 13-17 Example of a total parenteral nutrition order.

TABLE 13-3 **Types of Parenteral Additives**

Abbreviation	Electrolyte	Concentration	Notes
KCL	Potassium chloride	2 mEq/mL	
KPO$_4$	Potassium phosphate	Potassium 2 mEq/mL; phosphate 3 mEq/mL	Always work out phosphate first
CaGluconate	Calcium gluconate	0.465 mEq/mL	
MgSO$_4$	Magnesium sulfate	1 mg/mL	
K Ac	Potassium acetate	2 mEq/mL	*Used to balance
NaAcetate	Sodium acetate	2 mEq/mL	*Used to balance
NaPO$_4$	Sodium phosphate	2 mEq/mL	
NaCL	Sodium chloride	2 mEq/mL	*Used to balance
Miscellaneous Additives			
MVI	Multivitamin		Comes in pediatric dosing
MTE	Multiple trace elements		Comes in pediatric dosing
Zn	Zinc		
Se	Selenium		
Regular insulin	Insulin		Can be added to TPN and PPN

Other Nonsupplements Added to TPN or PPN Solutions

Generic name	Trade	Concentration
Ranitidine	Zantac	40 mg/mL
Famotidine	Pepcid	20 mg/mL
Cimetidine	Tagamet	150 mg/mL

*To balance means the pharmacist determines the amount to be added.
TPN, Total parenteral nutrition; *PPN,* peripheral parenteral nutrition.

TPN is discarded down the drain. Most hyperalimentation preparations are tailor-made for each patient. Figure 13-17 gives an example of a protocol order.

ELECTROLYTES AND ADDITIVES

All TPN contains dextrose and amino acids; both ingredients help to nourish the body. Dextrose (sugar) allows quick energy for the body, whereas amino acids are the essential parts that the body uses to build needed enzymes and other important molecules. In addition, lipids commonly are added to give the body the necessary fat needed to metabolize important cell components such as cell walls. The rest of the additives are additional electrolytes such as those listed in Table 13-3. These components can be determined daily if the patient is in a hospital setting. Other medications—such as ranitidine, cimetidine, or famotidine (all histamine$_2$ antagonists)—that help patients with stomach problems also can be added to hyperalimentation. In addition to stomach medications, insulin often is added in quantities up to 100 units per bag. Only regular insulin is added to hyperalimentation preparations.

Compatibility Considerations of Parenteral Medications

Many different types of medications are prepared in an intravenous room. Some medications must be protected from light, whereas others must be kept in bottles (as discussed before). Refer to Table 13-4 for additional considerations in the preparation of parenteral drugs. All intravenous rooms have reference

```
HOME INFUSION PHARMACY

Patient A                          Date: 03/26/07
RX#37856


Amino*Acids 10%=425 ml  Dextrose*70%=357 ml
Ster*Water=400 ml  Lipids*20%=125 ml
MVI=10 ml/day  *Additives per liter*
Sod*Chlor=35 mEq  Pot*Phos=15 mM  Calcium=
5 mEq  Magnesium=5 mEq


Qty#      TPN 40–51GM Protein+Lipids
Infuse nightly 8pm to 8am thru IV PICC line via sigma
pump.  *****Add 10 units Humulin-R to each bag just
prior to infusion***** **Note: contains TPN soln+lipids:
rate adjusted** Settings: rate=104 ml/hr
volume=1248 ml


              ***REFRIGERATE***

Expiration date: 04/01/07
```

FIGURE 13-18 Example of an intravenous medication label.

TABLE 13-4 Additional Considerations for the Preparation of Drugs

Medication	Special instructions
Insulin	NS or $\frac{1}{2}$NS
Amiodarone	D_5NS
Nitroglycerin	D_5NS or NS
Ciprofloxacin	Protect from light
Lorazepam	Protect from light; stable longer in glass than in plastic

NS, Normal saline; D_5NS, 5% dextrose in normal saline.

books one can use to find special instructions for all types of parenteral medications. The intravenous technician must become familiar with the idiosyncrasies of medications to ensure that all solutions he or she makes are effective and safe.

Components of a Label for Intravenous Medication

The final step in preparing parenteral medications is the application of the label. First check the label against the medication and the doctor's orders to make sure that the right medication is being given to the patient. Although each pharmacy prepares its own label, all labels require the same minimum information. Figure 13-18 shows an example of a label for intravenous medication.

All labels produced for parenteral medications must be initialed by the technician who prepares them. Labels get their final check from a registered pharmacist. Many pharmacy labels rely on the Julian date for determining the expiration date of the medication. If the medication does not get used, perhaps because of a discontinued order, it is recycled for use on another patient. The Julian date is the actual consecutive day of the year. For example, January 1 is day 1, whereas after January 31, February begins and the days continue in sequence with 32, 33, 34, and so on until day 365, which is December 31. Determining an expiration date is easier when using the Julian date instead of a traditional month/day/year system. However, if a computer system is used that relies on the calendar date, it should indicate the expiration date as well.

After the label has been applied, the intravenous preparations are set out for the pharmacist to check along with the vial or container of medication used to make the intravenous preparation. Once this is done, the intravenous preparations are loaded onto a cart or delivery vehicle that delivers them to their destinations. In a home health setting, a delivery service may be used to transport the medications to the patient's home. Within a hospital, this task normally is done by the technician. When the intravenous preparations are placed in the correct nursing unit, all unused intravenous preparations are obtained and are returned to the pharmacy for recycling. As long as the intravenous preparations are within their expiration dates and are kept at proper temperature, they can be used to fill new orders.

Chemotherapeutic Agents

A vertical flow hood and additional supplies are needed to prepare chemotherapy medications. Many facilities do not require a technician to wear a gown when preparing parenteral medications. However, when preparing chemotherapy agents, you must wear a gown and gloves. Also, the chemotherapy supplies must be disposed of in appropriate containers. Specially marked plastic pails clearly identified as "Hazardous Waste" containers are kept inside the hood. After thoroughly washing hands and arms to the elbows, the technician should put on the first pair of gloves, followed by a full gown. The gowns typically have Velcro tabs or ties to secure them. Once the gown is on, the technician dons a second pair of gloves over the cuff of the chemotherapy gown. This is to prevent any contamination of chemotherapy agents, if they should come into contact with the gloves. This also protects the technician from contamination. If contamination should occur, the outside pair should be removed and discarded appropriately. Goggles normally are not worn by technicians working with a chemotherapy hood because there is the added protection of the Plexiglas shield that does not allow any solution to come out of the hood toward the face or eyes.

BARRIER CHEMOTHERAPY HOODS

As discussed previously, newer hoods are being produced to ensure the sterility of the product being prepared. In the case of a chemotherapeutic agent, the hood not only must keep the agent sterile but also must keep the fumes from entering the room. This is accomplished by use of a highly sophisticated filtering system (Figure 13-13, *B*). Otherwise, this type of hood is similar to its counterpart hood as mentioned before in this chapter. An additional feature that this type of hood provides is the protection to the technician preparing the cytotoxic agent. With a conventional hood there is still a chance of spilling or squirting medication (cross-contamination) under the shield out into the intravenous room. A glove barrier hood greatly reduces this type of accident.

PROPER DISPOSAL OF CHEMOTHERAPEUTIC AGENTS AND SUPPLIES

When the chemotherapeutic agent preparation is done, it is important to discard the wrappings, needles, syringes, and the gown and gloves in appropriate containers. Most chemotherapy hoods contain a small sharps container in which all needles, syringes, and the remains of chemotherapy agents should be discarded. When these receptacles are two thirds full, they should be discarded following the pharmacy protocol. Many hospital pharmacies have environmental services collect the receptacle when it is full.

When preparation is complete, the gloves, gown, and all paper products, such as the outside wrappings of alcohol prep pads, should be placed within a plastic

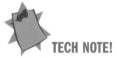

TECH NOTE!

Keep a sterile 4 × 4-inch gauze pad inside the chemotherapy hood just in case you have a minor spill. You can cover the spill with the gauze pad, decreasing the aerosolization of vapors and isolating the spill until you clean it up. Remember that all products discarded from the chemotherapy hood must be placed in an appropriate container.

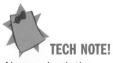

TECH NOTE!

Always check the pharmacy protocol regarding the disposal of sharps containers. This information can be found in the policies and procedures handbook.

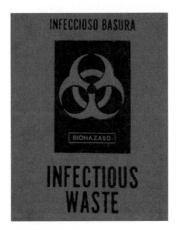

FIGURE 13-19 Biohazard symbol.

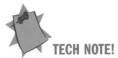

TECH NOTE!

You should always know the location of the cleanup kit for hazardous waste spills and should review the policies and procedures in case of a chemotherapy spill.

ziplock bag identified as hazardous waste. The bag then is disposed of inside a large waste receptacle that is marked "hazardous chemicals, dispose of properly." This too should be taken away by environmental services or per protocol when two-thirds full. All containers should be marked with a biohazard symbol (Figure 13-19).

DO YOU REMEMBER THESE KEY POINTS?

- The major responsibilities of a hospital technician
- The types and sizes of syringes available in an intravenous room
- The parts of a syringe and needle
- The important aspects of aseptic technique and when they should be used
- How to determine the Julian date
- Different types of parenteral medications and when they are used
- Different equipment and supplies used in an intravenous area
- The types of solutions used to mix various antibiotics and parenteral medications
- The main routes of administration

MULTIPLE CHOICE QUESTIONS

1. Which of the skills listed is the *most* important aspect of preparing sterile products?
   A. Aseptic technique
   B. Working in a horizontal flow hood
   C. Using 70% isopropyl alcohol to wipe down the hood
   D. Filter needles

2. A male/female adapter is used for which of the following reasons?
   A. To attach a needle to a syringe
   B. To attach syringes to tubing
   C. To attach syringes to syringes
   D. To attach two intravenous bags together

3. The smallest filter that can be used is a _____.
A. Filter straw
B. Filter needle
C. 5-μm filter
D. 0.22-μm filter

4. Which of the following sizes of syringes is not commonly found in an intravenous room?
A. 3 mL
B. 4 mL
C. 5 mL
D. 10 mL

5. Which of the following sizes of needles is not commonly used in an intravenous room?
A. 16 gauge
B. 18 gauge
C. 19 gauge
D. 25 gauge

6. Hands should always be washed or sanitized when _____.
A. Entering the intravenous room
B. Before working in the horizontal flow hood
C. Before working in a vertical flow hood
D. All of the above

7. Laminar flow hoods should be cleaned _____.
A. With 70% isopropyl alcohol
B. At least 30 minutes before using
C. At least once a day
D. All of the above

8. Chemotherapeutic agents should be disposed of _____.
A. In a plastic chemotherapy bag
B. In a sharps container
C. Only at the end of a shift
D. By a biohazard team of professionals

9. HEPA stands for _____ and traps particles larger than _____
A. Heated environmental parenteral air filter; 2 μm
B. High-environmental particulate air filter; 0.2 μm
C. Horizontal-efficiency particulate air filter; 0.2 μm
D. High-efficiency particulate air filter; 0.2 μm

10. You may find all of the following medications in a hyperalimentation preparation except _____.
A. Heparin
B. Insulin
C. Ranitidine
D. Ampicillin

TRUE/FALSE   If the statement is false, then change it to make it true.

_____ **1.** Intravenous stock ordering should be done weekly.

_____ **2.** NPO means nothing by mouth.

_____ **3.** Vials and intravenous bag ports should be wiped from front to back.

_____ **4.** Syringes normally are made of glass.

_____ **5.** Needles are made of aluminum or stainless steel.

_____ **6.** As the syringes increase in size, the calibration is less accurate.

_____ **7.** Laminar flow hoods should be checked monthly.

_____ **8.** You may recap syringes if they have been used only once.

_____ **9.** You must wear goggles when preparing chemotherapy agents.

_____ **10.** A sharps container must be replaced when it is full.

TECHNICIAN'S CORNER

The pharmacy receives an order for patient R. Jones.

Allergies: PCN, sulfa, morphine

Dx: Sepsis, diabetes

Transcribe the following order into lay terms and determine whether any of the orders should be brought to the attention of a pharmacist; if so, explain why.

#1 Unasyn 3 g q6h in 100 mL NS

#2 Vancomycin 1 g in 100 mL D_5NS

#3 NPH insulin "rainbow coverage" or "sliding scale"

BIBLIOGRAPHY

American Society of Health-Systems Pharmacists: *Manual for pharmacy technicians,* Bethesda, Md, 1993, The Society.

Ballington DA: *Pharmacy practice for technicians,* ed 3, St Paul, Minn, 2006, EMC/Paradigm.

Elkin MK, Perry AG, Potter PA: *Nursing interventions & clinical skills,* ed 3, St Louis, 2003, Elsevier.

NuAire Marketing Dept., Plymouth, Minn.

Potter PA, Perry AG: *Fundamentals of nursing,* ed 6, St Louis, 2004, Elsevier.

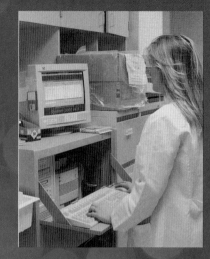

Pharmacy Stock and Billing

Objectives

UPON COMPLETING THIS CHAPTER, YOU SHOULD BE ABLE TO DO THE FOLLOWING:

- Explain the function of a drug formulary.

- List the primary types of insurance companies and how they manage drug coverages.

- Describe the differences between generic and trade drugs and how they affect cost to the patient and pharmacy.

- Differentiate between Medicaid and Medicare programs and who is eligible.

- Explain the purpose of worker's compensation.

- Describe three main ordering systems available in a pharmacy to keep stock levels constant.

- List the types of automated dispensing systems.

EVERYONE WORKING IN THE PHARMACY is responsible for maintaining the inventory stock. This is an essential part of the daily tasks of pharmacy staff. As stocks are depleted, it is important that replacement inventories be ordered. Although there are many different systems available for ordering stock, the task of ordering can be delegated to a specific person within the pharmacy. It then falls on the rest of the staff to inform the inventory control person of decreasing stock levels.

Along with ordering stock, pharmacy technicians often are placed in charge of the billing process. Proper knowledge of billing procedures is a skill that normally is learned over time as one works in the pharmacy. Because each pharmacy may accept different insurance claims, the technician must become acquainted with the normal billing procedures of that pharmacy. However, common types of billing practices are covered in this chapter that may help you understand the proper information needed to file a claim for reimbursement.

In addition, there is basic information on the major types of insurance coverage of which every technician should be aware. A firm knowledge of formulary must be in place for the proper ordering and billing practices. This chapter begins with the formulary and the necessary knowledge needed concerning insurance companies. Then pharmacy inventory, some major types of devices used to keep track of inventory, and how to handle special obstacles as they occur are discussed.

Formulary

A formulary is analogous to a backbone. The formulary is a list that describes all the medications covered under insurance plans. It also offers alternative medications if the first choice is not covered. For medications to become part of a formulary, they must meet certain requirements such as effectiveness and cost. Formularies are not the same at all pharmacies. A pharmacy can have an "open" formulary, which means any drug can be ordered and stocked for patient use, whereas a "closed" formulary limits the drugs that are ordered and can be used by patients.

Pharmacist's Perspective
BY SUSAN WONG, PharmD

Drug Utilization and Formulary Selection Process

Today's health care is in crisis. Health insurance companies and plans come and go. Ownership and management of hospitals and pharmacy benefits are in a state of flux. One of the greatest contributors to this instability is rising drug costs. The last few years have seen double-digit increases in annual drug costs. As medicine evolves and progresses, the average life span of Americans becomes longer and longer. But as we live longer, we need more medicines to treat our ills and keep us alive. Drug companies spend a great deal of time and money to develop and market their new drugs. They must recoup these investments during the patent life of a drug.

During the time in which a drug is under patent, its rights and exclusivity are under the sole ownership of usually one, sometimes more than one, drug company. The company has the right to price this new medicine in relation to its use, its costs over time, and what the market will bear. Not until the patent expires and all efforts to lengthen the patent life are exhausted will drug company competitors be allowed to manufacture a generic version, thereby lowering the retail cost through open competition.

In the past decade there also has been an explosion of "me-too" drugs. These drugs are in the same or a similar chemical class, have the same or similar action, but have slight modifications in their chemical structures. These slight differences might affect the side effect profile of a drug or its half-life (length of activity), or the different chemical structures may not have any variations in action at all. The slight variation in chemical structure allows the different drugs to be registered and licensed as separate drug entities within a drug class. Many of the drugs commonly used today for heart disease, hypertension, diabetes, hyperlipidemia, and others have brother or sister drugs that are in the same class (or family) and have the same action—hence the name "me-too" drugs.

All of these factors have necessitated the use of the formulary system for many organizations such as insurance companies, health maintenance organizations, and others. A formulary is a list of medicines that are preferred agents and provides a way of managing the use of drugs so that they are the most cost-effective for a given organization. The goal for any health care organization is to use the right medicine in the right amount at the right time to achieve a favorable outcome (i.e., health). The formulary system employs a team of professionals to review all the possible medicines for a given use and their costs to an organization for an average patient, and then to encourage or regulate the use of a preferred agent or agents for a given class or type of drug. The formulary review process also includes periodic reevaluations of medicines as new drugs come to market or as problems arise with old drugs.

The next time you go to the supermarket and go down the laundry soap aisle, look at how many types, sizes, colors, additives, and so on there are on the shelves for laundry soap. Now I would be willing to guess that they all clean your clothes pretty well. Some have fresh scents, some have no scent, some have bleach alternatives, and some claim to save the colors in your clothes. Some may cost $5, some may cost $15. But they all clean your clothes. You might buy the brand that cleans your clothes for the most economical price. Some folks may need certain brands or formulations because of allergies. Most will buy the bigger sizes (because they get more for their hard-earned cash). Choosing a preferred medicine for a formulary is a similar process (but a bit more scientific). If a patient has an allergy to or has failed therapy with the preferred agent, the patient may need to use a non-formulary medicine. In this instance, the pharmacy may have to specially order a nonpreferred medicine for the patient.

As a pharmacy technician you may be involved with the recording or billing of medicine that a patient has received. Or you may be involved with procuring a medicine that is not on the formulary and is used infrequently. Accuracy is the key because the misrecording of a medicine can affect what a patient must pay for the medicines and what your employer is reimbursed from the patient's insurance plan. Accuracy also can affect your employer if you are involved in supply chain management or inventory/stocking of your supplies. It is crucial for all involved to use the medicines that do the job and are most cost-effective. This helps patients spend their health care dollars wisely. ■

Many formulary drugs are generic. These drugs are as effective as the brand-name drugs but are less expensive. A committee composed of pharmacists, physicians, and other health care administrators reviews drugs that have been approved by the Food and Drug Administration (FDA) and that are cost-effective. In addition, consideration may be given to drug companies that bid or give rebates when their drug is chosen. This decrease in price to the pharmacy ultimately saves money for the insurance company and the patient. Although most insurance companies cover most of the cost of a generic drug, some do allow the patient to choose the brand-name drug. However, if the patient selects the brand-name drug, the patient must pay the difference between the generic and brand-name drug and also may be responsible for any copay required. For example, if the normal copay is $5 per prescription and the patient chooses a brand-name medication that costs $10 more than the generic equivalent, then the patient must pay $15. Finally, formularies are not permanent by any means. If and when new generic drugs come into the market, cost and other factors are reviewed again. Typically, the types of drugs not included on a formulary are new drugs, uncommon drugs, and extremely expensive drugs. However, if a non-formulary drug can be justified as a medically necessary substitution by the physician, it may be approved.

Generic versus Trade Drugs

The terms *trade, brand,* and *proprietary* are used interchangeably to refer to the name of the drug that was first patented and marketed by the owner or manufacturer. After a certain amount of time passes, the patent runs out. Eventually, other drug companies can apply for the right to produce the same drug. These drugs produced by other companies are considered "generic." Although the FDA approves generic drugs as equivalent to the trade name drug, they may have different appearances because of different manufacturing procedures. Brand-name drugs generally have between 17 to 20 years of protection before patents expire (CDER).[1] Once generic competition is introduced, prices can drop 50% to 80%. Drug price competition and patent term restoration expedite the availability of less costly generic drugs by permitting FDA to approve applications to market generic versions of brand-name drugs without repeating the research done to prove them safe and effective. At the same time, the brand-name companies can apply for up to 5 years of additional patent protection for the new medicines they developed to make up for time lost while their products were going through the FDA approval process.[2]

Third-Party Billing

The term *third-party billing* refers to the third part of the three parties—patient, pharmacy, and insurance company—involved in the overall payment process, that is, the insurance company. After the patient has paid his or her portion of the drug cost, the pharmacy must submit an invoice for the remaining cost for payment to the insurance company. This chapter begins by listing the primary types of insurance, followed by their common traits and the problems that may arise when processing medication claims.

TYPES OF INSURANCE

The technician must know the type of insurance, if any, each patient has for billing purposes. Learning about all of the different insurance policies is nearly impossible, especially because their guidelines change regularly. Therefore, this chapter covers the most basic information that can be applied to the major types of billing. The four types of insurance plans in use today are the following:

Health maintenance organization (HMO)
Preferred provider organization (PPO)
Government programs: Medicare and Medicaid
Worker's compensation

HEALTH MAINTENANCE ORGANIZATION

An HMO has specific features that set it apart from traditional insurance programs. An HMO is an effective method of controlling health care costs. Blue Cross, United Healthcare, Pacificare, Champus Tricare Program, and Kaiser are just five examples of the many insurance companies that offer HMO coverage. Special features of HMOs include the following:

1. Primary care physician: The insurance company allows the patient to choose a main physician rather than having to be seen by the physician on duty.
2. Independent physician association: The provider offers a discounted rate to the patient through the contract made with the insurance company. In return, the doctor accepts a lesser amount than normally is charged for the procedure performed. These are considered contracted providers; examples of contracted providers are certain hospitals, clinics, and medical groups.
3. Copay: The insurance company requires a predetermined amount to be paid by the patient for office visits, emergency room visits, and drugs, regardless of the final cost. The rate varies depending on the type of coverage the patient has. The insurance company is responsible for the remainder of the cost.

What If Your Patient Has HMO Insurance?

If a patient has HMO insurance, the technician must obtain information from the patient such as address, date of birth, insurance number, and full name. If the pharmacy accepts the patient's insurance, the technician charges the patient the copay per medication filled. The pharmacy in turn bills the insurance company for the remaining balance of the cost of the medication. The patient is responsible for the entire cost only if the insurance company denies coverage based on eligibility or authorization not received before service. An HMO may require prior authorization on certain medications per their formulary guidelines. State regulations regarding the types of forms used to approve such medications may vary.

PREFERRED PROVIDER ORGANIZATION

The difference between HMOs and PPOs is that the patient usually pays more out-of-pocket expenses for PPOs. The benefit is that the patient can choose a physician from the insurance plan list of contracted providers or may choose any physician a patient wants. There are no requirements for a primary care physician.

PPOs are offered by Blue Shield, Blue Cross, United Healthcare, State Farm Insurance, and others. As you can see, some insurance companies offer PPOs and HMOs. This is why it is important for the patient to choose the right insurance plan.

Patients choosing a PPO may have a copay for their visits, the copay tends to be higher, and PPOs may have a deductible (the amount that the patient must pay before the insurance company pays). The insurance then pays a certain percentage of the medical expenses and medication bills if the patient's claims meet the criteria (i.e., charges were incurred by a contracted provider and the service provided was within the allowed amount of the PPO). This helps control the cost to the insurance company because the patient pays everything that the insurance company does not pay.

What If Your Patient Has PPO Insurance?

You must find out whether the patient has medication coverage through the PPO plan. In addition, you must find out whether the patient pays upfront for the medication or has a copay. This is determined from the information on the patient's health insurance card. After the information is transmitted to the provider, an approval code is sent to the pharmacy. If the claim is rejected, the technician may instruct the patient to call the provider to rectify major problems.

GOVERNMENT-RUN INSURANCE PROGRAMS

Programs such as Medicare and Medicaid are examples of state and federal medical insurance plans. Each person who works pays the government a percentage of his or her income toward Medicare. A percentage of each state budget is applied toward Medicaid. Each plan has specific guidelines that must be followed to the letter for patients to qualify for reimbursement.

Medicare

Medicare is a federally run program for seniors, the disabled, and dialysis patients. Medicare works much like an HMO and a PPO. The patient must go to a provider that accepts Medicare, but the patient has a yearly deductible and a percentage share of cost. The share of cost is similar to a deductible and copay put together. The patient is responsible for paying up to a certain amount in a hospital setting. At present, Medicare pays outpatient costs with the exception of some diabetic supplies and equipment. Some major drug companies offer drug programs to the elderly and the disabled that will provide medications to those who use specific products. Before 2006, Medicare did not offer any prescription drug coverage. That has changed and is now called Medicare Part D.

The following is a brief overview of the types of Medicare levels that are available:

Medicare Part A	Hospital stays, skilled nursing facilities, hospice, and various therapies
Medicare Part B	Doctor visits, laboratory diagnostics, outpatient mental health, physical therapy, and certain medical equipment
Medicare Part D	Coverage of medicine primarily; also diabetic insulin and syringes

More on Medicare Part D. "Medicare is a Health Insurance Program for people 65 years of age and older, some disabled people under 65 years of age, and people with End-Stage Renal Disease (permanent kidney failure treated with dialysis or a transplant)" as outlined in Medicare overview. Medicare Part D was intended to help certain persons with their prescription drug costs but not everyone. Due to the language of the plan and the multitude of medical insurance companies has made it difficult to know whether to sign up for Part D. This can only be determined by the specific needs of the patient; therefore, there is not any clear information on what is the best choice. An important note, however, is that each plan may vary considerably in specific coverages. At this time the maximum deductible for any plan cannot exceed $265 per year. The two types of coverage are basic and enhanced. Again each has variable deductibles that apply. The basic coverage has a higher deductible than the enhanced coverage.

Other guidelines for seniors to consider when choosing the Medicare Part D plan can be found on the Medicare website at *www.Medicare.gov*. Examples include the following:

1. Medicare drug plans benefit certain groups of persons such as the following:
   a. Low-income families
   b. Those with Medigap coverage
   c. Those individuals who have more than $750 annually in drug costs
2. Those individuals with multiple prescriptions may benefit from this plan, but there are considerations that must be taken into account:
   a. Certain prescriptions that tend to lean toward formulary drugs rather than nonformulary ones.

3. Those individuals who are in good health or who spend less than $750 annually may benefit by waiting to find a drug plan that may be as good as Part D through another company.
4. Not all generic drugs are bioequivalent to the name brand. Also, not all brand drugs are available in generic form. This can make a huge difference in the choice of drug for the patient.
5. Check the formulary of each plan. Note, however, that each plan can change in the future.
6. Ask about any restrictions on certain medications.
7. Also important is to know whether the plan uses "step therapy." (This means that the drug company makes the patient take the cheapest drug first; if that does not work, then the company approves the second cheapest drug and so on until the company finds something that works.)

As patients cross over into Medicare Part D, they may experience a glitch in the system such as the following:

1. No coverage showing in the computer for their medications
2. A change in what they have been taking
3. Because of changing medications, they may experience a change in health

How does all of this information affect the pharmacy in general?

1. This change will increase the consultations of pharmacists as they explain different interactions caused by a change in medications.
2. The pharmacies may not be able to fill prescriptions for patients who have always had their medications filled there. This is because of the time it will take to get the patient into the database.
3. Pharmacies must apply for a National Provider Identifier (NPI) from the Centers for Medicare and Medicaid Services. All providers who bill electronically must use an NPI (Health Insurance Portability and Accountability Act rules). The deadline is May 2007.
4. Any pharmacist who provides services such as consultation and does not bill for this time under a pharmacy with an NPI will need his or her own NPI.
5. If a patient is not in the system yet and the physician has ordered a drug that is not covered, the pharmacist may call the doctor for a substitute if possible or the patient may pay out of pocket for the medication and try for reimbursement when he or she is in the system.

An important "bottom line" approach to consider is this:

The patient will not be able to continue using the brand-name drug but will be given a generic name drug in its place. The overall use of generic drugs will increase greatly under Medicare Part D. This can make a huge difference to the patient because not all generic drugs are bioequivalent to the brand drug. Also, not all brand drugs are available in generic form. Many pharmacists, doctors, and other caregivers are concerned about what might happen as drugs that currently are working for their patients are replaced by less expensive (generic) drugs.

Many times pharmacists must explain the types of benefits, and there is little doubt that technicians will be drawn into this whirlpool. This is especially true for technicians who work at a pharmacy counter or who are in charge of the billing. Many patients will need help in where to go or how to deal with medication changes or other problems. Technicians will need to keep themselves updated on any new changes in the system in order to help their patients.

The deadline for sign-up was in May 2006. The next window was in November 2006 with the coverage starting up in January 2007. In addition, late fees will be charged.

Medicaid

Each state has its own Medicaid program for low-income residents. This also includes uninsured pregnant women and those with certain disabilities. Federal funding accounts for only a small portion of the revenue. Medicaid can be used with Medicare if the person qualifies. In addition, each state may have many different programs that help defer the cost of health care and medication. The following are the three major levels of coverage within the Medicaid system:

1. The patient may not be responsible for any cost.
2. Share of cost. In the share of cost level, the patient's plan requires that the patient pay a deductible (i.e., a specific dollar amount must be met before the insurance company pays). For instance, the patient may be responsible for the first $1000, but any remaining amount is paid by Medicaid.
3. Geographical managed care program. A geographical managed care plan allows patients to belong to a medical group with which Medicaid has a contractual agreement. This includes HMOs, thus allowing patients to have benefits similar to benefits offered by HMOs. (Regulations of each state may vary.)

What If Your Patient Has Medicaid Insurance?

You must know whether the patient has medication benefits. If so, you need a copy of the patient's insurance card. This card identifies the program under which the patient is covered. These plans include county-run programs as well. Each program differs in the patient's coverage.

WORKER'S COMPENSATION

Worker's compensation is a type of insurance paid by employers to cover fully the injuries suffered by employees while on the job. The federal government requires employers with a certain number of employees to offer worker's compensation. Insurance coverage is paid to private insurance carriers.

Anyone who works for a company that pays into worker's compensation may be eligible to use this insurance if he or she has a work-related injury. The patient does not have to pay anything. Instead, claims are filed electronically or in paper copy to the insurance companies.

BILLING THE INSURANCE COMPANY

The information that insurance companies must know to process a claim from the pharmacy or to reimburse the patient is the same as the requirements on a pharmacy label plus date of birth, insurance group, and identification numbers. All information must be verified before the medication is dispensed. Once the patient's information is in the pharmacy computer system, it is important to keep that information updated for the pharmacy and the insurance company.

Minimum information required by the insurance company includes the following:

Required by the Insurance Company	Reason
Patient's name	To verify the insurance coverage
Date medication is filled	May be important to process claim
Pharmacy name and address	The insurance company must pay the pharmacy
Medication prescribed	To verify whether the drug is on the formulary
Dosage	Determines the cost of the medication
Date of birth	Verification
Identification number	Authorization

Each plan has its own formulary, limitations, and exclusions. In addition to these variances, each pharmacy has certain insurance that it accepts or rejects.

This means, if the pharmacy accepts the copayment as payment in full, the pharmacy will bill the insurance company for the cost of the medication. Otherwise, the pharmacy may not accept the insurance based on the limits of payment.

Patient Profiles

Each pharmacy has its own specific computer system, which details each patient's profile. This profile must be kept updated for proper billing. Basic information that can be viewed on this computer system includes the following:

- Patient's name
- Date of birth
- Address
- Phone number
- Gender
- Allergies
- Insurance provider's information, including provider's phone number and insurance number

If the information contains a mistake, the insurance claim may be rejected.

If the patient does not have insurance, he or she must pay full price for prescriptions. The cost of a prescription can vary greatly. Many pharmacies offer coupons on new prescriptions. The use of generic drugs can reduce the price of a medication greatly.

If the patient has insurance, determining the guidelines of the program is of primary importance if the pharmacy is to receive reimbursement. The process by which all claims are processed over a computerized system is referred to as adjudication. The insurance determines the amount of coverage per medication based on various criteria such as the following:

1. Average wholesale price: The average wholesale price can be found in *Drug Topics Red Book*. Use *Red Book* or *Blue Book* to determine the price of a medication based on the manufacturer's price.
2. Copay: The insurance company pays a certain amount based on the patient's copay. This also depends on whether the patient uses an HMO, PPO, or a government-run program. Processors, companies that work for insurance companies, are responsible for the approval of drug coverage, collecting and processing claims, and payment.

Processing Claims

When handling a patient's medication claim, the pharmacy is responsible for relaying the necessary information about each patient. Because each insurance company needs specific information, the technician must know the specific needs of each insurance company. The general types of information required may include the following:

- Processor, typically the insurance company
- Member's identification number, usually the Social Security number, or an assigned number of the policy owner
- Group number (if applicable)
- Plan code (if applicable)
- Insurance carrier

Claim Problems

A prescription may not be covered for the insured patient for many reasons. This can be a frustrating time for the patient and the technician who is trying to get a prescription covered, as well as for the insurance company representative. The most common reasons that a prescription may not be covered are as follows:

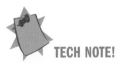

- Coverage has expired
- Coverage limits have been exceeded
- National Drug Code (NDC) is not covered
- Patient is trying to refill a prescription too soon
- The cardholder's information does not match the processor's information
- Doctor is not the primary care physician

Coverage Expiration Policy for Drugs

If the patient has lost his or her coverage, the claim is rejected. Following Health Insurance Portability and Accountability Act regulations in 2003, the pharmacy does not have access to information regarding reason for rejection and is disclosed only a termination date. Patients often are unaware of why this has happened and may want the pharmacy to investigate. Pharmacy personnel are not allowed to call the patient's insurance carrier regarding these types of inquiries. Patient confidentiality would be breached, and legal action could result. The only recourse is to explain to the patient that he or she must contact the insurance company to resolve the issue. In the meantime, the patient must pay full price for the medications. If there has been an error, reimbursement is made after the insurance company corrects the problem.

Limitation of Plan Exceeded

This problem of exceeding the limitations of a plan can arise for several reasons. One reason is that the drug is not covered in the insurance plan formulary (i.e., nonformulary). In this case, a special authorization form must be submitted to the insurance company from the physician explaining why the patient must have a specific (nonformulary) medication. Another reason is that the prescription calls for a greater amount of the drug than is allowed by the insurance plan. For example, some government insurance plans limit the number of prescriptions that can be filled per month or per year. If the prescription calls for a specific quantity of medication that exceeds the maximum amount to be filled per day, the prescription is rejected and the patient must contact the insurance company for special permission to obtain the drug.

Some patients are exempt from these types of limitations because of their illness. These include persons who suffer from diabetes or those who have been diagnosed with human immunodeficiency virus or acquired immune deficiency syndrome. Those persons suffering from diabetes require a continuous refill of lancets and blood-testing strips to monitor their blood glucose. In addition, they must refill their insulin syringes monthly. In the case of persons being treated for human immunodeficiency virus or acquired immunodeficiency syndrome, the medication is expensive and they usually have to take many medications simultaneously. When a claim is rejected because limits are exceeded, the technician must explain the problem and adhere to the maximum limit permitted by the insurance company. The patient is ultimately responsible for contacting the insurance company to dispute the problem.

Handling Nonformulary Drugs or Noncovered National Drug Codes

Formularies tend to be specific. This includes the decision of which drugs are included on the member's plan. These drugs are identified by their NDC, a code assigned to every drug in the United States. If the code submitted is not in the formulary, the claim is rejected by the insurance company. In pharmacy, these types of medications are referred to as nonformulary drugs. In this case, two options can be explored. First, the pharmacist can contact the doctor and request that the prescription be changed to a drug that is covered under the patient's insurance plan.

The other option is to submit a prior authorization form to the insurance company indicating why the patient must take the nonformulary drug. The type

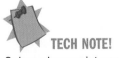

of prior authorization form varies depending on insurance company guidelines. Physicians normally fill out and submit the prior authorization form for approval. This approval process can take up to 2 weeks. The patient must pay upfront for the medication, or he or she can wait to have the prescription filled after the approval or rejection is given by the insurance company. If the patient pays upfront and the medication is approved, the patient is reimbursed by the insurance company after the pharmacist fills out a reimbursement form for the patient. The form is sent to the insurance company to reimburse the patient for the covered drug cost.

Filling a Prescription too Soon

Patients attempt to get their prescription refilled before they run out for several reasons. Most of the time it is not a problem to call in for a refill on the last week of the drug supply; however, there are instances in which the patient may call in as early as only 1 week after receiving the prescription. The patient may be leaving the country for an extended time and wants to make sure that he or she has enough medication to last until return. In this case, the pharmacist can decide to fill a prescription depending on the type of medication. If the patient's insurance will not pay, the patient is responsible for the cost of the medication. Prescriptions normally are written for a 30-day supply or more, depending on the condition being treated. Mail-order companies usually fill a 90-day supply. The amount of medication supplied may be related directly to safety issues that surround a specific medication. Because certain medications are dangerous, they may not be filled more than 30 days. These include schedule II drugs and also a specific drug called isotretinoin (Accutane; acne medication), which has been linked to teratogenicity in pregnant women. Many insurance plans allow additional savings if refills are ordered via mail-order pharmacies that are on their list of participating pharmacies.

Sometimes a physician instructs the patient to increase the dosage, thus forcing the refill process before its allotted time. In this case a new prescription order must be submitted to the insurance company. In some cases the technician must call the insurance company help desk to explain the circumstances of the prescription change. However, some insurance companies may require a direct response from the patient's physician before giving approval.

Nonidentification Match

Probably one of the most common problems is when the cardholder's information does not match up to the processor's information, thus resulting in a claim rejection. To determine whether this is the case, the technician should always recheck the information submitted to the insurance company. Items to double-check include the following:

- Health plan card number, identification number, and insurance number
- Patient's name, date of birth, and relationship to the insured person

The relationship of the patient to the cardholder is important because he or she may be a new spouse or adopted child or other changes may have been made. In this case the technician may be able to ask for a new insurance card for the member through the insurance help desk.

Pharmacy Stock

Each pharmacy orders drugs that include formulary drugs and some nonformulary drugs. The established level of medication stock kept on hand at any given time is referred to as the periodic automatic replenishment level. This is the minimum amount of medication that should be maintained in the pharmacy

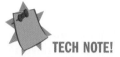

TECH NOTE!

If the patient received two 30-day supplies, then reimbursement may not be sent until three fourths of the prescription has been taken.

at any given time. Just as insurance billing has become a common task of pharmacy technicians, so has the responsibility of ordering medications. Different systems are available that can keep a running inventory of medications and order them. This can be done several ways, such as at the point of sale (POS), by order cards, or by handheld inventory computers. Because there are so many different types of systems in use today, this chapter explores the main idea behind these various systems and looks into when and how stock arrives to the pharmacy. This also includes proper storage of all drugs. In addition, this chapter discusses how recalls are handled and how returns are processed.

Although some pharmacies may contract out the job of writing up returns and sending them back to the manufacturer, this usually is done by a pharmacy technician who is an employee of the pharmacy. This technician typically is in charge of all aspects of ordering, restocking, and returning stock within the pharmacy.

ORDERING SYSTEMS

Maintaining a periodic automatic replenishment level in the pharmacy in important for several reasons. Many manufacturers do not fill orders on the weekend or holidays. This means the pharmacy could run out of stock during the weekend. The pharmacy may have to wait until the following delivery day to receive the necessary stock. This is serious if a patient cannot obtain an essential medication because the pharmacy is out of stock. Patients visiting a community pharmacy may be able to go elsewhere to have prescriptions filled, but hospitalized patients rely on the hospital pharmacy to stock medications.

In cases when stock is not going to arrive until the following Monday or Tuesday, the only recourse is to express-deliver the medication or to borrow it from another pharmacy. Express delivery can range from a courier delivering the medication to having the medication flown in from a long distance. Of course, this is used only in case of an emergency when all other options will not work. Express delivery also is expensive and in many cases unnecessary if the pharmacy staff understands when to reorder a specific drug. Shipping time varies depending on the type of drug ordered. This is when pharmacy personnel must show their teamwork. To assume it is someone else's job is not proper or appropriate.

More pharmacies rely on computerized systems that know when to order medications. This is by far one of the best ways to maintain appropriate stock levels, although not all pharmacies have this system. Three main systems are discussed in this chapter, although there are many more types. All systems are similar to those discussed in the following sections.

BAR CODING

Most manufacturers identify their products with bar codes that can be scanned. This process speeds up the input of information because one pass of the bar code device identifies the drug, strength, dosage form, quantity, cost, package size, and any other information. Pharmacies can use these bar codes as well. The medication is scanned at the register, called the point of sale, and electronically is taken off the computerized inventory list. When the in-stock quantity drops to a certain level (periodic automatic replenishment level), it is reordered automatically. Other devices used to scan drugs are handheld components that identify the necessary drug information. The operator (the technician) only needs to put in the quantity to be ordered. The information from this handheld set then is transferred to the main computer ordering system.

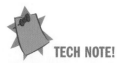

AUTOMATED DISPENSING SYSTEMS

For the pharmacy to determine the necessary stock levels, there has to be a way to inventory the stock that is not on the stock shelves but is in use or in a different location. For example, computerized dispensing units of community pharmacies keep track of the inventory as tablets and capsules are dispensed into a drug vial. As the pills pass a beam of light, they automatically are taken off the inventory. An example of this type of system is a Baker Cell System. Systems of this type are being developed constantly, and they work similarly.

In a hospital, the pharmacy is responsible for supplying various clinics and nursing units with stock. To avoid everyone needing stock at the same time and having a shortage of stock on hand to fill the orders, dispensing systems that link the nursing units to the pharmacy computer system allow the stock levels to be viewed at any time. Each time the nurse indicates the type and amount of drug taken from these drug cabinets, it is deducted from the current stock levels in the cabinet and this information then is transferred electronically to the pharmacy unit. Various reports can be run from this centralized unit, which can give an overall stock inventory for a specific drug. In addition to the inventory status, such units also monitor controlled substance use and inventory. All persons adding drugs to or taking drugs from the unit are identified, and a log is kept of all users. This also ensures the proper use of controlled substances and detects any discrepancies. Examples of this type of automated dispensing systems are PYXIS (see Chapter 8) and OMNICELL.

MANUAL ORDERING

Although manual ordering is being eliminated slowly as the main ordering technique, it is still important in the continued monitoring of stock levels. Many pharmacies visually note that stock is getting low or use ordering cards that stay inside the medication box. These cards list the drug information, including the ordering number and the necessary periodic automatic replenishment levels to aid the technician in ordering the proper amount. The card system or simply writing down the right amount of stock to be ordered depends on the technician knowing which drugs fall into which of the following categories:

- Formulary: Nonformulary drugs normally are kept at a lower level because they are not ordered often. In hospitals, they may not be kept at all, depending on the preferences of management.
- Fast mover: These drugs typically are kept in a separate area from the normal stock because of the high volume of use. These must be ordered in larger quantities, keeping the overstock nearby, or must be ordered more often.
- Slow mover: These drugs are prescribed regularly by a few doctors but are not commonly prescribed. These drugs must be checked before ordering and periodically to ensure that the drugs are not close to expiring.
- Special orders: These typically are drugs that are used by only a few patients, but they may be important for proper treatment. It is easy to forget to order these drugs because of their infrequent use. Usually they are ordered at the time of use.
- Time of year: The drugs that fall into this category vary depending on the time of year. Many medications that are fast movers during a particular time of year may need their periodic automatic replacement levels raised during that period. For example, albuterol inhalers are normally fast movers in the spring, when allergies increase. At this time of year there may be many more persons diagnosed with asthma or respiratory problems, which may double normal periodic automatic replacement levels. All pharmacy staff must be aware of the types of medications used during different times of the year and how they fluctuate.

Responding early when a trend is seen is a skill that takes time and experience. When stock begins to run low, it is everyone's responsibility to make sure that the stock is ordered.

NEW STOCK

Stock may arrive daily to the pharmacy. For billing purposes, it is important that all stock be checked completely against the invoice when first received. The following is a step-by-step approach that should be used when receiving stock:

1. Retrieve the manufacturer or warehouse invoice.
2. Account for all boxes. For example, if the invoice indicates there are five boxes, your first task is to verify that there are five boxes.
3. If any box is marked refrigerate or freeze, you must comply with the instructions immediately to avoid product damage.
4. All information must be checked against the invoice. For example, check the following:
   Name of drug
   Strength or dosage
   Dosage form
   Quantity
   Expiration date of product*
5. Compare the invoice with the order form to make sure that only what was ordered was sent.
6. Then sign and date the invoice and send it for processing per pharmacy protocol.
7. Once the received order has been confirmed as correct, the technician may put the stock away. Rotating stock is another important priority. New stock typically has later expiration dates and should be placed behind the existing stock that expires sooner. All stock should be rotated in this manner to avoid accumulation of expired drugs, which may be used accidentally.
8. Finally, it is important to return inventory cards to the medication box for future use.

Inventory may not sound difficult. However, marking stock shelves clearly ultimately affects the probability of drug errors. For example, if a drug is accidentally put in a box intended for a different drug with a similar-sounding name, it may be used to fill a prescription for the soundalike drug and make its way into the patient's possession.

PROPER STORAGE

As stock arrives it is important to follow the manufacturer's requirements for storage. Certain medications must be frozen, refrigerated, light-protected, or stored at room temperature. If these guidelines are not followed the medication is then compromised, rendering it unusable. Just as it is important to put unused stock back into place when being returned from the nursing floors (in hospital pharmacy) it is essential that the pharmacy technician places new stock into their respective areas of storage as soon as possible. Chemicals such as phenol and other toxic materials are usually kept behind cabinet doors and low to the ground. It is not wise to leave these types of materials out in the open, as they are toxic. Read the packaging on all medications and follow the manufacturer's requirements for storage. Storing medications in the right place is the responsibility of everyone working in pharmacy.

TECH NOTE!
You should not allow any medication into the pharmacy unless it has good dating on it. "Good dating" means that the expiration date is long enough to make it likely that the drug will be used before expiration. Most pharmacies use a 3-month expiration time. This means that a drug that expires in 3 months or less may expire before use unless it is a fast mover and may be sent back to the manufacturer for a refund.

---

*Checking the expiration date is important. Drugs that are used rarely and have short expiration dates may sit on the shelf and expire before use.

RETURNS

Medication is sent back to the warehouse or manufacturer for three main reasons. Depending on the reason, certain paperwork must accompany the medication. Pharmacy policies and procedures should list the steps involved for returns. Except for scheduled drugs that fall under the jurisdiction of the Drug Enforcement Administration (DEA), most medications can be sent back by the technician without a pharmacist's signature. The three reasons for returning drugs to the manufacturer are as follows:

1. Drug recalls
2. Damaged stock
3. Expired stock

Drug Recalls

Manufacturers are required by law to recall any product that has been found to violate any of the following guidelines:

1. Labeling is wrong.
2. Product was not packaged or produced properly.
3. Drug batch was contaminated.
4. Any other change occurs that causes the drug to fall outside the FDA or manufacturer's guidelines.

Recall notices may arrive by mail or fax and identify the necessary information about the drug or device in question and how to handle the recall procedure. This information includes the drug name and why it is being recalled. One of the most important pieces of information given is the lot number of the drug. This is the key to identifying the recalled medication. Technicians are responsible for checking all of the drug stock throughout the pharmacy and facility to make sure that the recalled drug is not in stock. If this is the case, the recall form is initialed to indicate that the item is not in stock. If pharmacy stock does include a drug with the recalled lot number, the pharmacist must be notified in case a patient has been issued one of these products. Any patient who may have been issued a recalled item should be notified by phone so that he or she may check the lot number of the drug or device. All recalled items must be sent back to the manufacturer as indicated. If all of the stock of a particular drug at a pharmacy is recalled, more stock must be reordered immediately, possibly from another manufacturer. All of these tasks may be performed by the pharmacy technician.

Damaged Stock

If you notice that some drugs were damaged en route to the pharmacy but you did not catch it at the time of delivery, it is still not too late to send the damaged stock back to the manufacturer. It may be necessary to call first and get an approval code to send back the damaged goods.

Expired Stock

Many pharmacies have a policy to pull any medication that will expire in 3 months or less. This ensures that there are no drugs on the shelves close to their expiration date. Depending on the contract between the pharmacy and the manufacturer, it may be allowable to send back items as long as they can be bundled into a minimum package size rather than partials. For instance, if the stock of cimetidine expires within 3 months, the manufacturer may allow it to be returned for full or partial credit if a box of 100 tablets can be returned at one time. Following manufacturer's guidelines for returns is important. Hazardous chemicals, including cytotoxic agents, must be repackaged carefully to avoid breakage during transport.

TABLE 14-1 Difference in Ordering from Manufacturers, Wholesalers, and Warehouse Repackaging Plants

Factors to consider	Manufacturer warehouse	Wholesaler/vendor repackaging plant	Warehouse
Supplier cost	No shipping fees	Lower per contract	Lowest cost
Supplier has electronic inventory control mechanism	No	Yes	Yes
Supplier able to stock large supplies when ordering	Yes	No	No
Supplier provides special delivery service	Varies by manufacturer	Yes	Yes
Supplier handles special orders	Yes	Some special orders must be done through the manufacturer	Some special orders must be done through the manufacturer

Automated Return Companies

Some companies have the sole job of processing returns for hospitals, wholesalers, pharmacy chain stores, and independent retailers. They are responsible for all records, recalled items, and disposal of hazardous waste.

NONRETURNABLE DRUGS AND THEIR DISPOSAL

Many items are not taken back by manufacturers. Any drug that is reconstituted or compounded within the pharmacy may not be returned to the manufacturer. Partially used bottles of medication normally are not taken back, nor are any drugs that have been repackaged by the pharmacy. These drugs, including most reconstituted agents such as amoxicillin suspension, can be dumped in the pharmacy garbage, but in most cases, especially in chain pharmacies, the drugs are sent to a central location for destruction or return to manufacturer for credit. Many agents must be disposed of carefully. Cytotoxic agents must be disposed of in a sharps container marked "hazardous waste." Nontoxic intravenous agents should be disposed of in a regular sharps container marked for proper disposal. Controlled substances must be counted and cosigned by a pharmacist before they are destroyed. Before any scheduled medications are destroyed, the DEA must be contacted for specific instructions for destruction. Controlled substances disposal is the only task for which the pharmacist must be present, must cosign the disposal of the drug, and must return information required by the DEA. The DEA issues a receipt for schedule II merchandise destroyed. This receipt must be kept for 5 years with the schedule II inventory.

SUPPLIERS

When ordering stock for the pharmacy, the technician orders from a centralized warehouse that the pharmacy owns, from a wholesaler, or directly from the manufacturer.

Each of these suppliers has pros and cons. As seen in Table 14-1, the benefits of using wholesalers compared with dealing directly with the manufacturer differ mostly in the amount of stock that must be ordered and kept as overstock and the difference in cost. The final column describes a warehouse situation in which a company orders high volumes of drugs from the manufacturer and may repackage the medications into more suitable sizes for the ordering physician. This serves several purposes, such as easier handling, increased productivity, and lower cost. Large-quantity bottles are hard to handle. They are more likely to be dropped, spilling the contents. Medications may be prepackaged in smaller, easy-to-handle containers to eliminate the bulkiness of the larger bottles. If the pharmacy warehouse prepackages common dosages, it speeds up the labeling process. For example, sulfamethoxazole/trimethoprim (Septra) normally is ordered to be taken twice daily for 10 days or twice daily for 15 days. These tablets are prepackaged in bottles of 20 and 30, eliminating the time it takes to count out the proper amount at the pharmacy counter. The technician must check the label against the prescription to determine the appropriate drug and quantity, and the prescription is ready to be checked by the pharmacist and dispensed. Finally, because the volume of drugs is much higher than what a normal pharmacy can stock, pharmacies have contracts with these warehouses that save the pharmacy a substantial amount of money. This ultimately keeps the cost lower for the consumer.

SPECIAL ORDERING CONSIDERATIONS

Special considerations must be given to a host of drugs ordered by pharmacy. Some of these include controlled substances, investigational drugs, cytotoxic drugs, and hazardous substances. Each of these types of medications require special ordering, inventory, handling, and return paperwork. The FDA requires special forms to be completed for ordering schedule II controlled substances and for returning them (see Chapter 2). In addition, controlled substances need to be inventoried daily by a trained pharmacy staff person. Usually, the ordering technician does not have this additional task.

Investigational drugs typically come with paperwork that must be completed and returned to the manufacturer each time a medication is given. Cytotoxic drugs do not need special paperwork, but they should be handled with great care and placed in a safety cabinet under the guidelines of the manufacturer. Some cytotoxic agents must be refrigerated and should be well marked to separate them from other agents. Most pharmacies stock certain chemicals that are considered hazardous. You must know where the material safety data sheets of your pharmacy are located in case of a spill. Agents such as phenol should be kept behind cabinet doors to protect persons from accidentally knocking the bottle off a shelf and inhaling the toxic fumes.

DO YOU REMEMBER THESE KEY POINTS?

- Why pharmacy formularies are important
- The major types of insurance and the differences between them
- The differences between government insurance programs
- The necessary information that patients must provide to the pharmacy for billing prescriptions to third parties
- The types of problems that often arise associated with insurance claims
- The importance of the National Drug Code and how to decipher it
- The responsibilities of a pharmacy technician concerning stock levels and ordering stock for the pharmacy
- Common types of automated dispensing systems and where they are used
- The set of steps that should be used when receiving stock
- How to return expired or recalled stock
- The importance of storing stock at the appropriate temperature

MULTIPLE
CHOICE
QUESTIONS

MULTIPLE CHOICE QUESTIONS

1. All of the following are types of insurance except _____.
   A. HMO
   C. Medicaid
   B. PPO
   D. FDA

2. Medicare is a government-run insurance program that covers all of the following except _____.
   A. Senior citizens
   C. Children
   B. Patients using dialysis
   D. Persons who are disabled

3. Medicaid covers all of the following persons except _____.
   A. Persons who are disabled
   B. Persons with low income
   C. Women who are pregnant
   D. Single working persons with above-average income

4. Geographical managed care can be best described as _____.
   A. A medical group that is covered under Medicare and works much like an HMO
   B. A program that belongs to a medical group covered by Medicare and works much like an HMO
   C. A program that belongs to a medical group covered by Medicaid and works much like an HMO
   D. An HMO program that covers general medical groups

5. Information required by insurance companies does not include _____.
   A. Date medication is filled
   C. Name and dosage form of drug
   B. Name of pharmacy filing the prescription
   D. Name of technician

6. Insurance claims that are transmitted electronically to the insurance provider are called _____.
   A. E-mail
   C. Adjudication
   B. NDC claims
   D. Copay

7. Of the automated systems listed, which is used most commonly to manage controlled substances levels?
   A. PYXIS
   C. Bar coding
   B. Baker Cell Systems
   D. Both A and C

8. Various types of drugs ordered for a pharmacy may include _____.
   A. Formulary drugs
   C. Cytotoxic drugs
   B. Hazardous substances
   D. All of the above

9. The proper storage of medications is the responsibility of _____.
   A. The inventory technician
   B. The pharmacist in charge
   C. The technician
   D. Everyone working in the pharmacy

10. An inventory system that automatically orders stock as it is used is called _____.
    A. PYXIS
    C. MSDS
    B. POS
    D. Inventory cards

TRUE/FALSE **If a statement is false, then change it to make it true.**

_____ 1. Trade and generic drugs cost the pharmacy the same price.

_____ 2. If a patient's drug claim is rejected by the insurance company, the technician may call the help desk and attempt to reactivate it.

_____ 3. Periodic automatic replacement levels are levels of drugs that should be kept at a predetermined level in the pharmacy.

_____ 4. All drug recall notifications must be initiated by the Food and Drug Administration.

_____ 5. The sole responsibility of the pharmacy inventory technician is to keep all drugs and pharmacy supplies in stock.

_____ 6. Drug companies never allow pharmacies to return drugs.

_____ **7.** The only drug return that requires a pharmacist's signature is controlled substances return.

_____ **8.** All hazardous substances should be kept behind cabinet doors for safety purposes.

_____ **9.** MSDS stands for *medication safety drug sheets* and gives descriptions of drugs.

_____ **10.** Drugs that expire within 3 months may (in many cases) be pulled and returned to the manufacturer.

TECHNICIAN'S CORNER

The pharmacy technician accidentally fills the quinine stock box with quinidine. What is the difference between these two medicines? As a technician, what can you do to avoid confusion between these two drugs?

REFERENCES

1. CDER]www.fda.gov/cder/about/smallbiz/patent_term.htm
2. [Consumer Reports] Prescription Drug coverage: Things to consider. www.medicare.gov/pdp-things-to-consider.asp#Coverage
3. Medicare overview.www.medicare.gov/MedicareEligibility/home

WEBSITES

www.medicare.gov
www.ConsumerReports.org
www.Webmd.com
www.drugtopics.com
www.accesstobenefits.org
www.nlm.nih.gov
www.fda.gov

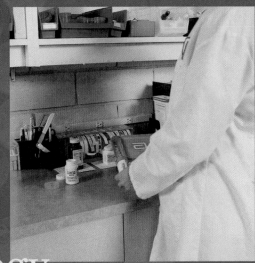

Psychopharmacology

Objectives

UPON COMPLETING THIS CHAPTER, YOU SHOULD BE ABLE TO
DO THE FOLLOWING:

- List the major medications used for each of the conditions described in this chapter.

- List the most common side effects of each of the drugs discussed.

- Describe the main emotional conditions affecting the brain.

- Differentiate between a normal depression and a severe depression.

- List the types of insomnia that can occur and why.

- Differentiate between older and newer treatments for the mentally disabled.

- Distinguish the capabilities of a psychologist versus a psychiatrist.

- List the differences between the uses of monoamine oxidase inhibitors (MAOIs), tricyclic antidepressants (TCAs), and selective serotonin reuptake inhibitors (SSRIs).

- Explain the reasons for the use of SSRIs over MAOIs and TCAs.

- Describe the differences between the uses of phenothiazines and thioxanthenes.

- Describe the types of nondrug therapy available for patients suffering from various mental disorders.

Anxiety *Feelings of apprehension, dread, and fear, with characteristics including tension, restlessness, tachycardia, dyspnea, and a sense of hopelessness*

Bipolar disorder *Depressive psychosis, alternating between excessive phases of mania and depression; formerly known as manic-depressive*

Depression *A mental state characterized by sadness, feelings of loss and grief, and loss of appetite and that may include suicidal thoughts*

Dystonia *Symptoms that include twisting, repeated jerking movements, and/or abnormal posture*

Extrapyramidal *Symptoms of taking antipsychotic medications that include parkinsonism, dystonia, and tremors*

Insomnia *Difficulty falling or staying asleep*

Mania *A form of psychosis characterized by excessive excitement, elevated mood, and exalted feelings*

Neurosis *Mental illness arising from stress or anxiety in the patient's environment without loss of contact with reality; phobias can be listed in this category*

Psychosis *A mental illness characterized by loss of contact with reality*

Schizophrenia *A group of mental disorders characterized by inappropriate emotions and unrealistic thinking*

Tardive dyskinesia *Unwanted side effects of taking phenothiazines that include slow, rhythmical, involuntary movements that are generalized or specific to a muscle group*

Tourette's syndrome *A disorder characterized by multiple motor tics, lack of muscle coordination, and involuntary, purposeless movements that are accompanied by grunts and barks*

PSYCHOTHERAPEUTIC MEDICATIONS

Trade Name	Generic Name	Pronunciation	Trade Name	Generic Name	Pronunciation
Antipsychotic Agents			Stelazine	trifluoperazine	(try-flew-**pear**-ah-zeen)
Abilify	aripiprazole	(a-rip-ip-**pra**-zol)	Thorazine	chlorpromazine	(klor-**pro**-ma-zeen)
Compazine	prochlorperazine	(pro-klor-**pear**-ah-zeen)	Trilafon	perphenazine	(per-**fen**-ah-zeen)
Eskalith	lithium	(**lith**-e-um)	Zyprexa	olanzapine	(oh-**lan**-zah-peen)
Geodon	ziprasidone	(zi-**praz**-ih-dohn)			
Haldol	haloperidol	(ha-low-**pear**-i-doll)	**Antidepressants**		
Loxitane	loxapine	(**lock**-sah-peen)	Anafranil	clomipramine	(klo-**mip**-ra-meen)
Mellaril	thioridazine	(thy-oh-**rid**-ah-zeen)	Asendin	amoxapine	(ah-**mox**-ah-peen)
Navane	thiothixene	(thy-oh-**thick**-seen)	Celexa	citalopram	(cit-**al**-o-pram)
Orap	pimozide	(**pim**-oh-zyde)	Cymbalta	duloxetine	(du-**lox**-uh-teen)
Prolixin	fluphenazine	(flew-**fen**-ah-zeen)	Desyrel	trazodone	(**trah**-zoe-doan)
Risperdal	risperidone	(ris-**pear**-ih-doan)	Effexor	venlafaxine	(ven-**la**-facks-een)
Seroquel	quetiapine	(kwe-**tie**-a-peen)	Elavil	amitriptyline	(am-eh-**trip**-tah-leen)

PSYCHOTHERAPEUTIC MEDICATIONS—cont'd

Trade Name	Generic Name	Pronunciation	Trade Name	Generic Name	Pronunciation
Nardil	phenelzine	(**fen**-el-zeen)	Ativan	lorazepam	(lor-**az**-ah-pam)
Norpramin	desipramine	(deh-**sip**-rah-meen)	BuSpar	buspirone	(bew-**spear**-on)
Pamelor	nortriptyline	(nor-**trip**-tah-leen)	Equanil	meprobamate	(meh-**pro**-bah-mate)
Parnate	tranylcypromine	(tran-ill-**sip**-roe-meen)	Librium	chlordiazepoxide	(klor-dye-az-eh-**pox**-ide)
Paxil	paroxetine	(par-**ox**-eh-teen)			
Prozac	fluoxetine	(flew-**ox**-eh-teen)	Serax	oxazepam	(ox-**az**-eh-pam)
Remeron	mirtazapine	(mer-**ta**-za-peen)	Sonata	zaleplon	(**zal**-e-plon)
Sinequan	doxepin	(**dock**-seh-pin)	Tranxene	clorazepate	(klor-**az**-eh-pate)
Tofranil	imipramine	(ih-**mip**-rah-meen)	Valium	diazepam	(dye-**az**-eh-pam)
Wellbutrin	bupropion	(bew-**pro**-pe-on)	Vistaril	hydroxyzine pamoate	(high-**drok**-seh-zeen **pam**-oh-ate)
Zoloft	sertraline	(**sir**-tra-leen)			
			Xanax	alprazolam	(al-**pra**-zoe-lam)
Antianxiety Agents			**Miscellaneous Agents**		
Atarax	hydroxyzine hydrochloride	(high-**drok**-seh-zeen high-dro-**klor**-ide)	Ambien	zolpidem	(zole-**pi**-dem)
			Dalmane	flurazepam	(flure-**az**-e-pam)

O VER THE COURSE OF HISTORY, one of the most difficult studies of medicine has been the study of the brain because of its complexities—specifically, what makes individuals behave the way they do? Historically, a person suffering from mental illness who did not "fit" into "normal" society easily could have been institutionalized for life. Families would try to forget or hide their knowledge of a mentally ill relative. The traditional treatments used ranged from electric shocks, straight jackets, and isolation to physical punishment. Few medications were known to help a mental disease. Even after some medications were discovered, most of them treated the illness by sedating the patient so that he or she could not "act out." It was not until the 1960s that advancements were made in psychopharmacology.

Many different specialists are trained in the study of human emotions, feelings, and behavior, such as psychiatrists, psychologists, and counselors. Psychiatrists are medical doctors who have completed a residency in the field of psychiatry. A psychologist has a doctoral degree in psychology. Unlike psychiatrists, psychologists (at this time) cannot write prescriptions, but they are trained extensively in the treatment of mental illness through counseling. There are certain states that are considering allowing psychologists the right to prescribe certain medications under the approval of a doctor. In addition to psychiatrists and psychologists, other professionals are available to treat individuals with emotional problems, such as family counselors and clergy. For many persons, this type of therapy may be adequate for help through difficult times. A person suffering from a severe emotional, behavioral, or biological instability involving the emotional portion of the brain may need to be seen by a psychiatrist for proper diagnosis and treatment. Depending on the diagnosis, a patient also may need to see a neurologist, a specialist of the nervous system. Many mental illnesses are caused by neuronal disturbances within the nervous system, such as twitching, or emotional problems stemming from a brain tumor or other physical problem.

Emotional Health

Emotional and behavioral instability often can be linked to functions of the body. A physician must evaluate the central nervous system (CNS) and the

TABLE 15-1 Conditions and Available Treatments

Examples of conditions	Specialist	Special notes
Mild depression, anxiety	Psychologist	Cannot prescribe drugs
Mild family problems, stress, child-rearing problems	Psychologist, family counselor, or support group	Cannot prescribe drugs
Psychosis, schizophrenia, manic-depressive disorders, major phobias	Psychiatrist (medical doctor)	Can prescribe drugs if necessary

environment in which a person lives. The CNS can be divided into two main functions, autonomic and somatic. The autonomic system works without conscious control, whereas the somatic system is under conscious control (see Chapter 17). The nervous system is an intricate network of chemical reactions that causes specific responses when activated. If any chemicals within the nervous system are out of balance or cease to produce, symptoms can appear as inappropriate behavior.

Nondrug Treatments

Because of the wide range of mental health conditions that exist, many alternative nondrug treatments are available. In the case of disorders that involve addictions or behavior disorders, many group therapies are available through nonprofit groups, such as Alcoholics Anonymous, or for-profit groups, such as Weight Watchers. Both groups give the patient a safe place where he or she can speak freely and not feel guilty. For more serious conditions or in cases in which the person does not feel comfortable speaking in front of others, a person can see a psychologist or counselor. For conditions that affect the whole family or a child, many family counselors specialize in group therapy within the family unit. For persons suffering from more severe crises, psychiatrists are able to meet one on one to discuss problems. If the psychiatrist feels that medication is appropriate, he or she can write prescriptions, unlike psychologists or family counselors. Table 15-1 lists mental health professionals and their scopes of practice.

Medication Therapy

Schizophrenia, mania, and psychotic depression often are treated with antipsychotic drugs and/or tranquilizers. These agents reduce the symptoms that often accompany these conditions. Mania, schizophrenia, and even psychotic depression tend to induce high-stress states in the patient. Antipsychotic agents and tranquilizers sedate the patient and produce a calming effect, lessening anxiety and depression.

ANTIPSYCHOTIC AGENTS

The two main classifications of antipsychotic drugs are phenothiazines and thioxanthenes. They differ in their lengths of effectiveness. Long-acting medications are called decanoates and are dosed monthly. In addition to the decanoates, there are the short-acting daily doses of the same type of drug. For instance, haloperidol can be dosed daily or on an as-needed basis. In addition to this type of dosing, the patient may be given a monthly dose of injectable haloperidol decanoate. The following medications are available as long-term decanoates.

LONG-ACTING DECANOATES

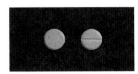

GENERIC NAME: haloperidol decanoate
TRADE NAME: Haldol
INDICATIONS: psychoses; Tourette's syndrome
STRENGTH: 50-mg injection, 100-mg injection; 0.5- to 5-mg tablets
ROUTE OF ADMINISTRATION: injection, oral
COMMON DOSAGE: 10 to 15 times the normal daily dose every month (maximum dose should not exceed 100 mg). Most daily oral doses range between 5 and 20 mg per day in divided doses
AUXILIARY LABELS:
- Do not drink alcohol.
- May cause dizziness and drowsiness.

GENERIC: fluphenazine decanoate
TRADE NAME: Prolixin
INDICATION: psychotic disorders
STRENGTH: 25 mg/mL
ROUTE OF ADMINISTRATION: injection
COMMON DOSAGE: 10 to 15 times the normal daily dose every month
AUXILIARY LABELS:
- Do not drink alcohol.
- May cause dizziness and drowsiness.

Side effects of decanoates include respiratory depression, tardive dyskinesia, drowsiness, orthostatic hypotension, and dry mouth.

Drug Action of Phenothiazines and Thioxanthenes

The drug action as it relates to the mechanism of action for the agents within two common classes of antipsychotics (phenothiazine and thioxanthene) is the inhibition of dopamine within the CNS. This antianxiety effect is caused by the effects on the brainstem area. These agents can cause blood pressure to drop but also (as a side effect) can decrease nausea and vomiting via their antiemetic effects. It can take up to 6 weeks or longer before the desired effects of these agents are obtained. If a change in medication is necessary, doses must be tapered slowly.

The main indications for these agents are psychosis, nausea, and vomiting. They can be given orally or parenterally (intravenously or intramuscularly). Side effects of these agents include drowsiness, confusion, insomnia, hypotension, and dry mouth. Alcohol and monoamine oxidase inhibitors (MAOIs) may potentiate (increase) CNS depression, whereas antacids and antidiarrheals can reduce the absorption rate of phenothiazines and thioxanthenes. One adverse reaction that can occur while taking these types of agents is tardive dyskinesia. The symptoms include involuntary movement of the facial muscles, tongue, jaw, and head. If these symptoms appear, the medication must be stopped immediately because these effects can be irreversible. Another type of adverse effect that is related to overdosing is extrapyramidal effects that mimic Parkinson's disease, causing the hands and head to shake. Drooling and a shuffling gait are present as well. These symptoms usually disappear if the medication strength is lowered or medication is stopped. Following are the shorter-acting agents listed under their respective classifications:

PHENOTHIAZINES

GENERIC NAME: prochlorperazine
TRADE NAME: Compazine
INDICATION: psychotic disorders; nausea and vomiting

ROUTE OF ADMINISTRATION: oral, injection, rectal
COMMON DOSAGE (ORAL): 5 to 10 mg (for nausea) 1q6 or q8hprn
AUXILIARY LABELS:

- May cause dizziness and drowsiness.
- Do not take if you become pregnant.
- Do not drink alcohol.

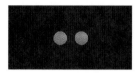

GENERIC NAME: thioridazine
TRADE NAME: Mellaril
INDICATIONS: psychotic disorders; anxiety, agitation, depression, sleep disturbances
ROUTE OF ADMINISTRATION: oral
COMMON DOSAGE: 10 mg bid (twice a day) or tid (three times a day)
AUXILIARY LABELS:

- May cause dizziness and drowsiness.
- Do not take if you become pregnant.
- Do not drink alcohol.

GENERIC NAME: perphenazine
TRADE NAME: Trilafon
INDICATIONS: psychotic disorders, nausea and vomiting, hiccups
ROUTE OF ADMINISTRATION: oral, injection
COMMON DOSAGE: 4 to 8 mg tid
AUXILIARY LABELS:

- May cause dizziness and drowsiness.
- Do not take if you become pregnant.
- Do not drink alcohol.

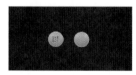

GENERIC NAME: chlorpromazine
TRADE NAME: Thorazine
INDICATION: manic-depressive reactions, hyperactivity in children
ROUTE OF ADMINISTRATION: oral, injection, rectal
COMMON DOSAGE: 25 mg tid up to 400 mg qd (every day)
AUXILIARY LABELS:

- May cause dizziness and drowsiness.
- Do not take if you become pregnant.
- Do not drink alcohol.

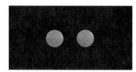

GENERIC NAME: trifluoperazine
TRADE NAME: Stelazine
INDICATION: psychotic disorders, anxiety
ROUTE OF ADMINISTRATION: oral, injection
COMMON DOSAGE: 1 to 5 mg qd or bid
AUXILIARY LABELS:

- May cause dizziness and drowsiness.
- Do not take if you become pregnant.
- Do not drink alcohol.

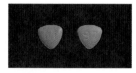

GENERIC NAME: fluphenazine
TRADE NAME: Prolixin
INDICATION: psychotic disorders, emesis
ROUTE OF ADMINISTRATION: oral, injection
COMMON DOSAGE: 0.5 to 10 mg qd
AUXILIARY LABELS:

- May cause dizziness and drowsiness.
- Do not take if you become pregnant.
- Do not drink alcohol.

The side effects of phenothiazines are drowsiness, dizziness, extrapyramidal symptoms, dry mouth, and tardive dyskinesia.

ANTIPSYCHOTIC

GENERIC NAME: thiothixene
TRADE NAME: Navane
INDICATION: psychotic disorders
ROUTE OF ADMINISTRATION: oral, injection
COMMON DOSAGE: 2 mg tid to 15 mg qd
AUXILIARY LABELS:
- May cause dizziness and drowsiness.
- Avoid alcohol.

The side effects of thioxanthenes are extrapyramidal symptoms, dry mouth, akathisia, dystonia, and tardive dyskinesia.

Alternative Antipsychotic Agents

Alternative antipsychotic agents are used to treat psychotic patients who do not respond well to phenothiazines or thioxanthenes or who have adverse reactions to them. Many of these agents are new on the market, and their drug actions are not entirely understood. A list of the most common agents are given in the following.

DIBENZAPINE DERIVATIVES

GENERIC NAME: loxapine
TRADE NAME: Loxitane
INDICATION: psychotic disorders
ROUTE OF ADMINISTRATION: oral, injection (intramuscular)
COMMON DOSAGE: 10 mg bid up to 50 mg qd (in divided doses)
AUXILIARY LABELS:
- May cause dizziness and drowsiness.
- Do not drink alcohol.
- Do not take if you become pregnant.

BENZISOXAZOLE DERIVATIVES

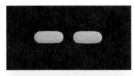
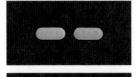
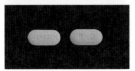

GENERIC NAME: risperidone
TRADE NAME: Risperdal
INDICATION: psychotic disorders and agitation in elderly persons
ROUTE OF ADMINISTRATION: oral
COMMON DOSAGE: 1 mg bid up to 8 mg qd to bid
AUXILIARY LABEL: none

The side effects of dibenzapines are drowsiness, hyperactivity, seizures, and tardive dyskinesia.

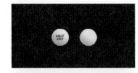

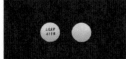

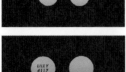

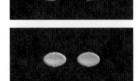

GENERIC NAME: olanzapine
TRADE NAME: Zyprexa
INDICATION: psychotic disorders
ROUTE OF ADMINISTRATION: oral
COMMON DOSAGE: 5 to 10 mg qd
AUXILIARY LABEL: none

The side effects are headache, agitation, insomnia, and constipation.

BUTYROPHENONE

GENERIC NAME: pimozide
TRADE NAME: Orap
INDICATION: Tourette's syndrome; psychosis
ROUTE OF ADMINISTRATION: oral
COMMON DOSAGE: 1 to 2 mg qd
AUXILIARY LABEL:

- Avoid grapefruit juice.

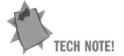

TECH NOTE!

All patients taking lithium must have their blood levels monitored regularly for toxicity. Because lithium toxicity levels are close to the necessary therapeutic levels, lithium therapy should be started only if the lithium levels can be monitored closely.

ANTIMANICS

The word *mania* is derived from the word *manic*. This form of psychosis is characterized by excessive mood swings that range from manic (high) to depressive (low) states, which also is known as bipolar disorder, indicating the extreme mood swings. Lithium is used to treat the manic phase. Although the complete mechanism for lithium is not understood fully, it is believed to alter behavior by enhancing uptake of serotonin and norepinephrine by nerve cells (see Chapter 17). This sets lithium apart from all the other psychiatric drugs, because it does not cause any major CNS changes such as sedation, feelings of euphoria, or depression. The effects of lithium are more powerful in older adults; therefore, it is important that their lithium levels be monitored more closely. It may take several weeks to see the desired effect of this agent.

ANTIMANIC

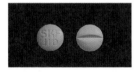

GENERIC NAME: lithium
TRADE NAME: Eskalith
INDICATION: mania, depression
ROUTE OF ADMINISTRATION: oral
COMMON DOSAGE: for acute mania; 600 mg tid or 900 mg bid; doses vary based on laboratory results of serum lithium levels
AUXILIARY LABELS:

- Do not drink alcohol.
- May cause dizziness and drowsiness.
- Take with food or milk.
- Drink plenty of water.

The side effects include dizziness, drowsiness, ataxia, hypotension, slurred speech, and weight gain.

ANTIDEPRESSANTS

Everyone is depressed at one time or another during his or her lifetime. Most persons who experience depression do not seek medical help and recover within a short period. However, for those persons in whom the depression does not subside within a few weeks, professional attention may be necessary.

Many drugs are used for depression. This mental state can range from prolonged feelings of extreme sadness to thoughts of suicide. Patients with manic depression fluctuate between the two extremes. Three closely related agents commonly are used to treat depression. These are the tricyclic antidepressants (TCAs), MAOIs, and selective serotonin reuptake inhibitors (SSRIs). Each of these agents increases the norepinephrine, serotonin, and dopamine chemicals of the brain, which elevates the mood of the patient. However, each type of agent accomplishes this by a different drug action.

Tricyclic Antidepressants

TCAs are used for depression, obsessive-compulsive disorders, and in some cases for chronic pain. These agents inhibit (stop) the reuptake (the cells taking back excess amounts) of norepinephrine and serotonin. A wide range of concerns surrounds TCAs in general. One of the main concerns with taking TCAs is the possibility of tardive dyskinesia. Worsening of symptoms in patients with heart disease, schizophrenia, seizure disorders, and renal or hepatic problems is also a concern. Because of these problems, TCAs are not the first line of treatment for depression. However, for some persons, they work well when all other medications fail. Side effects differ among the various types of TCAs and are described in the following.

TRICYCLIC ANTIDEPRESSANTS

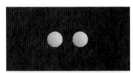

GENERIC NAME: amitriptyline
TRADE NAME: Elavil
INDICATION: depression
ROUTE OF ADMINISTRATION: oral, injection
COMMON DOSAGE: 75 to 100 mg qd (divided doses) up to 300 mg qd
AUXILIARY LABELS:

■ May cause dizziness and drowsiness.
■ Take with food.

GENERIC NAME: doxepin
TRADE NAME: Sinequan
INDICATION: depression, anxiety
ROUTE OF ADMINISTRATION: oral, cream*
COMMON DOSAGE: 50 to 150 mg qd
AUXILIARY LABELS:

■ May cause dizziness and drowsiness.
■ May cause sensitivity to sunlight.

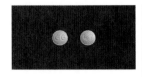

GENERIC NAME: imipramine
TRADE NAME: Tofranil
INDICATION: depression, enuresis (bed-wetting)
ROUTE OF ADMINISTRATION: oral (pamoate and hydrochloride), injection (hydrochloride only)
COMMON DOSAGE: oral, 75 to 150 mg qd†

---

*Cream is indicated for dermatological pruritus, alopecia, or rashes.
†In children the dosage is determined by the child's weight.

TABLE 15-2 Foods That Contain Tyramine

Foods	Additive
Cheese	Bacteria and fungi
Sour cream	Bacteria
Beer	Yeast
Wine	Yeast
Avocados	Bacteria
Soy sauce	Fungi
Yogurt	Bacteria
Chocolate	Caffeine
Tea	Caffeine
Coffee	Caffeine

AUXILIARY LABELS:
- May cause dizziness and drowsiness.
- Do not drink alcohol.

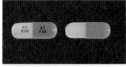
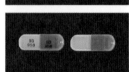
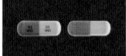

GENERIC NAME: clomipramine
TRADE NAME: Anafranil
INDICATION: obsessive-compulsive disorder, depression
ROUTE OF ADMINISTRATION: oral
COMMON DOSAGE: 25 mg qd up to 100 mg qd (divided doses)
AUXILIARY LABELS:
- May cause dizziness and drowsiness.
- Do not drink alcohol.

The side effects of TCAs include drowsiness, dry mouth, blurred vision, orthostatic hypotension, dizziness, and headache.

Monoamine Oxidase Inhibitors

MAOIs mostly differ from TCAs and SSRIs by their side effects. Patients taking MAOIs can exhibit hypertension. Many food interactions occur with MAOIs as well. Certain foods containing tyramine, such as red wine, can be extremely dangerous to a patient taking MAOIs. In addition to wine, in general, foods that use bacteria or other microbes in their processing cause interactions. Produce such as raisins, bananas, avocados, and papaya can cause adverse reactions also. Table 15-2 gives a sample list of foods with microbial ingredients.

Because of the many food interactions with MAOI agents, they are reserved for use in patients who do not respond to TCAs or SSRIs or who have a reaction to them. The following drugs are MAOIs.

MONOAMINE OXIDASE INHIBITORS

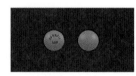

GENERIC NAME: tranylcypromine
TRADE NAME: Parnate
INDICATION: depression
ROUTE OF ADMINISTRATION: oral
COMMON DOSAGE: 30 mg qd (divided doses) up to 60 mg qd
AUXILIARY LABELS:
- Take with food.
- Do not drink alcohol.

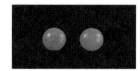

GENERIC NAME: phenelzine
TRADE NAME: Nardil
INDICATION: depression
ROUTE OF ADMINISTRATION: oral
COMMON DOSAGE: 15 mg tid up to 60 mg qd
AUXILIARY LABEL:

■ Do not drink alcohol.

The side effects of MAOIs include gastrointestinal upset, insomnia, drowsiness, hypotension, dry mouth, and anorexia.

Selective Serotonin Reuptake Inhibitors

SSRIs act specifically on keeping higher levels of serotonin in the brain. When serotonin is increased, mood is elevated. These agents work differently than the MAOIs and TCAs. Because SSRIs have fewer side effects, they are preferable to treat depression and obsessive-compulsive disorders. The doses that follow are the maximum doses. Patients may be started at a lower dose initially, and the dose may be increased gradually to the maximum dosage. An important note is that patients cannot take MAOIs and SSRIs concurrently. There have been reports of death caused by this dangerous combination. Typically, these medications can take up to 6 weeks to work at their full potential.

SELECTIVE SEROTONIN REUPTAKE INHIBITORS

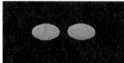

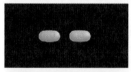

GENERIC NAME: citalopram
TRADE NAME: Celexa
INDICATION: antidepressant
ROUTE OF ADMINISTRATION: oral
STRENGTH: tablet, 20 mg, 40 mg, 60 mg; solution, 10 mg/5 mL
COMMON DOSAGE: oral, 20 mg qd
AUXILIARY LABEL:

■ May cause dizziness and drowsiness.

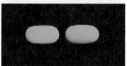

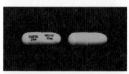

GENERIC NAME: paroxetine
TRADE NAME: Paxil
INDICATION: depression, obsessive-compulsive disorder
ROUTE OF ADMINISTRATION: oral
COMMON DOSAGE: depression, 10 mg qd; obsessive-compulsive disorder, 40 mg qd
AUXILIARY LABELS:

■ Take with food.
■ Do not drink alcohol.

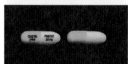

GENERIC NAME: fluoxetine
TRADE NAME: Prozac
INDICATION: depression, obsessive-compulsive disorder
ROUTE OF ADMINISTRATION: oral
COMMON DOSAGE: 60 mg qd maximum; usually 10 to 20 mg daily
AUXILIARY LABELS:

■ Take with food.
■ Do not drink alcohol.
NOTE: Drug may increase suicidal tendencies.

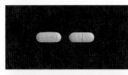

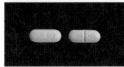

GENERIC NAME: sertraline
TRADE NAME: Zoloft
INDICATION: depression, obsessive-compulsive disorder
ROUTE OF ADMINISTRATION: oral
COMMON DOSAGE: 50 mg qd up to 200 mg qd
AUXILIARY LABEL:

■ Do not drink alcohol.

The side effects of SSRIs include insomnia, nausea, dizziness, drowsiness, sexual dysfunction, headache, constipation, dry mouth, and anorexia.

Additional Antidepressants

The antidepressants discussed next do not fit into the previous categories because they do not have the same drug actions as the other antidepressants. In some cases the exact drug action is not known; however, they work well for some patients.

OTHER ANTIDEPRESSANTS

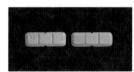

GENERIC NAME: trazodone
TRADE NAME: Desyrel
INDICATION: depression
ROUTE OF ADMINISTRATION: oral
DRUG ACTION: inhibits serotonin uptake mechanism
COMMON DOSAGE: 150 mg qd up to 600 mg qd (divided doses)
SIDE EFFECTS: dizziness, drowsiness, shortness of breath, chest pain, tachycardia
AUXILIARY LABELS:

■ Take with food.
■ May cause dizziness and drowsiness.
■ Do not drink alcohol.

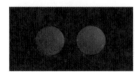

GENERIC NAME: bupropion*
TRADE NAME: Wellbutrin, Zyban (Wellbutrin is well known for its treatment for depression but it also can be used in addition for smoking cessation, whereas Zyban has been approved exclusively as an aid to quit smoking.)
INDICATION: depression; bupropion (Wellbutrin)* usually is given in two or three daily doses. When used for smoking cessation, bupropion usually is started at 150 mg once daily for 3 days, and then the dose is increased if the patient tolerates the starting dose. Smoking should be discontinued at least 2 weeks after starting bupropion therapy. Wellbutrin SR is given as two daily doses. Wellbutrin XL is given as one dose daily.
ROUTE OF ADMINISTRATION: oral
DRUG ACTION: a weak blocker of the uptake mechanism of serotonin and norepinephrine, as well as dopamine to an extent
COMMON DOSAGE: 100 mg tid or 150 mg bid
SIDE EFFECTS: dizziness, drowsiness, hallucinations, blurred vision
AUXILIARY LABELS:

■ Do not drink alcohol.
■ May cause dizziness and drowsiness.

---

*Has been known to cause seizures when dosage is greater than 450 mg per day.

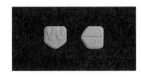

GENERIC NAME: venlafaxine
TRADE NAME: Effexor
INDICATION: depression
COMMON DOSAGE: 75 to 225 mg/day in split dosages given twice daily or 3 times daily
ROUTE OF ADMINISTRATION: oral
DRUG ACTION: This agent inhibits the dopamine inhibitors, thus increasing dopamine levels in the brain.
SIDE EFFECTS: dry mouth, elevated blood pressure, dizziness, drowsiness, sweating, sexual dysfunction
AUXILIARY LABELS:

- Do not drink alcohol.
- May cause dizziness and drowsiness.

SEDATIVE AND HYPNOTIC AGENTS

Sedative and hypnotic agents affect the CNS. The difference between the two types of agents is the degree to which they affect the CNS. Because sedatives affect the CNS to a lesser degree than do hypnotics, they are used to relax and ease a nervous or irritated person by producing a soothing effect. For example, sedatives sometimes are given to relax patients before a procedure, such as a magnetic resonance imaging or computed tomography scan. Hypnotics affect the CNS to a higher degree than sedatives, causing sleepiness. Examples of use of hypnotics include inducing sleep before surgery or inducing sleepiness for those who suffer from insomnia. Insomnia can occur for many reasons, including side effects of drugs, whether they are over-the-counter (OTC) or prescription. Older persons commonly suffer from insomnia because of pain or physiological changes. Another major cause of insomnia is stress. Listed in Table 15-3 are three types of insomnia and their specific descriptions.

For persons suffering from mild cases of insomnia there are many OTC drugs available. Table 15-4 lists some of the most popular agents.

The main ingredient in OTC sedative and hypnotic agents is diphenhydramine. Diphenhydramine (Benadryl) is classified as an antihistamine. The main side effect of this agent is sleepiness, which in the case of insomnia is the desired effect. Acetaminophen or magnesium salicylate are additive analgesics used to treat insomnia caused by pain resulting from injury or illness. OTC sedatives are meant to treat short-term insomnia and work well. However, if the insomnia continues over a longer period, a stronger medication may be needed, such as a prescription sedative-hypnotic agent.

The first two classes of drugs that are discussed are the barbiturates and benzodiazepines. These two drug classes are not considered a permanent solution to insomnia. One negative effect of using certain hypnotics is the hangover effect the following morning. Because both agents are controlled substances (schedule IV), they have an ability to become addictive; therefore, they normally are used for short-term treatment. Each class of drug has different indications, drug actions, dosing, and side effects that are discussed next.

TABLE 15-3 Types and Description of Insomnia

Types	Description
Initial insomnia	Difficulty falling asleep
Intermittent insomnia	Difficulty staying asleep
Terminal insomnia	Waking early and unable to fall back to sleep

TABLE 15-4 Over-the-Counter Agents to Treat Insomnia

Trade name	Generic name	Common dosage
Nytol	Diphenhydramine	25 mg
Excedrin PM	Diphenhydramine/acetaminophen	38 mg/500 mg
Sominex Caps	Diphenhydramine	50 mg
Nighttime Pamprin	Diphenhydramine/acetaminophen	50 mg/650 mg
Extra Strength Doan's PM	Diphenhydramine/magnesium salicylate	25 mg/500 mg

Barbiturates

Barbiturates are controlled substances that have been used for many years for sedation of persons suffering from different conditions such as seizures and insomnia and as a hypnotic before surgery. Barbiturates are differentiated by the time it takes them to work. They range from short- to long-acting and are listed in Table 15-5.

Drug action. Barbiturates act on the brainstem area, reducing nerve impulses to the cerebral cortex. Because barbiturates affect the respiratory system, nerves, and smooth muscles, their effects cause relaxation and sleep. If a low dose is given, barbiturates produce a mild sedative effect, whereas a high dose causes anesthesia. Examples of these agents include thiopental and methohexital, which are used in surgery to keep the patient under general anesthesia.

Side effects

Several side effects are associated with the use of barbiturates, such as drowsiness, dizziness, nausea, vomiting, constipation, and a hangover effect after the drug wears off. Because of the effect barbiturates have on the CNS and the respiratory system, barbiturates can cause death if the patient takes an overdose. Because of the many side effects produced by barbiturates, benzodiazepines are prescribed more often.

Benzodiazepines

Benzodiazepines have several effects on the body system. They are known to affect parts of the brain, decreasing convulsions and affecting emotional stability. Effects within the spinal cord cause muscle relaxation, and benzodiazepines can cause sedation. Because these agents affect the CNS, they can decrease breathing rate. Their main use is as hypnotic agents to induce sleep. Other common uses include seizure control and as muscle relaxants.

The benzodiazepines are lipid (fat) soluble. This means that they can enter into and through cells and areas within the body system that are made of lipids or are protected by a lipid barrier. The brain is a delicate and important area that must be protected from foreign bodies. The brain is protected by a blood-brain barrier that stops many chemicals from passing into the brain. Drugs that are lipid-soluble can pass through the blood-brain barrier, which is why mental function is changed after taking the medication. Excretion is through the urine. All the benzodiazepines are legend (prescription) drugs and are labeled controlled substances (schedule IV). A list of commonly prescribed benzodiazepines follows.

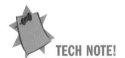

TECH NOTE!

Pharmacy technicians have the knowledge of classifications of drugs and personal patient information. It is important to remember that all medical information should be kept private. If patient confidentiality is broken, the consequences possibly can be devastating to the patient. Never disclose to anyone what medication the patient is taking or the condition the patient has.

TABLE 15-5 Common Barbiturates

Schedule	Generic name	Trade name	Common dosage	Length of action	Route of administration
C-IV	Phenobarbital	Luminal	Sedative: 30-120 mg qd Seizures: 60-120 mg qd	Long acting	PO, IV, IM
C-IV	Mephobarbital	Mebaral	Sedative: 32-100 mg tid/qid Seizures: 400-600 mg qd	Long acting	PO
C-III	Butabarbital	Butisol	Sedation: 15-30 mg tid/qid Sleep: 50-100 mg Pre-op: 50-100 mg	Intermediate	PO, IV
C-II	Secobarbital	Seconal	Sleep: 100 mg Pre-op: 200-300 mg	Short acting	PO, IV IM
C-II	Pentobarbital	Nembutal	Sedation: 20 mg tid/qid Insomnia: 100 mg qhs Pre-op: 1-3 mg/kg	Short acting	PO, IV, IM PR

qd, every day; *PO,* oral; *IV,* intravenous; *IM,* intramuscular; *tid,* 3 times a day; *qid,* 4 times a day; *qhs,* at bedtime; *pre-op,* preoperative; *PR,* per-rectal.

BENZODIAZEPINES

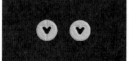
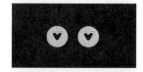

GENERIC NAME: diazepam
TRADE NAME: Valium
INDICATION: anxiety, acute alcohol withdrawal, muscle relaxant, anticonvulsant
ROUTE OF ADMINISTRATION: oral, injection
COMMON DOSAGE: anxiety, 2 to 10 mg; alcohol withdrawal, 10 mg tid or qid; muscle spasms, 15 to 30 mg qd
AUXILIARY LABELS:
■ May cause dizziness and drowsiness.
■ Do not drink alcohol.

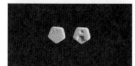

GENERIC NAME: lorazepam
TRADE NAME: Ativan
INDICATION: anxiety, insomnia
ROUTE OF ADMINISTRATION: oral, injection
COMMON DOSAGE: anxiety, 2 to 6 mg qd; insomnia, 2 to 4 mg qhs (at bedtime)
AUXILIARY LABELS:
■ May cause dizziness and drowsiness.
■ Do not drink alcohol.

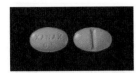
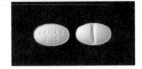

GENERIC NAME: alprazolam
TRADE NAME: Xanax
INDICATION: anxiety, panic disorders
ROUTE OF ADMINISTRATION: oral
COMMON DOSAGE: 0.25 to 0.5 mg tid
AUXILIARY LABELS:

- May cause dizziness and drowsiness.
- Do not drink alcohol.

GENERIC NAME: oxazepam
TRADE NAME: Serax
INDICATION: anxiety, tension, alcohol withdrawal
ROUTE OF ADMINISTRATION: oral
COMMON DOSAGE: anxiety, 10 to 15 mg tid or qid; alcohol withdrawal, 15 to 30 mg tid or qid
AUXILIARY LABELS:

- May cause dizziness and drowsiness.
- Do not drink alcohol.

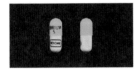

GENERIC NAME: chlordiazepoxide
TRADE NAME: Librium
INDICATION: anxiety, acute alcohol withdrawal
ROUTE OF ADMINISTRATION: oral, injection
COMMON DOSAGE: 5 to 10 mg tid or qid
AUXILIARY LABELS:

- May cause dizziness and drowsiness.
- Do not drink alcohol.

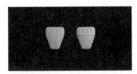

GENERIC NAME: clorazepate
TRADE NAME: Tranxene
INDICATION: anxiety, alcohol withdrawal
ROUTE OF ADMINISTRATION: oral
COMMON DOSAGES: anxiety, 30 mg qd (divided doses); alcohol withdrawal, 1 mg qd up to 30 mg qd
AUXILIARY LABELS:

- May cause dizziness and drowsiness.
- Do not drink alcohol.

BENZODIAZEPINE-LIKE

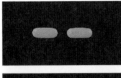
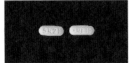

GENERIC NAME: zolpidem
TRADE NAME: Ambien
INDICATION: insomnia
DRUG ACTION: nonbenzodiazepine hypnotic; does not have muscle relaxant or anticonvulsant properties
ROUTE OF ADMINISTRATION: oral
COMMON DOSAGE: 5 to 10 mg qhs (at bedtime) for 5 to 7 days
AUXILIARY LABEL:

- May cause dizziness and drowsiness.

The side effects of benzodiazepines include drowsiness, dizziness, blurred vision, dry mouth, and fatigue.

MISCELLANEOUS ANTIANXIETY AGENTS

Each of the following antianxiety agents has a different drug action. Most, if not all, of the agents that affect certain parts of the CNS produce anticholinergic effects. This includes the drying out of secretions throughout the body, which can involve dry mouth, dry eyes, and constipation. Each type of agent causes these side effects to one degree or another.

ANTIANXIETY

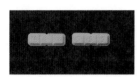

GENERIC NAME: buspirone
TRADE NAME: BuSpar
INDICATION: anxiety
ROUTE OF ADMINISTRATION: oral
COMMON DOSAGE: 15 mg per day
DRUG ACTION: unknown
SIDE EFFECTS: none
AUXILIARY LABEL:
- Take as directed.

ANTIHISTAMINE

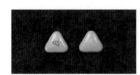

GENERIC NAME: hydroxyzine hydrochloride; hydroxyzine pamoate
TRADE NAME: Atarax; Vistaril
INDICATION: anxiety, pruritus resulting from allergic reactions, preoperative sedation
ROUTE OF ADMINISTRATION: oral; injectable form
DRUG ACTION: affects the CNS, producing muscle relaxation, analgesia, and
    anticholinergic effects
COMMON DOSAGE: anxiety or nausea, 25 to 100 mg tid or qid; pruritus, 25 mg tid or qid
SIDE EFFECTS: drowsiness, dry mouth
AUXILIARY LABELS:
- May cause dizziness and drowsiness. Alcohol intensifies these effects.

ANTIANXIETY

GENERIC NAME: meprobamate
TRADE NAME: Equanil, Miltown
INDICATION: anxiety, muscle relaxant, and for insomnia
ROUTE OF ADMINISTRATION: oral
DRUG ACTION: affects the CNS and also inhibits spinal reflexes, causing overall
    relaxation
COMMON DOSAGE: 400 mg tid to qid
SIDE EFFECTS: drowsiness, dizziness, dry mouth
AUXILIARY LABELS:
- May cause dizziness and drowsiness.
- Do not drink alcohol.

NOTE: Antianxiety/antipsychotic medications are schedule IV medications.

Medications and the Elderly

Keep in mind that older persons are much more sensitive to medications because their bodies are not in the same condition as when they were younger. Because of the loss of muscle tissue and changes in the functions of the organs, certain medications can become concentrated much easier than in a younger person. Organs such as the liver and kidneys take much longer in breaking down chemicals. In addition, it is reported that the average older person is taking more than four prescription medications at the same time plus two OTC medications.[1] Because it is common for the elderly to take many medications at the same time, be sure to tell patients to inform the pharmacist of all the medication they are taking, including OTC drugs.

DO YOU REMEMBER THESE KEY POINTS?

- The main causes of insomnia
- Various treatments for depression, including the types of agents used
- The differences between MAOIs, TCAs, and SSRIs
- Under what circumstances might a decanoate agent be used
- The method of action of phenothiazines
- The major side effects of TCAs
- How long most antidepressants must be taken before they are effective
- What foods contain tyramine and what importance they have when one is taking MAOIs
- Why MAOIs are normally less popular than SSRIs and TCAs for treating depression
- What major OTC drugs are available for treating insomnia
- What barbiturates are prescribed for and their schedules
- What benzodiazepines are prescribed for and their schedules

MULTIPLE CHOICE QUESTIONS

1. The blood-brain barrier protects the brain from _____.
   A. Toxins
   B. Drugs
   C. Large molecules
   D. All of the above

2. A prescription can be written by _____.
   A. A psychiatrist
   B. A psychologist
   C. A family counselor
   D. All of the above

3. A type of nondrug therapy for emotional problems may include _____.
   A. Family counseling
   B. Group therapy
   C. Visiting a psychologist
   D. All of the above

4. The illness that is marked by extremes in elevated and depressed moods is defined as _____.
   A. Schizophrenia
   B. Bipolar disorder
   C. Depression
   D. All of the above

5. Long-acting decanoates are given _____.
   A. Every other day
   B. Every week
   C. Every month
   D. In any of these combinations

6. The main neurotransmitters of the brain that are affected by benzodiazepines are _____.
   A. Dopamine
   B. Norepinephrine
   C. Epinephrine
   D. All of the above

7. Extrapyramidal effects that include shaky hands and head are caused mainly by _____.
   A. Overdosing MAOIs
   B. Overdosing TCAs
   C. Overdosing SSRIs
   D. All of the above

8. _____ is (are) the main drug(s) used for the treatment of manic phases of persons with bipolar disorder.
   A. TCAs
   B. SSRIs
   C. Lithium
   D. Diphenhydramine

9. The antidepressant class that has the mildest side effects and is used for depression is _____.

    A. SSRIs   C. TCAs

    B. MAOIs   D. Benzodiazepines

10. SSRIs inhibit the reuptake inhibitors within the neuronal transmission, which increases the levels of _____.

    A. Norepinephrine   C. Serotonin

    B. Epinephrine   D. Dopamine

TRUE/FALSE   If the statement is false, then change it to make it true.

_____ 1. Tardive dyskinesia is a mental illness.

_____ 2. Short-acting phenothiazines include oral fluphenazine (Prolixin), thioridazine (Mellaril), chlorpromazine (Thorazine), and trifluoperazine (Stelazine).

_____ 3. Decanoate dosage forms include oral and parenteral.

_____ 4. Persons taking SSRIs should avoid foods that contain tyramine.

_____ 5. MAOIs are used less than SSRIs and TCAs because of their side effects.

_____ 6. Most antidepressants must be taken for up to 1 week before the desired effects can be seen.

_____ 7. Two of the most common auxiliary labels for benzodiazepines are "Take with plenty of water" and "Take with food."

_____ 8. TCAs, MAOIs, and SSRIs can be used to treat bipolar behavior.

_____ 9. Bipolar behavior also is referred to as a manic-depressive disorder.

_____ 10. Hypnotic agents often are used to relax patients before procedures such as computed tomography scans.

TECHNICIAN'S CORNER

The doctor has ordered Tofranil for a child who is 5 years old and weighs 45 lb. He orders 1.5 mg/kg per day to be given 3 times daily.

Is this dosage safe according to the *Drug Facts and Comparisons* recommendations?

How much drug per day would this child be given based on the dose ordered?

How much drug per dose would be given based on the dose ordered?

Is there a generic equivalent to Tofranil; if so, what other companies manufacture this drug?

REFERENCE

1. Medications and older people, *FDA Consumer* Sept-Oct 1997 (Pub No FDA 03-1315C). Retrieved April 2006 from www.fda.gov/fdac/features/1997/697_old.html

BIBLIOGRAPHY

Medications and older people, *FDA Consumer* Sept-Oct 1997 (Pub No FDA 03-1315C). Retrieved April 2006 from www.fda.gov/fdac/features/1997/697_old.html

Medications: generic name—bupropion, MedicineNet.com. Retrieved April 2006, from www.medicinenet.com/bupropion/article.htm

Mosby's 2006 drug consult for nurses handheld software [CD-ROM], St Louis, 2006, Mosby.

WEBSITES

www.medterms.com
www.drugtopics.com/drugtopics
www.dr-bob.org/tips/
www.psycom.net/depression.central.drugnames.html

SECTION two

Body Systems

CHAPTER

16

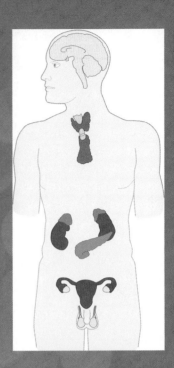

Endocrine System

Objectives

UPON COMPLETING THIS CHAPTER, YOU SHOULD BE ABLE TO
DO THE FOLLOWING:

- Write the generic and trade names for all drugs discussed in this chapter.

- List classifications and indications of each drug discussed.

- Name the major glands of the body.

- Write the location and function of the glands discussed.

- Differentiate between the endocrine and exocrine glands.

- Explain the role of iodine in the metabolism of hormones of the thyroid gland.

- Explain the role of calcium in bones.

- Describe the causes and symptoms of osteoporosis.

- Describe the conditions caused by improper gland functioning.

- List the main hormones that are produced in women and men.

- Explain the uses of androgens in men and women.

- List the causes of diabetes mellitus.

- Describe the differences between insulin-dependent diabetes mellitus and non–insulin-dependent diabetes mellitus.

- Explain the relationship between the central nervous system and the release of hormones from the adrenal gland.

- List the primary side effects of the medications discussed in the chapter.

- List the auxiliary labels required when filling prescriptions for hormones.

Addison's disease *Condition resulting in a decrease in adrenocortical hormones, such as mineralocorticoids and glucocorticoids, that causes symptoms including muscle weakness and weight loss*

Autocrine *Denoting a mode of hormone action in which a hormone binds to receptors on and affects the function of the cell type that produced it*

Autoimmune disease *Condition in which a person's tissues are attacked by his or her immune system; abnormal antigen-antibody reaction*

Cretinism *Condition in which the development of the brain and body is inhibited by congenital lack of thyroid secretion*

Cushing's disease *Syndrome causing an increase in secretion of the adrenal cortex that includes symptoms such as a moon face and deposits of fat (buffalo hump)*

Exophthalmos *Prominence of the eyeball caused by increased thyroid hormone*

Glucose *Simple sugar*

Goiter *Condition in which the thyroid gland is enlarged because of a lack of iodine, known as simple goiter, or because of a tumor, known as toxic goiter*

Graves' disease *Condition caused by hypersecretion of thyroid with diffuse goiter, exophthalmos, and skin changes*

Homeostasis *The equilibrium pertaining to the balance of the body with respect to fluid levels, pH level, and chemicals*

Hormones *Chemical substances produced and secreted by an endocrine duct into the bloodstream or duct that result in a physiological response at a specific target tissue*

Hypercalcemia *Unusually high concentration of calcium in the blood*

Hyperglycemia *Abnormally high glucose content circulating in the bloodstream*

Hypocalcemia *Low concentration of calcium in the blood*

Hypoglycemia *Abnormally low glucose content circulating in the bloodstream*

Myxedema *Condition associated with a decrease in overall thyroid function in adults; also known as hypothyroidism*

Neuroblastomas *Tumors of the neural crest; neuroblastomas often consist of cells morphologically*

NIDDM *Non–insulin-dependent diabetes mellitus*

Osteoporosis *Condition associated with the decrease of bone mass and softening of bones, resulting in the increased possibility of bone fractures*

Paget's disease *Condition that affects older adults in which the density of the bones decreases, resulting in softening and weakening*

Paracrine *Denoting a type of hormone function in which hormone synthesized in and released from endocrine cells binds to its receptor*

Pheochromocytomas *Tumors of the adrenal gland that produce excess adrenaline*

PTH *Parathyroid hormone*

Simmonds' disease *A pituitary disorder that is a form of hypopituitarism in which all pituitary secretions are deficient*

Spermatogenesis *The process of producing sperm with half the number of chromosomes*

Thyroxine *Known as T₄; contains four ions of iodine*

Triiodothyronine *Known as T₃; contains three ions of iodine*

DRUGS

Trade Name	Generic	Pronunciation	Trade Name	Generic	Pronunciation
Thyroid Replacement			**Estrogens**		
Armour Thyroid	desiccated thyroid	(**des**-eh-kate-ed **thigh**-roid)	Diethylstilbestrol	diethylstilbestrol	(dye-eth-ill-still-**best**-roll)
Cytomel	liothyronine	(lie-oh-**thigh**-row-neen)	Estinyl	ethinyl estradiol	(**eth**-in-ill ess-tra-**dye**-ole)
Synthroid, Levoxyl	levothyroxine	(lee-vo-**thigh**-rox-een)	Estrace	estradiol	(ess-tra-**dye**-ole)
			Estrovis	quinestrol	(kwye-**ness**-troll)
Thyrolar	liotrix	(**lee**-ow-tricks)	Premarin	conjugated estrogens	(**kon**-juh-gat-ed **ess**-troe-jens)
Hyperthyroidism			Prempro	combined estrogen/ progestin	(**ess**-troe-jen/pro-**jess**-tin)
Propyl-Thyracil	propylthiouracil	(pro-pull-thigh-oh-**your**-ah-sill)			
Tapazole	methimazole	(meth-**em**-ah-zoll)	**Progestins**		
Thyro-Block	potassium iodide	(poh-tas-ee-um **eye**-oh-dyed)	Aygestin	norethindrone acetate	(nor-**eth**-in-drone **as**-see-tate)
			Megace	megestrol acetate	(me-**jess**-trall **as**-see-tate)
Calcium Regulator			Prometrium	progesterone	(pro-**jess**-tur-own)
Calcimar	calcitonin-salmon	(**cal**-sit-toe-nen **sam**-men)	Provera	medroxyprogesterone	(me-drock-see-pro-**jess**-tur-own)
Didronel	etidronate disodium	(eh-tea-**droh**-nate dy-**sow**-dee-um)			
Skelid	tiludronate disodium	(ti-**loo**-drue-nate dy-**sow**-dee-um)	**Insulin**		
			Humalog	insulin lispro	(**in**-su-lin **lis** pro)
Bisphosphonates			Humulin N	normal insulin	
Aredia	pamidronate	(pa-mi-**droe**-nate)	Humulin R	regular insulin	
Fosamax	alendronate	(a-**len**-drone-ate)			
			Oral Antidiabetic Drugs		
Calcium			Actos	pioglitazone	(pye-oh-**glit**-ah-zone)
Os-Cal	calcium carbonate	(**kal**-see-um **car**-bone-ate)	Amaryl	glimepiride	(gly-**mep**-er-ide)
	calcium gluconate	(**kal**-see-um **glue**-ko-nate)	Avandia	rosiglitazone	(roes-i-**glit**-ah-zone)
PhosLo	calcium acetate	(**kal**-see-um **as**-see-tate)	Diabinese	chlorpropamide	(klor-**pro**-pah-myde)
	calcium lactate	(**kal**-see-um **lack**-tate)	Glucophage	metformin	(met-**four**-men)
			Glucotrol	glipizide	(**glip**-eh-zyed)
Adrenal Corticosteroids			Glyset	miglitol	(mig-**lee**-tall)
Acthar	corticotropin	(**kore**-tye-co-troe-pin)	Micronase, DiaBeta	glyburide	(**glye**-burr-eyed)
Cortrosyn	cosyntropin	(koe-sin-**troe**-pin)			
Florinef	fludrocortisone acetate	(floo-droe-**kor**-ti-sone **as**-see-tate)	Orinase	tolbutamide	(toll-**butte**-ah-myde)
			Prandin	repaglinide	(re-**pag**-lih-nide)
			Precose	acarbose	(**ay**-car-bose)
Synthetic Adrenocorticosteroid			Starlix	nateglinide	(na-**teg**-lin-ide)
Aristocort	triamcinolone	(trye-am-**sin**-oh-lone)	Tolinase	tolazamide	(toll-**laze**-ah-myde)
Decadron	dexamethasone	(dex-ah-**meth**-ah-sone)			
Glucocorticoids					
Cortef	hydrocortisone	(hye-droe-**kor**-ti-sone)			
Deltasone	prednisone	(pred-**nis**-oh-lone)			
Solu-Medrol	methylprednisolone	(meth-il-pred-**nis**-oh-lone)			

T HE ENDOCRINE SYSTEM ENCOMPASSES the production and secretion of hormones from the glands. The Greek word *orme* means "to excite." This is exactly what hormones do. They activate specific target cells, causing a response. Many different types of hormones are produced in different glands. Doctors who specialize in the study of glands and hormones of the body are endocrinologists. In this chapter we look at the location and function of the major glands of the body. Major conditions affecting the endocrine system are discussed along with the types of agents used to treat them.

Endocrine Anatomy

Three glands are located in the head: the pituitary gland, hypothalamus, and pineal gland. These glands play an important role in hormone production. The pituitary gland produces hormones that affect other glands and specific organs of the body as shown in Figure 16-1. The hypothalamus, located above the pituitary gland, is a bridge between the nervous system and hormone system. The hypothalamus secretes hormones that affect the pituitary gland. The pineal gland, located behind and below the hypothalamus, is responsible for control-

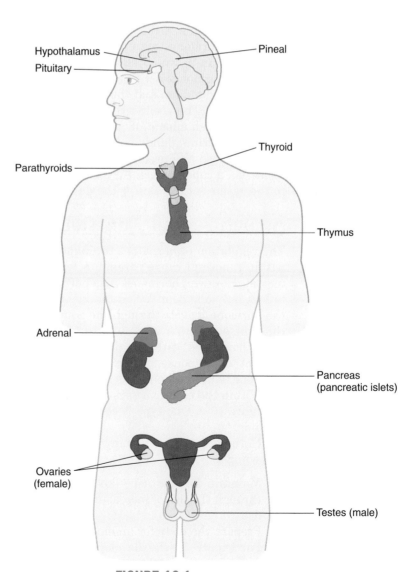

FIGURE 16-1 Endocrine anatomy.

ling the circadian rhythms, sexual growth, and other body functions, which are discussed later in this chapter.

Located at the base of the neck, the thyroid gland is responsible for hormones that participate in metabolism. The parathyroid glands, positioned slightly behind and above the thyroid gland, secrete hormones that help the body keep the calcium levels adequate. Located lower in the chest is the thymus, which secretes hormones that play an important role in the defense system of the body. The adrenal glands are located in the abdominal area right above the kidneys and secrete specific hormones linked to the stress level of the body.

The largest gland is the pancreas, located behind the left kidney at the back of the abdominal wall. The pancreas is responsible for the production and secretion of different types of hormones and digestive juices. Two major hormones produced are insulin and glucagon. Glands that are specific to reproduction are the ovaries in women and the testes in men. In women the ovaries secrete hormones such as progesterone and estrogen. In men the main hormone secreted is testosterone. Each of these hormones is also responsible for gender characteristics.

Description of Hormones

Hormones are responsible for many different human functions, including emotions, in women and men. Hormones are classified by the distance they travel. Autocrine hormones act on the same cell from which they are secreted, such as interleukin-2, which stimulates T cells (part of the immune system). The paracrine hormones act on cells that are in proximity to the target cells such as with prostaglandins, and the endocrine hormones act on cells that are located farther away. These endocrine hormones are the focus of this chapter. Glands have two mechanisms of action—endocrine or exocrine. Hormones produced within endocrine glands enter into the bloodstream to reach their target site, whereas those produced in the exocrine glands are sent to the target organ or tissue via a tube or duct. An example of a tube or duct that secretes outwardly to the surface of the skin is the duct of the sweat glands.

Structure and Function of Hormones

The regulation of hormones throughout the body is kept in balance constantly within a normal range through a feedback system similar to your home thermostat. However, hormones in general can be thought of as specialized keys that unlock only one door. When the key enters the lock, a reaction takes place. As the hormone travels through the body, it does not react with any keyhole other than the one it was made to fit. Homeostasis is disrupted if glands secrete too many hormones; rather, a delicate balance must be kept to produce the right amount of response. When a gland stops producing or secretes too much hormone, various conditions of the endocrine system may result.

Within the endocrine system are two different types of hormones, as shown in Figure 16-2. One type is composed of proteins, and the other is composed of steroids.

Hormones perform many functions throughout the body, including the following:

- Maintain homeostasis—keep the body within normal physiological limits through the use of increasing and decreasing blood glucose levels for energy use
- Prepare the body for an emergency situation—"fight or flight" reaction
- Participate in the development and reproductive system of the human body—sexual maturity and reproductive functions, such as menstruation and pregnancy

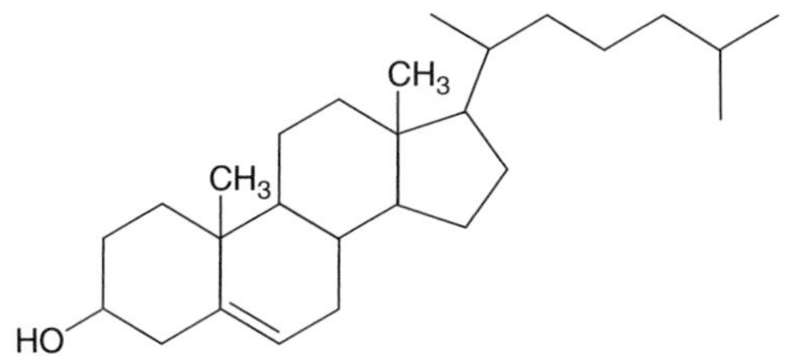

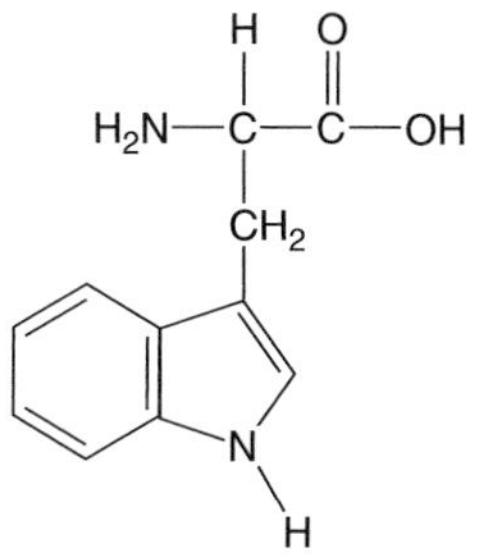

Cholesterol—a steroid   Tryptophan—a protein

FIGURE 16-2 Anatomy of a steroid and protein.

Mechanism of Action

Receptor sites are located inside and outside of cells. Protein hormones fit into receptor sites outside cells, whereas steroid hormones enter into and attach to receptor sites inside the cell. Both mechanisms cause a reaction. The following are the three systems that influence the endocrine system:

1. Negative feedback is the first way in which hormones are produced and secreted. For example, if the level of sugar drops below a certain point in the body, it triggers the secretion of the specific gland. The gland secretes hormones (the key) that target organs (the door lock) to bring the glucose level back up to the necessary level.
2. The second response system is by hormonal chemicals that also may participate in a chain reaction. For example, a chemical response may initiate the first set of hormones to be released from the pituitary gland that interact with the receptors on the adrenal glands; in turn this response releases hormones into the bloodstream.
3. The third response system is via the nervous system. Stressful situations can alter the production and secretion of specific hormones that, when released, prepare the body for the situation. For example, if a person is in an emergency situation, the body requires more energy; therefore, chemicals such as epinephrine may be released, giving the body an extra boost of energy.

Functions of the Endocrine Glands

HYPOTHALAMUS

Located in the brain below the thalamus, the hypothalamus is a small organ that links the nervous system to the endocrine system. The hypothalamus plays a key role in the regulation of several functions such as water balance, metabolism of fat and carbohydrates, body temperature, appetite, and emotions. This organ also produces hormones that regulate the anterior pituitary gland to various degrees. Although the hypothalamus is responsible for the production of two hormones, oxytocin and antidiuretic hormone (ADH), they are stored in the posterior section of the pituitary gland. The hypothalamus stimulates the pituitary gland by neuronal impulses. The pituitary gland then releases oxytocin, which stimulates the ovaries, or ADH (also known as vasopressin), which affects the kidneys. The hypothalamus also produces and secretes two substances known as releasing or inhibiting hormones. The target organ of these hormones is the anterior lobe of the pituitary gland, where they stimulate or inhibit the release of other hormones.

TABLE 16-1 Hormonal Production of Anterior and Posterior Pituitary Gland

Abbreviation	Hormone	Target tissue	Result
Anterior Pituitary Gland			
ACTH	Adrenocorticotropic hormone	Adrenal glands	Secretes glucocorticoids and adrenocortical hormones
FSH	Follicle-stimulating hormone	Ovaries in women; testes in men	Estrogen secretion in women; sperm production in men
GH	Growth hormone	Tissues and bones throughout the body	Growth throughout childhood
LH	Luteinizing hormone	Ovaries in women; testes in men	Progesterone production in women; testosterone production in men
	Prolactin	Mammary glands in women	Produces milk for lactation
TSH	Thyroid-stimulating hormone	Thyroid gland	Causes the thyroid gland to produce thyroid hormones
Posterior Pituitary Gland			
ADH	Antidiuretic hormone	Kidneys	Causes resorption of water back into the bloodstream
	Oxytocin	Uterus	Causes contraction of the smooth muscle; also stimulates anterior pituitary lobe to produce prolactin

PINEAL GLAND

The pineal gland is responsible for the production and secretion of melatonin. Melatonin is a chemical substance that helps to regulate the sleep-wake cycle. The target tissue of melatonin is the hypothalamus. Although this gland is small in adults, it is larger in small children. As a person ages, the pineal gland becomes smaller in relation to other structures and also begins to function less. The gland is affected by light and secretes melatonin more during the night and less during the daytime. The effects of melatonin have been linked to the beginning of puberty and the menstrual cycle.

PITUITARY GLAND

The pituitary gland is like the control tower of the endocrine system. The pituitary gland commonly is called the master gland of the body system. The gland is composed of two portions, the anterior and posterior lobes. Although small, the anterior lobe makes the hormones that stimulate many different organs (listed in Table 16-1). The posterior lobe also contains hormones that regulate the kidneys via reabsorption (ADH), and oxytocin is responsible for uterine contractions initiating labor and milk production (lactation) in postpartum women. This entire system is regulated via negative feedback control from the nervous system (specifically the hypothalamus) and other hormone glands.

THYROID GLAND

The thyroid gland is located at the base of the neck. This gland is responsible for producing and secreting three hormones: thyroxine (T_4), triiodothyronine (T_3), and calcitonin. Iodine is necessary within the thyroid gland to synthesize T_4 and T_3; each is named to indicate the number of atoms of iodine contained. T_4 and T_3 are transported via the bloodstream along with plasma proteins; the hormones pass through target cells into the interior of the cell where they bind to a specific protein. This ultimate reaction helps trigger the rate of metabolism of proteins, fats (lipids), and sugars (carbohydrates) throughout the body; therefore, T_3 and T_4 play an important role in the growth and homeostasis of the body. Calcitonin plays an active role in the regulation of calcium. Calcium is the major mineral found in bones. Calcium is also important for the proper functioning of muscle contractions, nerve impulses, and blood clotting. A constant level is maintained by three different hormones, including calcitonin. The function of calcitonin is to inhibit the resorption of calcium from the bone and kidney. Vitamin D and parathyroid hormone (PTH) are the two other hormones that help regulate calcium and are discussed in other sections of the chapter.

PARATHYROID GLANDS

Located behind the thyroid gland are the parathyroid glands (*para* meaning "across"). The parathyroid organ is composed of two sets of secreting glands. These glands are the main regulators of calcium levels in the blood through the release of PTH. The glands can draw calcium out of the bone when needed to increase the concentration of calcium in the extracellular fluid of the body. Along with the calcium increase, they affect the concentration of phosphate by lowering it, thus allowing more calcium to be used.

ADRENAL GLANDS

Located directly on top of each of the two kidneys, the adrenal glands participate in the activities of the kidneys. The adrenal glands secrete steroids and catecholamines. If the adrenal glands are dissected in a cross section, two layers of tissue can be seen: the medulla (located in the center) and the cortex (outer portion) of the gland. Each of the two layers within the adrenal gland is specific to its function.

The adrenal medulla synthesizes and secretes catecholamines, norepinephrine, and epinephrine. These hormones are stored in the adrenal medulla until activated by the sympathetic nervous system. As mentioned previously, one of the functions of the endocrine system is to stimulate the "fight or flight" reaction. For instance, when one comes into contact with a stressful situation such as when one is scared, the body prepares itself for fighting or running, depending on the situation. The heart rate increases and the veins dilate to allow more blood to reach all muscles and to increase blood flow to the brain. Stored glucose is released into the bloodstream to fuel the body. The secretion of epinephrine accounts for approximately 70% to 80% and norepinephrine is 20% to 30%.

The cortex of the adrenal glands produces three types of hormones: the glucocorticoids, mineralocorticoids, and the sex hormones (androgens or estrogens). Table 16-2 lists the adrenal hormones and their effects.

Glucocorticoids affect the metabolism of lipids, carbohydrates, and proteins (meats). Glucocorticoids produce a reaction opposite to the effect of insulin produced by the pancreas. They increase glucose levels. They also reduce

TABLE 16-2 Adrenal Hormones and Their Effects on the Body

Class of hormones	Specific hormone	Produced and secreted	Effects
Glucocorticoids	Cortisol	Adrenal cortex	Increases blood sugar concentration; also has antiinflammatory and antiallergy effects
Mineralocorticoids	Aldosterone	Adrenal cortex	Increases urinary output, including potassium and hydrogen while retaining sodium; keeps blood volume at par
Sex hormones	Androgens in men	Adrenal cortex	Affects male and female characteristics such as hair growth and sex drive
	Estrogens in women	Adrenal cortex	Affects female sex drive, fat deposition, and bone formation

inflammation and increase the capacity to cope with stressful situations. Mineralocorticoids also are produced within the cortex but within a different layer than the glucocorticoids. Their function is to regulate the secretion of water and salt by the kidney.

PANCREAS

The pancreas is the largest organ of the endocrine system. The function of the pancreas is to maintain energy homeostasis throughout the body. The gland does this by secreting glucagon and insulin, inhibiting the release of somatostatin. Glucagon is secreted in response to low blood glucose. This hormone triggers the liver to release stored glucose for use by the body when levels are low. The hormone also triggers fatty acids to be released by adipose (fat) tissue for energy use. When blood glucose is high, insulin is released into the bloodstream. This hormone targets tissues such as the liver, muscle, and adipose tissues to take up excess glucose from the bloodstream, where it can be stored for later use. Somatostatin, secreted by the hypothalamus, inhibits the release of insulin and glucagon.

OVARIES

The two ovaries in women are responsible for production (oogenesis) and secretion of one or, rarely, two eggs or more (ovulation) each month. Located on either side of the uterus, the ovaries sit above the uterus and are attached to the fallopian tubes, which connect the two organs. Although the ovulation of eggs begins at puberty, it is not possible to become pregnant until the menstrual cycle begins. The ability to have children ends as the hormones responsible, such as estrogen, decline until the ovarian cycle stops. The ovaries also secrete the hormones estrogen and progesterone. The function of estrogen is the development of breasts and genitals and the menstrual cycle, which prepares the female for pregnancy. The anterior pituitary gland releases follicle-stimulating hormone that triggers estrogen levels to increase, which causes luteinizing hormone (another pituitary hormone) to be secreted. The combination of these two hormones causes ovulation.

TESTES

The two testes in men are responsible for the production and secretion of sperm (spermatogenesis). The testes are located within the scrotum. Sperm production begins before the age of puberty and decreases with age, although most men produce sperm throughout their lifetime. Follicle-stimulating hormone is released as puberty begins and causes the stored sperm to divide. Each sperm contains one half of the genetic material that will be contributed to a new life. The production of testosterone (also from the testes) is responsible for the growth of adjacent organs: prostate gland, seminal vesicles, vas deferens, and others. Testosterone is also responsible for changes in the voice pitch as a boy enters puberty and for muscle development. This hormone also affects the differences in the physiques of men and women.

Conditions of the Endocrine System and Their Treatments

Many different types of conditions and illnesses can affect the endocrine system. Causes can range from the effects of aging and genetic factors to those that result from a condition affecting another part of the body. The failure of the endocrine system to perform correctly affects other areas of the body such as heart, brain, and kidney function. Table 16-3 lists the common conditions and illnesses that affect the endocrine system.

CONDITIONS OF THE PITUITARY GLAND AND HYPOTHALAMUS AND THEIR TREATMENTS

Hyperfunction of the pituitary gland can be caused by various tumor growths. Giantism and acromegaly are two conditions that involve an increase in growth hormone. If this condition is present in children, it is referred to as giantism. The bones elongate, resulting in heights that have reached 8 feet. If this condition arises in adulthood, it is called acromegaly and symptoms involve increased size of the head, tongue, nose, hands, feet, and toes. This excess of growth hormone also can cause more serious conditions such as hyperglycemia and hypercalcemia. Treatment involves removal of the tumor, although any bone growth preceding removal cannot be reversed. These tumors tend to be benign.

Hypofunction of the pituitary gland causes a decrease of hormones to secondary target organs. A congenital defect of the pituitary gland can cause dwarfism. Tumors also can disturb the functioning of the pituitary gland and hypothalamus. Simmonds' disease affects adults, causing a lack of menstruation in women and impotence in men. Oxytocin is a hormone released by the posterior pituitary gland that has a direct effect on the uterus and is responsible for the beginning stages of labor. Oxytocin commonly is used as a medication in hospitals to help induce labor or to abort a fetus. Oxytocin is administered parenterally only.

Diabetes insipidus can be caused by a lack of ADH resulting from lesions, tumors, or an infection in or on the hypothalamus or posterior pituitary gland. Treatment for this type of diabetes and diabetes mellitus is discussed later.

CONDITIONS OF THE THYROID GLAND AND THEIR TREATMENT

The two main conditions of the thyroid gland are hyperthyroidism and hypothyroidism. Hyperthyroidism is caused by an excess of thyroid hormones. This can be caused by autoimmunity, as in Graves' disease. An autoimmune disease is one in which the body attacks itself; in Graves' disease the body produces antibodies to thyroid-stimulating hormone receptors. When this happens, the

TABLE 16-3 Endocrine Conditions with Corresponding Glands and Hormones

Glands/hormones	Condition/disease	Possible treatments
Thyroid/T_3, T_4, calcitonin	Hyperthyroidism (Graves' disease)	Medication, surgery
	Hypothyroidism (myxedema, cretinism)	Medication
Parathyroid	Hyperparathyroidism	Reduce calcium intake, diuresis
	Hypoparathyroidism	Calcium and vitamin D replacements
Pituitary		
Anterior pituitary		
	Deficiency	
TSH, ACTH, FSH, LH	Sexual dysfunction, metabolism imbalance, sterility	Hormone replacement therapy
Growth hormone	Dwarfism	Growth hormone replacement
	Overproduction	
TSH	Giantism (child) Acromegaly (adult)	Radiation, surgical intervention
Posterior pituitary		
	Deficiency	
Vasopressin (antidiuretic hormone)	Diabetes insipidus	Medication (desmopressin [DDAVP])
Adrenal		
	Deficiency	
Mineralocorticoids (aldosterone)	Body chemical imbalance	Medication for hormone replacement
Glucocorticoids (cortisol)	Addison's disease	Hormone replacement
Gonadocorticoids (androgens/estrogens/ progestins)	Sexual immaturity/dysfunction	Hormone replacement
	Overproduction	
Mineralcorticoids/ glucocorticoids	Cushing's syndrome	Surgery, medication
Pancreas		
Insulin		
	Deficiency	
	Diabetes mellitus, IDDM	Insulin, diet
	NIDDM (insulin resistance)	Oral medication, diet, insulin
	Gestational diabetes	Insulin during pregnancy
	Overproduction	
	Hypoglycemia	Diet, lifestyle changes

TABLE 16-3 Endocrine Conditions with Corresponding Glands and Hormones—cont'd

Glands/hormones	Condition/disease	Possible treatments
Testes Testosterone		
	Deficiency Stunted sexual growth, sexual dysfunction	Hormone replacement therapy
	Overproduction Precocious puberty	Female hormones, treatment of cause
Ovaries Estrogen/progesterone		
	Deficiency Stunted sexual growth	Hormone replacement therapy
	Menopause	Hormone replacement therapy
	Overproduction Precocious puberty	Male hormones, treatment of cause

TSH, Thyroid-stimulating hormone; *ACTH,* adrenocorticotropic hormone; *FSH,* follicle-stimulating hormone; *LH,* luteinizing hormone; *IDDM,* insulin-dependent diabetes mellitus; *NIDDM,* non–insulin-dependent diabetes mellitus.

thyroid gland is triggered to produce more hormones, which results in the enlargement of the glands behind the eye, known as exophthalmos. Other symptoms of Graves' disease include restlessness, nervousness, sweating, weight loss, and tachycardia.

A goiter is caused by the lack of iodine, which is needed for thyroid hormone production, and by tumors that can cause overproduction of hormone. Goiters also are caused by excessive amounts of T$_3$ and T$_4$, causing enlargement of the thyroid gland. This gives the appearance of an enlarged neck and usually is caused by a tumor. Goiter is not commonly found in developed countries because of the addition of iodine to salt.

Treatment of hyperthyroidism includes removal of the tumor, if that is the cause. Antithyroid agents can be used in Graves' disease, and radioactive iodine is used to decrease nodules in goiters. Radiation also may be used to destroy part of the thyroid gland.

AGENTS USED TO TREAT HYPERTHYROIDISM

GENERIC NAME: propylthiouracil (PTU)
TRADE NAME: Propyl-Thyracil
INDICATION: hyperthyroidism
COMMON DOSAGE: 300 to 450 mg qd
SIDE EFFECTS: nausea, headache, urticaria
AUXILIARY LABEL:
■ Take as directed.

> **GENERIC NAME:** methimazole
> **TRADE NAME:** Tapazole
> **INDICATION:** hyperthyroidism
> **COMMON DOSAGE:** 5 to 15 mg qd
> **SIDE EFFECTS:** fever, rash, itching
> **AUXILIARY LABEL:**
> ■ Take as directed.

Hypothyroidism occurs when the thyroid gland is unable to secrete enough T_3 and T_4. This can be caused by congenital deficiencies referred to as thyroid aplasia. A lack of iodine in the diet can cause a deficiency because iodine is necessary for the synthesis of T_3 and T_4. Inflammation of the thyroid gland, known as thyroiditis, also can be caused by an autoimmune effect. Thyroid aplasia affects children who are not born with a thyroid gland. The lack of the thyroid gland affects the growth of the child's body and nervous system. If the condition is not discovered early, the child's growth will be stunted (dwarfism), and the child will develop mental retardation (cretinism). Once diagnosed, thyroid medication is given for life, although any retardation that has occurred cannot be reversed.

Hypothyroidism in adults causes the condition myxedema. Symptoms include skin that appears puffy. The overall deficiency of thyroid hormones has a dramatic effect on all the organs of the body. This results in an overall decrease in energy and mental alertness. Tumors that affect the thyroid gland are usually benign (adenomas) and rarely are malignant (carcinoma). The main treatment for these types of tumors is removal. Thyroid hormone replacement agents need to be taken for life (one dose a day) because there are no other available treatments. Because the metabolism of the body is at its highest in the morning, doctors advise patients to take their thyroid medications in the morning at the same time daily.

AGENTS USED TO TREAT HYPOTHYROIDISM

> **GENERIC NAME:** thyroid (desiccated)
> **TRADE NAME:** Armour Thyroid
> **INDICATIONS:** hypothyroidism, thyroid cancer
> **COMMON DOSAGE:** 60 to 120 mg qd
> **SIDE EFFECTS:** no major effects if correct dosage is taken
> **AUXILIARY LABEL:**
> ■ Take as directed.

> **GENERIC NAME:** levothyroxine sodium
> **TRADE NAME:** Synthroid, Levothroid
> **INDICATION:** hypothyroidism
> **COMMON DOSAGE:** 0.2 mg qd*
> **SIDE EFFECTS:** no major effects if correct dosage taken
> **AUXILIARY LABEL:**
> ■ Take as directed.

> **GENERIC NAME:** liothyronine sodium
> **TRADE NAME:** Cytomel
> **INDICATION:** hypothyroidism
> **COMMON DOSAGE:** 25 mcg qd up to 100 mcg qd
> **SIDE EFFECTS:** no major effects if correct dosage taken
> **AUXILIARY LABEL:**
> ■ Take as directed.

---

*Dosage may vary depending on weight of patient and extent of illness.

GENERIC NAME: liotrix
TRADE NAME: Thyrolar, Euthroid
INDICATION: hypothyroidism
COMMON DOSAGE: 60 to 120 mg qd
SIDE EFFECTS: no major effects if correct dosage taken
AUXILIARY LABEL:
- Take as directed.

CONDITIONS OF THE PARATHYROID GLANDS AND THEIR TREATMENT

Two parathyroid glands sit on each side of the thyroid gland. Hyperparathyroidism is a condition in which there is an increase of PTH secreted into the bloodstream; it can arise from just one of the four glands. The most common cause of this condition is benign tumors. Another condition closely related is secondary parathyroid hyperplasia, in which all four glands are enlarged; this is linked to chronic renal disease.

Symptoms of these two conditions are similar; this includes increase of calcium because the increased levels of PTH promote the release of calcium into the bloodstream, which leads to bone weakening with an increase in possibility of fractures. This softening of the bones resulting from the loss of calcium may lead to Paget's disease and commonly causes osteoporosis in postmenopausal women. Also, the increase of calcium in the blood causes a buildup of the calcium salts in the kidneys, which can cause kidney stones. Other side effects of hypercalcemia include muscle weakness, lethargy, and heart conduction changes.

Treatment depends on the underlying cause. If the hyperparathyroidism is caused by improper kidney function, then transplantation may be necessary to stop the problem. If transplantation does not work, removal of the glands may be necessary. Following are the common drugs used for replacement therapy for hyperparathyroidism.

BONE METABOLISM REGULATOR

GENERIC NAME: calcitonin-salmon
TRADE NAME: Calcimar
INDICATIONS: Paget's disease, hypercalcemia, postmenopausal osteoporosis
COMMON DOSAGE: Paget's disease, 50 units qd; hypercalcemia, 4 units/kg q12h; osteoporosis (injected intramuscularly or subcutaneously) 100 units qd or 200 units qd intranasal for osteoporosis
SIDE EFFECTS: nausea, vomiting, diarrhea, facial flushing
AUXILIARY LABEL: none

BISPHOSPHONATES

GENERIC NAME: etidronate sodium
TRADE NAME: Didronel
INDICATION: Paget's disease
COMMON DOSAGE: 5 to 10 mg/kg per day (may be given orally for 6 months or intravenously for 3 to 7 days)
SIDE EFFECTS: headache, gastrointestinal upset
AUXILIARY LABEL:
- Oral: Take as directed. (Intravenous form is administered in hospital.)

GENERIC NAME: alendronate
TRADE NAME: Fosamax
INDICATIONS: Paget's disease, postmenopausal osteoporosis
COMMON DOSAGE: Paget's disease, 40 mg qd PO; osteoporosis, 10 mg qd or 70 mg every week
SIDE EFFECTS: Headache, gastrointestinal upset
AUXILIARY LABELS:
- Take 30 minutes before breakfast.
- Take with full glass of water.

GENERIC NAME: pamidronate
TRADE NAME: Aredia
INDICATIONS: hypercalcemia, Paget's disease, osteolytic bone lesions resulting from myelomas
COMMON DOSAGE: hypercalcemia, 60 to 90 mg IV over 24 hours; Paget's disease, 30 mg qd IV over 3 days; osteolytic lesions, 90 mg over 2 hours every 3 to 4 weeks
SIDE EFFECTS: headache, gastrointestinal upset
AUXILIARY LABEL:
- None; administered in hospital as medicine in IV only

OSTEOPOROSIS MANAGEMENT AND TREATMENTS

The aforementioned medications, such as Fosamax and Calcimar, are two agents used to treat osteoporosis. These agents have been used for many years. Research into osteoporosis is helping Americans improve their risk against this disease with new treatments. The Surgeon General reported in 2004 that approximately 10 million Americans over 50 years of age have osteoporosis, costing more than $18 billion annually.[1] It has been found that prevention against this disease must be started early in life through lifestyle changes such as exercise, diet, and smoking cessation. Exercise helps to increase bone density, as does calcium and vitamin D. Calcium requirements can be met by drinking milk, eating cheese, or by taking calcium tablets. New studies have shown that only 15 minutes of direct sunlight twice weekly (without the use of sunscreen) can supply enough vitamin D for the body. If this cannot be done, then multivitamins that contain vitamin D may replace the sun treatment. Long-term use of medications such as corticosteroids, medroxyprogesterone, and excessive thyroid hormones actually can promote osteoporosis. Several medications are being used to treat osteoporosis, including the following:

Trade Name	Generic Name	Normal Oral Dosage
Actonel	risedronate	5 mg qd/35 mg every week
Evista	raloxifene	60 mg qd
Forteo	teriparatide (SQ)	20 mcg qd
Fosamax	alendronate plus vitamin D	5 mg qd/35mg every week
Miacalcin	calcitonin-salmon (nasal spray)	1 spray, alternate nostril, every day

Osteoporosis Prevention

For prevention of osteoporosis, the following agents are used (these should not be taken if one is pregnant or breast-feeding):

Trade Name	Generic Name	Normal Oral Dosage
CombiPatch	estradiol/norethindrone acetate (patch)	1 mg qd
Estrace	estradiol	0.5 mg qd (23 days on/5 days off)
Ogen	estropipate	0.75 mg qd for 25 out of 31 days
Premarin	conjugated estrogens	0.625 mg qd

TABLE 16-4 Hyperfunction of Three Types of Adrenal Hormones

Condition	Common name	Increased secretion	Specific steroid
Hyperaldosteronism	Conn's syndrome	Mineralocorticoids	Aldosterone
Hypercortisolism	Cushing's syndrome	Glucocorticoids	Cortisol
Adrenogenital syndrome	Adrenogenital syndrome	Sex steroids	Androgens

Hypoparathyroidism

Hypoparathyroidism involves the malfunctioning of the parathyroid glands and can occur after removal of the parathyroid glands; in rare cases it may be congenital or an autoimmune disease. The result is hypocalcemia, which is the decrease in or lack of calcium. Symptoms include muscle spasms, irregular heart contractions, and alteration of normal nerve conduction. Treatment is limited to replacement therapy with calcium supplements listed as follows:

Generic Name	Trade Name	Normal Dosage for Replacement
Calcium acetate	PhosLo	250 mg to 1 g PO qd
Calcium carbonate	Tums, Os-Cal	500 mg to 1.5 g PO qd
Calcium chloride		10% IV
Calcium citrate	Citracal	950 mg PO qd
Calcium gluconate		500 mg to 1 g qd; 10% IV

CONDITIONS OF THE ADRENAL GLANDS AND THEIR TREATMENT

The adrenal glands are divided into the cortex and the medulla. Diseases of the adrenal cortex range from overproduction to underproduction of steroids. The cortex can be subdivided into three separate areas, each with its own specialized functions. Conditions affecting the cortex can be within one or more of the three areas. The three types of steroids include mineralocorticoids, glucocorticoids, and sex steroids. A decrease in secretion of any of these steroids can affect the levels of sodium, potassium, and chloride within the body (Table 16-4). Carbohydrate metabolism may be affected, or sexual problems may result.

The most common syndrome of those listed in Table 16-4 is Cushing's syndrome, or Cushing's disease. Most cases of Cushing's syndrome are caused by the oversecretion of glucocorticoids. This overproduction of adrenocorticotropic hormone often results from tumors of the pituitary gland. The remaining conditions occur from other tumors located in the lungs or tumors of the adrenal cortex. Cushing's syndrome also can be caused by overmedication with steroids. The adrenal glands enlarge, and symptoms develop that can include obesity, flushing of the face, hypertension, and thick, scaling skin. Other symptoms include overall weakness and fatigue. Treatment may include the use of aminoglutethimide, or surgery may be used to remove tumors.

Hypofunction of the adrenal cortex can be caused by autoimmune disease, infections, or tumors that cause the destruction of the gland. In approximately 70% of persons suffering from Addison's disease, the condition is caused by an autoimmune disease. Addison's disease results in the total necrosis of the adrenal cortex. Symptoms include fatigue, weight loss, nausea, and syncope. Treatment consists of replacement therapy of glucocorticoids and mineralocorticoids.

MINERALOCORTICOID

GENERIC NAME: fludrocortisone acetate
TRADE NAME: Florinef
INDICATION: Addison's disease
COMMON DOSAGE: 0.1 mg qd
SIDE EFFECTS: gastrointestinal upset
AUXILIARY LABEL:
■ Take as directed.

An overexuberant, inflammatory response can result in more serious conditions. Under certain conditions, glucocorticoids can help the healing process of an inflamed, injured area. Following are glucocorticoid agents used for Addison's disease and for inflammation.

GLUCOCORTICOIDS

GENERIC NAME: hydrocortisone
TRADE NAME: Cortef
INDICATIONS: adrenal deficiency, inflammation
COMMON DOSAGE: 20 to 240 mg qd
SIDE EFFECTS: gastrointestinal upset
AUXILIARY LABELS:
■ Take as directed.
■ Take with food.

GENERIC NAME: methylprednisolone sodium succinate, methylprednisolone acetate
TRADE NAME: Solu-Medrol, Depo-Medrol
INDICATIONS: Addison's disease, inflammation
COMMON DOSAGE: 10 to 40 mg IV or IM (maximum 3 days)
SIDE EFFECTS: gastrointestinal upset
AUXILIARY LABEL: none

GENERIC NAME: prednisone
TRADE NAME: Deltasone
INDICATION: inflammation
COMMON DOSAGE: 5 to 60 mg qd
SIDE EFFECTS: gastrointestinal upset
AUXILIARY LABELS:
■ Take as directed.
■ Do not stop taking abruptly.
■ Take with food or milk.

GENERIC NAME: triamcinolone, triamcinolone hexacetonide, triamcinolone acetonide
TRADE NAME: Aristocort (PO), Aristospan (IV), Kenalog-40 (IV)
INDICATIONS: adrenocortical deficiency, respiratory diseases
COMMON DOSAGE: adrenal, 4 to 12 mg qd; respiratory, 16 to 48 mg
SIDE EFFECT: gastrointestinal upset
AUXILIARY LABELS:
■ Take as directed.
■ Take with food.

GENERIC NAME: dexamethasone
TRADE NAME: Decadron
INDICATION: allergic disorders

COMMON DOSAGE: 0.75 to 9 mg qd
SIDE EFFECTS: gastrointestinal upset
AUXILIARY LABELS:
- Take as directed.
- Take with food.

Adrenal Medulla

Most of the conditions that affect the adrenal medulla result from tumor growths. The two main tumors are neuroblastomas and pheochromocytomas. Although neuroblastomas are known to grow rapidly and metastasize, they can be treated with chemotherapy, radiation, and surgical removal. Pheochromocytomas usually are benign and can cause hypertension. With surgical removal, the hypertension is relieved and the patient's prognosis is good.

CONDITIONS OF THE PANCREAS GLAND AND THEIR TREATMENT

One of the most well-known conditions that can affect the pancreas is diabetes mellitus. Two categories of diabetes are insulin-dependent diabetes mellitus (IDDM) and non–insulin-dependent diabetes mellitus (NIDDM). These two forms of diabetes have many differences: Most persons with IDDM are affected during childhood and require subcutaneous injections of insulin for the rest of their lives (hence the name insulin-dependent). The reason is that their body is unable to produce enough insulin. In contrast, NIDDM is responsible for 90% to 95% of all cases of diabetes. This condition results from insulin resistance and deficiency. Causes range from age, obesity, lack of exercise, family history of diabetes, and/or gestational diabetes and ethnicity. Non–insulin-dependent diabetes rates are highest (at 80%) with those persons who are obese. The first line of treatment is lifestyle changes including losing weight and exercising. In the past, are older persons (over 40 years) would be most prone to NIDDM, but there have been more cases of younger persons with NIDDM or pre-NIDDM.

The cause of diabetes is the inability of the pancreas to secrete insulin or a resistance to insulin that affects the levels of glucose. The result is hyperglycemia. Diabetes mellitus can lead to renal disease, blindness, and even gangrene, which can lead to amputations of extremities. Two main types of insulin are used for IDDM: natural insulin, which is taken from animals such as pigs or cows, and synthesized human insulin, which is made in a laboratory and is chemically identical to human insulin. Persons who are newly diagnosed with IDDM are given the newer DNA recombinant human insulin, but some persons continue to take insulin derived from animals. Injected insulin helps maintain the glucose levels of the blood. Short- and long-acting insulins are used to keep the metabolism of the body in homeostasis. Typical insulins prescribed are listed in Table 16-5. Two types of dosage forms for injectable insulins are prefilled syringes or vials. Insulins such as NPH are clear liquids, whereas mixtures of insulin combine two types of solutions that form a suspension. These latter include Lente, isophane, and others. A suspension is formed when solutions such as zinc are mixed with crystalline-type insulin, which precipitates and forms a milky mixture. Clear insulins do not need to be mixed before use, but suspensions need to be mixed. Also, all insulins, while kept in the refrigerator in the pharmacy, should be at room temperature before being administered to the patient. Figure 16-3 shows a sample of the two types of insulin labels.

The first line of treatment for patients with NIDDM is a change of lifestyle. Incorporating diet, exercise, and oral medications may take care of the problem. In more severe cases, insulin may be necessary. The drugs listed in Table 16-6 are a sample of hypoglycemic agents used to treat NIDDM.

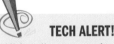

TECH NOTE!

The terms *rainbow coverage* and *sliding scale* refer to the varying doses of insulin that should be given depending on the reading of the blood glucose meter.

TECH ALERT!

All insulin suspensions must be mixed before administration; they cannot be shaken but must be rolled between the hands several times in order to mix the solution before use. Insulin should never be shaken because this will break down the proteins and the insulin will become unusable. Also, when checking insulin stock, always check for proper consistency, clarity, and color. If there is any clumping or unusual coloration, alert the pharmacist before dispensing.

TABLE 16-5 Commonly Prescribed Insulins for Insulin-Dependent Diabetes Mellitus

Generic Name	Trade Name	Human/animal	Length of action
Insulin injection	Regular Iletin I	Beef or pork	Rapid
	Regular Iletin II	Purified pork	Rapid
	Novolin R	Human	Rapid
Isophane insulin	NPH Iletin I	Beef or pork	Intermediate
	Humulin N	Human	Intermediate
Isophane insulin suspension and insulin injection	Humulin 70/30	Human	Intermediate
Isophane insulin suspension and insulin injection	Humulin 50/50	Human	Intermediate
Insulin zinc suspension	Lente L	Purified pork	Intermediate
	Humulin L	Human	Intermediate
Insulin zinc suspension; extended Lente	Humulin Ultralente	Human	Long acting
Insulin analog injection	Humalog	Human	Rapid
Insulin glargine	Lantus	Human	Long acting

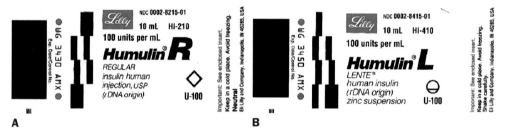

FIGURE 16-3 A, Humulin R (fast-acting). **B,** Humulin L (intermediate-acting).

Newer oral agents in use to treat NIDDM include the following agents. Because so many new agents are making their way into the pharmacy, it is important for technicians always to stay abreast of the new agents being used.

ORAL HYPOGLYCEMICS

GENERIC NAME: glimepiride
TRADE NAME: Amaryl
COMMON DOSAGE: 1 to 2 mg qd
AUXILIARY LABEL:
■ Take with meals.

GENERIC NAME: miglitol
TRADE NAME: Glyset
COMMON DOSAGE: 25 mg tid
AUXILIARY LABEL:
■ Take with meals.

TABLE 16-6 **Oral Antidiabetic Agents for Non–Insulin-Dependent Diabetes Mellitus**

Generic Name	Trade Name	Normal dosage
Oral Antidiabetic Agents		
Biguanides		
Metformin	Glucophage	500-1000 mg qd
Sulfonylureas		
Acetohexamide	Dymelor	250-500 mg qd
Chlorpropamide	Diabinese	100-250 mg bid
Glimepiride	Amaryl	1-4 mg qd
Glipizide	Glucotrol	5-10 mg qd
Glyburide	Micronase	1.5-20 mg qd
Tolazamide	Tolinase	100-500 mg qd
Tolbutamide	Orinase	500 mg qd
Antidote for Antidiabetic Agents or to Treat Hypoglycemia		
Glucagon	Glucagon	1 mg oral to 10 mL by injection

GENERIC NAME: nateglinide
TRADE NAME: Starlix
COMMON DOSAGE: 120 mg tid
AUXILIARY LABEL:
- Take before each meal.

GENERIC NAME: pioglitazone
TRADE NAME: Actos
COMMON DOSAGE: 15 to 30 mg qd
AUXILIARY LABEL:
- Finish all this medication unless otherwise directed by prescriber.

GENERIC NAME: acarbose
TRADE NAME: Precose
COMMON DOSAGE: 50 to 100 mg tid maintenance dose*
AUXILIARY LABEL:
- Finish all this medication unless otherwise directed by prescriber.

GENERIC NAME: repaglinide
TRADE NAME: Prandin
COMMON DOSAGE: 0.5 to 4 mg bid, tid, or qid maintenance dose*
AUXILIARY LABEL:
- Finish all this medication unless otherwise directed by prescriber.

GENERIC NAME: rosiglitazone
TRADE NAME: Avandia
COMMON DOSAGE: 4 mg qd or 2 mg bid maintenance dose*
AUXILIARY LABEL:
- Finish all this medication unless otherwise directed by prescriber.

*These doses are recommended after initial doses are given; initial doses vary.

New Combination Agents

A movement in the therapy for type 2 diabetes is toward multiple drug therapy. This therapy is considered advantageous to those persons suffering from NIDDM who may not be able to control their condition by exercise and diet alone. Four new combination drugs have been approved by the Food and Drug Administration, with more to follow. These agents are the following:

- Glucovance (metformin/glyburide), approved by the Food and Drug Administration in 2000, was the first of its kind. Glucovance is indicated as initial therapy in addition to diet and exercise to improve glycemic control in patients with type 2 diabetes whose hyperglycemia cannot be managed satisfactorily with diet and exercise alone. Glucovance also is used as a second-line therapy when diet, exercise, and initial treatment with a sulfonylurea or metformin do not result in adequate glycemic control in patients with type 2 diabetes.
- Metaglip (glipizide/metformin) was approved in 2002. Metaglip is available in several dosage strengths: 2.5 mg/250 mg, 2.5 mg/500 mg, and 5 mg/500 mg tablets.
- Avandamet (rosiglitazone/metformin) was approved in 2002. Avandamet comes in 1 mg/500 mg, 2 mg/500 mg, and 4 mg/500 mg tablets.
- Actoplus Met (pioglitazone/metformin was approved in 2005. Actoplus Met, for example, is available in 15 mg pioglitazone plus 500 mg metformin or 15 mg pioglitazone plus 850 mg metformin tablets.

Two more combination drugs waiting for approval via the Food and Drug Administration are Avandaryl (rosiglitazone/glimepiride) and a yet unnamed combination (pioglitazone [Actos]/glimepiride [Amaryl]).

One concern over these combination drugs is the limited dosage strength in which they are available. This lessens the possible dosage strengths the physician can prescribe for a patient, thus the problems with correct dosing may lengthen the time it takes to treat the patient correctly.

Blood Glucose Meters

Patients with diabetes must monitor their blood glucose levels by blood draw, often several times daily. Small needles called lancets are placed into a device that is used to collect a drop of blood, which then is compared with a color-coded strip of paper. Reading the amount of glucose by checking the glucose content of urine is another commonly used method. When the strip comes into contact with glucose in the urine, the strip changes color. The resulting color is compared with the chart provided, which indicates the amount of glucose in the blood or urine and the amount of insulin necessary. From the determination made, the patient can take the proper amount of insulin necessary to balance his or her system. Table 16-7 lists common diagnostic devices used for monitoring glucose levels.

HORMONES SECRETED BY THE OVARIES AND THEIR USES

Many important hormones regulate the female reproductive system. Within the ovaries, many hormones are produced that are responsible for the secondary sex characteristics of the female body and for reproduction. The two main hormones produced are estrogen and progesterone. Estrogen is primarily responsible for the development of female organs, breasts, and female body contours caused by fat distribution. Estrogen also stimulates growth of epithelial cells that line the uterus. Progesterone is secreted toward the halfway mark in the menstrual cycle and is responsible for changes in the uterus that prepare it for normal menstrual periods.

TABLE 16-7 Common Diagnostic Devices Used for Monitoring Glucose Levels in Patients with NIDDM

Name	Type	Sizes available
Urinalysis		
Chemstrip bG	Strips	100 per bottle
Clinistix	Strips	50 per bottle
Diastix	Strips	50 and 100 per bottle
Clinitest	Tablets	36 and 100 per bottle
Blood Analysis		
Glucostix	Strips	50 and 100 per bottle
One Touch	Strips	25, 50, and 100 per bottle*
First Choice	Strips	25, 50, and 100 per bottle†

*Used with One Touch brand meter.
†Used with First Choice brand meter.

Treatment with estrogen is indicated for the following:

- To correct estrogen deficiency; estrogen deficiency results in abnormal uterine bleeding, hypogonadism, decreased ovarian functioning, and post-menopausal osteoporosis
- For cancer therapy in the breast or advanced prostatic carcinomas

Treatment with progesterones is indicated for the following:

- To correct female hormonal imbalance that may cause amenorrhea, dysmenorrhea, or endometriosis
- To prevent pregnancy

See Chapter 23 for drugs used with these hormones.

CONDITIONS OF THE TESTES AND THEIR TREATMENT

For men, the main hormone secreted is androgen; testosterone is one of the main androgens. Testosterone regulates the secondary development of the male sex characteristics. Testosterone also influences protein development to the musculoskeletal system and the development of sperm.

Treatment with testosterone is indicated for the following:

- Testosterone deficiency resulting from a formation of a cyst or removal of the testicles
- Treatment of delayed onset of puberty
- Certain types of breast carcinoma in women
- Certain types of anemia

See Chapter 23 for drugs used with this hormone.

DO YOU REMEMBER THESE KEY POINTS?

- The main glands of the endocrine system
- The main function of the thyroid gland, pituitary gland, hypothalamus, adrenal glands, and pancreas
- The common diseases associated with the organs of the endocrine system
- The effect melatonin has on the body and what gland produces it
- How hormones regulate the reproductive system
- Types of replacement therapies available to treat conditions of the reproductive system
- Where the main regulators of calcium are located and where secretion takes place
- The cause and types of diabetes
- The treatments of diabetes
- The differences between types of insulin

MULTIPLE CHOICE QUESTIONS

1. Three glands located in the head are the _____.
   A. Pineal, pituitary, and pancreas
   B. Hypothalamus, pituitary, and pineal
   C. Pituitary, exocrine, and endocrine
   D. None of the above

2. _____ hormones act on the same cell from which they are secreted, whereas _____ hormones must travel to their target organ in the blood.
   A. Endocrine; autocrine
   B. Autocrine; paracrine
   C. Paracrine; endocrine
   D. Autocrine; endocrine

3. T_4 and T_3 are secreted from the _____.
   A. Thymus
   B. Adrenal gland
   C. Thyroid gland
   D. Pituitary gland

4. The endocrine system keeps the body in balance by a mechanism known as _____.
   A. Endocrine mechanism
   B. Exocrine mechanism
   C. Homeostasis mechanism
   D. Negative feedback mechanism

5. Thyroid-stimulating hormone, follicle-stimulating hormone, and adrenocorticotropic hormone are secreted from the _____.
   A. Hypothalamus
   B. Anterior pituitary gland
   C. Posterior pituitary gland
   D. Thyroid gland

6. The essential ions necessary for T_3 and T_4 production are _____.
   A. Proteins
   B. Carbohydrates
   C. Fatty acids
   D. Iodines

7. The endocrine gland(s) that help(s) regulate the kidneys and secrete(s) epinephrine and norepinephrine is(are) the _____.
   A. Parathyroid glands
   B. Pituitary gland
   C. Pancreas
   D. Adrenal glands

8. The most common causes of conditions affecting the endocrine system are _____.
   A. Tumors
   B. Cancer
   C. Congenital factors
   D. Smoking

9. The condition that affects children suffering from hypothyroidism is known as _____.
   A. Aphasia
   B. Cretinism
   C. Myxedema
   D. None of the above

10. The cause of diabetes is _____.
- A. The inability of the pancreas to secrete enough insulin to regulate glucose
- B. A resistance to insulin that can affect the metabolism of glucose
- C. Other factors such as blindness or renal failure
- D. Both A and B

TRUE/FALSE **If the statement is false, then change it to make it true.**

_____ **1.** Acromegaly is a childhood disease caused by a deficiency of growth hormone.

_____ **2.** The hypothalamus links the central nervous system to the endocrine system.

_____ **3.** Hormones are produced in the primary gland and secreted from the target gland.

_____ **4.** Graves' disease is marked by the enlargement of the neck region.

_____ **5.** Types of insulin can be long- or short-acting.

_____ **6.** Aphasia is another term for hyperthyroidism.

_____ **7.** Persons with non–insulin-dependent diabetes mellitus usually need to make lifestyle changes, whereas those with insulin-dependent diabetes mellitus need insulin injections for life.

_____ **8.** Insulin helps maintain glucose levels in the pancreas.

_____ **9.** The two main hormones secreted by the ovaries are estrogen and progesterone.

_____ **10.** The hormone androgen is responsible for the secondary development of the male and also affects women's sex drives.

TECHNICIAN'S CORNER

Using *Drug Facts and Comparisons,* find out whether there are any drug interactions between the following drugs:

Calcium carbonate (Os-Cal) 500 mg qd
Levothyroxine (Synthroid) 0.1 mg qd
Aspirin, enteric-coated, 325 mg qd
Glipizide (Glucotrol) 5 mg qd

REFERENCE

1. www.suregongeneral/news/speeches/10142002.htm. Bone Health and Osteoporosis: A report of the Surgeon General. Issued 10-14-2004.

BIBLIOGRAPHY

Damjanov I: *Pathology for the health professions,* ed 3, Philadelphia, 2005, Saunders.
Drug facts and comparisons, ed 60, St Louis, 2005, Wolters Kluwer.
Gebhart F: Combination products offer alternative for type 2 diabetes patients, *Drug Topics* Oct 2005. Retrieved from www.drugtopics.com/drugtopics/article/articleDetail.jsp?id=184895
National Osteoporosis Foundation, www.NOF.org
Rosenthal WM: *New insights into osteoporosis management,* New York, 2004, Power$_X$-Pak CE/Jobson Publishing.
Salerno E: *Pharmacology for health professionals,* St Louis, 2003, Mosby.
Thibodeau GA, Patton KT: *Structure & function of the body,* ed 11, St Louis, 2000, Mosby.
Voet D, Voet J: *Biochemistry,* New York, 1990, John Wiley & Sons.

WEBSITES

www.diabetes.org
www.healthybodyhealthymind.com

Nervous System

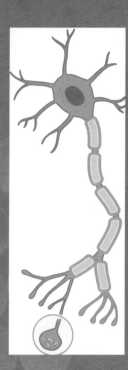

Objectives

UPON COMPLETING THIS CHAPTER, YOU SHOULD BE ABLE TO
DO THE FOLLOWING:

- Describe the main functions of the nervous system.

- Identify the main parts of a neuron.

- Describe how nerves function in transmitting impulses.

- List the main neurotransmitters of the nervous system.

- Describe the differences between the central nervous system and
  the peripheral nervous system.

- Explain how the efferent system functions as opposed to the
  afferent system.

- Describe the main neurotransmitters of the peripheral nervous
  system and the central nervous system.

- Identify the types of drugs affecting the nervous system.

- Identify the differences between cholinergics, adrenergics, and
  their blocking agents.

- Give examples of conditions that affect the nervous system and
  how they are treated.

- List the drugs that affect the nervous system, their methods of
  action, and normal dosing.

- Identify the auxiliary labels for the drugs discussed.

Afferent *The direction of neuronal impulse from the body toward the central nervous system*

Autonomic *Self-controlling or involuntary*

Autonomic nervous system *Division of the nervous system that controls the involuntary body functions; consists of sympathetic and parasympathetic divisions*

Axon *The part of a nerve cell that conducts impulses away from a cell body*

Blood-brain barrier *A barrier formed by special characteristics of capillaries to prevent certain chemicals from moving to the brain*

Cell body *The main part of a neuron from which axons and dendrites extend*

Central nervous system *Brain and spinal cord*

Cerebrospinal fluid *A fluid that fills the ventricles of the brain and also lies in the spaces of the brain or spinal cord and the arachnoid layer of the meninges*

Cervical *Neck region*

Dendrite *The part of a neuron that branches out to bring impulses to the cell body*

Efferent *The conduction of electrical impulses away from the central nervous system to the body*

Lumbar *The region of the back that includes the area between the ribs and the pelvis; the area around the waist*

Monoamine oxidase *An enzyme (includes MAO-A and MAO-B) found in the nerve terminals, the neurons, and liver cells; it inactivates chemicals such as tyramine, catecholamines, serotonin, and certain medications*

Nerve terminal *The end portion of the neuron where nerve impulses cause chemicals to be released; these cross a small space, called a synaptic cleft, to carry the impulse to another neuron*

Neuron *The functional unit of the nervous system, which includes the cell body, dendrites, axon, and terminals*

Parasympathetic nervous system *Division of the autonomic nervous system that functions during restful situations; "breed or feed" part of the autonomic nervous system*

Peripheral nervous system *The division of the nervous system outside the brain and spinal cord*

Somatic *The motor neurons that control voluntary actions of the skeletal muscles*

Sympathetic nervous system *Division of the autonomic nervous system that functions during stressful situations; "fight or flight" part of the autonomic nervous system*

Thoracic *Relates to the thorax area or the chest*

CENTRAL NERVOUS SYSTEM DRUGS

Trade Name	Generic Name	Pronunciation
Muscle Relaxants		
Dantrium	dantrolene	(**dan**-tro-lean)
Flexeril	cyclobenzaprine	(sigh-klo-**benz**-ah-preen)
Lioresal	baclofen	(**back**-low-fen)
Norflex	orphenadrine	(or-**fen**-ah-dreen)
Parafon	chlorzoxazone	(klor-**zocks**-ah-zone)
Robaxin	methocarbamol	(meth-o-**kar**-ba-mol)
Soma	carisoprodol	(kar-i-soe-**proe**-dole)
Neuromuscular Blocking Agents		
Anectine	succinylcholine	(suck-si-nill-**koe**-leen)
Pavulon	pancuronium	(pan-kur-**roe**-nee-um)
Zemuron	rocuronium	(row-kur-**oh**-nee-um)
Anticonvulsants		
Cerebyx	fosphenytoin	(fos-**fen**-i-toyn)
Depakene	valproic acid	(val-**pro**-ic **as**-id)
Dilantin	phenytoin	(**fen**-i-toyn)
Klonopin	clonazepam (C-IV)	(kloe-**naz**-e-pam)
Luminal	phenobarbital (C-IV)	(fee-no-**bar**-bi-tall)
Mebaral	mephobarbital (C-IV)	(mep-oh-**bar**-bi-tall)
Mysoline	primidone	(**prim**-i-don)
Neurontin	gabapentin	(gab-a-**pen**-tin)
Tegretol	carbamazepine	(kar-ba-**maz**-e-peen)
Valium	diazepam (C-IV)	(dye-**az**-eh-pam)
Zarontin	ethosuximide	(eith-oh-**suks**-ah-mide)
Parkinson's Disease Agents		
Artane	Trihexyphenidyl	(try-heks-ah-**fen**-a-dill)
Cogentin	benztropine	(benz-**tro**-peen)
Eldepryl	selegiline	(se-**lej**-a-leen)
Larodopa	levodopa	(lee-vo-**doe**-pa)
Mirapex	pramipexole	(pra-mi-**pex**-ole)
Parlodel	bromocriptine	(bro-mo-**krip**-teen)
Permax	pergolide	(**pur**-go-lide)
Requip	ropinirole	(row-**pin**-ah-roll)
Sinemet	carbidopa/levodopa	(car-bih-**doe**-pa/lee-vo-**doe**-pa)
Symmetrel	amantadine	(ah-**man**-tie-deen)

Trade Name	Generic Name	Pronunciation
Multiple Sclerosis Agents		
Avonex	interferon β_{1a}	(in-tur-**fear**-on **bay**-ta won aye)
Betaseron	interferon β_{1b}	(in-tur-**fear**-on **bay**-ta won bee)
Amyotrophic Lateral Sclerosis		
Rilutek	riluzole	(**ril**-you-zole)
Alzheimer's Disease Agents		
Aricept	donepezil	(don-**nay**-pa-zil)
Cognex	tacrine	(**tac**-kreen)
Exelon	rivastigmine	(ri-vas-**tig**-meen)
Reminyl	galantamine	(ga-**lan**-ta-meen)
Myasthenia Gravis Agents		
Eserine	physostigmine	(phi-zo-**stig**-meen)
Mestinon	pyridostigmine	(pie-rid-o-**stig**-meen)
Prostigmin	neostigmine	(knee-oh-**stig**-meen)
α- and β-Adrenergics		
Levophed	norepinephrine	(nor-ep-i-**nef**-rin)
Yutopar	ritodrine	(**ri**-toe-dreen)
α- and β-Adrenergic Blocking Agents		
Brevibloc	esmolol	(**es**-mo-lol)
Cardura	doxazosin	(dok-**sah**-zo-sin)
Hytrin	terazosin	(tur-**ah**-zoh-sin)
Minipress	prazosin	(**pra**-zoe-sin)
Normodyne	labetalol	(la-**bay**-ta-lol)
Regitine	phentolamine	(fen-**toll**-ah-meen)
Sympathomimetics or Adrenergic Agents		
Adrenalin	epinephrine	(ep-i-**nef**-rin)
Intropin	dopamine	(doe-**pah**-meen)
Yutopar	ritodrine	(**ri**-toe-dreen)

THE NERVOUS SYSTEM is a complex system controlling and coordinating the movements and many functions of the body. This includes activities that we usually do not think about consciously, such as walking or running. Nerves also enable the body to perform internal functions involuntarily, such as the heart beating, the digestive system breaking down a meal, or the brain interpreting visual awareness. We take much for granted when it comes to the nervous system; however, if we lost a simple function, such as moving our eyes along a page of a book, it would be a devastating event in our lives. The nervous system is better understood when broken down into divisions and specific functions of those divisions. We begin with a generalized overview of the nervous system and its main branches, working through some of the basic functions of each. An understanding of the nervous system and how drugs affect the various levels is important. Some conditions that affect the nervous system are discussed along with the medications that treat those conditions.

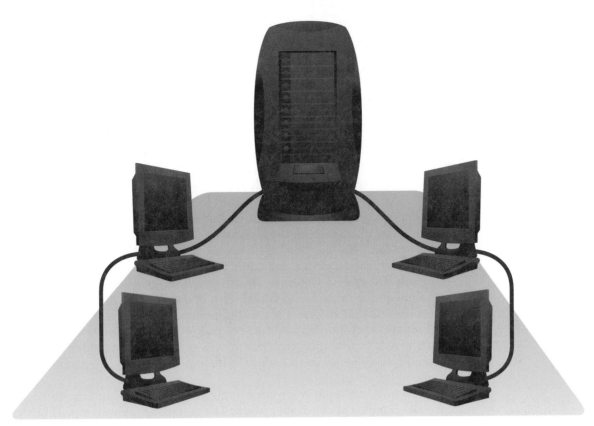

FIGURE 17-1 Computer mainframe with extensions to other computers.

Nervous System

The nervous system has four main functions. One function consists of impulses sent to the central nervous system (CNS); a second function sends impulses from the CNS. A third function coordinates activities of all parts of the nervous system (those functions that rely on outside stimulation), and the fourth function, a sensory function, detects various changes of the body. The many functions of the nervous system serve to keep the body in a balanced mode, which is referred to as homeostasis. The nervous system can be described as a complex mainframe computer system with its network of nerves connected to the body much like the Internet is connected to millions of homes. The mainframe (CNS) is connected to computers (target sites) that interpret the signals; likewise, the computer extensions can send messages to the mainframe computer (CNS) where it can be interpreted, and a response then is sent back (Figure 17-1).

The nervous system (the mainframe) is composed of the CNS (brain and the spinal cord) and the peripheral nervous system (PNS). The PNS has four distinct functions composed of two efferent and two afferent nerve tracts. The two efferent functions serve as the highways for motor impulses traveling from the CNS to the muscles of the body and two sensory afferent functions that travel from the body to the CNS. The two efferent branches are called the somatic and the autonomic branches. Each efferent branch reaches out to specific areas of the body and relays motor messages from the CNS. The somatic branches make contact with skeletal muscles throughout the body, whereas the autonomic branches make contact with the cardiac (heart) and smooth muscles such as those in the blood vessels, stomach, and other large organs. The branches that represent the afferent system carry impulses from the soft tissue areas and

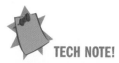

involuntary muscles of the body and other organs back to the CNS via visceral branches and the somatic branches. The various branches of the PNS allow the CNS to work at an optimal level because each area of the nervous system is in charge of a specific type of motor action or sensory response (Figure 17-2).

Recall that all the components of the nervous system are considered one system. We begin with the smallest functional part of the CNS, the neuron.

The Neuron

The smallest unit of the nervous system is the neuron. Billions of neurons make up the nervous system. This highly sophisticated circuitry is analogous to a computer chip that is responsible for relaying information within a computer system. The computer chip is small and carries a massive amount of information; similarly, millions of nerves run throughout our bodies and carry messages back and forth from the CNS.

The cell body, dendrites, axon, and the nerve terminal compose the four main sections of a neuron. As neurons branch out, forming a network of relay stations, they allow nerve impulses to travel from one neuron to another. The dendrites are extensions that receive electrical impulses. The cell body processes the electrical message before it enters the axon. A specialized insulation called a myelin sheath wraps around the axon. The myelin sheath is composed of the same fatty material that is found in the white matter of the brain. The myelin helps with impulse conduction (Figure 17-3).

Nerves are not separate from one another in the PNS but form bundles made of axons. Bundles of cell bodies are called ganglions. However, within the CNS the terminology differs—the axons are called tracts and the cell bodies are called nuclei or ganglia. The electrical nerve impulses are transmitted from one neuron to another by various chemicals called neurotransmitters. Many different neurotransmitters are used, each responsible for a different message. The most common neurotransmitters are listed in Table 17-1, along with their type of response. When the impulse is activated by a neurotransmitter, a series of actions take place to transmit the nerve impulse.

Nerve Transmission

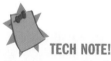

A neuron has three main states. These states are polarized, depolarized, and repolarized. When the cell is in a resting state, there is an overall negative charge inside the neuron that is made up of potassium (positive) and chloride ions (negative). The outside of the neuron is more positive, with sodium as the positive charge. At this point the cell is considered polarized and waiting to be excited. When a neurotransmitter activates the cell membrane, an influx of outside sodium ions rushes through channels, changing the negative charge inside to a positive charge, as shown in Figure 17-4. This is called depolarization. The cell restores the resting state by allowing the inside positive charges (potassium ions) to escape. As the transition back to the resting state is made, the cell actively transports the sodium back to the outside and allows the potassium to reenter the cell. This repolarizes the cell, bringing the cell full circle and back to the resting stage again.

Central Nervous System

THE BRAIN

The brain is composed of two types of matter. Gray matter is made up of neuron cell bodies and dendrites, and the white matter is made up of bundles of nerve fibers (myelinated axons). These fibers are woven in a pattern, making up the contents of the brain. Several sections of the brain serve specific functions of the

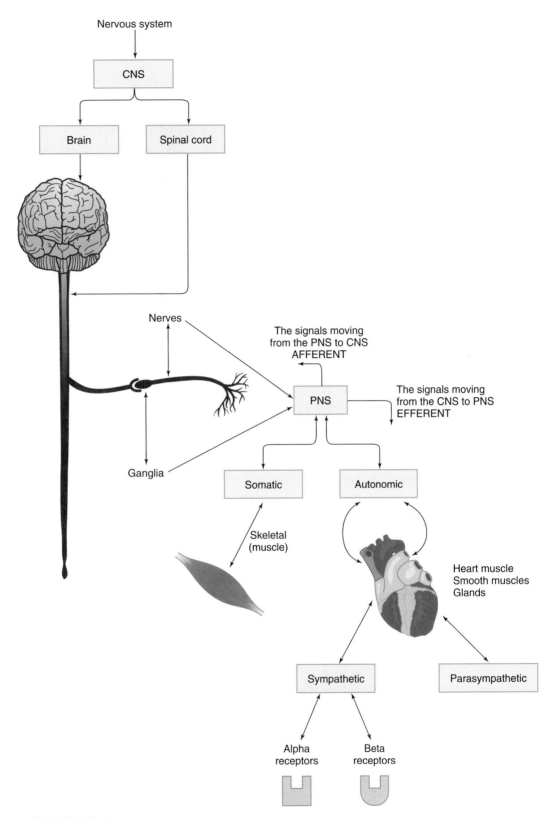

FIGURE 17-2 The nervous system: the divisions include the somatic and autonomic branches.

body. The largest area of the brain is the cerebrum. This area deals with the ability to reason, remember, speak a language, and create. The cerebrum is divided into two hemispheres: the right hemisphere, which controls logical thinking processes, and the left hemisphere, which controls creativity. Each of the two hemispheres can be divided further into four different lobes, each having

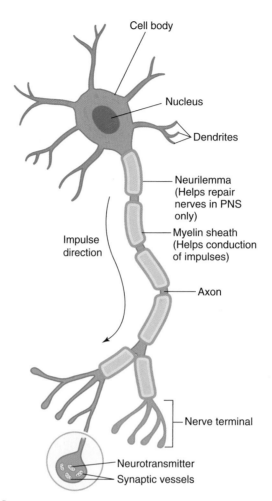

FIGURE 17-3 Complete neuron and cell membrane of efferent (motor) nerve.

TABLE 17-1 **Neuronal Transmitters, Their Most Important Clinical Locations, and Some of Their Actions**

Neurotransmitter	Type of response
Acetylcholine (PNS)	Excitatory (skeletal muscles, gastrointestinal muscles); inhibitory (decreases heart rate)
Norepinephrine (PNS)	Excitatory (increases heart rate)
Epinephrine (PNS)	Inhibitory (bronchodilator); excitatory (increases heart rate)
Dopamine (CNS)	Helps to inhibit involuntary movement
Serotonin (CNS)	Helps to inhibit pain perception

PNS, Peripheral nervous system; *CNS,* central nervous system.

its own function. These functions cover the six senses—hearing, vision, balance, taste, touch, and smell—and motor functions to muscles. The next largest segment is the cerebellum, located at the base of the brain, which helps control most of the muscle functions and precise movements of the body. This control includes balance, posture, and overall coordination. The brainstem connects the brain to the spinal cord and consists of three main areas: the midbrain, pons, and medulla oblongata. These three areas are linked to many of the nerves within the brain. Each area serves as a control center with specific functions (Figure 17-5).

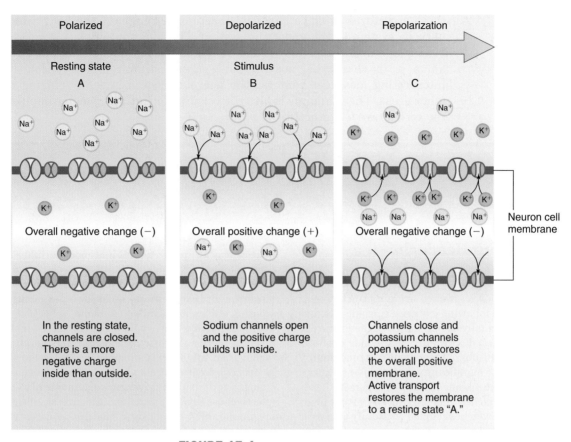

Polarized	Depolarized	Repolarization

Resting state
A

Stimulus
B

C

Overall negative change (−)

Overall positive change (+)

Overall negative change (−)

Neuron cell membrane

In the resting state, channels are closed. There is a more negative charge inside than outside.

Sodium channels open and the positive charge builds up inside.

Channels close and potassium channels open which restores the overall positive membrane. Active transport restores the membrane to a resting state "A."

FIGURE 17-4 Neuronal impulse transfer.

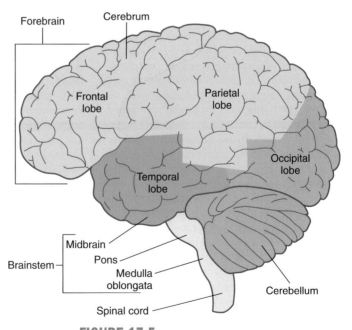

FIGURE 17-5 Anatomy of the brain.

The midbrain and pons are a collection of nerves that branch off into other areas and serve as an intersection, whereas the medulla oblongata controls breathing or respiration, cardiac rate, the force of contraction of the heart, and dilation of blood vessels. Wedged between the midbrain and the cerebrum are two other parts of the brain, the thalamus and hypothalamus. When activated, these structures produce chemical reactions throughout the body, linking the nervous system to the endocrine system. The hypothalamus is a built-in thermostat and appetite center; it also relays messages to the thalamus. The thalamus is in charge of most of our sensory stimuli and is responsible for interpreting messages sent via the nervous system and for relaying them to other areas. The thalamus is also responsible for initiating motor impulses from the cortex (see Chapter 16).

Pharmacist's Perspective

BY SUSAN WONG, PharmD

What's New in Headache Management?

Many persons say, "I've got a migraine." What is a migraine headache? Migraines are a distinct type of headache with the following features: episodic, not continuous or daily, usually on one side of the head, may or may not be associated with aura, autonomic dysfunction (nausea, vomiting, photophobia), strong family history, and may be significantly disabling—not "just a headache." Daily throbbing headaches are more likely to be rebound headaches than migraines. Daily or near-daily throbbing headaches coupled with daily analgesic use are likely analgesic rebound headaches. Rebound headaches typically occur in patients who have been initially diagnosed with migraine and get caught up in a cycle of frequent and excessive analgesic use. Management includes educating the patient about the cause of analgesic rebound, initiating preventive therapy, and tapering the patient off analgesics over several weeks.

The primary goal of management of migraine headaches is prevention. This involves identifying and eliminating risks or triggers for headaches such as fatigue, noise, bright lights, certain foods, and other lifestyle factors. Simple analgesics (aspirin, nonsteroidal antiinflammatory drugs) work well for acute attacks, especially in patients with mild to moderate pain in whom risks and trigger factors are under control. Antiemetics, such as metoclopramide or prochlorperazine, are useful additions if nausea is a prominent symptom. Analgesic combinations (e.g., Fiorinal or Midrin) and ergots (e.g., ergostat or Cafergot) are usually effective for more severe migraines. Dihydroergotamine injectable or more recently dihydroergotamine nasal spray (Migranal) has been a mainstay of migraine treatment.

The "triptans"—sumatriptan (Imitrex), rizatriptan (Maxalt MLT), zolmitriptan (Zomig), and naratriptan (Amerge)—are useful for patients whose migraines do not respond to or who are intolerant of other classes of agents. Compared with sumatriptan (Imitrex), the new triptans are more selective 5-hydroxytryptamine (serotonin) agonists and offer greater oral bioavailability, a potentially improved risk-to-benefit ratio, and a potentially greater therapeutic benefit through a combination of peripheral and central effects.

Preventive drug therapy is indicated when a patient has frequent (two or more) headaches per month that create significant disability at home, school, or work (e.g., cancelled plans), causing significant emotional distress, or when a patient requires large quantities of medications to stop the pain quickly. Prevention should be part of a treatment plan that emphasizes behavioral changes and should be given an adequate trial to assess effectiveness (usually 2 to 3 months unless side effects are intolerable). Prescribing inadequate doses of preventive medications for brief periods is a major cause of therapeutic failure. β-Blockers and tricyclic antidepressants remain the drugs of choice for prevention. Propranolol is found to be the most effective agent but may cause a slow heart rate; it should be used with caution in patients with asthma. Failure of one β-blocker does not preclude success with another. A number of over-the-counter alternatives may be effective; they include riboflavin (400 mg/day) or magnesium (500 to 700 mg/day for adults and 7 mg/kg for children). Magnesium supplementation also may improve the efficacy of triptan medications. Diarrhea and intestinal cramping are rare side effects at these doses; caution is necessary in renal impairment or disease.

Your role as a technician is to be aware of what a patient tells you or asks for. If it seems like the same patient is asking for over-the-counter pain or headache medicine in a large quantity or regularly, it should be a red flag, causing you to ask, "How often do you need to take this type of medicine? Are you using it for headaches or other pain? Does it help?" If any of the answers are more than just on an occasional basis, tell the pharmacist. Sometimes chronic use of over-the-counter medicines can be a problem because they can interfere with some of the prescription medicines, they can worsen or cause other problems, and in the case of headaches, they actually can contribute to having them (hence the description of analgesic rebound). A patient may ask you for single-agent supplements such as riboflavin or magnesium. Make sure he or she speaks with the pharmacist to prevent drug interactions or adverse effects from too much of a certain substance. ■

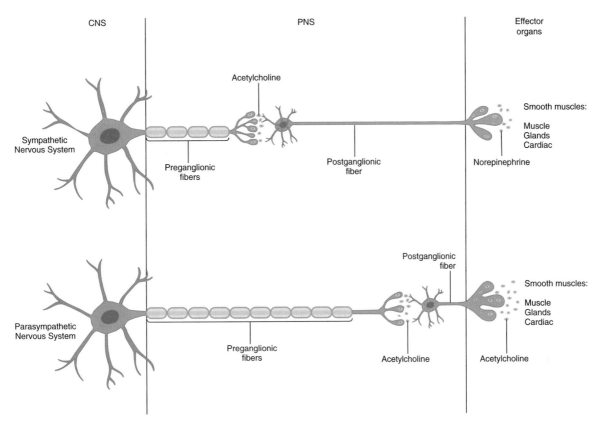

FIGURE 17-6 The afferent and efferent nerves and the areas attached by the sympathetic and parasympathetic systems. Preganglionic and postganglionic nerves and cell bodies with the axon for both are shown. Efferent and afferent neurons also are included.

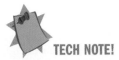

TECH NOTE!

The nerves of the brain crisscross so that the left side of the brain controls the right side of the body. Thus persons suffering from a stroke (blocked blood flow) on one side of the brain can lose the ability to move parts of the body located on the opposite side.

AFFERENT (SENSORY) NEURONS

The main functions of the afferent branch include transferring information via electrical impulse from the peripheral area (outside the CNS) back to the CNS. The afferent, or sensory, branch is composed of neurons that have long axons (the dendrites at the ends of the axon going to the cell body) and a short axon. The cell body is located within the PNS axon that enters the CNS.

EFFERENT (MOTOR) NEURONS

After the CNS receives a message, a response via nerve impulse is sent through the efferent branch to a target muscle. The neurons, which compose the efferent branch, have short dendrites and a long axon. The dendrites and cell body of these efferent neurons are located within the CNS, and the axon becomes part of the PNS (Figure 17-6).

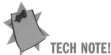

TECH NOTE!

The brain and spinal cord make up the CNS. The brain has three main areas: the cerebrum, cerebellum, and brainstem. The brain is composed of gray and white matters that contain neurons. The meninges, cerebrospinal fluid, and the blood-brain barrier protect the brain and spinal cord. The afferent nerves bring messages from our body to the CNS, and the efferent nerves send messages back to the muscles of the skeleton, organs, and other tissues in response to the stimulus. The axon synapses are located in the CNS in the afferent system, whereas the axon synapses are located in the CNS and PNS in the efferent system.

Peripheral Nervous System

SOMATIC SYSTEM

The somatic system is a network of nerves that relay messages to the CNS from the outside world and return messages back to the body. The spinal and cranial nerves are part of the somatic system. This system is part of the PNS and regulates the motor nerves that control voluntary actions of the skeletal muscles and impulses from sensory receptors. Receptor sites are sensitive to a stimulus and include smell, taste, touch, and hearing.

SPINAL CORD NERVES

The spinal cord is composed of an inner gray matter that houses many nerve cells and an outside white matter containing nerve fibers. The meninges, a thin covering lining the inside of the bones, separates and protects the brain and the spinal cord from the bony structure of the skull and spinal column. The brain and spinal cord also are cushioned by a watery liquid called the cerebrospinal fluid. This combination of the meninges and fluid serves to protect and cushion the CNS.

The brain and spinal cord are protected by a barrier called the blood-brain barrier. This barrier is another protectant that allows only certain types of very small molecules to pass into the brain. This includes some drugs. Most drugs that can pass through the blood-brain barrier are lipid soluble (i.e., they dissolve in fat).

The spinal cord is divided into sections, each identified by its attachment location along the spinal cord. The five main areas of the spinal cord include the cervical (neck), thoracic (chest), lumbar (lower back), sacral (below lower back), and coccygeal (Figure 17-7).

CRANIAL NERVES

As shown in Figure 17-8, there are 12 pairs of cranial nerves that originate within the brain matter. These nerves have specific functions that are labeled by Roman numerals and name. The numbers represent the order in which the fibers are located within the brain from front to back. Most of these nerves have sensory and motor fibers, with three sets having sensory fibers only. Table 17-2 lists the primary functions for each set of cranial nerves from I to XII.

AUTONOMIC SYSTEM

A subdivision of the PNS, the autonomic branch is called the autonomic nervous system because it controls automatic functions. These are the functions that you do not have to think about consciously, such as heartbeat. The autonomic nervous system is called the involuntary nervous system and is subdivided further into two branches called the sympathetic and parasympathetic nervous systems. Both of these systems serve to regulate organs, tissues, and blood vessels. They can perform this function in response to outside and inside stimuli with the use of specific neurotransmitters. The sympathetic and parasympathetic systems are made of nerves and ganglia. Both systems have neurons of approximately the same length that carry impulses from the CNS to target tissue. The ganglia is the area where the synapse (relay) is located. The nerve fibers are considered to be preganglionic or postganglionic, depending on whether the nerve fibers come before or after the ganglia. Each neurotransmitter has its own specific receptor that it contacts opposite the synapse (the lock-and-key mechanism; Figure 17-9).

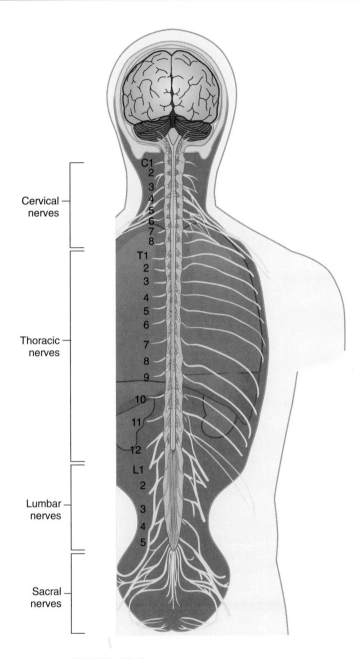

Cervical nerves

Thoracic nerves

Lumbar nerves

Sacral nerves

C1
2
3
4
5
6
7
8
T1
2
3
4
5
6
7
8
9
10
11
12
L1
2
3
4
5

FIGURE 17-7 Segments of the spinal cord.

SYMPATHETIC SYSTEM

The areas of the CNS where the sympathetic nerves emerge are the thoracic and lumbar regions of the spinal cord. The function of the sympathetic division is to respond to stressful situations, such as the "fight or flight" response. During the fight-or-flight stress response, the sympathetic system shuts down the nonessential systems of the body. This redirects energy to other areas such as the muscular system. The nerves that are responsible for this type of behavior are composed of preganglionic neurons imbedded into the gray matter of the spinal cord. As the impulses travel through this gray matter, they synapse with postganglionic neurons that go out into the body systems. The sympathetic preganglionic neurons synapse and affect many postganglionic neurons. This massive transfer to many areas of the body allows human beings to respond quickly and

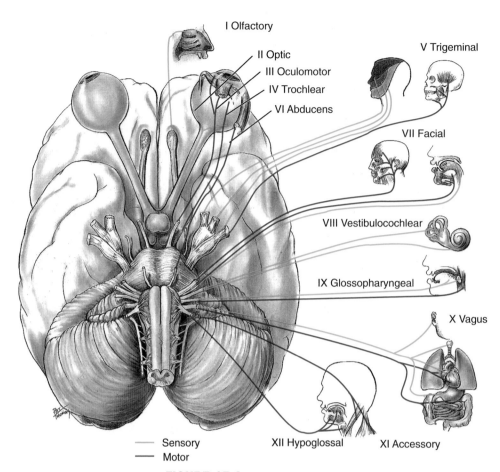

FIGURE 17-8 Cranial nerves.

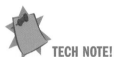

TECH NOTE!

Drugs that mimic the sympathetic system are called adrenergic drugs; those that block the actions of the sympathetic system are called adrenergic blockers. Drugs that mimic the parasympathetic system are called cholinergic drugs; those that block the actions of the parasympathetic system are called anticholinergics. Monoamine oxidase enzymes are responsible for destroying excess neurotransmitters. Activators such as adrenergics and cholinergics increase the amount of neurotransmitters or stop the monoamine oxidase enzymes from destroying the neurotransmitters. When blockers are used, they block the receptor sites of the neurotransmitters so that they cannot connect and cause a response.

powerfully to a situation. The sympathetic system also sends impulses to various organs and tissues for other emotional situations such as anxiety, hate, and even stress. When you go for an interview and your palms get sweaty, your heart rate increases, and breathing becomes quick and shallow, you are experiencing a sympathetic reaction but to a lesser degree than a person having a panic attack or who is in fear for his or her life. Whether you are in a life-threatening situation or in minor stress, the sympathetic nervous system keeps the body in homeostasis through its fight-or-flight responses. Table 17-3 shows the response of each major organ when affected by the sympathetic system. All of the nonessential energy-consuming functions, such as urination or digestion, are placed on hold while blood flow to large muscles, the release of glucose from the liver, the heart rate, and other functions are increased. This sympathetic response is one that is not mentally activated but is an instinctive or autonomic reaction.

Adrenergic Agents and Adrenergic Blockers

The main neurotransmitters of the sympathetic system are norepinephrine and epinephrine. Dopamine is a precursor for norepinephrine and is found as a neurotransmitter within the CNS, specifically the basal ganglia. Persons suffering from Parkinson's disease have low levels of dopamine, causing tremors and other physiological problems.

Within the nerve ending are enzymes that destroy excess norepinephrine or take it up to be reused. One of the enzymes responsible for this action is called monoamine oxidase. Destruction of excessive amounts of norepinephrine is important because overexcitement can cause unwanted effects.

Four types of receptors are found opposite the sympathetic postganglionic fiber endings. α_1-Receptors are located in peripheral blood vessels, the heart,

TABLE 17-2 Primary Functions of Cranial Nerves

Name	Type of fiber	Functions
I (olfactory)	Sensory	Smell
II (optic)	Sensory	Vision
III (oculomotor)	*Motor	Eye and eyelid movement
IV (trochlear)	*Motor	Eye movements
V (trigeminal)	Sensory/motor	Sensory fibers (over face area, scalp and teeth)
Motor Fibers of the Face (Such as Chewing Food)		
VI (abducens)	*Motor	Eye movements
VII (facial)	Sensory/motor	Sensory fibers for taste
Motor Fibers for Facial Expression and Lacrimal and Salivary Glands		
VIII (vestibulocochlear)	Sensory	Hearing and equilibrium (balance)
IX (glossopharyngeal)	Sensory/motor	Sensory fibers for taste
Motor Fibers for Muscles Used in Swallowing and Salivary Glands		
X (vagus)	Sensory/motor	Sensory fibers for pharynx, larynx (speech), esophagus, and visceral organs
Autonomic Motor Fibers (Heart/Heart Rate, Respiration, Blood Pressure, Smooth Muscles, Glands Related to Gastric Motility)		
Somatic Motor Fibers for the Muscles of the Pharynx and Larynx		
XI (accessory)	*Motor	Neck muscles: Trapezius muscle (a triangular muscle that covers the posterior neck and shoulder) Sternocleidomastoid muscle (a straplike muscle that wraps obliquely over the neck area that is responsible for flexing and rotating the head)
XII (hypoglossal)	*Motor	Movement of tongue muscles

*These cranial fibers are primarily motor but not exclusively.

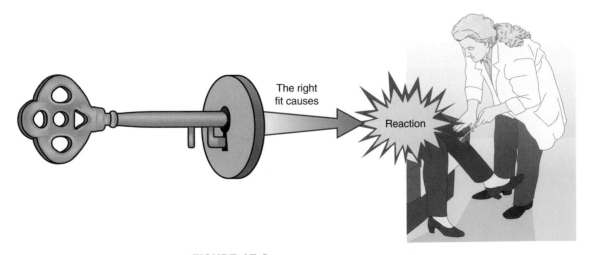

FIGURE 17-9 Lock-and-key mechanism.

TABLE 17-3 Major Organ Response When Sympathetic System Is Activated

Organ/tissue	Sympathetic response
Heart	Increases force of contraction, speed of conduction within the heart, and rate
Lung	Bronchi and bronchioles become dilated; secretions are suppressed
Blood vessels	Constricts all surface areas so person looks pale; increases circulation to areas where blood is most needed, such as the gastrointestinal system, muscles, heart, and brain
Digestive system	Inhibition; decreases gastrointestinal motility, and gastrointestinal secretions are suppressed
Urinary system	Bladder wall relaxes; sphincter contracts
Liver	Increases release of glucose
Eyes	Pupils dilate for better vision; ciliary muscle relaxes for far vision
Adrenal medulla	Epinephrine is released into the blood
Sweat glands	Increases secretion

TABLE 17-4 α- and β-Receptors and Their Effects on the Body Systems

Receptors	Effects
α_1	Heart contraction increases
	Eyes (pupils) dilate
	Peripheral vasoconstriction occurs
α_2	Smooth muscles contract
β_1	Heart rate increases
β_2	Bronchial muscles dilate
	Uterus relaxes

and the eyes. α-Receptors are located on the smooth muscle; β_1 receptors are located on the heart muscle; and β_2 receptors are located in the respiratory system and elsewhere. Drugs that mimic natural sympathetic neurotransmitters are referred to as sympathomimetics or adrenergics, and the drugs used to block them are called sympatholytics or are named after the specific receptor they block. The adrenergic agents that mimic the sympathetic nervous system are epinephrine and norepinephrine. Table 17-4 lists some uses for α- and β-sympathomimetics with their effects.

SYMPATHOMIMETICS OR ADRENERGIC AGENTS

GENERIC NAME: epinephrine
TRADE NAME: Adrenalin
DRUG ACTION: activates α_1 and β_1 sites, causing vasoconstriction and increasing the heart rate
INDICATION: low blood pressure; used to treat heart attacks and shock
ROUTE OF ADMINISTRATION: injection
COMMON DOSAGE: 1 mg/mL
SIDE EFFECTS: headache, tachycardia, and high blood pressure

GENERIC NAME: dopamine
TRADE NAME: Intropin
DRUG ACTION: stimulates α_1 (but only at high rates of infusion) and β_1 receptors
INDICATIONS: In low dosages, dopamine causes vasodilation and increased urine output; in moderate doses, it releases norepinephrine, which affects β_1 receptors, increasing heart contractions; in high doses, it is used for patients suffering from shock.
ROUTE OF ADMINISTRATION: injection
COMMON DOSAGE: 1 to 5 µg/kg per minute up to 50 mg/kg per minute
SIDE EFFECTS: tachycardia, headache, vomiting

GENERIC NAME: ritodrine
TRADE NAME: Yutopar
MODE OF ACTION: activates β_2 receptors that inhibit contraction of the uterine muscles
INDICATION: premature labor
ROUTE OF ADMINISTRATION: injection
COMMON DOSAGE: 50 to 100 µg/min
SIDE EFFECTS: bradycardia, nausea, and vomiting

PARASYMPATHETIC SYSTEM

The sympathetic and parasympathetic systems have many differences. The parasympathetic system can be thought of as the opposite or counterbalance to the sympathetic system. In the parasympathetic system, nerves emerge from the brainstem and the sacral part of the cord. Another important difference is the location of the preganglionic nerves. In the parasympathetic system these nerves are located in the gray matter of the brainstem or spinal cord. They exit the CNS and have a long preganglionic fiber. The impulse moves to the target organ, creating a response. One of the main functions of the parasympathetic system is activation of the digestive system. This function includes secreting acidic juices, increasing peristalsis, and inducing hormonal secretion of insulin. The parasympathetic system also slows the heart rate. The parasympathetic system works while we rest and is inhibited only when the sympathetic system takes over during periods of intense stress. Table 17-5 describes the organs and effects of the parasympathetic system.

Cholinergic Agents and Cholinergic Blockers
The main neurotransmitter of the parasympathetic system is acetylcholine. Acetylcholine is important in the CNS and PNS. Acetylcholine works quickly and has a short duration of action. Two types of cholinergic agents are those that mimic acetylcholine and those that stop the destruction of acetylcholine by

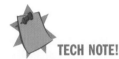

TECH NOTE!
The autonomic system is an involuntary branch of the PNS. The autonomic system is divided into sympathetic and parasympathetic systems. The sympathetic system releases the neurotransmitter norepinephrine when we are stressed, and the parasympathetic system releases acetylcholine when we are at rest. Sympathetic ganglions synapse with many postganglionic fibers for a widespread effect, whereas parasympathetic preganglionic fibers synapse with fewer postganglionic fibers.

TABLE 17-5 Response of the Body Systems to Parasympathetic Stimulation

Organ/tissue	Parasympathetic response
Heart	Slows
Lungs	Dilates bronchi
Blood vessels	None
Digestive system	Increased motility; digestion takes place
Urinary system	Urinary bladder muscle contracts; sphincter relaxes
Liver	None
Eyes	Pupils constrict; ciliary muscle contraction for near vision
Adrenal medulla	None
Sweat glands	None

the enzyme acetylcholinesterase. Because these cholinergic drugs mimic the parasympathetic system, they are referred to as parasympathomimetics, whereas drugs that inhibit the cholinergic reaction by blocking the receptor most commonly are called anticholinergics. The main side effects of anticholinergics are dry mouth and an inhibition of urine output.

Parasympathetic receptors, which respond to the neurotransmitter acetylcholine, are located on smooth and cardiac muscle cells. Cholinergic blockers stop the response. They prevent acetylcholine from combining with the receptor, causing the nerve impulse to stop. This is useful when patients must be sedated or when their eyes have to be dilated by the optometrist. Anticholinergic drugs have many uses, including for many of the conditions that are discussed later.

Conditions of the Nervous System and Their Treatments

Many disorders involve inappropriate or excessive muscle contractions. Some muscular disorders involve the wasting away of the muscles. Many of the following conditions are still without cures, and researchers still are trying to find the causes. Some conditions are hereditary, whereas others may be random genetic mutations. Other disorders are being investigated to determine whether environmental conditions may increase the incidence of their occurrence. Because there are so many conditions, disorders, and diseases that can affect the brain and nervous system, only a sample of the major disorders is examined. For a list of these and additional disorders along with informational websites, see Box 17-1.

BOX 17-1 COVERED AND ADDITIONAL DISEASES AFFECTING THE NERVOUS SYSTEM, WITH WEBSITES FOR ADDITIONAL INFORMATION

Alzheimer's disease	www.alz.org
Amyotrophic lateral sclerosis	www.alsa.org
Aphasia	www.aphasia.org
Ataxia	www.ataxia.org
Birth defects	www.birthdefects.org
Brain tumors	http://hope.abta.org/site/PageServer
Cerebral palsy. Office of Rare Diseases	http://rarediseases.info.nih.gov/html/reports/ fy1998/ord.html
Epilepsy	www.epilepsyfoundation.org
Lupus	www.lupusny.org
Multiple sclerosis	www.msaa.com
Muscular dystrophy	www.mdausa.org
Myasthenia gravis	www.myasthenia.org
Pain, chronic	www.theacpa.org
Parkinson's disease	www.pdf.org
Pediatric brain tumor	www.braintumorkids.org
Pediatric strokes	www.pediatricstrokenetwork.com
Psychological disorders	www.apa.org
Polio	www.post-polio.org
Rare disorders	www.rarediseases.info.nih.gov
Restless leg syndrome	www.rls.org
Sleep disorders	www.sleepfoundation.org
Spinal cord injuries	www.spinalcord.org
Stroke	www.stroke.org
Stuttering	www.stutteringhelp.org
Vestibular disorders	www.vestibular.org

GENERAL NERVOUS SYSTEM DISORDERS

Skeletal Muscle Pain

Pain in the muscles is a warning signal from the body. Although everyone experiences some pain at one time or another, severe injury or chronic pain may need additional care. Treatments include surgery followed by physical therapy or drug therapy. Other causes of pain related to the nervous system include headaches, migraines, and various bone conditions affecting the skeletal system. Analgesics and nonsteroidal antiinflammatory drugs used to treat head pain are discussed in Chapter 24. For chronic muscle pain that cannot be identified, the patient may be treated only with skeletal muscle relaxants. Two main types of these drugs are used—central acting and direct acting.

Central-Acting Medications

Although the drug actions of central-acting medications are not well known, the result of the medications is well documented. One of most important effects of these agents is the depression of the CNS. These drugs affect the brainstem, thalamus, basal ganglia, and the spinal cord. Side effects include dizziness, drowsiness, blurred vision, and headaches. These agents are not meant for long-term use. These drugs are classified as smooth muscle relaxants. The main drugs used as smooth muscle relaxants follow, along with their primary indication, drug action, and necessary auxiliary labels. In several instances the specific drug action currently is not known; therefore, a general drug action is supplied. Auxiliary labels are placed on certain prescription bottles and contain brief information about the drug for the patient's reference. The information usually refers to side effects. For instance, if an auxiliary label states, "Take with food," the medication can cause stomach upset.

SMOOTH MUSCLE RELAXANTS

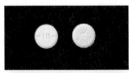
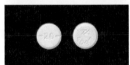

GENERIC NAME: baclofen
TRADE NAME: Lioresal
DRUG ACTION: inhibits synaptic reflexes at CNS level
INDICATION: spasticity associated with multiple sclerosis or spinal cord injury
ROUTE OF ADMINISTRATION: oral, injection
COMMON DOSAGE: oral dosage ranges from 5 mg tid to 80 mg maximum per day
AUXILIARY LABELS:

■ Take with food or milk.
■ May cause dizziness or drowsiness.

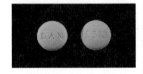

GENERIC NAME: carisoprodol
TRADE NAME: Soma
DRUG ACTION: blocks neuron activity at CNS level
INDICATION: acute muscle pain
ROUTE OF ADMINISTRATION: oral
COMMON DOSAGE: 350 mg tid or qid
SIDE EFFECTS: dizziness, drowsiness, vertigo, upset stomach, headache
AUXILIARY LABELS:

■ May cause dizziness or drowsiness.
■ Take with food.

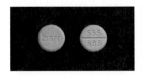

GENERIC NAME: chlorzoxazone
TRADE NAME: Parafon Forte DSUBCUT
DRUG ACTION: reduces multisynaptic impulses at CNS level
INDICATION: discomfort caused by muscle pain and spasms

ROUTE OF ADMINISTRATION: oral
COMMON DOSAGE: ranges from 250 mg tid to qid to 750 mg tid to qid, tapering off dose as pain decreases
SIDE EFFECTS: dizziness, drowsiness, and stomach upset
AUXILIARY LABELS:
- May cause dizziness or drowsiness.
- Take with food.

GENERIC NAME: cyclobenzaprine
TRADE NAME: Flexeril
DRUG ACTION: decreases muscle spasms without loss of muscle function
INDICATION: acute muscle pain
ROUTE OF ADMINISTRATION: oral
COMMON DOSAGE: 10 mg tid; maximum length of time, 3 weeks
SIDE EFFECTS: dizziness, drowsiness, blurred vision, dry mouth
AUXILIARY LABELS:
- May cause dizziness or drowsiness.
- Avoid alcohol.

GENERIC NAME: methocarbamol
TRADE NAME: Robaxin
DRUG ACTION: general CNS depression
INDICATION: acute muscle pain and muscle pain associated with tetanus
ROUTE OF ADMINISTRATION: oral, injection
COMMON DOSAGE: oral dosage, 1.5 g qid up to 8 g per day in severe cases
SIDE EFFECTS: drowsiness, dizziness; urine may change color to black, brown, or green
AUXILIARY LABELS:
- May cause dizziness or drowsiness.
- Avoid alcohol.
- Urine may change color.

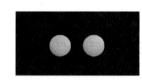

GENERIC NAME: orphenadrine
TRADE NAME: Norflex
DRUG ACTION: acts at the brainstem using analgesia
INDICATION: acute muscle pain and bedtime leg cramps
ROUTE OF ADMINISTRATION: oral, injection
COMMON DOSAGE: oral dosage, 100 mg bid
SIDE EFFECTS: dizziness, drowsiness, blurred vision, fainting, dry mouth
AUXILIARY LABELS:
- May cause dizziness or drowsiness.
- Avoid alcohol.

Direct-Acting Agents

Direct-acting agents work directly on the muscles by inhibiting calcium release, which results in decreased muscle response. Side effects include fatigue, dizziness, drowsiness, diarrhea, and respiratory depression. (The medication dantrolene is listed under multiple sclerosis.) Commonly used oral agents are listed next. These are samples of combinations of agents that include a variety of popular analgesics and antiinflammatories.

MUSCLE RELAXANTS WITH ANALGESICS/ANTIINFLAMMATORIES

GENERIC NAME: carisoprodol/aspirin
TRADE NAME: Soma Compound
COMMON DOSAGE: 200 mg, one to two tablets 4 times daily

SIDE EFFECTS: Dizziness, drowsiness
AUXILIARY LABELS:
- May cause drowsiness.
- Do not drink alcohol.

GENERIC NAME: carisoprodol/aspirin/codeine
TRADE NAME: Soma Compound with codeine
COMMON DOSAGE: 16 mg codeine, one to two tablets 4 times daily
SIDE EFFECTS: Dizziness, drowsiness
AUXILIARY LABELS:
- May cause drowsiness.
- Do not drink alcohol.

GENERIC NAME: orphenadrine/aspirin/caffeine
TRADE NAME: Norgesic
COMMON DOSAGE: 25 mg/385 mg/30 mg, one to two tablets every 6 to 8 hours
SIDE EFFECTS: Dizziness, drowsiness
AUXILIARY LABELS:
- May cause drowsiness.
- Do not drink alcohol.

Conditions Affecting the Peripheral Nervous System

MYASTHENIA GRAVIS

Myasthenia gravis is a rare autoimmune disorder in which electrical messages from the CNS to muscles throughout the body, especially the muscles of the throat and eyes, are affected. The immune system attacks and destroys the receptors that normally receive neuronal impulses. A tumor within the thymus sometimes may be the cause. Although the muscles in the face, eyes, and mouth areas are affected, other areas can be affected as well. Vocal and vision difficulties often occur, and drooping of the eyelids is a common side effect seen in persons suffering from this autoimmune disease. Muscles tire easily and take a much longer time to recover. This is a chronic disease that worsens over time. Eventually the respiratory system may be affected and death results. Myasthenia gravis affects more women than men; only 3 in 100,000 persons are affected in the United States. Drugs that block the destruction of acetylcholine, called anticholinesterases, most often are used for treatment. Surgery is performed to remove the thymus if a thymic tumor is found. Of persons with myasthenia gravis, 8 out of 10 can be helped; only rare cases result in death when the respiratory system fails. No cure for myasthenia gravis has been found, except in those cases in which the cause is a tumor in the thymus (15% of cases).

Drug Treatments
The class of drugs used for treating myasthenia gravis is cholinergics. The drug action is to block the destruction of the neurotransmitter acetylcholine by the enzyme acetylcholinesterase. Side effects of the medications may occur because of overstimulation that can result in nausea, vomiting, diarrhea, and severe abdominal pain.

CHOLINERGIC AGENTS

> **GENERIC NAME:** neostigmine
> **TRADE NAME:** Prostigmin
> **INDICATION:** myasthenia gravis
> **ROUTE OF ADMINISTRATION:** oral, injection
> **COMMON DOSAGE:** oral dosage ranges from 15 mg to 375 mg qd

> **GENERIC NAME:** pyridostigmine
> **TRADE NAME:** Mestinon
> **INDICATION:** myasthenia gravis
> **ROUTE OF ADMINISTRATION:** oral, injection
> **COMMON DOSAGE:** oral dosage ranges from 70 mg to 1.5 g per day

Disorders of the Brain and Spinal Cord

EPILEPSY

Epilepsy is a seizure disorder in which there is a hyperexcitability in some of the nerve cells in the brain. Diagnosis normally is based on an electroencephalogram. For an electroencephalogram, electrodes are attached to the head of the patient, and the electrical impulses corresponding to brain waves are transferred onto paper strips that can be read by a physician. The two types of seizures are partial or generalized. Partial seizures affect only one hemisphere of the brain and may result in only a twitching of a limb without any loss of consciousness. Generalized seizures affect both hemispheres and have different levels of intensity ranging from petit mal (the least violent) to grand mal seizures that are longer and more intense. Children often have petit mal seizures, causing them to stare off into space for a time. In grand mal seizures, also known as tonic-clonic seizures, the person loses consciousness and falls to the ground; there are widespread muscle spasms (tonic phase) followed by muscle relaxation (clonic phase). The person can be injured depending on where and when he or she has the seizure. The person having the seizure does not remember the episode. Other causes for seizure include skull fracture or tumor, although often no cause is found. Treatment can range from drugs to surgery in the case of an operable tumor. Anticonvulsants are the types of drugs used for epilepsy. Often the dosage or type of medicine must be adjusted to help the patient become seizure-free. For the patient to take the medication on time every day is important to avoid the possibility of seizures.

Drug Treatment

Anticonvulsants inhibit abnormal impulses within the CNS by inhibiting one or more of the ions such as sodium, calcium, or potassium within the nervous system. When dosed correctly, these agents stop seizures from occurring. The various agents used for treatment of seizures—hydantoins, barbiturates, succinimides, and benzodiazepines—and their maintenance dosing is discussed.

HYDANTOIN ANTICONVULSANTS

> **GENERIC NAME:** phenytoin
> **TRADE NAME:** Dilantin
> **DRUG ACTION:** inhibits seizure activity at the motor cortex; decreases sodium ion gradient
> **INDICATION:** most often tonic-clonic seizures and partial seizures
> **ROUTE OF ADMINISTRATION:** oral, injection

COMMON DOSAGE: oral dosage is 100 mg tid, although the dosage can range widely
AUXILIARY LABELS:

- May cause dizziness or drowsiness.
- Avoid alcohol.

GENERIC NAME: fosphenytoin
TRADE NAME: Cerebyx (intravenous only; because phenytoin given intravenously irritates and burns the vein, fosphenytoin, a different form of phenytoin, is given instead; after it enters the body, it converts into phenytoin; note that the drug action and trade name are the same as phenytoin).

SUCCINIMIDE ANTICONVULSANT

GENERIC NAME: ethosuximide
TRADE NAME: Zarontin
INDICATION: absence (petit mal) seizures
ROUTE OF ADMINISTRATION: oral
COMMON DOSAGE: 250 mg qd
AUXILIARY LABEL:

- May cause dizziness or drowsiness.

CNS ANTICONVULSANT

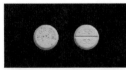
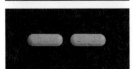

GENERIC NAME: carbamazepine
TRADE NAME: Tegretol; Tegretol-XR
INDICATION: all types of seizures
ROUTE OF ADMINISTRATION: oral
COMMON DOSAGE: 200 to 1200 mg; 200 mg bid for XR
AUXILIARY LABELS:

- May cause dizziness or drowsiness.
- Avoid alcohol.
- Take with food.

BARBITUATE ANTICONVULSANT

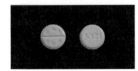

GENERIC NAME: primidone
TRADE NAME: Mysoline
INDICATION: all types of seizures
ROUTE OF ADMINISTRATION: oral
COMMON DOSAGE: 250 mg tid or qid
AUXILIARY LABELS:

- May cause dizziness or drowsiness.
- Take with food.

CNS ANTICONVULSANTS

GENERIC NAME: valproic acid, valproic sodium, divalproic sodium
TRADE NAME: Depakene (valproic acid), Depakene syrup (divalproex sodium), Depacon (valproate), Depakote, Depakote ER, and Depakote sprinkles (divalproex sodium)
INDICATION: all types of seizures
ROUTE OF ADMINISTRATION: oral, injection
COMMON DOSAGE: oral dosing, 30 to 60 mg/kg per day tid or qid

AUXILIARY LABELS:
- Take with food or milk.
- Do not crush or chew.
- May cause dizziness or drowsiness.

GENERIC NAME: gabapentin
TRADE NAME: Neurontin
INDICATION: all types of seizures
ROUTE OF ADMINISTRATION: oral
COMMON DOSAGE: 900 mg to 1.8 g tid
AUXILIARY LABEL:
- May cause dizziness or drowsiness.

BARBITURATES (CONTROLLED SUBSTANCES)

GENERIC NAME: phenobarbital
TRADE NAME: Luminal
DRUG ACTION: depresses the sensory cortex
INDICATION: partial and generalized seizures; also used for sedation and other effects
SIDE EFFECTS: nausea and vomiting; also can cause respiratory depression if overdosed
ROUTE OF ADMINISTRATION: oral, injection
COMMON DOSAGE: oral dosage varies from 60 to 100 mg qd

GENERIC NAME: mephobarbital
TRADE NAME: Mebaral
ROUTE OF ADMINISTRATION: oral
COMMON DOSAGE: 400 to 600 mg qd
- Drug action, indication, and side effects are the same as for phenobarbital.

BENZODIAZEPINES (CONTROLLED SUBSTANCES)

DRUG ACTION: stops seizures by affecting areas of the brain such as the thalamus, cortex, and limbic areas
INDICATIONS: anxiety and insomnia (diazepam and clonazepam are indicated additionally for seizures)
GENERIC NAME: diazepam
TRADE NAME: Valium
INDICATIONS: seizures, antianxiety
ROUTE OF ADMINISTRATION: oral, injection
COMMON DOSAGE: oral dosage 2 to 10 mg bid to qid
SIDE EFFECTS: drowsiness
AUXILIARY LABELS:
- Do not drink alcohol.
- Not to be used as sole treatment for seizures. Parenteral dose is for control of acute seizures.

GENERIC NAME: clonazepam
TRADE NAME: Klonopin
INDICATIONS: seizures, antianxiety
ROUTE OF ADMINISTRATION: oral
COMMON DOSAGE: ranges from 1.5 mg tid up to a maximum of 20 mg qid to control seizures
- Indications and side effects are the same as for diazepam.

TECH NOTE!

All benzodiazepines are controlled substances. Although these agents can work well, they are schedule IV controlled substances and usually are not used for long-term treatment but instead are used with other anticonvulsants or in emergency situations. The main side effect of these drugs is CNS depression.

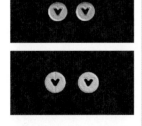

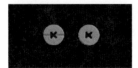

ALZHEIMER'S DISEASE

Alzheimer's disease affects millions of elderly persons, including some famous persons such as former President Ronald Reagan and actor Charlton Heston. Alzheimer's disease is a degenerative brain condition that progresses as one ages but can occur in younger persons. Because of the loss of neuronal synapses, the transfer of electrical stimuli is stifled; the memory banks cannot process information, and memory loss occurs. Brain cells are replaced with deposits of protein that can be described as tangles and knots. The brain begins to shrink in size, and memory is affected.

Most persons lose some memory as they age; however, an abnormal loss of memory and basic mental function is called dementia. Other symptoms include inability to perform normally familiar tasks, difficulty talking, and disorientation in familiar surroundings. Alzheimer's disease affects approximately 7% of persons younger than 65 years; incidence rises to 30% for persons older than 85. Researchers are getting closer to the possible causes of this condition, and it is now known that most persons suffering from Alzheimer's disease lack the neurotransmitter acetylcholine, which is needed to transmit impulses properly. Many hypotheses have been proposed for the cause of Alzheimer's disease, including viruses, immunizations, and tainted water. The disease has been shown to run in families as well. In addition to the use of drugs to help slow the advancing progression of this disease, patients usually need 24-hour care in skilled nursing facilities if their families cannot take on the responsibility.

Drug Treatment
Although the main therapy for Alzheimer's disease tends to be cholinesterase inhibitors, other agents such as nimodipine and physostigmine may help delay the progression of the disease.

CHOLINESTERASE INHIBITORS

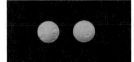

GENERIC NAME: donepezil
TRADE NAME: Aricept
DRUG ACTION: inhibits acetylcholinesterase, which is responsible for destroying acetylcholine; therefore, it allows a higher concentration of acetylcholine to activate receptors
INDICATION: mild to moderate Alzheimer's disease
ROUTE OF ADMINISTRATION: oral
COMMON DOSAGE: 5 to 10 mg qd
SIDE EFFECTS: nausea, vomiting, and diarrhea with initial dosing

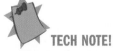

TECH NOTE!
Tacrine is associated with liver damage and is dosed 4 times daily rather than once, as is donepezil. Therefore, tacrine is not used as often.

GENERIC NAME: tacrine
TRADE NAME: Cognex
DRUG ACTION: elevates acetylcholine concentrations in the cerebral cortex
INDICATION: mild to moderate Alzheimer's disease
ROUTE OF ADMINISTRATION: oral
COMMON DOSAGE: varies depending on status of disease; initial dose, 10 mg qid
SIDE EFFECTS: most effects are caused by high dosage; nausea, vomiting, and diarrhea

MULTIPLE SCLEROSIS

Multiple sclerosis involves deterioration of the myelin sheath as shown in Figure 17-10.

The insulating myelin sheaths that surround neurons help in the conduction of electrical current as the impulses travel. With multiple sclerosis the body begins to attack the myelin sheaths, destroying this important material. The sheaths are replaced by plaques of sclerotic (hard) tissue. When this happens,

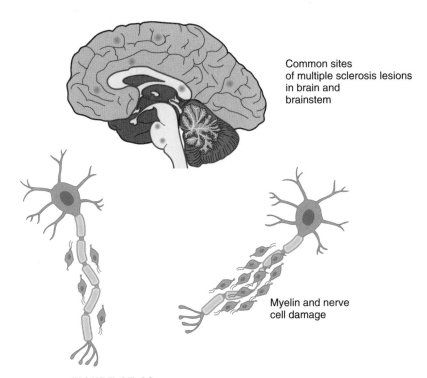

Common sites of multiple sclerosis lesions in brain and brainstem

Myelin and nerve cell damage

FIGURE 17-10 Normal versus abnormal basal ganglia.

the electrical impulses cannot pass from one neuron to another, and the person fails to complete the movement he or she wishes to make. The average age of onset is in the early 30s. Some symptoms include muscle weakness, abnormal sensations such as numbness or tingling over any part of the body, vision change, and loss of coordination. Many persons experience a period of remission followed by attacks of loss of function. The cause is considered an autoimmune response to some unknown stimulus.

Drug Treatment
Currently, only autoimmune stimulants (interferons) are used to treat multiple sclerosis specifically, although other medications are used to treat the symptoms.

ANTISPASMODIC MEDICATION

GENERIC NAME: baclofen
TRADE NAME: Lioresal
DRUG ACTION: inhibits synaptic reflexes at CNS level
INDICATION: spasticity in multiple sclerosis and some spinal cord injuries
ROUTE OF ADMINISTRATION: oral
COMMON DOSAGE: increasing dosage over several weeks from 5 mg tid to 20 mg qid
AUXILIARY LABEL:
■ May cause dizziness or drowsiness.

CENTRAL-ACTING SMOOTH MUSCLE RELAXANT; ANTISPASMODIC

GENERIC NAME: dantrolene
TRADE NAME: Dantrium
INDICATION: (antispastic) multiple sclerosis, cerebral palsy, and cerebrovascular accident
ROUTE OF ADMINISTRATION: oral
COMMON DOSAGE: 25 mg qd

INTERFERONS

GENERIC NAME: interferon β_{1a}
TRADE NAME: Avonex
INDICATION: multiple sclerosis
ROUTE OF ADMINISTRATION: injection
COMMON DOSAGE: 30 µg intramuscularly every week
AUXILIARY LABEL:
- Avoid sunlight.

GENERIC NAME: interferon β_{1b}
TRADE NAME: Betaseron
INDICATION: multiple sclerosis
ROUTE OF ADMINISTRATION: injection
COMMON DOSAGE: 0.25 mg subcutaneously qod
AUXILIARY LABEL:
- Avoid sunlight.

PARKINSON'S DISEASE

Parkinson's disease is a condition that has affected millions of people, including famous persons such as Michael J. Fox and Muhammad Ali. This condition is another progressive disease that is a disorder of the basal ganglia and is associated with the loss or deficiency of dopamine. The basal ganglia is a group of cells (gray matter) located in the medulla (white matter) of the cerebrum. The function of the basal ganglia is to regulate skeletal muscle tone and overall body movement. Dopamine is a natural chemical produced in the brain that inhibits movement. Acetylcholine activates the neurons, and dopamine inactivates them. If dopamine is lacking, then there is movement without ending. The overall degeneration of dopamine-producing neurons brings about the symptoms of Parkinson's disease (Figure 17-11).

The severity of symptoms increases over months to years. The most common symptoms include tremors, muscle rigidity, loss of balance, and hypokinesia and bradykinesia. Hypokinesia results in a decrease in the range of motion, and bradykinesia involves an overall slowing of motion and performing of simple tasks such as buttoning a shirt or eating. As this disease progresses, the patient's movement slows and eventually stops; the person becomes wheelchair bound. Swallowing may become difficult, and speech may be slurred. Signs of Parkinson's disease develop at approximately 60 years of age. The cause is unknown; although researchers have found a genetic defect in some cases, whether the disease is genetic or environmental or a combination of both is still unclear. Diagnosis is difficult because the disease can progress slowly. Doctors usually order computed tomography scans or magnetic resonance imaging to rule out other possibilities. Often, administration of anti-Parkinson's agents is used to make the correct diagnosis of Parkinson's disease. Treatments include surgery, physical therapy, and drugs. Various drugs increase the dopamine and acetylcholine levels in the brain, which are responsible for fine motor movements, and improve balance. However, these drugs have major side effects. Following is a list of some of the most common drugs.

Drug Treatment

The following drugs are classified as anti-Parkinson's agents. Most of these agents increase the neurotransmitter dopamine in one way or another.

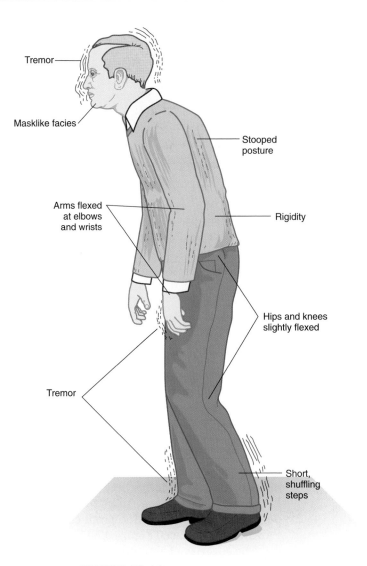

FIGURE 17-11 Signs of Parkinson's disease.

ANTIPARKINSONISM DRUGS; ANTICHOLINERGICS

GENERIC NAME: amantadine
TRADE NAME: Symmetrel
DRUG ACTION: stimulates dopamine receptors, relieving tremors and rigidity
INDICATION: Parkinson's disease
ROUTE OF ADMINISTRATION: oral
COMMON DOSAGE: 10 to 40 mg per day
SIDE EFFECTS: may cause insomnia if taken late in the day

GENERIC NAME: selegiline
TRADE NAME: Eldepryl
DRUG ACTION: inactivates monoamine oxidase, which is responsible for destroying dopamine; therefore, it increases the amount and duration of dopamine
INDICATION: Parkinson's disease
ROUTE OF ADMINISTRATION: oral
COMMON DOSAGE: 5 mg bid along with other anti-Parkinson agents such as levodopa/carbidopa (Sinemet)
SIDE EFFECTS: most adverse effects happen only when an overdose is given

GENERIC NAME: levodopa/carbidopa
TRADE NAME: Sinemet
DRUG ACTION: Levodopa is a precursor of dopamine (which is decreased in Parkinson's disease); in this form it can cross the blood-brain barrier and is converted into dopamine in the brain; carbidopa is given only with levodopa to extend the life and transport of dopamine by inhibiting the transformation into dopamine outside of the blood-brain barrier; because carbidopa cannot cross the blood-brain barrier, once inside the brain, the levodopa can convert easily to dopamine.
INDICATION: Parkinson's disease
ROUTE OF ADMINISTRATION: oral
COMMON DOSAGE: doses range from 25 mg/100 mg tid to 25 mg/250 mg tid
SIDE EFFECTS: dystonic movements, anorexia, nausea and vomiting, dry mouth, dizziness, headache, weakness, fatigue
AUXILIARY LABELS:
- May cause dizziness or drowsiness.
- Do not crush tablet.
- Take with food.

ANTICHOLINERGICS

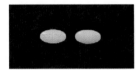

GENERIC NAME: benztropine
TRADE NAME: Cogentin
DRUG ACTION: prolongs the effects of dopamine by inhibiting the reuptake mechanism
INDICATION: Parkinson's disease, normally used with other anti-Parkinson's agents
ROUTE OF ADMINISTRATION: oral, injection
COMMON DOSAGE: oral dosages range from 0.5 to 6 mg per day
AUXILIARY LABELS:
- May cause dizziness or drowsiness.
- Take with food.
- No alcohol.

GENERIC NAME: trihexyphenidyl
TRADE NAME: Artane
DRUG ACTION: prolongs the effects of dopamine by inhibiting the reuptake mechanism
INDICATION: Parkinson's disease, normally used with other anti-Parkinson's agents
ROUTE OF ADMINISTRATION: oral
COMMON DOSAGE: 2 to 5 mg bid to tid
AUXILIARY LABELS:
- May cause dizziness or drowsiness.
- Take with food.
- No alcohol.

AMYOTROPHIC LATERAL SCLEROSIS

Amyotrophic lateral sclerosis (ALS) stands for *without* (a) *spinal cord* (myo) *degeneration* (trophic) *sides* (lateral) and *hardening* (sclerosis). Although this disease was first discovered in the mid-1800s, it is known in the United States as Lou Gehrig's disease, after the famous baseball player who contracted ALS. ALS is a progressive degeneration of the motor tract in the spinal cord. One theory is that it may be caused by the excitatory neurotransmitter glutamate at the synapse, and that this causes cell death.

Although the motor functions of the body decrease, the mind is left unaffected. Those who suffer from this fatal disease describe it as being trapped inside a dying body. The cause for this disease is unknown, but it affects more men than women and usually begins between the ages of 50 and 60 years. Only

10% of patients can be expected to live 10 years or more, and approximately 50% of persons die within 18 months of diagnosis. Initially, the symptoms include weakness in the skeletal muscles and, toward the end, difficulty swallowing and talking. The respiratory muscles become affected, and dyspnea (shortness of breath) occurs. The patient is eventually wheelchair bound and ultimately dies by choking because he or she can no longer swallow. Treatment is limited to a few agents, such as muscle relaxants, to help the side effects, which include muscle spasm, depression, muscle cramping, and excessive salivation.

Drug Treatment

Only riluzole has been developed specifically for treating ALS, and it only slows the progression of the disease. There is no cure.

ANTISPASMODIC

GENERIC NAME: riluzole
TRADE NAME: Rilutek
DRUG ACTION: inhibits glutamine release and decreases the influx of sodium
INDICATION: ALS
ROUTE OF ADMINISTRATION: oral
COMMON DOSAGE: 50 mg q12h
SIDE EFFECTS: nausea, dizziness, diarrhea, and abdominal pain

MISCELLANEOUS MUSCLE AGENTS

Neuromuscular Blockers

Neuromuscular blocking agents are used with anesthetics when a patient is having surgery. They are not used outside of the hospital setting. Many hospitals prepare "conscious sedation packs" of various medications, including neuromuscular blocking agents. The reason for this terminology is that although these agents almost instantly paralyze a patient, they do not sedate or affect any pain levels. The pharmacy technician is responsible for preparing, delivering, and refilling these packs.

Paralyzing Agents

Paralyzing agents are used as adjunctive agents with anesthetics. The result is a complete loss of muscle skeletal function. Most of the agents are short acting and are useful when intubating a patient. Intubation is necessary when a person is placed on a ventilator; these types of agents keep patients stationary so they do not fight the breathing rhythm of the ventilator.

GENERIC NAME: pancuronium
TRADE NAME: Pavulon
INDICATION: muscle rigidity; patient should be under anesthesia before use because pancuronium has no effect on pain levels
ROUTE OF ADMINISTRATION: intravenously only
DOSAGE FORMS: 1 mg/mL, 2 mg/mL, in volumes of 2-, 5-, and 10-mL vials and 2- and 5-mL ampules and syringes

GENERIC NAME: rocuronium
TRADE NAME: Zemuron
INDICATION: muscle contractions during procedures; patient should be under anesthesia before use because rocuronium has no effect on pain levels
ROUTE OF ADMINISTRATION: intravenously only
DOSAGE FORMS: 10 mg/mL, 5-mL vials

TABLE 17-6 Agents Used for Various Conditions of the Nervous System

Disease	Generic name	Trade name	Mode of action/effect
Myasthenia gravis	Pyridostigmine	Regonol	Cholinergic
Multiple sclerosis	Baclofen	Lioresal	Skeletal muscle relaxant
	Interferon β_{1a}	Avonex	Immune modulator
	Interferon β_{1b}	Betaseron	Immune modulator
	Dantrolene	Dantrium	Skeletal muscle relaxant
	Riluzole	Rilutek	Benzathiazol
Parkinson's disease	Amantadine	Symmetrel 1	Dopaminergic
	Benztropine	Cogentin	Anticholinergic
	Bromocriptine	Parlodel	Dopaminergic
	*Carbidopa/levodopa	Sinemet	Dopaminergic
	*Ropinirole	Requip	Dopaminergic
	Diphenhydramine	Benadryl	Anticholinergic
	Dopamine	Intropin	Dopaminergic
	Levodopa	Larodopa	Dopaminergic
	*Pergolide	Permax	Dopaminergic
	*Pramipexole	Mirapex	Dopaminergic
	Trihexyphenidyl	Artane	Anticholinergic
	Selegiline	Eldepryl	Dopaminergic
Alzheimer's disease	Donepezil	Aricept	Cholinesterase inhibitor
	Tacrine	Cognex	Cholinesterase inhibitor
Epilepsy	Carbamazepine	Tegretol	Anticonvulsant
	Fosphenytoin	Cerebyx	Anticonvulsant
	Gabapentin	Neurontin	Anticonvulsant
	Mephobarbital	Mebaral (schedule IV)	Anticonvulsant
	Phenobarbital	Luminal (schedule IV)	Anticonvulsant
	Phenytoin	Dilantin	Anticonvulsant
	Primidone	Mysoline	Anticonvulsant
	Divalproex DR	Depakote	Anticonvulsant

*Lower doses of these medications are used in treating restless leg syndrome.

TABLE 17-7 Miscellaneous Agents That Affect the Central Nervous System

Treatment	Class of drug	Effect
Analgesic	Controlled substances	Reduce pain
Antiemetic/antivertigo	Anticholinergics	Decrease secretions
Antianxiety	Monoamine oxidase inhibitors	Antidepressant
Sedative/hypnotic	Benzodiazepines	Antianxiety, anti-insomnia
Anesthetic	Barbiturates	Inhibit pain perception
Diet aid	Stimulants	Reduce hunger

TECH ALERT!

Remember the following soundalike/look-alike drugs:

Dopamine versus dobutamine

Levodopa versus methyldopa

Clonazepam, lorazepam, and clorazepate

Esmolol versus Osmitrol

Trandate, and Tridrate

Depolarizing Agents

GENERIC NAME: succinylcholine

TRADE NAME: Anectine

INDICATION: intubation and during surgical procedures (currently the only depolarizing agent)

ROUTE OF ADMINISTRATION: intravenously only

DOSAGE FORMS: 20-mg/mL vials, 50-mg/mL ampules, 100-mg/mL in 5- and 10-mL vials, Powder for injection in 500 mg and 1 gm vials.

Table 17-6 lists some of the conditions affecting the nervous system and the agents used in treating those specific diseases. Other drugs that affect the CNS are listed in Table 17-7. These are discussed under their respective chapters within this textbook.

DO YOU REMEMBER THESE KEY POINTS?

- Generic and trade names of drugs covered in this chapter
- The divisions of the nervous system (nervous system tree)
- The major divisions of the brain covered in this chapter and their primary functions
- Conditions in which the sympathetic or parasympathetic systems are stimulated
- Medications that directly affect the sympathetic or parasympathetic system
- Composition of a neuron
- The anatomy of the ganglionic neuronal system with respect to the CNS
- The importance of the blood-brain barrier with respect to medications
- The major classifications of medications used on the sympathetic system and their side effects
- The major classifications of medications used on the parasympathetic system and their side effects
- Major conditions that affect the CNS
- Commonly used medications to treat conditions covered in this chapter

MULTIPLE CHOICE QUESTIONS

1. Cholinergic agents are stimulants of which system?
   A. Nervous system
   B. Sympathetic system
   C. Parasympathetic system
   D. None of the above

2. Afferent and efferent fibers have the function of _____.
   A. Relaying messages to and from the central nervous system
   B. Running the central nervous system
   C. Stimulation
   D. Inhibiting neuronal impulse transfers

3. Neurons are made of the following components except _____.
   A. Dendrites
   B. Cell body
   C. Nerve terminals
   D. Amino acids

4. The area where a neurotransmitter crosses over to another neuron is called _____.
   A. The nerve ending
   B. The axon
   C. The cell body
   D. The synapse

5. All of the following are neurotransmitters except _____.
   A. Dopamine
   B. Norepinephrine
   C. Serotonin
   D. Succinylcholine

6. Which of the following drugs is not used as a smooth muscle relaxant?
   A. Baclofen
   B. Cyclobenzaprine
   C. Cerebyx
   D. Soma

7. Which of the following system activities is not increased during a sympathetic response?
   A. Digestive system
   B. Heart
   C. Lung
   D. Liver

8. The part of the brain that controls memory, reason, and language skills is the
_____.

    A. Medulla oblongata   C. Cerebrum

    B. Cerebellum   D. Brainstem

9. The area that controls breathing and cardiac functions is the _____.

    A. Medulla oblongata   C. Left hemisphere

    B. Right hemisphere   D. Thoracic spinal cord

10. The hypothalamus functions as the _____ of the body.

    A. Thermostat   C. Memory

    B. Appetite relay center   D. Both A and B

11. Which of the following medications used for Parkinson's disease can pass the blood-brain barrier?

    A. Dopamine   C. Carbidopa

    B. Levodopa   D. Both A and B

12. Which of the statements describing dopamine is inaccurate?

    A. Dopamine is a naturally occurring substance within the body.

    B. Dopamine allows for smooth movements of the muscle system.

    C. Dopamine can be injected to replace low levels within the basal ganglia.

    D. Dopamine is a precursor to norepinephrine.

13. Which of the following classes of drugs is used most often for epileptic seizures?

    A. Barbiturates   C. Hydantoins

    B. Benzodiazepines   D. All of the above may be used

14. Which of the types of seizures listed normally is caused by not taking medications?

    A. Tonic-clonic   C. Atonic type seizures

    B. Absence seizures   D. None of the above

15. The most common reason neuromuscular blocking agents are used is to _____.

    A. Keep the patient asleep during an operation

    B. Keep the patient from fighting a respirator (ventilator)

    C. Stop all pain and movement while the patient is being intubated

    D. Both B and C

16. _____ is converted into norepinephrine within the _____ system.

    A. Acetylcholine, sympathetic   C. Acetylcholine, parasympathetic

    B. Epinephrine, sympathetic   D. Dopamine, central nervous system

17. Which of the following statements is not true concerning the sympathetic system?

    A. When activated, glucose is released from the liver.

    B. All parasympathetic system functions stop.

    C. It is responsible for the fight-or-flight reaction.

    D. Drugs that activate this system are called cholinergics.

18. Of the components listed, which one is not housed in the brainstem?

    A. Hypothalamus and thalamus

    B. Pons

    C. Midbrain

    D. Medulla oblongata

19. The name of the enzyme that is responsible for destroying norepinephrine is
_____.

    A. Anticholinergic   C. Acetylcholine

    B. Antiadrenergic   D. Acetylcholinesterase

20. _____ affect the sympathetic system, whereas _____ affect the parasympathetic system.

    A. Cholinergics, anticholinergics

    B. Cholinergics, adrenergics

    C. Adrenergics, antiadrenergics

    D. Adrenergics, cholinergics

TRUE/FALSE **If a statement is false, then change it to make it true.**

_____ **1.** Gray matter makes up the brain, and white matter makes up the spinal cord.

_____ **2.** Homeostasis is when the body is in a sympathetic response mode.

_____ **3.** The peripheral nervous system can be divided into two divisions.

_____ **4.** The thalamus and hypothalamus link the nervous system to the endocrine system.

_____ **5.** The blood-brain barrier serves to prevent large molecules (such as toxins) from passing into the central nervous system.

_____ **6.** Carbidopa is an ingredient added to Sinemet to extend the life of the drug.

_____ **7.** Amyotrophic lateral sclerosis is a degenerative disease of the motor cells of the central nervous system that affects the myelin sheaths surrounding the neuronal axon.

_____ **8.** Tonic seizures involve stiffening of the muscles, whereas clonic is rapid jerking.

_____ **9.** Neuromuscular blocking agents block pain perception and muscle movement.

_____ **10.** Drugs that mimic the cholinergic neurotransmitters of the sympathetic system also are called sympathomimetics.

TECHNICIAN'S CORNER Mr. Perkins was just diagnosed with Parkinson's disease. He comes into the pharmacy with a new prescription for levodopa. What auxiliary labels are necessary? (Use *Drug Facts and Comparisons* for reference.)

BIBLIOGRAPHY

Applegate E: *The anatomy and physiology learning system,* ed 2, Philadelphia, 2000, WB Saunders.

Drug facts and comparisons, ed 53, St Louis, 1999, Wolters Kluwer.

McCuistion LE, Gutierrez K: *Real-world nursing survival guide: pharmacology,* Philadelphia, 2002, WB Saunders.

Potter PA, Perry AG: *Fundamentals of nursing,* ed 5, St Louis, 2001, Mosby.

Thibodeau GA, Patton KT: *Structure and function of the body,* ed 11, St Louis, 2000, Mosby.

Respiratory System

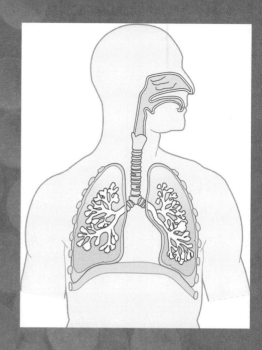

Objectives

UPON COMPLETING THIS CHAPTER, YOU SHOULD BE ABLE TO DO THE FOLLOWING:

- Define all terms used in this chapter as they pertain to the respiratory system.

- List the functions of the respiratory system.

- Describe the act of respiration in transferring oxygen for carbon dioxide.

- Identify the components of the respiratory system outlined in this chapter.

- Differentiate between emphysema, asthma, and bronchitis.

- List the most common conditions that affect the lungs and the types of medications used to treat them.

- List both generic and trade drug names covered in this chapter.

- List the classification and indication for each of the drugs described in this chapter.

- Choose the appropriate auxiliary labels when filling prescriptions for respiratory conditions.

- List the most common side effects for medications discussed in this chapter.

Antitussive *A drug that can decrease the coughing reflex of the central nervous system*

Asthma *A condition in which narrowing of the airways impedes breathing*

Chronic obstructive pulmonary disease *A disease process in which the lungs have decreased ability for gas exchange; also known as emphysema and chronic bronchitis*

Cough reflex *Response of the body to clear air passages of foreign substances and mucus by a forceful expiration*

Cystic fibrosis *An inherited disorder that causes production of very thick mucus in the respiratory tract and affects the pancreas and sweat glands; the patient experiences difficulty breathing and has frequent respiratory infections*

Decongestants *Drugs that reduce swelling of the mucous membranes by constricting dilated blood vessels; they reduce blood flow to nasal tissues, thus reducing nasal congestion*

Expectorant *Chemical that causes the removal of mucous secretions from the respiratory system; it loosens and thins sputum and bronchial secretions for ease of expectoration*

Influenza *A respiratory tract infection caused by an influenza virus*

Metered dose inhaler *A device for supplying medications to the lungs through inhalation*

Nonproductive cough *Cough that does not produce mucous secretions from the respiratory tract*

Productive cough *Cough that expectorates mucous secretions from respiratory tract*

Prophylaxis *Treatment given before an event to prevent the event from happening*

Sputum *Fluid coughed up from the lungs and bronchial tissues*

Viscosity *The thickness of a solution or fluid (e.g., corn syrup is very viscous)*

RESPIRATORY MEDICATIONS

Trade Name	Generic Name	Pronunciation	Trade Name	Generic Name	Pronunciation
Antitussives			**Expectorant**		
Benylin DM	dextromethorphan	(dex-troh-meh-**thor**-fan)	Hycotuss	hydrocodone/ guaifenesin	(hye-droe-**koe**-done)
Robitussin DM	guaifenesin/ dextromethorphan	(gwi-**fen**-ah-sin/dex-troe- me-**thor**-fan)	Robitussin	guaifenesin	(gwi-**fen**-ah-sin)
Tessalon Perles	benzonatate	(ben-**zoe**-na-tate)	**Antihistamines**		
			Benadryl	diphenhydramine	(dye-fen-**hi**-dra-meen)
Analgesic/Antitussives			Chlor-Trimeton	chlorpheniramine	(klor-fen-**air**-ah-meen)
Tussionex	hydrocodone/ chlorpheniramine	(hi-droe-**koe**-deen/ klor-fen-**air**-ah-meen/	Claritin	loratadine	(lo-**rat**-ah-dean)

RESPIRATORY MEDICATIONS—cont'd

Trade Name	Generic Name	Pronunciation	Trade Name	Generic Name	Pronunciation
Mucolytic			**Xanthines**		
Mucomyst	acetylcysteine	(a-sea-till-**sis**-teen)	Phyllocontin	aminophylline	(am-in-**off**-eh-lin)
			Theo-Dur	theophylline	(thee-**off**-ah-lin)
Decongestants					
Sudafed	pseudoephedrine	(sue-doe-e-**fed**-dren)	**Leukotriene Receptor Antagonists**		
Neo-Synephrine	phenylephrine	(fen-ill-**ehf**-rin)	Singulair	montelukast	(mon-tea-**lu**-cast)
Afrin	oxymetazoline	(ox-e-met-**taz**-o-leen)	Accolate	zafirlukast	(zay-**fur**-lu-cast)
			Zyflo	zileuton	(zi-**leu**-ton)
Antituberculosis					
Laniazide	isoniazid	(eye-soe-**nye**-a-zid)	**Corticosteroids**		
Myambutol	ethambutol	(e-**tham**-byoo-tole)	Beclovent	beclomethasone	(beck-low-**meth**-the-sewn)
Rafadin	rifampin	(rif-**am**-pin)	Azmacort	triamcinolone	(try-am-**sin**-oh-lone)
	streptomycin	(strep-toe-**mye**-sin)	AeroBid	flunisolide	(flew-**nis**-oh-lide)
Bronchodilators			**Bronchodilator/Steroid Inhaler (Combination)**		
Proventil, Ventolin	albuterol	(al-**bu**-ter-all)	Advair Diskus	fluticasone/ salmeterol	(flu-**tick**-ah-sewn/sal-**met**-er-ol)
Tornalate	bitolterol mesylate	(bye-**tole**-ter-ole **mess**-ah-late)	**Anticholinergics**		
Adrenalin	epinephrine	(ep-i-**nef**-rin)	Atrovent	ipratropium bromide	(ih-prah-**trow**-pea-um **bro**-mide)
Isuprel	isoproterenol	(eye-so-pro-**tear**-in-all)			
Alupent	metaproterenol	(met-a-pro-**tear**-in-all)	Intal, Nasalcrom	cromolyn	(**krom**-oh-lin)
Maxair	pirbuterol	(pur-**bu**-ter-all)			
Serevent	salmeterol	(sal-**met**-er-ol)			

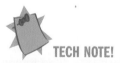

TECH NOTE!

The average respiration rate for adults is 12 to 18 breaths per minute, whereas a child's rate is 40 breaths per minute.

THE RESPIRATORY SYSTEM plays an important role in the body, working to keep us alive and well. The respiratory system is one function of which we become acutely aware when it is not working properly. As seen in Figure 18-1, the respiratory system is composed of many organs, each having specific functions. For example, the lungs enable the body to extract oxygen from the atmosphere when inhaling and to remove carbon dioxide from the body when exhaling. The respiratory system also works to remove unwanted particles from the air before they enter the body system through fine hairs of the nose and the mucosal lining of the bronchi. In addition, the nose helps to heat and humidify cold, dry air so that it is more compatible with our body temperature. This chapter discusses respiration, form and function, and the conditions that affect the respiratory system, including medications to treat them. The drug action, normal dosages, and any auxiliary labels that need to be affixed to prescriptions also are listed in this chapter.

Structure of the Respiratory System

Imagine a large tree with many branches, hollow it out, and invert it, and you have an idea of what the respiratory system looks like. The large trunk is analogous to the trachea, and the two main branches represent the bronchi. The smaller branches are the bronchioles, and the leaves are the alveolar sacs where gas exchange takes place (Figure 18-2). Let's begin to take a more in-depth look at the respiratory tract, starting with the upper respiratory system.

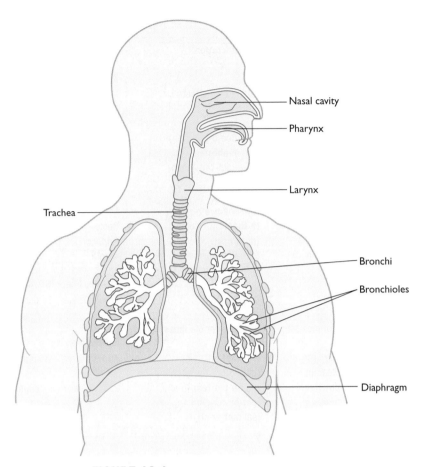

Nasal cavity

Pharynx

Larynx

Trachea

Bronchi

Bronchioles

Diaphragm

FIGURE 18-1 Diagram of respiratory system.

UPPER RESPIRATORY SYSTEM

The upper respiratory system is composed of the nose, pharynx, larynx, and nasal cavities. A mucosal lining covers the inside of the respiratory tract. More than 125 mL (approximately $\frac{1}{2}$ cup) of mucus is produced each day by the body, which forms a protective blanket over much of the respiratory tree. The mucus also serves as an air purification mechanism by trapping inhaled irritants such as dust and pollens. The nasal septum separates the interior of the nose into two distinct cavities. The cavities also are lined by a mucous membrane with small microscopic hairlike structures called cilia. The function of the mucous membrane is to warm and moisten inhaled air. The cilia catch small dust particles in the air that we breathe. Other functions of the nose include the sense of smell and a drain system for tears from the eye. The pharynx is a tube approximately 5 inches long that is shared with the digestive system. Food goes into the esophagus and air goes to the trachea, also known as the windpipe. The tonsils, composed of lymphatic tissue, are located in the pharynx.

LOWER RESPIRATORY SYSTEM

The lower respiratory system is composed of the trachea, bronchial tree, and lungs. The trachea is lined with a mucous membrane that traps airborne particles, and cilia (fine microscopic hairlike structures) that move the particles upward where they are swallowed. The trachea branches off into the right and left bronchi. In turn, each bronchus branches off into smaller and smaller bronchi and into smaller and smaller bronchioles. The function of the bronchi-

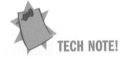

TECH NOTE!

Years ago, doctors quickly removed inflamed tonsils in children. Recently, it was discovered that the tonsils, which are part of the lymphatic system, help the body fight off disease. Now doctors are less quick to use removal as a treatment for inflamed tonsils.

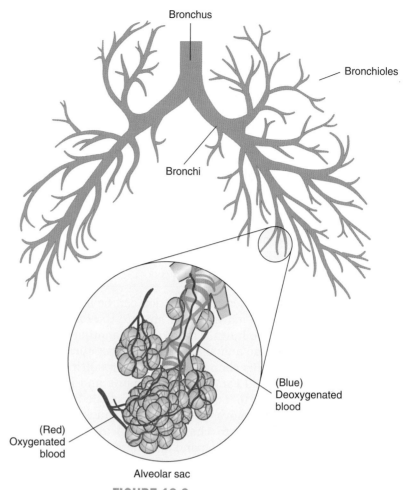

Bronchus

Bronchioles

Bronchi

(Blue)
Deoxygenated
blood

(Red)
Oxygenated
blood

Alveolar sac

FIGURE 18-2 Bronchial tree.

oles is to provide oxygen distribution and a passageway for air to reach the alveoli. The bronchioles end in millions of clusters of microscopic alveolar sacs deep in the lungs.

The pleural cavity is composed of moist, smooth, slippery membranes that line the chest cavity and cover the outer surface of the lungs. This lining is called the pleura and serves to reduce friction between the lungs and the chest wall during breathing.

The larynx also is known as the voice box, because it is responsible for the sounds that we produce. Men and women have a larynx, although it is much smaller in women and does not protrude from the neck as it does in men. This cartilage (usually only visible in men) is referred to as the "Adam's apple." The vocal cords are in the larynx. They provide air distribution and voice production.

The epiglottis, a thin leaf-shaped structure, is located at the entrance of the larynx. Its function is to close off the trachea automatically when swallowing takes place to keep food, liquid, and saliva from going down the airway. If food enters the trachea rather than the esophagus, choking occurs. The epiglottis is formed by one piece of cartilage.

The trachea (windpipe) is approximately $4\frac{1}{2}$ inches long and also has a mucosal lining. At the lower end it branches off into two tubes called bronchi that lead to the right and left lungs, respectively. The right bronchus is bigger than the left because the heart displaces some of the left side of the chest. The trachea has incomplete rings of cartilage reinforcing it so that it will not collapse when the neck is bent.

At the base of the chest cavity is a muscle called the diaphragm. This large muscle layer separates the chest cavity from the abdominal area. In the chest cavity, within the alveoli sacs that are surrounded by tiny capillaries, oxygen is picked up and carbon dioxide is released and exhaled. The lungs fill the chest cavity, except for the space occupied by the heart and large vessels. The lungs are divided into lobes: three in the right lung and two in the left. The right lung has a greater volume capacity, whereas the left lung is longer and has less capacity. The consistency of the lung is like that of a sponge because of the millions of alveolar sacs and connective tissue surrounding them. The lungs are separated from each other by the mediastinum, which is where the heart is located. The left lung has a notch, called the cardiac notch, where the left side of the heart is located. The main function of the lungs is breathing, also known as pulmonary ventilation.

Respiration

The act of respiration can be broken down into two distinct phases: inspiration, the movement of air into the lungs, and expiration, the movement of air out of the lungs. The thorax is another name for the chest cavity. The changes in the size and shape of the thorax during respiration cause a change in air pressure. This change in pressure, resulting from expansion and contraction of the chest wall caused by the raising and lowering of the diaphragm (breathing), causes air to move into and out of the lungs. As a person actively inhales (inspiration), air moves into the lungs causing the muscles of the diaphragm and intercostal areas to change. Specifically, the diaphragm flattens while the intercostal muscles expand and increase the size of the thoracic cavity. This increase in the size of the chest cavity reduces pressure inside so that air can enter the lungs. Expiration is a passive response because, unlike inspiration, it does not use any energy to perform. As the chest relaxes during expiration, the thorax returns to its resting size and shape. The reduction in the size of the thoracic cavity causes the pressure within the thorax to increase, and air leaves the lungs (Figure 18-3).

Exchange of Gases

The air we breathe is composed of approximately 21% oxygen, 79% nitrogen, and less than 0.5% carbon dioxide. As we breathe, the lungs exchange inspired oxygen for carbon dioxide (waste) carried by the blood to the lungs. This waste then is expelled from our lungs. An average adult inhales approximately 250 mL of oxygen and produces approximately 200 mL of carbon dioxide per minute at rest, using a type of diffusion (transfer) to accomplish this function.

After air travels through the bronchioles, it enters more narrow corridors (the alveolar sacs). In the alveolus, each oxygen molecule is able to move across the thin membrane into the waiting blood cells that are passing closely by on the other side of the membrane. The moving blood cells drop off the carbon dioxide before picking up the oxygen molecule. The carbon dioxide molecule then moves out of the lung capillary blood supply into the alveolar sacs and out of the body via expired air. The fully saturated blood moves into larger veins where it returns to the left atrium of the heart via four pulmonary veins. From the left atrium it moves into the left ventricle where it is pumped back out through the body via the arteries, replenishing oxygen to all tissues and organs.

The regulation of respiration permits the body to adjust to varying demands for oxygen supply and carbon dioxide removal. This is done efficiently with the help from the respiratory center within the medulla. The medulla is situated in

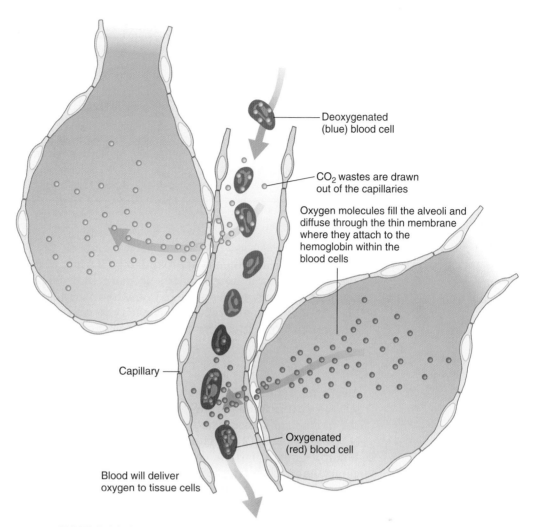

FIGURE 18-3 Inhalation/exhalation for exchange of oxygen and carbon dioxide.

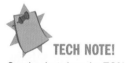

TECH NOTE!

Our body takes in 79% nitrogen but does not use it. Nitrogen is sent back into the air along with the carbon dioxide and leftover oxygen molecules.

the brainstem and is influenced by various inputs or receptors located in other body areas. The exchange of oxygen and carbon dioxide also helps keep our blood pH balanced. The body uses some of the carbon dioxide to make bicarbonate, which maintains the blood pH either by reducing the amount of hydrogen in the blood, causing the pH to become more alkaline, or by increasing the amount of hydrogen, making the blood more acidic. The blood pH must remain close to 7.4 to sustain life (see Figure 18-3).

Breathing

Breathing is an involuntary mechanism. This means you do not have to think about it; the body automatically exhales and inhales when needed. This response is partly because of the respiratory control center located in the medulla in the brain. As the lungs fill with air, nerve impulses originating in the stretch receptors of the lungs are transferred to the respiratory center, which begins a series of neuronal impulses to the respiratory muscles to relax them, resulting in expiration. Impulses then are sent via the respiratory center in the brain that causes the muscles to contract, causing inspiration.

Depending on the size of the person, breathing rates will vary: the smaller the size, the faster the breathing. The breathing rates of small children can be twice as fast as those of adults. The normal amount of air expelled from the

TABLE 18-1 Types of Breathing Dysfunctions

Condition	Symptoms
Apnea	Respiration stops as in heart failure
Bradypnea	Slow breathing
Cyanosis	Lack of oxygen causes skin to turn blue-gray
Dyspnea	Labored or difficult breathing
Hyperventilation	Deep and rapid breathing
Hypopnea	Shallow, inadequate breathing
Orthopnea	Labored or difficult breathing while lying down
Tachypnea	Rapid breathing

lungs in a typical exhale is approximately 500 mL, or 0.5 L, for an average adult, although the total lung capacity is more than 5 L of air. When a person is running, the body needs more oxygen than when sitting or sleeping. The elasticity of the lungs allows for the capacity to vary widely depending on the need for oxygen. Table 18-1 lists common breathing problems.

SNEEZING

A common reflex action that occurs is sneezing. Breathing irritating materials, such as dust or dander, into the respiratory passageway causes the body to expel the foreign substance. The three mechanisms that cause someone to sneeze are (1) ciliary action, (2) peristaltic motion of the bronchioles, and (3) cough reflex. When a foreign particle comes into contact with the sensory receptors of the ciliary hairs, they trigger the reflex of deep inspiration, which then is followed by closure of the vocal cords. The vocal cords remain closed until the actual sneeze is underway, at which point the outward push of air expels the foreign material from the passageways, usually accompanied by a loud noise. Other examples of air movement include coughing, yawning, hiccuping, sighing, crying, and laughing.

Disorders of the Upper Respiratory System

Many conditions affect the respiratory system. Some may be genetic, and others may be contracted because of other factors, such as contagious infections, habits such as smoking, and other environmental factors. One common condition that affects the respiratory system periodically is respiratory colds. Colds are caused by viruses. Because there are more than 140 cold viruses, the common cold has remained an untreatable illness; although recently there have been breakthroughs in the research for finding a cure. Symptoms include coughing, congestion, and sometimes wheezing within the upper respiratory system. Common treatments include decongestants and antihistamines. Other symptoms that accompany colds are rhinitis (inflammation of the lining of the nose), pharyngitis (sore throat), or rhinorrhea (a runny nose).

Hoarseness is another problem that affects the vocal cords and may be caused by several conditions that cause a loss of voice. Laryngitis is the temporary loss of speech resulting from an inflammation, irritation, or infection of the larynx. A more severe type of cold, also caused by viruses, commonly is known as the flu or influenza. This is a viral illness that strikes millions of persons each year; each strain of virus usually is named after the region where it was first detected. Influenza is responsible for millions of dollars of lost wages and health care costs annually. Influenza can be deadly, especially to those who are older or those with weakened immune systems. Influenza vaccinations normally are given each winter season to those at high risk of infection, especially older adults and health care workers.

Another infection common to the upper respiratory tract is rhinitis. Colds, influenza, or allergies produce this nasal inflammatory condition. The common cold also referred to as influenza is caused by a virus that makes it difficult to fight with medications. Allergies are one of the most common types of respiratory problems and are experienced by millions of persons. Allergies range from sensitivity to pollens, animals, textiles, and more. The most common cold remedies include antitussives, expectorants, and decongestants. Allergy medications include oral and nasal decongestants and antihistamines. Most allergy medications can be obtained without a prescription as an over-the-counter (OTC) drug In addition, more anti-drowsy medications are becoming available over the counter for use against colds and allergies.

Disorders of the Lower Respiratory Tract

Pneumonia is an infection that causes acute inflammation in lung airways that become blocked with thick mucus. The cause for this infection can be bacterial, viral, fungal, chemical, or in rare cases, parasitic. Older adults are at high risk, especially after an injury that requires them to remain in bed. Viral pneumonia is not preventable because there are no vaccines available that can be used as a prophylactic. A vaccine is available, Pneumovax, that gives immunity for 14 common bacterial pneumonia infections. This injection is given only once in a lifetime. Persons with a weakened immune system are at a higher risk than most, but pneumonia can strike anyone.

ACUTE AND CHRONIC CONDITIONS

Acute bronchitis is an inflammation of the bronchi and the trachea caused by infection. In some individuals bronchitis can become chronic. When this happens, the repeated inflammation of the bronchioles causes them to become narrow. Smokers commonly contract chronic bronchitis. Chronic bronchitis can progress to emphysema. Either disorder is considered a chronic obstructive pulmonary disease (COPD).

The three types of COPD are chronic bronchitis, emphysema, and bronchiectasis. Emphysema is a condition that causes the destruction of the alveolar walls that eventually leads to a loss of elasticity of the lungs and heart failure. This can be caused by smoking, environmental hazards such as asbestos and fiberglass, or in rare cases, by a genetic predisposition. Because normal exhalation requires elastic recoil of the lungs, the affected lungs allow air to get in but cannot expel all the air. The condition worsens as the surface area of the lungs becomes further reduced because of destruction of the alveolar walls. Bronchiectasis is less common than chronic bronchitis or emphysema and is not discussed.

Asthma

Millions of persons suffer from asthma. Asthma is a major childhood respiratory problem. Asthma is an obstructive airway disease that can be caused by genetic defects or a chronic allergic reaction to irritating substances in the environment. Asthma is classified as an inflammatory disease. The muscles around the bronchioles contract, narrowing the air passages so that air cannot be inhaled properly. In addition to this increase of resistance to airflow, the condition is worsened by edema and secretion of mucus of the airway. This causes the crackling sound heard during an asthma attack. In severe cases, the end result is equivalent to suffocation as the brain is deprived of oxygen. Although many medications can prevent or reverse asthma attacks, deaths are reported from asthma. Usually these deaths occur because many asthmatic persons do not have their medication available when an attack occurs or they delay going to an emergency room for treatment. Treatments for bronchitis, emphysema, and asthma include bronchodilators, corticosteroids, xanthenes, and leukotriene receptor antagonists.

Tuberculosis

Worldwide, tuberculosis is the most common bacterial disease affecting the pulmonary system. This highly contagious lung infection is characterized by an infection within the lining of the lungs by a bacterium that needs oxygen to survive. The lungs provide an environment that is extremely oxygenated where the causative bacteria, *Mycobacterium tuberculosis,* may reside for an extended time with few or no symptoms. When the immune system becomes weakened, the bacteria multiply and symptoms appear (Figure 18-4). Tuberculosis has been on the rise for several years because of the emergence of drug-resistant strains. This occurs partly because many persons with tuberculosis do not complete their course of treatment once they feel better, allowing the bacterium not only to return but also to mutate, making it resistant to traditional drugs. Persons at high risk are those in a confined living space, such as a prison.

Emergency Disorders of the Lungs

The following conditions affect the lungs and their lining, usually requiring hospitalization: pneumothorax, pulmonary embolism, and hemothorax. Pneumothorax can be caused by COPD, tuberculosis, and chest wounds. Pneumothorax is characterized by a collapse of the alveoli resulting from air escaping into the pleural space. A pulmonary embolism results when an embolus (small blood clot that breaks away from origin) blocks a branch of the pulmonary artery that goes from the heart to the lungs. Hemothorax is the collapse of a lung resulting from blood leaking into the pleural space. All of these examples are serious conditions that need to be treated immediately, or death may result. Cancer of the respiratory tract can occur in any part of the respiratory system. Persistent hoarseness is one of the first signs of laryngeal cancer. Persons who smoke pipes, cigars, or cigarettes or those who have inhaled chemicals that contain hazardous particles are at higher risk than most. Treatments may include surgery, chemotherapy, radiation, or a combination of these. Table 18-2 lists other conditions that can affect the respiratory system.

Cardiopulmonary resuscitation. If cardiopulmonary resuscitation (CPR) is started immediately when someone stops breathing, there is a good chance of reviving him or her. Persons who collapse from cardiac arrest or respiratory arrest and children who have accidentally fallen into water and are not breathing are some of the types of victims who have been saved from death through the use of CPR. Most hospitals train pharmacy staff to learn CPR, free of charge. CPR training is in the best interest of all pharmacy technicians because they are in contact with the sick and with older adults daily.

Treatment of Respiratory Disorders

The following drugs are listed in order of their indication with a brief description that includes their drug action, normal adult dosage, common side effects, and auxiliary labels most commonly used.

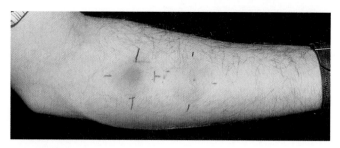

FIGURE 18-4 Positive result of a tuberculosis test.

TABLE 18-2 Conditions of the Respiratory System

Condition	Definition
Pleurisy	Inflammation of the lining of the lungs and lung cavities
Croup	A childhood condition that causes obstruction of the larynx, a barking cough, and noisy breathing
Whooping cough	Also known as pertussis, this bacterial infection is contagious; it affects the larynx and trachea, and produces coughing spasms
Pulmonary edema	Caused by fluid filling the respiratory air sacs (alveoli) and bronchioles

TREATMENTS FOR THE COMMON COLD AND SORE THROAT

GENERIC NAME: zinc combinations
TRADE NAME: Halls Zinc Defense
DRUG ACTION: unknown
INDICATION: to decrease the duration of the common cold and sore throat
ROUTE OF ADMINISTRATION: oral
COMMON DOSAGE: 5-mg lozenges as needed
SIDE EFFECTS: vomiting
AUXILIARY LABEL:
■ OTC; none needed

LOCAL ANESTHETICS FOR THROAT

GENERIC NAME: benzocaine/menthol
TRADE NAME: Chloraseptic relief strips
DRUG ACTION: deadens nerve endings
INDICATION: for the relief of sore throats
ROUTE OF ADMINISTRATION: oral
COMMON DOSAGE: as needed
SIDE EFFECTS: vomiting
AUXILIARY LABEL:
■ OTC; none needed

GENERIC NAME: benzocaine, cetylpyridium chloride
TRADE NAME: Cepacol
DRUG ACTION: deadens nerve endings
INDICATION: for the relief of sore throats

ROUTE OF ADMINISTRATION: oral
COMMON DOSAGE: as needed
SIDE EFFECTS: vomiting
AUXILIARY LABEL:

- OTC; none needed

Cough Suppressants: Antitussives

Antitussives are agents that suppress coughing. Types of medications include controlled substances such as codeine and hydrocodone. Usually each is prescribed as a liquid combination with other agents to treat coughing. For instance, codeine with acetaminophen or codeine with promethazine is found in fixed combinations for coughs. Common OTC agents include guaifenesin/dextromethorphan. Common side effects may include nausea, vomiting, drowsiness, and constipation. All normal dosing regimens are based on the average adult dose.

OPIOID ANALGESIC, SCHEDULE III

GENERIC NAME: phenylpropanolamine/hydrocodone, hydrocodone/chlorpheniramine
TRADE NAME: Hycomine, Tussionex
DRUG ACTION: decreases the cough reflex by binding to opiate receptor sites located in the CNS
INDICATION: pain and coughing
ROUTE OF ADMINISTRATION: oral
COMMON DOSAGE: 5 to 10 mg every 4 to 6 hours
SIDE EFFECTS: drowsiness, constipation, nausea, and vomiting
AUXILIARY LABELS:

- Do not drink alcohol.
- Alcohol will intensify the effects.
- Take with food.
- Take with plenty of water.

NARCOTIC ANTITUSSIVE/EXPECTORANT SCHEDULE III

GENERIC NAME: hydrocodone and guaifenesin
TRADE NAME: Hycotuss Expectorant Syrup
DRUG ACTION: decreases the cough reflex by binding to opiate receptor sites located in the CNS
INDICATION: nonproductive cough (dry cough) and mild to moderate pain
ROUTE OF ADMINISTRATION: oral
COMMON DOSAGE: 10 to 20 mg every 4 to 6 hours
SIDE EFFECTS: drowsiness, constipation, nausea, and vomiting
AUXILIARY LABELS:

- Do not drink alcohol.
- Alcohol intensifies the effects.
- Take with food.
- Take with plenty of water.

NONNARCOTIC ANTITUSSIVE

GENERIC NAME: dextromethorphan
TRADE NAME: Benylin DM
DRUG ACTION: acts on the medulla (cough center) of the brain, decreasing the urge to cough
INDICATION: nonproductive coughs
ROUTE OF ADMINISTRATION: oral
COMMON DOSAGE: 10 to 20 mg every 4 hours or 30 mg every 6 to 8 hours
SIDE EFFECTS: drowsiness, constipation; avoid alcohol because it will intensify drowsy effects
AUXILIARY LABEL:
■ Drink plenty of water.

ANTIHISTAMINE

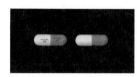

GENERIC NAME: diphenhydramine
TRADE NAME: Benadryl
DRUG ACTION: inhibits CNS, as well as binding to histamine receptor sites for the control of allergies
INDICATION: coughs caused by colds or allergies
ROUTE OF ADMINISTRATION: oral, topical, injection
COMMON DOSAGE: 12.5 to 25 mg every 4 hours (not to exceed 150 mg every 24 hours)
SIDE EFFECT: drowsiness
AUXILIARY LABEL:
■ May cause dizziness or drowsiness.

Expectorants

Expectorants are agents that break up thick mucous secretions of the lungs or bronchi so that they can be expelled from the system through coughing. The main example of an expectorant is guaifenesin. Following administration of expectorants, the patient should be told to increase fluid intake to assist with thinning of mucous secretions.

EXPECTORANT

GENERIC NAME: guaifenesin
TRADE NAME: Robitussin
DRUG ACTION: increases respiratory tract fluid, allowing for the removal of excess mucus; dry coughs become productive coughs, and there is an overall decrease in the amount of coughing
INDICATION: dry, nonproductive coughs
ROUTE OF ADMINISTRATION: oral
COMMON DOSAGE: 200 to 400 mg every 4 hours
SIDE EFFECTS: dizziness, headache, nausea, and vomiting
AUXILIARY LABELS:
■ May cause drowsiness.
■ Drink plenty of water.

Mucolytics

Mucolytics are agents that break up mucus that can obstruct the airway. Their mode of action is to act directly on the blockage, causing a breakdown of molecular linkages. This action causes the plug to become less viscous, thus allowing the mucus to be coughed up more easily or, if needed, to be suctioned out manually. Mucolytics are used in patients suffering from COPD and cystic fibrosis and those patients with a tracheostomy. This type of medication is limited to acetylcysteine.

MUCOLYTIC

GENERIC NAME: acetylcysteine
TRADE NAME: Mucomyst
DRUG ACTION: breaks the bonds between proteins responsible for mucus buildup; this decreases the viscosity of the mucus, allowing it to be expelled
INDICATION: COPD and cystic fibrosis; also overdoses of acetaminophen
ROUTE OF ADMINISTRATION: inhalation
COMMON DOSAGE: inhalant, 10% (3 to 5 mL) to 20% (6 to 10 mL) tid to qid
SIDE EFFECTS: nausea, vomiting, runny nose
AUXILIARY LABEL:
■ None (Most treatments are given in the hospital, although family members can be taught how to give treatments at home.)

TREATMENT OF ALLERGIES AND COLDS

Decongestants

Decongestants also help to clear respiratory passages but work more on the swollen nasal passages that usually accompany common colds or allergies. Most cold remedies are available over the counter and consist of oral liquids, tablets, capsules, or nasal inhalants. Examples of these agents include pseudoephedrine, phenylephrine, and oxymetazoline. Persons suffering from hypertension (high blood pressure) should not take decongestants because they raise blood pressure. This is the type of information about which a physician or pharmacist will notify the patient.

SYMPATHOMIMETIC, NASAL DECONGESTANT

GENERIC NAME: pseudoephedrine
TRADE NAME: Sudafed
DRUG ACTION: affects the adrenergic receptors of the vascular smooth muscle, causing vasoconstriction and a decrease in mucus
INDICATION: nasal congestion
ROUTE OF ADMINISTRATION: oral, nasal
COMMON DOSAGE: 60 mg every 4 to 6 hours
SIDE EFFECTS: insomnia, restlessness
AUXILIARY LABEL: none
NOTE: Pseudoephedrine is now a regulated drug. Because of the misuse of a key component used in making crack (street drug), its quantity is now limited. Refer to Chapter 2 for more information on this drug.

GENERIC NAME: phenylephrine
TRADE NAME: Neo-Synephrine
DRUG ACTION: affects the adrenergic receptors of the vascular smooth muscle, causing vasoconstriction of nasal arterioles
INDICATION: nasal secretions

ROUTE OF ADMINISTRATION: oral, nasal, injection, ophthalmic
COMMON DOSAGE: one to two sprays every 4 hours as needed
SIDE EFFECTS: nasal congestion, if used longer than a few days (rebound congestion)
AUXILIARY LABEL:
- For nasal use.

GENERIC NAME: oxymetazoline
TRADE NAME: Afrin
DRUG ACTION: affects the adrenergic receptors of the vascular smooth muscle, causing vasoconstriction of nasal arterioles
INDICATION: nasal congestion; allergic rhinitis
ROUTE OF ADMINISTRATION: nasal spray
COMMON DOSAGE: two or three sprays every 10 to 12 hours
SIDE EFFECTS: nasal congestion, if used longer than a few days (rebound congestion)
AUXILIARY LABEL:
- For nasal use.

TREATMENT OF CHRONIC OBSTRUCTIVE PULMONARY DISEASE

COPD includes conditions such as emphysema and chronic bronchitis that can progress to the point at which there is irreversible damage to the lung. The dosage forms used to treat COPD include liquids, syrups, inhalants, and in some instances, parenteral preparations. Examples of the types of agents used are bronchodilators, corticosteroids, xanthines, and sympathomimetics. In the following drug monographs, when several classifications have the same indications and side effects, these are outlined before the monographs.

Drug Action

For the following bronchodilator medications, the drug action is sympathomimetic. These agents produce bronchodilation by relaxing the smooth muscle of the bronchioles. Common side effects for this class of drugs are headache, nervousness, and shakiness. The one combination drug (Advair Diskus) provides corticosteroid action along with a long-acting bronchodilator and is used as a prophylactic treatment for persons with asthma. Most common side effects include upper respiratory infection, pharyngitis, and headaches.

SYMPATHOMIMETICS, BRONCHODILATORS

GENERIC NAME: salmeterol
TRADE NAME: Serevent
INDICATION: asthma
ROUTE OF ADMINISTRATION: inhalant disk
COMMON DOSAGE: two puffs bid (not meant for acute attacks)

GENERIC NAME: metaproterenol
TRADE NAME: Alupent
INDICATIONS: asthma, bronchitis, emphysema
ROUTE OF ADMINISTRATION: inhalant, oral
COMMON DOSAGE: liquid, 10 mg every 6 to 8 hours; metered dose inhaler (MDI), two to three puffs every 3 to 4 hours
SIDE EFFECTS: tremors, shakiness, nausea, and vomiting
AUXILIARY LABEL:
- Shake well.

GENERIC NAME: bitolterol mesylate
TRADE NAME: Tornalate
INDICATION: prophylaxis and treatment of bronchial asthma
ROUTE OF ADMINISTRATION: inhalant
COMMON DOSAGE: two puffs every 6 to 8 hours

GENERIC NAME: pirbuterol
TRADE NAME: Maxair
INDICATION: prophylaxis and treatment of bronchial asthma
ROUTE OF ADMINISTRATION: inhalant
COMMON DOSAGE: two puffs every 6 hours

COMBINATION: BRONCHODILATOR/STEROID INHALER

GENERIC NAME: fluticasone propionate/salmeterol
TRADE NAME: Advair Diskus
INDICATION: Prophylaxis for persons with asthma
ROUTE OF ADMINISTRATION: inhalant
COMMON DOSAGE: one blister dose as prescribed every 12 hours
AUXILIARY LABELS:
■ Can cause dizziness.
■ Use as directed

SYMPATHOMIMETICS

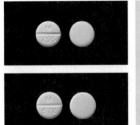
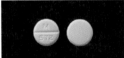

GENERIC NAME: albuterol
TRADE NAME: Proventil, Ventolin
INDICATION: COPD
ROUTE OF ADMINISTRATION: inhalant, oral, liquid for nebulizer
COMMON DOSAGE: syrup, 2 to 4 mg tid to qid; MDI, two puffs every 4 to 6 hours; tablets, 4 mg tid to qid
AUXILIARY LABELS:
■ (MDI: inhalants) Shake well.
■ Can cause dizziness.

GENERIC NAME: epinephrine
TRADE NAME: Adrenalin, Bronkaid
INDICATIONS: asthma, bronchitis, emphysema
ROUTE OF ADMINISTRATION: inhalant, injectable
COMMON DOSAGE: MDI, two puffs, waiting between 1 to 10 minutes between doses
AUXILIARY LABELS:
■ (Inhalants) Shake well.
■ Rinse mouth with water after inhalation.

Xanthine Bronchodilator Agents

Xanthine bronchodilator agents relax the smooth muscle of the bronchi and pulmonary blood vessels. Drugs under this heading include theophylline and aminophylline and dosage forms include tablets, capsules, liquids, syrup, and injectable forms. Indications for these agents include asthma and emphysema. Side effects include shakiness, restlessness, and trembling.

XANTHINE BRONCHODILATOR

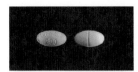

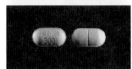

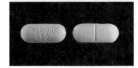

GENERIC NAME: theophylline, aminophylline
TRADE NAME: Theo-Dur, Slo-bid, Uni-Dur
ROUTE OF ADMINISTRATION: oral, inhalant, injection, rectal
COMMON DOSAGE: oral forms—16 mg/kg or approximately 400 mg every 6 to 12 hours; dose varies depending on whether it is sustained release; injection—dose varies based on weight and age of patient*
AUXILIARY LABEL:
- Drink plenty of water.

Leukotriene Receptor Antagonist Agents

Leukotriene receptor antagonist agents inhibit the mechanisms that produce symptoms including edema and smooth muscle constriction that lead to asthma attacks. These agents are used for prophylaxis and chronic treatment of asthma. Side effects include headache.

LEUKOTRINE RECEPTOR ANTAGONISTS

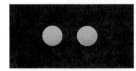

GENERIC NAME: zafirlukast
TRADE NAME: Accolate
ROUTE OF ADMINISTRATION: oral
COMMON DOSAGE: 20 mg 2 times daily
AUXILIARY LABEL: none

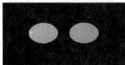

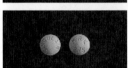

GENERIC NAME: montelukast
TRADE NAME: Singulair
ROUTE OF ADMINISTRATION: oral
COMMON DOSAGE: 10 mg once daily in the evening; 2-, 4-, and 5-mg chewable tablets for pediatric use
SIDE EFFECTS: Headache
AUXILIARY LABEL:
- Do not take aspirin.

Corticosteroid Agents

Corticosteroids are steroids. Inhalants often are used to treat severe asthma attacks. The drug action of corticosteroids includes acting as an antiinflammatory, thus lessening the constriction of the bronchial tubes. Corticosteroids also produce smooth muscle relaxation. These medications are indicated for chronic asthma and as a prophylactic agent. Side effects for corticosteroids are similar to glucocorticoids; these include weight gain, bruising, and possible reduction in growth rate in adolescence children (Figure 18-5).

CORTICOSTEROID AGENTS

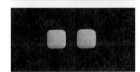

GENERIC NAME: beclomethasone
TRADE NAME: oral—Beclovent, Vanceril; nasal—Beconase AQ, Vancenase AQ
ROUTE OF ADMINISTRATION: oral, nasal
COMMON DOSAGE: oral inhalant, two puffs tid to qid; nasal inhalant, one spray into each nostril tid to qid
AUXILIARY LABELS:
- Shake well.
- Take as directed.

---

*Note that theophylline IV 400 mg/500 mL is equivalent to 500 mg/500 mL.

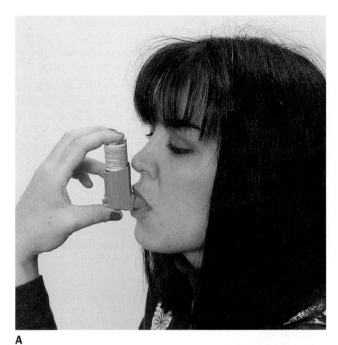

A

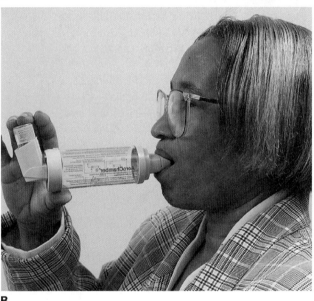

B

FIGURE 18-5 **A**, Proper usage of an inhaler. **B**, Inhaler with spacer (aka: aerochamber).

GENERIC NAME: triamcinolone acetonide*
TRADE NAME: Azmacort
ROUTE OF ADMINISTRATION: inhalation
COMMON DOSAGE: two puffs tid to pid
AUXILIARY LABELS:
- Shake well.
- Take as directed.

*Other triamcinolone agents differ by their additive ingredient: triamcinolone diacetate, triamcinolone hexacetonide, and plain triamcinolone.

GENERIC NAME: flunisolide
TRADE NAME: AeroBid, Nasalide
ROUTE OF ADMINISTRATION: inhalation, oral and nasal
COMMON DOSAGE: oral inhalant (AeroBid), two puffs bid; nasal inhalant (Nasalide), two sprays into each nostril, bid
AUXILIARY LABELS:

- Shake well.
- Take as directed.

GENERIC NAME: fluticasone
TRADE NAME: Flovent, Flonase
ROUTE OF ADMINISTRATION: Oral and nasal inhalant and topical
COMMON DOSAGE: oral inhalation (Flovent), two to four puffs bid; nasal inhalation (Flonase), two sprays per nostril qd
SIDE EFFECTS: Headache
AUXILIARY LABELS:

- Shake well.
- Take as directed.

Anticholinergic Agents

Anticholinergics inhibit the action of acetylcholine, thus relaxing smooth muscle of the bronchioles. Anticholinergics are indicated for bronchospasms resulting from COPD. Side effects include dryness of airway membranes.

ANTICHOLINERGIC AGENT

GENERIC NAME: ipratropium bromide
TRADE NAME: Atrovent*
ROUTE OF ADMINISTRATION: inhalant, oral and nasal
COMMON DOSAGE: oral inhalant, two puffs qid; nasal inhalant, two sprays into each nostril bid to tid
AUXILIARY LABEL:

- Shake well.

ANTIASTHMATIC, MAST CELL STABILIZER

GENERIC NAME: cromolyn
TRADE NAME: Intal, Nasalcrom, Crolom
ROUTE OF ADMINISTRATION: inhalant, oral, nasal, and ophthalmic
COMMON DOSAGE: oral solution (Intal), 20 mg qid; nasal inhalant (Nasalcrom), one spray into each nostril tid to qid
AUXILIARY LABEL:

- None (available as an OTC medication)

TREATMENT FOR TUBERCULOSIS

Most of the primary antituberculin agents are bactericidal. This means that they kill the bacterium that causes tuberculosis. These agents are used in combination for a course of treatment lasting many months. Although the medication used to treat tuberculosis is effective, many patients do not continue to take the medication once they are feeling better because they are unaware that the tuberculosis will return. Also, one of the many side effects is nausea, which can complicate the lengthy treatment. For this reason, patients must be educated by their physician

---

*Also available in combination with albuterol (Combivent).

about the importance of finishing their medication regimen to eradicate the bacteria completely from their system. The commonly used multiple medication treatment plans include isoniazid and rifampin given together as a daily dose. Another regimen includes isoniazid, streptomycin, and ethambutol. Another commonly used agent is pyrazinamide. Examples of the types of combination therapy are given in Table 18-3. These therapies can be given as a short or long course depending on the diagnosis. In the monographs that follow, specific side effects for each agent are listed along with the auxiliary labels and other drug information pertaining to that specific agent. To determine whether tuberculosis is cured entirely, sputum tests are required before treatment can stop.

ANTITUBERCULOSIS AGENTS

GENERIC NAME: isoniazid
TRADE NAME: Laniazid, Nydrazid
ROUTE OF ADMINISTRATION: oral, injection
SIDE EFFECTS: Gastrointestinal upset
COMMON DOSAGE: 300 mg qd 1 to 2 hours before or after meals (oral Laniazid)
SIDE EFFECTS: tremors, shakiness, nausea, and vomiting
AUXILIARY LABELS:
- Take on an empty stomach.
- Take as directed.
- Do not drink alcohol.
- Special instructions: Avoid alcohol because of the risk of hepatitis. Avoid certain foods such as fish or those containing tyramine, such as aged foods. Patient must not discontinue unless instructed to do so by physician.

GENERIC NAME: rifampin
TRADE NAME: Rifadin
ROUTE OF ADMINISTRATION: oral
SIDE EFFECTS: orange to reddish urine and other secretions
COMMON DOSAGE: 600 mg qd 1 to 2 hours before or after meals
SIDE EFFECTS: tremors, shakiness, nausea, and vomiting
AUXILIARY LABELS:
- Take on an empty stomach.
- Take as directed.
- Special instructions: Patient must not discontinue unless instructed to do so by physician. Treatment normally lasts 6 to 9 months or 6 months if sputum culture is negative.

GENERIC NAME: ethambutol
TRADE NAME: Myambutol
ROUTE OF ADMINISTRATION: oral
COMMON DOSAGE: 100 to 300 mg qd
SIDE EFFECTS: gastrointestinal upset, nausea, vomiting, fever, or decrease in visual acuity
AUXILIARY LABEL:
- Take with food.

GENERIC NAME: pyrazinamide
TRADE NAME: (no trade name)
ROUTE OF ADMINISTRATION: oral
SIDE EFFECTS: nausea, vomiting, anorexia, myalgia, gout
NORMAL DOSAGE: 500 mg qd for 2 months
AUXILIARY LABEL:
- Take as directed.

TECH ALERT!

Remember the following sound-alike/look-alike drugs:

Diphenhydramine versus dicyclomine or dimenhydrinate

Hydrocodone versus hydrocortisone

Epinephrine versus ephedrine

Alupent versus Atrovent

Albuterol versus atenolol

TABLE 18-3 Examples of Tuberculosis Regimens

Trade name	Generic name	Adult dosing	Comment
Regimen 1			Common regimes last 6 or 9 months in duration.
Laniazid	isoniazid	5 mg/kg/day	
Rifadin	rifampin	10 mg/kg/day	
Regimen 2			Streptomycin may be added to treatment if necessary although it is only available in injectable form
Laniazid	isoniazid	5 mg/kg/day	
Myambutol	ethambutol	15 mg-25 mg/kg/day	
Streptomycin	streptomycin	500 mg to 1 gm	Administered intramuscularly 3 times a week for the first 3 months. Given in severe cases of TB
Regimen 3			With four-medication regimen alternate combination drugs may be used to replace 2 (long-term) to 3 (short-term) of the drugs listed
Laniazid	isoniazid	5 mg/kg/day	
Myambutol	ethambutol	15 mg-25 mg/kg/day	
Pyrazinamide	pyrazinamide	20 mg-35 mg/kg/day	Dose can be taken four times daily if needed
Rifadin	rifampin	10 mg/kg/day	
Regimen 4			Rifapentine must be taken along with another TB agent such as ethambutol, isoniazid, pyrazinamide or streptomycin
Priftin	rifapentine	150 mg twice weekly for 2 months followed by once weekly for 4 months	Taken no less than 72 hours apart for the first two months
Combination/ Replacement drugs			Combination drugs help with compliance with long-term therapy. Each has its own specific time-frame of use as indicated
Mycobutin	rifabutin	300 mg capsule daily or 150 mg twice daily	Alternative drug to replace rifampin. Used for patients with HIV that are taking specific antiretroviral agents
Rifamate	isoniazid/ rifampin	2 capsules once daily	Not for initial therapy, may be taken for the additional 4 months after initial 2 months of isoniazid, pyrazinamide and rifampin
Rifater	isoniazid/ pyrazinamide/ rifampin	1 tablet daily	For first 2 months of initial therapy. Must be followed by additional 4 months of treatment with isoniazid and rifampin

DO YOU REMEMBER THESE KEY POINTS?

- The main functions of the respiratory system
- The major organs of the respiratory system
- Common upper respiratory conditions
- Common lower respiratory conditions
- Medications used to treat respiratory conditions
- Main side effects of the drugs discussed in this chapter
- Major auxiliary labels that should be affixed to the container
- Differences between emphysema, bronchitis, and asthma
- Special instructions given for patients who are taking antituberculin agents
- Types of contributing factors that can influence respiratory conditions

MULTIPLE CHOICE QUESTIONS

1. Which of the following statements is not true?
   A. Respiration is an involuntary response.
   B. Expiration is an active response.
   C. The diaphragm flattens while the intercostal muscles contract, increasing the thoracic cavity and allowing for inspiration.
   D. Two phases describe respiration: expiration and inspiration.

2. The act of gas exchange within the lungs takes place specifically in the _____.
   A. Brainstem   C. Medulla
   B. Brain   D. Alveoli

3. The main function(s) of the cilia within the upper respiratory tract is(are) _____.
   A. To smell   C. To warm and moisten air molecules
   B. To catch foreign material   D. Both A and C

4. The normal exhalation of air in an adult is _____.
   A. 0.25 L   C. 1 L
   B. 0.5 L   D. More than 5 L

5. Which of the following symptoms are not common in a typical cold?
   A. Laryngitis   C. Wheezing
   B. Congestion   D. Coughing

6. Pneumonia can be described as _____.
   A. Viral or bacterial in origin
   B. An upper respiratory tract infection
   C. Contagious
   D. Both A and C

7. A patient diagnosed with asthma might receive which of the following drugs as a prophylaxis?
   A. Narcotic antitussive
   B. Bronchodilator
   C. Xanthines
   D. Leukotriene receptor antagonist

8. Persons who smoke are more likely to suffer from _____.
   A. Bronchitis and emphysema
   B. Emphysema and asthma
   C. Bronchitis and asthma
   D. All of the above

9. Tuberculosis is on the rise mostly because of _____.
   A. Noncompliance with drug regimen
   B. Lack of money to buy medication
   C. Living in close quarters
   D. Both A and C

10. The function of gas exchange includes all of the following except _____.
   A. Balancing the pH of the body
   B. Oxygenation of the bloodstream
   C. Discarding unused carbon dioxide
   D. Exchanging nitrogen for carbon dioxide

TRUE/FALSE **If the statement is false, then change it to make it true.**

_____ **1.** The highest percentage of gas in the air that we breathe is oxygen.

_____ **2.** The larynx also is known as the voice box.

_____ **3.** Colds can be caused by viruses, bacteria, or both.

_____ **4.** Influenza only strikes older adults.

_____ **5.** Allergies are caused by genetic traits.

_____ **6.** The main function of the epiglottis is to protect the vocal cords.

_____ **7.** Persons who smoke are not any more at risk of getting chronic obstructive pulmonary disease than nonsmokers.

_____ **8.** The overall effect of bronchodilators is vasodilation.

_____ **9.** Tuberculosis is caused by a bacterium and is not contagious.

_____ **10.** Asthma is caused by rupture of the alveolar sacs.

TECHNICIAN'S CORNER A 37-lb 4-year-old was admitted into the hospital, and the doctor wants the pharmacy to calculate enough doses of metaproterenol to medicate the child for a 3-day hospital stay based on the recommended dose. If the recommended dose is 1.3 to 2.6 mg/kg per day and you have metaproterenol sulfate syrup 10 mg/5 mL in stock, how many milliliters will you need to fill the dose for 1 day? How much for the whole course of treatment?

BIBLIOGRAPHY

Asperheim MK: *Introduction to pharmacology,* ed 10, St. Louis., 2005, Saunders.
Clayton BD, Stock YN: *Basic pharmacology for nurses,* ed 14, St Louis, 2006, Mosby.
Drug facts and comparisons, ed 60, St Louis, 2005, Wolters Kluwer.
Grollman S: *The human body: its structure and physiology,* New York, 1965, Collier-Macmillan Limited.

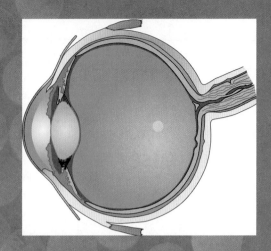

Visual and Auditory Systems

Objectives

UPON COMPLETING THIS CHAPTER, YOU SHOULD BE ABLE TO DO THE FOLLOWING:

- List both trade and generic drug names covered in this chapter.
- Describe the functions of the eyes and ears.
- List the major components of the eyes and ears.
- Explain the drug action of the medications listed.
- Describe what causes glaucoma.
- Describe the different types of conjunctivitis and their treatments.
- List the various infections that affect the eyes and ears.
- Explain how medications work to relieve glaucoma.

Accommodation *The change that occurs in the ocular lens when it focuses at various distances*

Aqueous humor *The fluid that is found in the anterior and posterior chambers of the eye*

Cataract *Loss of transparency of the lens of the eye*

Cones *Photoreceptors responsible for color (daylight vision)*

Cornea *The transparent tissue covering the anterior portion of the eye*

Miosis *Contraction of the pupil*

Mydriasis *Dilation of the pupil*

Myopia *Nearsightedness*

Ophthalmic *Pertaining to the eye*

Rods *Photoreceptors that respond to dim light and are responsible for black and white color (night vision)*

Acoustic nerve *The cranial nerve that controls the senses of hearing and equilibrium and eventually leads to the cerebellum and medulla*

Auditory canal *A 1-inch segment of tube that runs from the external ear to the middle ear*

Auditory ossicles *The set of three small bony structures in the ear: malleus, incus, and stapes*

Eustachian tube *A tubular structure within the middle ear that runs to the nasopharynx (throat)*

Labyrinth *A bony maze composed of the vestibule, cochlea, and semicircular canals of the inner ear*

Otic *Pertaining to the ear*

Tympanic membrane *A membranous skin that separates the external ear from the middle ear*

DRUGS USED FOR THE EYE

Trade Name	Generic Name	Pronunciation	Trade Name	Generic Name	Pronunciation
Anticholinergics			**Antiinflammatory**		
Cyclogyl	cyclopentolate	(sye-kloe-**pen**-toe-late)	Acular	ketorolac	(kee-toe-**role**-ak)
Isopto Atropine	atropine	(**a**-troe-peen)	Ocufen	flurbiprofen	(flure-**bi**-pro-fen)
Isopto Homatropine	homatropine	(hoe-**ma**-troe-peen)	Voltaren	diclofenac	(dye-**kloe**-fen-ak)
Isopto Hyoscine	scopolamine	(skoe-**poll**-a-meen)			
Mydriacyl	tropicamide	(troe-**pik**-a-mide)	**Antiinfectives**		
			Aminoglycosides		
Adrenergic Agonists			Genoptic	gentamicin	(jen-tah-**my**-sin)
OcuClear	oxymetazoline	(oxy-met-**tah**-zoe-leen)	Tobrex	tobramycin	(toe-bra-**my**-sin)
Propine	dipivefrin	(dye-**pihv**-eh-frin)			
Vasocon, Allerest	naphazoline	(naf-**az**-oh-leen)	***Antifungal***		
Visine	tetrahydrozoline	(tet-ra-hye-**droz**-oh-leen)	Natacyn	natamycin	(na-ta-**mi**-sin)

DRUGS USED FOR THE EYE—cont'd

Trade Name	Generic Name	Pronunciation	Trade Name	Generic Name	Pronunciation
Antivirals			**Cholinergics**		
Herplex	idoxuridine	(eye-docks-**yur**-eh-dean)	Eserine	physostigmine	(phi-zo-**stig**-meen)
Vira-A	vidarabine	(vi-**dar**-ah-bean)	Miochol-E	acetylcholine	(a-see-till-**kol**-leen)
Viroptic	trifluridine	(try-**floor**-eh-dean)	Miostat	carbachol	(**kar**-ba-kol)
			Pilocar, Ocusert	pilocarpine	(pye-low-**kar**-peen)
Macrolide					
Ilotycin	erythromycin	(eh-rith-roh-**my**-sin)	**Corticosteroids**		
			Betnesol	betamethasone	(beh-tah-**meth**-ah-sone)
Sulfonamide			Decadron	dexamethasone	(dex-ah-**meth**-ah-sone)
Bleph-10	sulfacetamide	(sull-fah-**see**-tah-mide)	FML	fluorometholone	(floor-oh-**meth**-oh-lone)
			Maxidex	dexamethasone	(dex-ah-**meth**-ah-sone)
β-Adrenergic Blocking Agents			Pred-Forte	prednisolone	(pred-**niss**-oh-lone)
Betagan	levobunolol	(lee-voe-**byoo**-noe-lol)			
Betaxon	levobetaxolol	(le-vo-be-**tax**-oh-lol)	**Prostaglandin Agonist**		
Betoptic	betaxolol	(be-**tax**-oh-lol)	Lumigan	bimatoprost	(bye-**mat**-oh-prost)
Ocupress	carteolol	(**car**-tee-oh-lol)	Travatan	travoprost	(**trav**-oh-prost)
OptiPranolol	metipranolol	(me-ti-**pran**-oh-lol)	Xalatan	latanoprost	(la-**tan**-oh-prost)
Timoptic	timolol	(**tye**-moe-lol)			
			Sympathomimetics		
Carbonic Anhydrase Inhibitors			Glaucon, Epifrin	epinephrine	(ep-i-**nef**-rin)
Azopt	brinzolamide	(brin-**zoh**-la-mide)	Propine	dipivefrin	(dye-**pihv**-eh-frin)
Neptazane	methazolamide	(meth-a-**zoe**-la-mide)			
Trusopt	dorzolamide	(dor-**zoe**-la-mide)			

DRUGS USED FOR THE EAR

Trade Name	Generic Name	Pronunciation	Trade Name	Generic Name	Pronunciation
Americaine	benzocaine	(**ben**-zoe-kane)	Otic Domeboro	acetic acid/aluminum acetate	(ah-**loom**-i-num sub-**ace**-ah-tate)
Cerumenex	triethanolamine polypeptide oleate-condensate	(tri-eth-ah-**noll**-am-in pol-e-**pep**-tide **oh**-lee-ate **kon**-den-sate)	Tridesilon	desonide, acetic acid	(**deh**-so-nide ah-**see**-tick **as**-id)
Chloromycetin Otic	chloramphenicol	(klor-am-**fen**-eye-chole)			
Cortisporin Otic	hydrocortisone/ neomycin/ polymyxin B	(hi-drow-**core**-tah-zone/ knee-oh-**my**-sin/ poll-ee-**mix**-in bee)			

W E RELY ON OUR SENSES from the moment we are born until we die. Although there are six main senses of the body system—sight, hearing, touch, smell, taste, and equilibrium—the two senses that can change a life the most dramatically are seeing and hearing. Every day from the moment we wake until the time we fall asleep, our senses are taking in new information, and our mind relies on the memories of sights and sounds. The ability to see enables us to navigate, whereas the ability to hear can prevent walking into an area where we might be harmed. The conditions that can affect the eyes and ears may not seem as important as other conditions; however, the

BOX 19-1   MAJOR STRUCTURES OF THE EYE

Structures	Eyebrows, eyelashes, orbit
Eyelid	Major structures such as the skin, muscle, connective tissue, and conjunctiva
Outer eye	Cornea, sclera
Middle eye	Ciliary body or muscle, iris, aqueous humor, pupil
Inner eye	Retina, optic disc
Chemicals	Rods, cones, rhodopsin
Glands	Lacrimal
Secretions	Vitreous humor, vitreous body
Nerves	Optic nerve
Muscles	Superior and inferior oblique; superior, inferior, medial, and lateral rectus

ramifications of neglecting these conditions can be earth-shattering. In this chapter, we cover the major components of the eyes and ears, as well as major conditions that can affect these two senses and their common treatments.

The Eyes

As one of the five main sensors of the body, the eyes link the outside world and the mind. As images are perceived, they are translated into impulses that create lasting memories in the mind. The three different levels or categories of persons who work in the field of eye care are opticians, optometrists, and ophthalmologists. Opticians are skilled in making lenses that compensate vision loss. Optometrists are trained to perform eye examinations. Ophthalmologists are medical doctors who treat major conditions affecting the eye, including performing surgery.

ANATOMY OF THE EYE

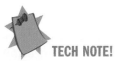

TECH NOTE!

When we cry, the lacrimal glands are activated directly by the parasympathetic nervous system.

The eye has several structures working in unison to help protect it, maintain its shape, and enhance vision. Box 19-1 lists the major structures of the eye that are defined in this chapter. The eyebrows shade the eyes from light. More than 2000 eyelashes work to catch debris, help keep the eyes moist, and help shade the eyes. The eye sits in a bony socket called the orbit. The position of the eyes allows for peripheral vision up to approximately 100 degrees. Covering the eyes are the eyelids, which are composed of four individual layers: the outer skin, the muscles, the connective tissue, and the conjunctiva. The muscles and the fibers of connective tissues are under the skin within the lid. They allow the eyelid to open and close. The natural reaction of blinking serves to protect the eye from foreign objects and allows lacrimal fluid to cleanse the eye. The conjunctiva is a thin, transparent layer that is composed of a mucous membrane that covers the anterior eye, the eyelids, and the sclera. The lacrimal gland is located within the orbit, secretes tears into the eye, and has ducts that lead into the nasal cavity. Tears contain an enzyme called lysozyme that has antimicrobial properties. An overview of the anatomy of the eye is shown in Figure 19-1.

The cornea is a bulged transparent cover that allows light into the eye for visual acuity. The cornea is composed of connective tissue and is covered in a thin coating of epithelium. The cornea does not contain blood vessels to provide nourishment; instead it is nourished by being bathed in a solution called the aqueous humor and from oxygen from the air. The aqueous humor is found within the anterior of the eye. Many nerve fibers within the cornea are sensitive to pain. The sclera is attached to the cornea but wraps around to the back

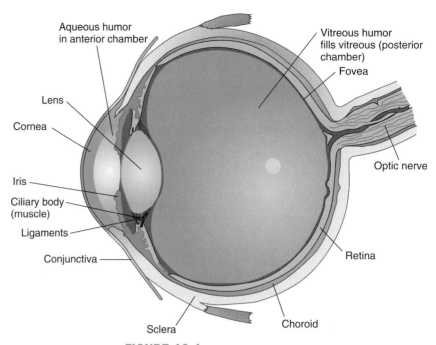

Aqueous humor in anterior chamber

Vitreous humor fills vitreous (posterior chamber)

Fovea

Lens

Cornea

Iris

Ciliary body (muscle)

Ligaments

Conjunctiva

Optic nerve

Retina

Sclera

Choroid

FIGURE 19-1 Anatomy of the eye.

of the eyeball. Unlike the cornea, however, it is not transparent. The sclera is the protective white portion of the eye, and it also contains many fibers and muscles. The optic nerve extends from the back of the eye through the sclera. The optic nerve sends images from the eye to the brain for interpretation.

The layer just inside the sclera is the choroid coat, followed by the inner-most layer, the fovea. The fovea is the area where the sharpest vision occurs. From the front of the eye the sclera joins with the iris and the ciliary body. The iris is responsible for the color of the eye. The iris filters light. The largest space of the eye is an area called the posterior cavity, which is surrounded by the lens, ciliary body, and retina. The ciliary body forms a ring around the front of the eye. The ciliary body is responsible for holding the lens in place. When certain fibers in the eye contract, the choroid coat is pulled forward, shortening the ciliary body. This in turn thickens the lens, allowing for up-close focusing. The area between the lens and the retina is filled with a jellylike substance called the vitreous humor. A function of the vitreous body is to hold the shape and form of the eye. The retina is a thin layer that contains layers of neurons, nerves, pigmented epithelium, and membranous tissues. Receptor cells (known as photoreceptors) of the retina are responsible for vision, and the neurons provide a path to the brain.

Six major muscles of the eye extend from the skeletal bone. These muscles are responsible for the movement of the eye. The direction of movements is shown in Figure 19-2. Other important muscles include those that close and open the eye and dilate and constrict pupils.

When focusing on a distant figure or in the dark, the pupil of the eye dilates (mydriasis), allowing more light in. When the eye is in extreme light, the pupil constricts (miosis). Through complicated connections, visual information is transferred to the nerve endings located at the back of the eye, which then send information to the brain, causing the necessary change in the lens to adjust to the incoming image, called accommodation. Aqueous humor is the watery fluid that plays an important function within the eye by keeping the eye moist so it maintains its shape. The aqueous humor provides the nutrients and oxygen to maintain the lens and cornea. As aqueous humor is formed, it must

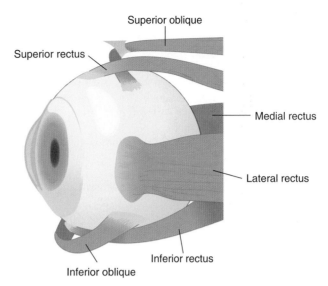

FIGURE 19-2 Eye muscles and direction of movement. Superior rectus rotates upward and inward; inferior rectus rotates downward and inward; medial rectus rotates inward; lateral rectus rotates outward; superior oblique rotates downward and outward; inferior oblique rotates upward and outward.

be released to maintain the pressure within the anterior chamber. Pressure is released by the built-in ducts called the canals of Schlemm. After the aqueous humor moves across the lens through the pupil and into the anterior chamber, it drains out of the eye through small openings located near the sclera and cornea. The retina contains the nerve endings that transmit electrical impulses to the brain. The retina also contains the components, rods and cones, that are responsible for color vision and for distinguishing the shapes of objects and darkness and light.

VISION

Each area of the eye has a specific function. As an image passes through the lens, it reaches the back of the eye, the retina. The rods and cones are located in the retina. Rods are responsible for sight in dim light and produce only an image in black and white. Cones detect color and can produce an image in bright light. As the rods and cones synapse (connect) with nerve endings, the signals are sent through the optic nerve to the brain. The occipital lobe is responsible for visual interpretation.

CONDITIONS THAT AFFECT THE EYE

A variety of conditions can affect the eye. Depending on the cause, treatment can range from medication to surgery. Over the past decade there have been many new developments made in corrective lens treatment. For conditions such as myopia, surgery is becoming an alternative to wearing glasses. For certain persons who are blind, a new surgical technique implants new lenses, allowing some individuals to see. As new techniques become available, many more eye conditions will be able to be treated and even cured. In this section, we cover commonly used medications for examinations and current treatments for the following common conditions of the eye:

- Glaucoma
- Conjunctivitis

BOX 19-2 TYPES OF GLAUCOMA*

Primary (Includes Angle-Closure or Open-Angle Conditions)
Acute congestive: Termed angle-closure, this refers to the closure of the anterior chamber, possibly resulting from genetic defects.

Chronic simple: Termed open-angle, this refers to the increase in intraocular pressure rather than a closed duct. About 90% of persons suffering from glaucoma have this type of condition.

Treatment: Correction by medication or surgery (laser).

Secondary
This condition may result from an existing eye condition or may happen following cataract extraction.

Treatment: Correction or control by medication.

Congenital
This condition exists because of genetic predisposition.

Treatment: Correction by surgery.

*See Table 19-1 for agents used to treat glaucoma.

- Congestion of the eye
- Viral infections
- Bacterial infections

Glaucoma

Glaucoma is a condition of the eye in which the pressure within the eye is higher than normal. This is referred to as increased intraocular pressure. Two main causes for this condition are overproduction of aqueous humor or blockage of the ducts that drain excess aqueous humor. Although glaucoma is easily treated, if left untreated, it can cause blindness. The three types or levels of glaucoma are listed in Box 19-2. Depending on the degree of severity, a wide range of medications and treatments are available.

Conjunctivitis

This condition is common in day care centers and is contagious. Also known as "pink eye," conjunctivitis is an acute inflammation of the conjunctiva. The cause can be viral, bacterial, or fungal infections or allergies. Major symptoms include inflammation, itching, burning, and a production of white mucus in the eye.

Color Blindness

As previously discussed, the cones are responsible for color perception. The cones produce three photopigments, each responsible for the identification of a different color: green, blue, and red. If a pigment is missing or abnormal, then detection of individual colors becomes difficult or impossible. This condition cannot be treated.

Blindness

Depending on the cause of blindness, new treatments are available that possibly can reverse the effects. For many persons, a corneal transplant may correct blindness. Another type of treatment for certain damaged corneal linings is stem cell transplant. This may reverse blindness through regeneration of a new membrane lining.

TABLE 19-1 **Commonly Used Agents for the Treatment of Glaucoma**

Classification of drug	Generic name	Trade name	Indication	Side effects
Beta-Adrenergic blocking agents	betaxolol	Betoptic	Open-angle glaucoma	Burning, stinging, eye irritation
	carteolol	Ocupress	Open-angle glaucoma	
	levobunolol	Betagan	Open-angle glaucoma	
	metipranolol	OptiPranolol	Open-angle glaucoma	
	timolol	Timoptic	Open-angle glaucoma	
Carbonic anhydrase inhibitors	dorzolamide methazolamide	Trusopt Neptazane	Lower IOP in open-angle or angle-closure glaucoma	
	brinzolamide dorzolamide	Azopt Trusopt	Lower IOP in open-angle or angle-closure glaucoma	
Miotics, intraocular	carbachol	Miostat	Open-angle or angle-closure glaucoma	Blurred vision, irritation, myopia, headache
	pilocarpine dipivefrin	Isopto-Carpine Propine	Glaucoma Elevated IOP	Burning, stinging, eye irritation
Sympathomimetics	epinephrine	Glaucon	Open-angle glaucoma	
	dipivefrin	Propine	Open-angle glaucoma	
Anticholinergics	atropine cyclopentolate homatropine	Isopto Atropine Cyclogyl Isopto Homatropine	Glaucoma Glaucoma Glaucoma	Stinging, increased IOP
	scopolamine tropicamide	Isopto Hyoscine Midriacyl	Glaucoma Glaucoma	
Prostaglandin agonist	latanoprost	Xalatan	Elevated IOP	

IOP, Intraocular pressure.

OPHTHALMIC AGENTS

Most ophthalmic medications are aimed at controlling glaucoma, controlling infection or inflammation, or manipulating dilation. For an overview of some of the more common agents used in treating the eyes for glaucoma, refer to Table 19-1.

Dosage forms used in treating the eyes include drops, suspensions, ointments, and in some cases, medicated disks or corrective lenses. Dosage forms and their method of action are discussed in the following section under each type of medication used in treatment.

Antiglaucoma Agents

Five classifications of drugs can be used topically to treat glaucoma: β-adrenergic blockers, carbonic anhydrase inhibitors, miotics, sympathomimetics, and prostaglandin agonists. The right diagnosis is important in order to prescribe the right medication because these drugs are specific in their actions. In many cases, more than one medication is used.

β-Adrenergic blockers

The β-adrenergic blockers are referred to as β-blockers. These medications lower the intraocular pressure in open-angle glaucoma. These medications are used topically as drops. Side effects of these ophthalmic drops are decreased vision after application and alteration of night or distance vision.

Drug action. These agents affect a specific site within the adrenergic system also known as the sympathetic system. The site they lock onto is the β-receptor. Because there are two different β sites available and it is not specified, it can be assumed that this medication will affect both β sites. When β sites are activated (agonistic effect), the response in many of the areas of the body is altered (see Chapter 17), including the constriction of the vessels in the eyes. This worsens glaucoma by increasing the intraocular pressure; therefore, if the β response can be blocked, then the vessels relax and the eyes can drain properly, decreasing the intraocular pressure.

β-ADRENERGIC BLOCKING AGENTS

GENERIC NAME: betaxolol
TRADE NAME: Betoptic, Betoptic S*
ROUTE OF ADMINISTRATION: ophthalmic
COMMON DOSAGE: one drop into eye(s) twice daily (1 gtt bid)
AUXILIARY LABEL:
■ For the eye.

GENERIC NAME: carteolol
TRADE NAME: Occupress
ROUTE OF ADMINISTRATION: ophthalmic
COMMON DOSAGE: 1 gtt bid
AUXILIARY LABEL:
■ For the eye.

GENERIC NAME: levobunolol
TRADE NAME: Betagan
ROUTE OF ADMINISTRATION: ophthalmic
COMMON DOSAGE: 1 gtt qd or bid into affected eye
AUXILIARY LABEL:
■ For the eye.

GENERIC NAME: metipranolol
TRADE NAME: OptiPranolol
ROUTE OF ADMINISTRATION: ophthalmic
COMMON DOSAGE: 1 gtt qd or bid into affected eye
AUXILIARY LABEL:
■ For the eye.

*If suspension is used, apply the label "Shake well before using."

GENERIC NAME: timolol
TRADE NAME: Timoptic, Timoptic XE
ROUTE OF ADMINISTRATION: ophthalmic
COMMON DOSAGE: 1 gtt qd or bid into affected eye
AUXILIARY LABEL:
- For the eye.

SPECIAL NOTE: Patient must be instructed to shake Timoptic XE once only before application. This is done by a pharmacist at the time of consultation.

Carbonic anhydrase inhibitors

Carbonic anhydrase inhibitors are medications used for open-angle glaucoma or preoperatively for procedures to treat angle-closure glaucoma. These medications sometimes are given along with other miotic and osmotic ophthalmic agents. Side effects include eye irritation, such as blurring, and a stinging sensation.

Drug action. These agents inhibit a specific enzyme, carbonic anhydrase, from increasing formation of the aqueous humor in the eye. By directly applying these medications to the eye, the intraocular pressure is reduced in persons suffering from chronic simple open-angle glaucoma. In persons suffering from secondary (angle-closure) glaucoma, carbonic anhydrase inhibitors can be used only for a short duration to lower the intraocular pressure in order to perform surgery.

CARBONIC ANHYDRASE INHIBITORS

GENERIC NAME: dorzolamide
TRADE NAME: Trusopt
ROUTE OF ADMINISTRATION: ophthalmic
COMMON DOSAGE: 1 gtt tid into affected eye
AUXILIARY LABEL:
- For the eye.

GENERIC NAME: brinzolamide
TRADE NAME: Azopt
ROUTE OF ADMINISTRATION: ophthalmic
COMMON DOSAGE: 1 gtt tid into affected eye
AUXILIARY LABELS:
- For the eye.
- Shake well before using.

GENERIC NAME: methazolamide
TRADE NAME: Neptazane
ROUTE OF ADMINISTRATION: oral
COMMON DOSAGE: 50 to 100 mg bid or tid
AUXILIARY LABEL:
- May cause drowsiness.

Miotics

Miotics are similar to carbonic anhydrase inhibitors regarding the types of glaucoma that they treat. Carbonic anhydrase inhibitors are used as a long-term treatment for open-angle glaucoma, whereas miotics are used only preoperatively for persons with angle-closure glaucoma. The side effects of these types of medications include headaches and decreased night vision.

Drug action. These medications reduce the intraocular pressure by increasing the outflow of aqueous humor from the eye. Within the classification of miotics are direct-acting agents and indirect-acting agents. Direct-acting agents lower the intraocular pressure by contracting the ciliary muscle around the eye, increasing the outflow of aqueous humor. Certain ophthalmic drugs are injectable and are used in eye surgery. Indirect agents inhibit an enzyme (cholinesterase) that brings about muscle contraction, reducing the resistance of the aqueous humor outflow. The result is the same in either case.

CHOLINERGICS—MIOTICS

GENERIC NAME: acetylcholine
TRADE NAME: Miochol-E
ROUTE OF ADMINISTRATION: ophthalmic
COMMON DOSAGE: 15 to 20 mg injection before or after suture is in place
SPECIAL NOTE: used for eye surgery

GENERIC NAME: carbachol
TRADE NAME: Miostat
ROUTE OF ADMINISTRATION: ophthalmic
COMMON DOSAGE: 1 to 2 gtt, max tid, into affected eye
AUXILIARY LABEL:
- For the eye.

GENERIC NAME: pilocarpine
TRADE NAME: Pilocar, Isopto-Carpine
ROUTE OF ADMINISTRATION: ophthalmic
COMMON DOSAGE: 1 to 2 gtt tid to qid into affected eye
AUXILIARY LABEL:
- For the eye.
SPECIAL NOTE: Pilocarpine has an ocular insert (Ocusert), which is a disk that is placed onto the eye to release the medication over 7 days.

GENERIC NAME: physostigmine
TRADE NAME: Eserine Sulfate
ROUTE OF ADMINISTRATION: ophthalmic
COMMON DOSAGE: Apply small amount (ointment) to inside of lower eyelid up to 3 times daily
AUXILIARY LABEL:
- For the eye.
SPECIAL NOTE: This medication must be prepared by reconstitution and is stable only 1 month if kept at room temperature. It is good for 6 months if refrigerated.

Sympathomimetics

The name *sympathomimetics* refers to mimicking or "acting like" the sympathetic system. The primary agent, phenylephrine, is used commonly along with miotics to treat glaucoma. Other uses include dilating the eye for examination and, in lower concentrations, as a decongestant for eye irritation. Most of the agents in this class are meant specifically for persons suffering from allergies and congestion in the eyes.

Drug action. When the sympathetic system is activated (among the changes in the body system), the vessels in the eyes contract, pupils dilate, and the ciliary muscle relaxes. The result is an increase in drainage and, with certain agents, a decrease in aqueous humor. These medications are used to treat open-angle glaucoma in addition to use of other antiglaucoma agents to reduce intraocular pressure. Common side effects include blurriness and, if overused, redness of the eyes.

SYMPATHOMIMETICS, OPHTHALMIC

GENERIC NAME: epinephrine
TRADE NAME: Glaucon, Epifrin
ROUTE OF ADMINISTRATION: ophthalmic
COMMON DOSAGE: 1 gtt qd or bid into affected eye
AUXILIARY LABEL:
■ For the eye.

GENERIC NAME: dipivefrin
TRADE NAME: Propine
ROUTE OF ADMINISTRATION: ophthalmic
COMMON DOSAGE: 1 gtt q12h into affected eye
AUXILIARY LABEL:
■ For the eye.

Prostaglandin agonist

Only one agent is indicated to treat glaucoma in this classification. The medication latanoprost is kept in the refrigerator, unlike other ophthalmic drugs. Latanoprost is used to treat open-angle glaucoma and can be used to decrease intraocular pressure in patients who have not responded to the other agents available. The side effects of this medication include a possible change in iris color (becomes darker).

Drug action. This medication reduces the intraocular pressure by increasing the outflow of the aqueous humor. Because this medication has not been used as long as the others discussed in this chapter, no long-term findings are available. The action of the drug is not clear. However, many unknown effects of this agent are yet to be discovered.

TECH ALERT!
Unopened Xalatan ophthalmic must be kept refrigerated. Once opened, it may be kept at room temperature for up to 1 month. Therefore, when you remove this medication from the refrigerator, you must write the date on the bottle of when it was removed.

GENERIC NAME: latanoprost
TRADE NAME: Xalatan
ROUTE OF ADMINISTRATION: ophthalmic
COMMON DOSAGE: 1 gtt qpm (once in the evening) into affected eye
AUXILIARY LABEL:
■ For the eye.

General information

Many combinations of ophthalmic medications are available by prescription. These combinations lessen the number of application times and agents that patients need. Keeping eye solutions sterile is imperative because foreign objects instilled into the eyes can cause damage or infection. Patients are counseled by the pharmacist to avoid touching the medication and contaminating it. In addition, most medications should not be instilled into the eyes while one is wearing contact lenses.

Antiinfective and Antiinflammatory Agents

The next classification of agents treats infections of the eye and other conditions that cause inflammation. A wide variety of conditions affect the eyes, such as bacterial, viral, and fungal infections and allergies. The course of treatment depends on identifying the microbe that has caused the infection. Box 19-3 lists the two types of drugs used to treat these conditions.

Antiinflammatory agents

Most of the agents used to decrease inflammation are solutions or suspensions. Suspensions need to be shaken well before use. Side effects include mild burning and/or stinging on instillation.

BOX 19-3 MAIN TREATMENTS FOR INFLAMMATION AND INFECTION*

Antiinflammatory Agents
Nonsteroidal antiinflammatory drugs
Corticosteroids
Decongestants and antihistamines (listed in Table 19-2)

Antiinfective Agents
Sulfonamides
Aminoglycosides
Erythromycins
Antifungals
Antivirals

*Antiinflammatories and antiinfectives use different classes of drugs to treat the condition depending on its cause.

Nonsteroidal antiinflammatory drugs. *Drug action.* Nonsteroidal antiinflammatory drugs inhibit the enzyme cyclooxygenase, which is responsible for the synthesis (creation) of prostaglandins. Prostaglandins are related directly to the mechanisms that are responsible for inflammation and pain associated with it. These agents are available as an ophthalmic in solution only. Flurbiprofen and suprofen are indicated for intraoperative miosis. Diclofenac and ketorolac may be used to treat postoperative inflammation after cataract surgery. Ketorolac also relieves itching resulting from allergies.

ANTIINFLAMMATORY, NONSTEROIDAL ANTIINFLAMMATORY DRUGS

GENERIC NAME: flurbiprofen
TRADE NAME: Ocufen
ROUTE OF ADMINISTRATION: ophthalmic
COMMON DOSAGE: one drop into affected eye every 30 minutes beginning 2 hours before surgery
AUXILIARY LABELS:
- For the eye.
- Use as directed.

GENERIC NAME: suprofen
TRADE NAME: Profenal
ROUTE OF ADMINISTRATION: ophthalmic
COMMON DOSAGE: two drops into affected eye at 3, 2, and 1 hour before surgery
AUXILIARY LABELS:
- For the eye.
- Use as directed.

GENERIC NAME: diclofenac
TRADE NAME: Voltaren
ROUTE OF ADMINISTRATION: ophthalmic
COMMON DOSAGE: one or two drops into affected eye within 1 hour before surgery; after surgery, one drop into affected eye 4 times daily for 2 weeks
AUXILIARY LABELS:
- For the eye.
- Use as directed.

GENERIC NAME: ketorolac
TRADE NAME: Acular
ROUTE OF ADMINISTRATION: ophthalmic
COMMON DOSAGE: ocular itching, 1 gtt qid; after cataract surgery, 1 gtt qid × 2 weeks
AUXILIARY LABELS:
■ For the eye.
■ Use as directed.

Corticosteroids. The corticosteroids are potent agents used to relieve inflammation resulting from infection or injury. They commonly are used postoperatively to decrease swelling. These agents should not be used too long because they can influence the length of time it takes to heal. The dosage forms include solutions, suspensions, and ointments. Side effects may include burning, blurred vision, eye pain, or headaches.

Drug action. Steroids have many actions on the body system, including decreasing macrophage movement, kinin release, and other functions associated with swelling and pain. If they are used over a long period, they can decrease antibody production.

ANTIINFLAMMATORY, CORTICOSTEROIDS

GENERIC NAME: prednisolone
TRADE NAME: AK-Pred (solution), Pred Forte* (suspension)
ROUTE OF ADMINISTRATION: ophthalmic
COMMON DOSAGE: 1 to 2 gtt bid to qid into affected eye
AUXILIARY LABEL:
■ For the eye.

GENERIC NAME: dexamethasone
TRADE NAME: Decadron Phosphate (solution and ointment), Maxidex* (suspension)
ROUTE OF ADMINISTRATION: ophthalmic
COMMON DOSAGE: one to two drops into affected eye(s) hourly during the daytime
    and every 2 hours at night until inflammation decreases; then decrease as
    directed
AUXILIARY LABELS:
■ For the eye.
■ Use as directed.

Decongestants and antihistamines. Decongestants and antihistamines are used to combat allergies. Antihistamines inhibit the release of histamine that results in common symptoms of itching and inflammation. Decongestants are used to dry out mucous secretions caused by allergies and hay fever. Table 19-2 lists decongestants and combination drugs that contain decongestants and antihistamines. These are indicated for allergies resulting from pollen or other allergens.

Drug action. Decongestants act on the specific receptors that cause constriction of the mucous membrane, thus lessening congestion. The drug action for antihistamines involves blocking the histamine receptors. Mast cells are responsible for histamine release when an allergen or antigen invades the body. By inhibition of the histamine receptors, the effects of seasonal allergies and other allergens can be lessened.

---

*Shake well before using

TABLE 19-2 Ophthalmic Decongestants and Combinations*

Generic name	Trade name	Availability
naphazoline	VasoClear A	Over the counter
naphazoline	Naphcon Forte	Prescription
naphazoline (decongestant) with pheniramine (antihistamine)	Naphcon A	Over the counter
oxymetazoline	Visine L.R., OcuClear	Over the counter
phenylephrine	Neo-Synephrine	Over the counter
tetrahydrozoline	Visine	Over the counter
olopatadine	Patanol	Prescription

*Patients must read the package insert and follow manufacturer's recommended dosage. Dangerous side effects may occur if ophthalmic over-the-counter agents are used by patients with glaucoma.

Antiinfective Agents

Agents used for conjunctivitis. The severe inflammation and discomfort of conjunctivitis can be treated with many different antibiotics. The physician determines the medication depending on the cause of the infection. If the infection is viral, an agent such as vidarabine may be used. If the infection is fungal, natamycin may be prescribed. If the infection is bacterial, a wide variety of antibiotics can be used depending on the specific microbe. For many bacterial infections a wide-spectrum antibiotic, such as gentamicin or ciprofloxacin, may be used. Other popular ophthalmic drugs used to treat conjunctivitis and other infections of the eye are discussed in the following sections.

Sulfonamides. Sulfacetamide and sulfisoxazole are the two primary agents used to treat bacterial infections. Dosage forms include solutions, suspensions, and ointments. Side effects may include stinging of the eye on application. Sulfa-type preparations are also available in different strengths of combinations with antiinflammatories or decongestants such as the following:

- Sulfacetamide sodium and fluorometholone (antiinflammatory)
- Sulfacetamide sodium and phenylephrine (decongestant)
- Sulfacetamide sodium and prednisolone (antiinflammatory)

The actions of sulfonamides are bacteriostatic. Their range of microbes includes gram-negative and gram-positive organisms. Sulfonamides block the formation of folic acid required by microbes.

OPHTHALMIC SULFONAMIDES

GENERIC NAME: sulfacetamide sodium
TRADE NAME: Bleph-10 (solution, ointment)
ROUTE OF ADMINISTRATION: ophthalmic
COMMON DOSAGE: one to two drops into lower eyelid every 1 to 4 hours initially; for ointment, apply a thin ribbon to lower eyelid for the same dosing as the solution
AUXILIARY LABELS:
- For the eye.
- Use as directed.

WARNING: This medication should not be used if the solution darkens. Avoid contamination.

Aminoglycosides. Aminoglycosides are a potent group of medications. Because of their wide spectrum of activity, they also can be used for some microbial-resistant strains. Side effects and adverse effects include burning, stinging, and photosensitivity.

The drug action is the inhibition of bacterial protein synthesis. Aminoglycosides are bactericidal and are used to treat gram-negative and gram-positive microbes. Because these agents are extremely strong, the physician must determine the correct dosage based on the weight of the patient and the severity of the infection.

OPHTHALMIC AMINOGLYCOSIDES

GENERIC NAME: gentamicin
TRADE NAME: Genoptic (solution), Garamycin (ophthalmic ointment)
ROUTE OF ADMINISTRATION: ophthalmic
COMMON DOSAGE: solution—instill one to two drops every 2 to 4 hours; ointment—apply
$\frac{1}{2}$ inch every 3 to 4 hours, 2 to 3 times daily
AUXILIARY LABELS:
- For the eye.
- Use as directed.

GENERIC NAME: tobramycin
TRADE NAME: Tobrex (solution and ointment)
ROUTE OF ADMINISTRATION: ophthalmic
COMMON DOSAGE: Solution—instill one to two drops every 4 hours; ointment—apply 2 to
3 times daily
AUXILIARY LABELS:
- For the eye.
- Use as directed.

Erythromycin. The antiinfective erythromycin comes only in ointment form. Side effects may include stinging, burning, itching, and inflammation.

This agent is a bacteriostatic but can be bactericidal if used in high doses. Erythromycin is used to treat mostly gram-positive and some gram-negative microbes. Erythromycin is used most often to treat conjunctivitis. The ophthalmic ointment also is used as a prophylaxis in the eyes of newborns to prevent infection.

OPHTHALMIC MACROLIDE

GENERIC NAME: erythromycin
TRADE NAME: Ilotycin
ROUTE OF ADMINISTRATION: ophthalmic
COMMON DOSAGE: Instill $\frac{1}{2}$ inch 2 to 8 times daily, depending on the type and severity
of the eye infection
AUXILIARY LABEL:
- For the eye.

Antifungals

Specific fungal infections must be treated with agents that can attack the specific metabolism of the invading fungus. The primary agent, natamycin, is an aminoglycoside and a fungicidal agent. The only noted adverse effect is a possible sensitivity to the formulation. Safety has not been established in children and pregnant or lactating women.

Drug action. The specific method of action involves the antifungal binding to cell membrane of the fungus. When this occurs, the stability of the membrane is jeopardized, and the cell membrane breaks down, killing the fungus.

GENERIC NAME: natamycin
TRADE NAME: Natacyn (suspension)
ROUTE OF ADMINISTRATION: ophthalmic
COMMON DOSAGE: To treat fungal conjunctivitis, four to six applications are all that may be necessary.
AUXILIARY LABELS:
- For the eye.
- Shake well before using.

Antivirals

The three most common viral infections of the eye are herpes simplex, keratitis, and conjunctivitis. The aim of antivirals is to interrupt or alter synthesis (the making) of new virions at a specific step, thus rendering the virion inactive. Many of the viruses that affect the eyes are more common in persons with immunodeficiency, such as those diagnosed with acquired immunodeficiency syndrome. Side effects may be sensitivity to light, stinging, or mild burning sensation.

Drug action. The general method of action for these antiviral agents is at the point where the attacking virus is using the host's DNA to replicate. This results in a malformation of various components necessary for properly working virions. Therefore, all agents are viricidal because they kill the virus.

OPHTHALMIC ANTIVIRALS

GENERIC NAME: idoxuridine
TRADE NAME: Herplex
ROUTE OF ADMINISTRATION: ophthalmic
COMMON DOSAGE: initally, one drop into eye(s) every hour during the day and every 2 hours at night; may decrease over time as determined by physician
AUXILIARY LABELS:
- For the eye.
- Take as directed.

GENERIC NAME: vidarabine
TRADE NAME: Vira-A (ointment)
ROUTE OF ADMINISTRATION: ophthalmic
COMMON DOSAGE: apply thin ribbon of ointment to lower eyelid 5 times daily at 3-hour intervals
AUXILIARY LABELS:
- For the eye.
- Use as directed.

GENERIC NAME: trifluridine
TRADE NAME: Viroptic (solution)
ROUTE OF ADMINISTRATION: ophthalmic
COMMON DOSAGE: one drop into affected eye every 2 hours while awake for a maximum of 9 drops, then treatment may decrease to 1 drop every 4 hours while awake (for 7 days) for a maximum of 7 drops per day
AUXILIARY LABELS:
- For the eye.
- Use as directed.
- Must be refrigerated.

BOX 19-4 PROPER USE OF EYE DROPS

Basic steps for use of eye drops are as follows:

1. Wash hands first.
2. Tilt head backward or lie down and gaze upward.
3. Gently pull lower eyelid down and away from the eye to form a pouch.
4. Place dropper directly over the eye. Avoid contact of the dropper with the eye or any other surface such as fingers.
5. Look upward just before applying a drop.
6. After instilling the drop, look downward for several seconds.
7. Release the lid slowly and close eyes gently.
8. With eyes closed, apply gentle pressure with fingers to the inside corner of the eye 3 to 5 minutes (this stops drainage of solution from the eye).
9. Do not rub the eye or squeeze the eyelid, and try not to blink.
10. Do not rinse the dropper.
11. If more than one eye drop is being used, wait at least 5 minutes before administering the second agent.
12. If it is too difficult to instill eye drops as described, another method is to close the eye while lying down. Place the drops on the eyelid in the inner corner of the eye, and then open the eye so that the drops fall into the eye by gravity.
13. For ointments, follow steps 1 to 3 and then apply $1/4$ to $1/2$ inch of ointment with a sweeping motion inside the lower eyelid by squeezing the tube gently and slowly release the eyelid. Close the eye for 1 to 2 minutes and roll the eyeball in all directions. Remove any excess ointment from around the eye with a tissue. If using more than one kind of ointment, wait 10 minutes before applying the second.

TABLE 19-3 Artificial Tear Products

Trade name	Manufacturer	Ingredients
Tear Drop	Parmed	Polyvinyl alcohol, NaCl, EDTA, benzalkonium chloride
Artifical Tears	Various manufacturers	Polyvinyl alcohol, povidone, NaCl, chlorobutanol
Cellufresh	Allergan	Carboxymethylcellulose, NaCl, KCl, sodium lactate
ReFresh	Allergan	Polyvinyl alcohol, povidone, NaCl
Just Tears	Blairex	Benzalkonium chloride, EDTA, polyvinyl alcohol, NaCl
Murine	Ross	Polyvinyl alcohol, povidone, benzalkonium chloride, dextrose, EDTA, NaCl, sodium bicarbonate, sodium phosphate

EDTA, Ethylenediaminetetraacetic acid.

Miscellaneous ophthalmic agents

Agents such as artificial tears commonly are bought over the counter. They are used for the relief of dry eyes and irritation that may occur. Their ingredients include sodium chloride, buffers to adjust for pH, and other additives to prolong their effects. The only dosage form is a solution, but they are available in various strengths and in combination with various ingredients. Although each tear product has somewhat different ingredients, all contain sodium chloride and all are used for the same reasons. Box 19-4 gives application techniques used for instillation of ophthalmic solutions.

Artificial tear inserts are also available by prescription for dry eye syndrome or severe keratoconjunctivitis by physician recommendation. Table 19-3 lists some of the most common types of artificial tears.

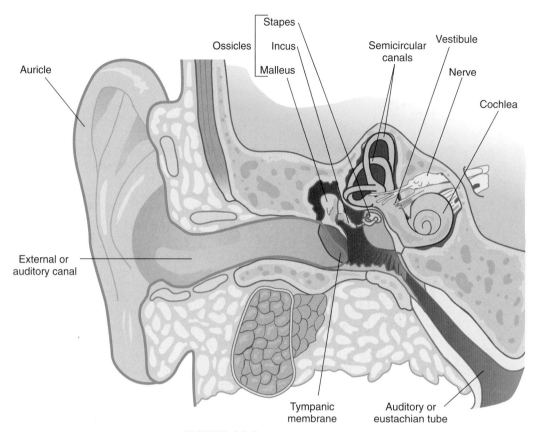

FIGURE 19-3 Anatomy of the ear.

The Ears

The human ear is not only responsible for hearing but also for balance, equilibrium, and many communication skills. The ear is composed of three major sections: the external, middle, and inner ear (Figure 19-3).

EXTERNAL EAR

Working from the outside in, we begin with the most exterior area of the ear, called the auricle. This area is composed of cartilage and skin and serves as an entrance for sound waves. The next section is the auditory canal. This canal, measuring approximately 1 inch long, leads to the tympanic membrane (eardrum) inside the ear. This membrane has two major functions:

- Protection of the middle ear from foreign objects
- Transmission of sounds to the middle ear

The transmission is possible because of the vibration caused when sound hits the membrane, much the same way a drum skin vibrates, carrying the sound when struck with a drumstick. Cerumen (a waxy substance) is produced by glands at the tympanic membrane.

MIDDLE EAR

Vibrations from the tympanic membrane are carried into the middle ear. This cavity (space) contains three small bony structures called auditory ossicles. These are as follows:

BOX 19-5 THREE MAIN AREAS OF THE INNER EAR AND THEIR FUNCTIONS

Cochlea
This area is coiled and composes three fluid-filled canals. Here the small, hairlike structures are connected to the nerve that runs to the brain. As the sound waves enter, the hairs bend and create impulses that are transmitted to the nerve.

Vestibule
The vestibule is located between the cochlea and membrane division and is responsible for equilibrium and balance. It does this by hair-type cells that are affected by gravity when moved. Nerves carry this information to the brain, specifically to the cerebellum and midbrain areas. Thus equilibrium is maintained. This gives human beings a sense of direction and orientation.

Semicircular Canal
Three semicircular canals are filled with a fluid that helps with the transfer of messages via the acoustic nerve. Small, hairlike fibers behave as sensors, moving back and forth as one moves forward, backward, or stops. The signals sent from two of these canals provide information to the brain about the orientation of the body when at rest, whereas the third canal sends information pertaining to the body when in motion.

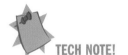

TECH NOTE!

When climbing altitudes in a car or plane, the eustachian tube relieves the decreased pressure from the outside by causing a pop of the ear. This brings equalization between the two pressure levels.

- Malleus (hammer)
- Incus (anvil)
- Stapes (stirrup)

These three small bones are connected to each other and pass on the sound waves that enter the cavity. Another area in the middle ear is the eustachian tube. This tube leads to the nasopharynx. When swallowing, yawning, or movement of the jaw occurs, the eustachian tube opens and relieves the change in pressure between the outside and inside atmosphere.

INNER EAR

After the transmission of sounds through the ossicles, the stapes (last bone) then continues the transfer of sound into the third section of the ear called the inner ear. This fluid-filled area is called the labyrinth and is composed of many components that process and transmit the audible sounds via nerve impulses to the brain where the sound then is interpreted. The two important areas or divisions of the labyrinth are the following:

Perilymph (bony labyrinth)	Composed of three main structures: cochlea, vestibule, and semicircular canal
Membrane division	Lines the bony division; areas include sacs and tubes that run throughout the inner ear and aid in sound wave transference

The three main structures within the bony division are in proximity to one another and have separate but important functions as described in Box 19-5 (Figure 19-4).

CONDITIONS AFFECTING THE EAR

Various conditions can affect the quality of hearing, including infections, ear wax accumulation, damage to the eardrum, and genetic defects. The following conditions are more common. The preparations that may be used to treat them follow.

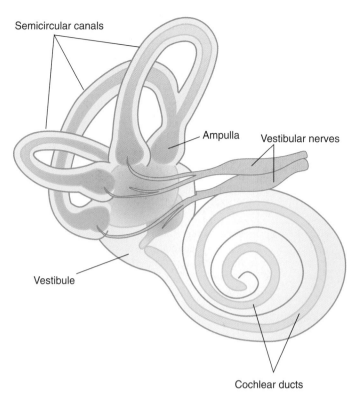

Semicircular canals

Ampulla

Vestibular nerves

Vestibule

Cochlear ducts

FIGURE 19-4 Anatomy of the inner ear.

Deafness

Deafness caused by factors other than genetic abnormalities include age and inflicted damage. A normal loss of hearing occurs as one ages, resulting from the effects of loud noises over the years. The small, hairlike structures in the middle ear can break with loud noise. Unfortunately, they do not regenerate, and over time a loss of hearing can occur. In the normal aging process the hairs become less able to bend, and transmission can be decreased. Although there is no medication that can increase hearing, there are hearing aids that can amplify sounds.

Otitis Media

Otitis media is an infection in the middle ear and often is associated with inflammation of the eustachian tube, which courses from the middle ear to the nasopharynx. The lining of the middle ear and nasopharynx are a single continuous membranous structure. This is why a sore throat can lead to a middle ear infection, as often is seen in children. Antiinfectives can treat the infection. However, many times because of recurring infections in children, pediatricians insert small tubes that allow drainage from the middle ear and eustachian tube, which lessens the occurrence of infections.

Cerumen Buildup

As mentioned previously, the glands at the tympanic membrane naturally build up a waxy substance referred to as cerumen. If excessive wax builds up or dries, it can impede hearing quality. It may be necessary for a doctor to remove this buildup to perform an examination or to improve hearing quality.

Ototoxicity

Certain medications can cause toxic levels within the lymph tissue of the ear that in turn may cause hearing damage (ototoxicity). This injury to the auditory

TABLE 19-4 Medications That Cause Ototoxicity

Class	Specific drugs
Aminoglycosides	gentamicin, tobramycin
Erythromycins	clarithromycin, erythromycin (macrolides)
Analgesics	aspirin, nonsteroidal antiinflammatory drugs
Loop diuretics	furosemide, bumetanide, ethacrynic acid
Antineoplastics	cisplatin
Antimalarials	quinine

TABLE 19-5 Ear Preparations*

Generic name	Trade name	Availability	Indication
acetic acid	Domeboro	Over the counter (OTC)	Used for external ear infections and prophylaxis of swimmer's ear
benzocaine, benzethonium chloride, glycerin, PEG 300	Americaine	OTC	Used for pain within the ear caused by swimmer's ear and infections
carbamide peroxide, glycerin, propylene glycol, sodium stannate	Debrox	OTC	Used to remove ear wax
chloramphenicol	Chloromycetin Otic	Prescription (Rx)	Used to treat ear infections caused by gram-negative and gram-positive microbes
desonide, acetic acid	Tridesilon	Rx	Used to treat ear infections of the external canal
triethanolamine polypeptide oleate-condensate	Cerumenex	OTC	Used to remove ear wax
hydrocortisone, neomycin, polymyxin	Cortisporin Otic	Rx	Used to treat superficial bacterial infections of the external auditory canal
isopropyl alcohol, anhydrous glycerin	Swim-Ear	OTC	Used for swimmer's ear

*Many of the otic preparations are combination drugs.

nerve may include a ringing or buzzing within the ears (tinnitus). This can progress to permanent ear damage if left untreated. Balance also may be affected. Specifically, aminoglycosides have been known to cause ear damage if given in high enough doses over a long period. This is specific only when parenteral drugs are administered. Drugs listed in Table 19-4 have been noted to have ototoxic side effects. Daily patient assessment is necessary when these drugs are used to avoid permanent damage yet effectively to fight off bacterial infections.

OTIC PREPARATIONS

Some of the conditions that affect the ears are infections. Most of these infections are bacterial. Depending on the type of infection affecting the ears, certain preparations are available that may be bactericidal or bacteriostatic. Bactericidal agents kill the bacteria (see Chapter 29), whereas bacteriostatic agents hold the bacteria in stasis or stop any continued growth. Drugs that cause stasis are used to assist the body in the battle against bacteria. Table 19-5 lists agents

TABLE 19-6 Major Ingredients in Otic Preparations

Agents	Classification	Indication
acetic acid	Antibacterial, antifungal	Infection
desonide	Steroid	Antiinflammatory
hydrocortisone	Steroid	Antiinflammatory
phenylephrine	Vasoconstrictor	Decongestant

BOX 19-6 PROPER USE OF EAR DROPS

1. Wash hands.
2. Avoid touching the dropper to any part of the ear or any other surface.
3. Hold container in hands to warm it up to room temperature.
4. If drops are in suspension, then shake well first before removing suspension.
5. For adults, hold the earlobe up and back; for children, hold the earlobe down and back.
6. Instill the prescribed number of drops directly into the ear; do not insert the dropper into the ear.
7. Keep the ear tilted for 2 minutes or plug ear with a soft cotton, whichever is recommended.

used on the ears and their indication. Almost all ear preparations contain several major ingredients. These include antibiotics, steroids, and other agents that help remove wax buildup. Table 19-6 gives the names of the additives and their active ingredient in some of the otic preparations.

All prescription agents used for the ear must be labeled with auxiliary labels "for the ear" and "external use only." Agents such as cerumenolytics should not be used by persons suffering from a perforated eardrum, swimmer's ear, or itching of the ear canal. As with all ear products, it is advisable to lie down on one side to allow the solution to enter into the ear canal. Box 19-6 lists application techniques used for instilling of otic solutions. Examples of common uses and dosages to treat various ear infections and/or inflammation are listed along with the indication.

STEROID AND ANTIBIOTIC COMBINATION

INDICATION: steroid and antibiotic
GENERIC NAME: neomycin/polymyxin B sulfate/hydrocortisone
TRADE NAME: Cortisporin
ROUTE OF ADMINISTRATION: otic
COMMON DOSAGE: three drops instilled 3 or 4 times daily
AUXILIARY LABEL:
- For the ear.

NOTE: This drug combination also is available in suspension. Use the additional auxiliary lable "Shake well before using."

MISCELLANEOUS OTIC PREPARATION

INDICATION: Anesthetic, analgesic
GENERIC NAME: antipyrine and benzocaine otic
TRADE NAME: Auralgan Otic

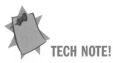

TECH NOTE!

Ophthalmic agents commonly are prescribed for ear treatment. This is acceptable because all ophthalmic preparations are sterile and can be used in the ear. However, otic preparations cannot be used in the eye because they are not sterile.

TECH ALERT!

Remember the following sound-alike/look-alike drugs:

Timoptic versus Viroptic
Tobrex versus TobraDex
Toradol versus Inderal, Torecan, tramadol, and Tegretol
Prednisone versus prednisolone
Carteolol versus carvedilol

ROUTE OF ADMINISTRATION: otic
COMMON DOSAGE: fill ear canal with two to four drops; insert saturated cotton pledget. Repeat 3 or 4 times daily, or up to once every 1 to 2 hours.
AUXILIARY LABEL:
- For the ear.

MISCELLANEOUS OTIC PREPARATIONS

INDICATION: antiinflammatory, antibacterial or antifungal
GENERIC NAME: ingredients—1% hydrocortisone, alcohol, propylene glycol, dermoprotective factor yerba santa, benzyl benzoate
TRADE NAME: EarSol-HC
ROUTE OF ADMINISTRATION: otic
COMMON DOSAGE: insert four to six drops into ear 3 to 4 times daily
AUXILIARY LABEL:
- For the ear.

MISCELLANEOUS OTIC PREPARATIONS

INDICATION: antifungal, antiinfective
GENERIC NAME: acetic acid 2% and aluminum acetate solution
TRADE NAME: Burow's solution
ROUTE OF ADMINISTRATION: otic
COMMON DOSAGE: four to six drops every 2 to 3 hours
AUXILIARY LABEL:
- For the ear.

DO YOU REMEMBER THESE KEY POINTS?

- Main structures of the eye
- The function of rods and cones
- Conditions that can affect the eye
- What glaucoma is and the medications used to treat it
- Agents used to treat infections of the eye
- Main structures of the ear
- The three bony structures that make up the labyrinth of the inner ear
- Conditions that affect the ear
- Why children suffering from colds and flu often get ear infections
- Ear preparations
- Which medications for eye and ear are available over the counter or by prescription
- What auxiliary labels are necessary for eye and ear medications
- Why ear drops cannot be used in the eye

MULTIPLE CHOICE QUESTIONS

1. The cornea is responsible for _____.
   A. The color of the eye
   B. Lubrication of the eye
   C. Protection of the eyeball
   D. Visual acuity

2. The substance that bathes the eye with nutrition is the _____.
   A. Conjunctiva
   B. Aqueous humor
   C. Sphincter
   D. Blood vessels

3. Glaucoma is a condition of the eye that results from _____.
   A. Narrowing of eye blood vessels
   B. A lack of aqueous humor
   C. Intraocular pressure
   D. Age

4. Glaucoma can be divided into three types; these are _____.
   A. Acute congestive, chronic simple, and congenital
   B. Primary, secondary, and congenital
   C. Angle-closure, open-angle, and chronic
   D. None of the above

5. Which of the medications that follow is not a β-adrenergic blocker?
   A. Blocadren
   B. Betoptic
   C. Betagan
   D. Trusopt

6. Miotics act by _____.
   A. Contraction of ciliary muscles, increasing outflow of aqueous humor
   B. Inhibition of β sites that then relax vessels allowing proper drainage of aqueous humor
   C. Inhibition of anhydrase, thus lessening the formation of aqueous humor
   D. The drug action is not clear

7. Of the various antiinfectives used to treat eye conditions, which works as a bacteriostatic at low doses and as a bactericidal at high doses?
   A. Aminoglycosides
   B. Sulfacetamide sodium
   C. Erythromycin
   D. Natacyn

8. The cavity of the middle ear contains all the following structures except _____.
   A. Cochlea
   B. Malleus
   C. Incus
   D. Stapes

9. The structure within the inner ear responsible for balance is the _____.
   A. Semicircular canal
   B. Vestibule
   C. Cochlea
   D. A and B

10. The following ingredients are used to treat inflammation of the ear except _____.
    A. Desonide
    B. Benzethonium chloride
    C. Phenylephrine
    D. Boric acid

TRUE/FALSE

If the statement is false, then change it to make it true.

_____ 1. The eye is located in an area called the socket.

_____ 2. The back of the eye is oxygen-rich through blood vessels.

_____ 3. The occipital lobe in the brain is responsible for interpretation of images.

_____ 4. Conjunctivitis is inflammation of the cornea.

_____ 5. Otic drugs may be prescribed to be used in the eye or ear.

_____ 6. The ossicles of the ear are located in the middle ear and are composed of four bones.

_____ 7. The eustachian tube connects the middle ear to the throat.

_____ 8. Debrox is an agent available over the counter for ear wax removal.

_____ 9. Otitis media is an infection or inflammation of the inner ear.

_____ 10. The tympanic membrane is a covering of the entrance of the middle ear.

TECHNICIAN'S CORNER Look up the following agents in *Drug Facts and Comparisons,* and list the following information on each one: Both generic and trade name, normal dosage, strength/s, indication, and auxiliary labels that each one would require.

Auralgan Otic
Blephamide
Neptazaine
Octicair
Timolol

BIBLIOGRAPHY

Drug facts and comparisons, ed 60, St Louis, 2005, Wolters Kluwer.
Edmunds M: *Introduction to clinical pharmacology,* ed 5, St Louis, 2005, Mosby.
Hitner N: *Basic pharmacology,* ed 4, New York, 1999, Glencoe.
McCuistion L, Gutierrez K: *Real world nursing survival guide: pharmacology,* Philadelphia, 2002, Saunders.
Salerno E: *Pharmacology for health professionals,* St Louis, 1999, Mosby.
Thibodeau GA, Patton KT: *Structure & function of the body,* ed 12, St Louis, 2004, Mosby.

Gastrointestinal System

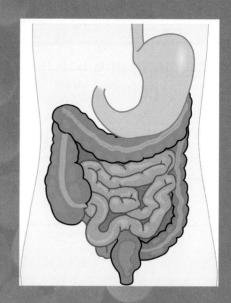

Objectives

UPON COMPLETING THIS CHAPTER, YOU SHOULD BE ABLE TO DO THE FOLLOWING:

- Identify the anatomy of the digestive system that is covered in this chapter.

- List the most common conditions affecting the digestive system.

- List both trade and generic names of drugs covered in this chapter.

- Explain the differences between stool softeners, laxatives, and bulk-forming laxatives.

- Describe the drug action of the medications covered in this chapter.

- Explain the types of treatments used for ulcers, including nonmedication treatments.

- Describe nonmedication treatments for ulcers.

- List common drug interactions between antacids and other medications.

- Distinguish between common ulcers and those caused by *Helicobacter pylori,* and explain why the treatments are different.

- Explain causes of diarrhea, constipation, flatulence, and emesis.

- List the different types of treatments for each of the conditions discussed.

Absorption *The taking in of nutrients from food and liquids*

Amino acids *Molecules that make up proteins*

Appendicitis *Inflammation of the appendix*

Carbohydrates *Chemical substances that include sugars, glycogen, starches, and cellulose with only a carbon, hydrogen, and oxygen makeup*

Chyme *The soupy consistency of food after mixing with stomach acids as it passes into the small intestines*

Constipation *Dry, hard stools that may be decreased in frequency*

Diarrhea *Frequent, watery, loose stools*

Digestion *The mechanical, chemical, and enzymatic action of breaking food into molecules that can be used in metabolism*

Emesis *Vomiting*

Excretion *Elimination of waste products through stools and urine*

Gastritis *Inflammation of the stomach lining*

Ingestion *The act of taking in food or liquid*

Peptic ulcer *An ulcerative condition of the lower esophagus, stomach, or duodenum, usually resulting from the bacterium Helicobacter pylori*

Peristalsis *The contraction and relaxation of the tubular muscles of the esophagus, stomach, and intestines that move food substances from the mouth to the anus*

Ulcer *A lesion on a mucous surface of the gastrointestinal tract*

GASTROINTESTINAL DRUGS

Trade name	Generic name	Pronunciation	Trade name	Generic name	Pronunciation
H₂ Antagonists			Dulcolax	bisacodyl	(by-saw-**co**-dill)
Axid	nizatidine	(nye-**zah**-tih-deen)	Glycerin	glycerin anhydrous	(**glis**-ir-in)
Pepcid	famotidine	(fa-**mo**-ta-deen)	Metamucil	psyllium	(**sill**-ee-um)
Tagamet	cimetidine	(sy-**met**-ta-deen)	Peri-Colace	casanthranol/docusate	(kah-**san**-thrah-nole/
Zantac	ranitidine	(ran-**nit**-ta-deen)			**dock**-you-sate)
			Senokot	senna	(**sen**-ah)
Proton Pump Inhibitors					
AcipHex	rabeprazole	(rah-**bep**-rah-zole)	**Antidiarrheals**		
Nexium	esomeprazole	(es-o-**mep**-rah-zole)	FiberCon	calcium polycarbophil	(**kal**-ce-uhm
Prevacid	lansoprazole	(lan-**sew**-prah-zole)			pol-ee-**kar**-bow-phyl)
Prilosec	omeprazole	(oh-**mep**-rah-zole)	Imodium	loperamide	(low-**pear**-ah-myde)
Protonix	pantoprazole	(pan-**tow**-prah-zole)	Kapectolin	kaolin/pectin	(**kay**-oh-lin/**peck**-tin)
			Lomotil	diphenoxylate/atropine	(die-fen-**ox**-i-late/
Anticonstipation Agents					**at**-row-peen)
Citrucel	methycellulose	(meth-ill-**cell**-you-lows)	Pepto-Bismol	bismuth subsalicylate	(**biz**-muth
Colace	docusate sodium	(**dock**-you-sate)			sub-suh-**li**-suh-late)

GASTROINTESTINAL DRUGS—cont'd

Trade name	Generic name	Pronunciation	Trade name	Generic name	Pronunciation
Antinausea Antiemetics			**Antiflatulence Agent**		
Antivert	meclizine	(**meck**-la-zeen)	Mylicon	simethicone	(sye-**meth**-i-cone)
Compazine	prochlorperazine	(pro-klor-**pear**-ah-zeen)	**Antiulcer Agent**		
Dramamine	dimenhydrinate	(die-men-**hi**-dra-nate)	Carafate	sucralfate	(soo-**kral**-fate)
Reglan	metoclopramide	(mea-toe-**clow**-prah-myde)			
Tigan	trimethobenzamide	(try-meth-oh-**ben**-za-mide)	**Over-the-Counter Treatments for Indigestion**		
Torecan	thiethylperazine	(thye-eth-ill-**per**-a-zeen)	Tums, Maalox,	calcium carbonate	(**kal**-see-um **kar**-bow-
Transderm-Scōp	scopolamine	(sko-**pole**-la-meen)	Mylanta		nate)
			Serotonin Receptor Antagonist		
Emetic			Zofran	ondansetron	(on-**dan**-see-tron)
Ipecac	Ipecac	(**ip**-eh-kak)			
Antispasmodic/Anticholergic					
Cystospaz	hyoscyamine	(hye-oh-**sigh**-a-meen)			

THE DIGESTIVE TRACT RUNS from the mouth to the end of the intestines and works to break down and absorb food and fluids. Foods are broken down from large items into small molecules that can be absorbed readily into the bloodstream and sent to areas of the body where they will be used for energy, synthesis of proteins, and enzymes for essential reactions. As food is broken down, nutrients are absorbed, and all nonessential food elements are excreted through the feces or urine. The common analogy used to describe the entire gastrointestinal system is as one long tube that runs through the body. This description is adequate for most of the functions that are covered in this chapter. However, a pharmacy technician should be aware of various important functions. These areas are covered more thoroughly as they pertain to medications. Many conditions that affect the gastrointestinal system (including digestion) are recognized immediately by the suffering patient, such as diarrhea. Many medications are available over the counter (OTC) to treat the symptoms of the digestive tract and the intestines. Because of the ease of self-treatment by purchasing OTC medications, many patients do not think it is necessary to ask their doctor or pharmacist about the possible interactions of these drugs and their legend (prescription) drugs. Many interactions need to be considered when filling new prescriptions for patients.

Form and Function of the Gastrointestinal System

The three main functions of the gastrointestinal system are digestion, absorption, and metabolism. Within the gastrointestinal tract, the various organs perform these functions 24 hours a day. The gastrointestinal system is controlled by the parasympathetic nervous system. The parasympathetic nervous system is the part of the nervous system that balances with the sympathetic system in controlling many of the functions of the body (see Chapter 17). When we are at rest, the parasympathetic nervous system is at work in body systems such as the gastrointestinal system. Each organ within the gastrointestinal tract completes a specific task. This chapter examines the gastrointestinal system from

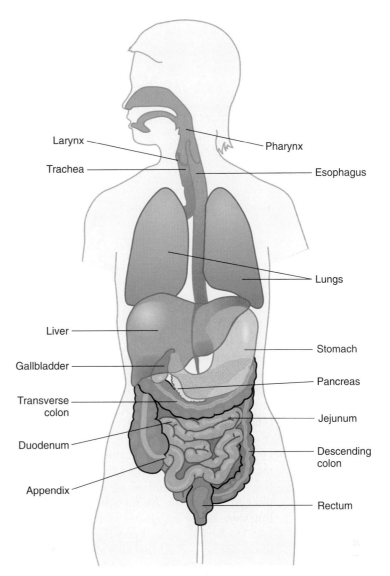

FIGURE 20-1 Anatomy of the gastrointestinal system (including mouth, pharynx, esophagus, stomach, and intestines).

the time food is ingested until it is expelled. This chapter also discusses additional organs, including the liver, pancreas, and gallbladder, that help the gastrointestinal tract complete its task.

ANATOMY OF THE GASTROINTESTINAL SYSTEM

The main organ one might think of when learning about the gastrointestinal system is the stomach, yet by the time food has arrived to this organ it has already begun its transformation from a solid food. Let's begin by looking at the overall system of the gastrointestinal tract (Figure 20-1). The organs discussed in this chapter, in sequence, are the mouth, salivary glands, pharynx, and esophagus (ingestion); followed by the stomach, small intestine, and large intestine (absorption); and finally the rectal area (excretion).

Ingestion

The mouth is the first apparatus of the human body where food is mixed manually. In addition to the action of the teeth chewing food into smaller pieces, sali-

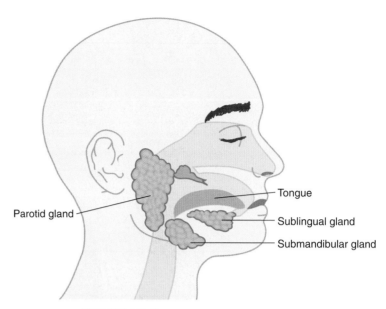

FIGURE 20-2 Major glands of the mouth.

vary glands begin to secrete an enzyme called amylase that initiates the chemical breakdown of food. The mouth has three pairs of salivary glands that are responsible for the beginning of food breakdown: sublingual, submandibular, and parotid. The sublingual and submandibular glands are located below the tongue and jaw, respectively. The parotid glands are just in front of the ear (Figure 20-2).

Another function of the saliva besides enzymatic breakdown of food is to moisten the esophagus so that food can be swallowed easily. With the help from the tongue, the food is swallowed and makes its way into the pharynx. The pharynx connects the mouth to the esophagus and contains the epiglottis. The function of the epiglottis is to close off the trachea so that food will not enter into the wrong tube. Food then makes its way to the stomach via peristalsis of the esophagus pushing and moving the food downward into the stomach. As the food arrives in the stomach, it enters into an acidic environment that will perform some of the chemical breakdown (Figure 20-3).

When activated by food, gastric juices are secreted in the stomach. The gastric juices are composed of intrinsic factor enzymes and hydrochloric acid, which has a pH of 2 in the stomach lumen. Thus the stomach contents are extremely acidic and would irritate your skin if you were to come into contact with them. To help balance this extremely acidic pH, the inner mucosal lining of the stomach is alkaline for protection. An additional protective mucosal lining prevents the acid from eating through the stomach wall. (Another function of the stomach muscles is to help with digestion by a churning action that mixes the food.) The extremely acidic environment kills bacteria that have been ingested and helps activate the enzymes that break down food. An important chemical produced, pepsinogen, becomes an active enzyme in the stomach called pepsin. When the churning and chemicals have broken down the solid substances into small bits, the acidic mixture left is referred to as *chyme*. The chyme then leaves the stomach and passes through the pyloric sphincter, the muscle that forms the division and opening into the small intestine. The pyloric sphincter must relax in order for the chyme to pass. This is a reflex action.

Absorption

Absorption of nutrients takes place from the food we eat. The vitamins and minerals move through the lining of the gut. Molecules of glucose, amino acids, and

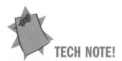

TECH NOTE!

Intrinsic factor is a chemical needed to absorb vitamin B$_{12}$. A person born without the ability to secrete intrinsic factor must take a supplement for his or her entire life.

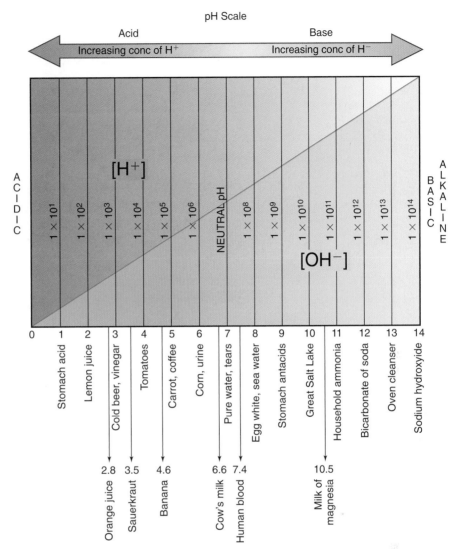

FIGURE 20-3 pH scale ranges from 1 (the most acidic) to 14 (the most basic). Normal human blood pH is about halfway between at 7.4 pH.

fatty acids begin to circulate into the body fluids. The blood becomes another avenue that nutrients must travel to reach their ultimate destination, the cells. Without the process of absorption, our cells would not be nourished and would die. The overall process is called metabolism. Nutrients are used for energy and as building blocks for larger complex chemicals. The act of building molecules is known as anabolism, whereas breaking down molecules to release energy is known as catabolism. Together they are known as metabolism (see Chapter 30).

The small intestine is about 6 m long and is responsible for the final steps in the digestion of food. The small intestine also begins to absorb nutrients and then sends the remains into the large intestine. The structure of the intestines works perfectly for what it must do—absorb nutrients from the foods we eat. To do this, it must be able to make contact with as much of the broken-down food as possible and for as long as possible. The intestine accomplishes this by being extremely long. Because there is limited space in a human body, it winds around, taking up much less space. In addition, the inside of the lining of the intestine is formed in such a way that it folds back and forth, again increasing the overall amount of surface area so that it has maximum exposure to the food (Figure 20-4).

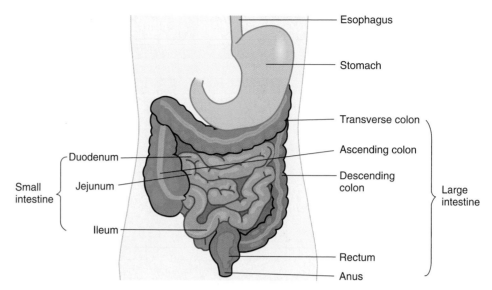

FIGURE 20-4 Intestinal tract (including duodenum, jejunum, and ileum).

TABLE 20-1 Foods and Enzymes That Digest Them

Food	Enzyme*
Proteins	Peptidase
Sugars	Maltase, sucrase, lactase
Fats	Lipase

*Words ending in -ase indicate that the substance is an enzyme.

The small intestine can be divided further into three sections: the duodenum, jejunum, and ileum. Each has its specific function and contribution to the breakdown and absorption of food. The duodenum is at the beginning of the small intestine and is about 25 cm long. The duodenum also is connected to the liver and pancreas from which it receives secretions that mix with the chyme from the stomach. The next section of intestine is the jejunum, which is much longer (about 2.5 m). The ileum is the last section, which measures about 3.5 m.

Within these three areas most of the food absorption takes place. Intestinal secretions have a more alkaline pH, allowing for better absorption of nutrients. Various enzymes continue to break down specific foods such as sugar, protein, and fat (Table 20-1). This enzymatic function of the stomach is important because it allows the intestines to absorb the nutrients and chemicals from the foods we eat into the body for metabolic processes. However, this acidic environment also destroys many medications that enter into the stomach, which is why several medications need special coating for protection or must be used in a different form, such as a parenteral preparation, so that they may bypass the stomach altogether.

The amount of secretions produced depends on how much food or chyme is present. In addition to the liver and pancreas, the gallbladder also helps in the digestion of food. The gallbladder releases the stored bile to help in the dispersion of fats.

Excretion

The large intestine follows the small intestine. Although the large intestine is much larger in circumference, it is not as long as the small intestine (only

1.5 m). The main sections of the large intestine include the cecum, colon, rectum, and anus. The colon takes up most of the length of the large intestine. Although absorption continues in the large intestine, it is limited to water and electrolytes. The substances moving through this portion of the intestine are not chyme but are transformed into solid fecal matter as water and electrolytes are absorbed into the bloodstream.

The rectum is the shortest section of the intestinal tract and connects to the anal canal. The rectum is usually empty except during defecation. The amount of time for normal passage of fecal material can range from 3 to 5 days. Within the anal canal, the sphincter is under involuntary control and is responsible for the urge to defecate. The external anal sphincter is voluntary, giving the person control of the bowels.

Auxiliary Organ Functions

The chemical contribution from the auxiliary organs (pancreas, liver, and gallbladder) is only one function of many that these organs have. All three organs have ducts that lead to the duodenum. In the duodenum the enzymes from the pancreas meet the contents from the stomach and actively break down various foods. Foods such as proteins, carbohydrates, and fats must be broken down from complex molecules into simple molecules. Proteins are large molecules that are broken down into peptides first by pepsin in the stomach and then by trypsin and chymotrypsin from the pancreas. Carbohydrates arrive in the stomach as large sugar molecules and are broken down into disaccharides, and in the duodenum they are broken down into monosaccharides and are absorbed and used for energy. Fats are not broken down much until they reach the duodenum, where they come into contact with bile produced by the liver and stored in the gallbladder. These long carbon chains of fat are more difficult to break down. They are first made water soluble by a process called emulsification and then are broken down further by enzymes called lipases.

The appendix, attached to the cecum of the large intestine, is a small worm-shaped lymphatic structure that has no apparent function within the digestive system. If the lining of the appendix becomes inflamed, appendicitis results, which requires removal of the appendix (appendectomy).

Conditions Affecting the Gastrointestinal System

Numerous conditions can affect the gastrointestinal system. These include commonly occurring and recurring conditions, such as heartburn, upset stomach, gastroesophageal reflux disease (GERD), gastritis, constipation, and occasionally diarrhea. More severe illnesses—such as Crohn's disease, ulcers, and others—can be caused by consistent stress, which can worsen these conditions of the gastrointestinal. Other gastrointestinal conditions can be caused by bacterial infections, food allergies, and tumors or may be caused by genetic defects, such as the lack of specific chemicals that are necessary for the proper function of this system. This section begins with a discussion of conditions of the mouth and then proceeds through the gastrointestinal tract. The drugs used to treat each specific condition follow the condition and the symptoms description.

MOUTH AND THROAT

The mouth is subject to many kinds of bacteria daily. The lack of good oral hygiene is the most common reason for conditions affecting the mouth. Ulcers or inflammation of the gums can occur within the mouth cavity, causing pain and discomfort. In addition, the condition of the teeth plays an important role in the initial breakdown of food. The throat may become inflamed because of

TABLE 20-2 Over-the-Counter Antacid Agents

Trade		Normal dose
Phillips' Milk of Magnesia	Magnesium hydroxide	5 to 15 mL qid
Alu-Cap	Aluminum hydroxide gel	1 cap tid prn
Tums	Calcium carbonate	1 to 2 tablets prn
Uro-Mag	Magnesium oxide	1 tid to qid
Combination Agents		
Gaviscon chewable tablets	Aluminum hydroxide, sodium bicarbonate	prn
Rolaids	Magnesium hydroxide, calcium carbonate	prn
Maalox Suspension	Aluminum hydroxide, magnesium hydroxide	prn
Titralac extra-strength tablets	Calcium carbonate, saccharin	prn
Mylanta Gelcaps	Calcium carbonate, magnesium carbonate	prn

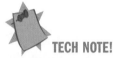

TECH NOTE!

The abbreviated term s/s means "swish and swallow" or can mean "swish and spit." This is a common order for a nystatin oral suspension used for ulcers of the mouth or throat.

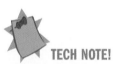

TECH NOTE!

The prescription counterparts of H₂ antagonists are usually twice the strength of their OTC counterparts. For instance, the OTC form of Zantac (ranitidine) is 75 mg. If you wanted the same drug in a 150-mg strength, it would require a prescription. Likewise, Tagamet (cimetidine) 100 mg is an OTC drug; the 300 mg strength is a legend drug. OTC remedies are not meant to treat ulcers or GERD but are for common heartburn.

colds or the flu or through straining the vocal cords. Symptoms of inflammation include sore throat and fever. Treatments for the mouth and throat include mouthwashes, sprays, lozenges, or troches. Many agents contain alcohol or phenol bases. These agents are antiseptics and are good at killing bacteria. Benzocaines, phenols, and menthol have anesthetic effects. Oral antibiotics may be swished and spit out or swallowed per doctor's orders.

STOMACH

The high acid content of stomach fluids causes a number of stomach conditions. These conditions are known more commonly as upset stomach, indigestion, or heartburn. Three main conditions affect the stomach: hyperacidity, GERD, and peptic ulcers resulting from the bacterium *Helicobacter pylori.*

Hyperacidity is the occurrence of excessive acid secretion within the stomach. Conditions caused by hyperacidity include peptic and duodenal ulcers. Hyperacidity can result from the overproduction of acidic secretions or the decrease of chemicals that help deactivate excessive acidic secretions between meals. Small areas within the stomach lining are eroded away, causing a sore that causes pain. GERD can occur when the cardiac sphincter (opening) at the top of the stomach relaxes. This allows acidic contents from the stomach to back up into the esophagus. This causes the burning sensation that most persons feel in their chest or throat. Antacids are the types of drugs normally used for both of these conditions (Table 20-2). These agents decrease the acid content of the stomach. Most remedies can be purchased OTC.

Many OTC medications contain simethicone along with antacids, because of the common occurrence of flatulence (gas) that accompanies gastric upsets (Table 20-3). Gas also can be a side effect of the carbonates that are major ingredients in antacids.

In addition to antacids, histamine₂ (H₂) antagonists are used to treat GERD and ulcers. Agents such as cimetidine and ranitidine block H₂ receptors located within the lining of the stomach. A third type of agent used for GERD is proton pump inhibitors. These agents inhibit gastric acid secretion within the stomach lining by blocking the last enzymatic reaction before acid secretion takes place.

TABLE 20-3 Over-the-Counter Antiflatulence Agents

Trade name	Generic name	Common dosage
Maalox extra-strength tablets	Aluminum hydroxide, magnesium hydroxide, simethicone	Usually taken after meals or as needed
Tempo tablets	Aluminum hydroxide, magnesium hydroxide, calcium carbonate, simethicone	Usually taken after meals or as needed
Mylanta liquid	Aluminum hydroxide, magnesium hydroxide, simethicone	Usually taken after meals or as needed

TABLE 20-4 Example of Anion and Cation Combination Drugs Used for the Relief of GERD or Indigestion

Ions	Combination agents	Trade name
Anions*		
Bicarbonate	Sodium bicarbonate	Alka-Seltzer
Carbonate	Calcium carbonate	Tums
Citrate	Sodium citrate	Citra pH
Cations		
Aluminum	Aluminum hydroxide	Alu-Cap
Magnesium	Magnesium hydroxide	Phillips' Milk of Magnesia

GERD, Gastroesophageal reflux disease.
*The anions listed normally are combined with one of the two listed cations.

This makes proton pump inhibitors effective; thus they usually are prescribed for more severe cases of GERD. Currently, all medications for the treatment of GERD are available by prescription only, although it may be just a matter of time before they too will get Food and Drug Administration (FDA) approval as an OTC drug.

Antacids Used to Treat Hyperacidity and GERD

Antacids include a variety of ion additives such as aluminum carbonate, sodium bicarbonate, calcium carbonate, magnesium hydroxide, and aluminum hydroxide. These ions each act in their own way to change the pH level in the stomach. Although aluminum and magnesium are metallic cations, they differ in their side effects. Aluminum tends to cause constipation, whereas magnesium causes diarrhea. Compounds containing cations act as buffers, decreasing acidity within the stomach. Side effects vary depending on the various concentrations of these compounds. Most antacids contain a combination of the previously mentioned ions, thus reducing the probability of side effects such as diarrhea or constipation. Table 20-4 gives an example of key anions used to alter pH. A common use of an OTC medication that does not contain magnesium is given next.

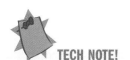

TECH NOTE!
Patients taking certain antibiotics such as tetracycline and ciprofloxacin should not take antacids containing magnesium or aluminum at the same time because they can decrease the absorption of the antibiotic.

GENERIC NAME: calcium carbonate
TRADE NAME: Tums, Maalox, Mylanta (all OTC)
ROUTE OF ADMINISTRATION: oral
INDICATION: for the relief of hyperacidity and GERD
DRUG ACTION: decreases acid secretions by binding to hydrogen ions
COMMON DOSAGE: as needed
SIDE EFFECTS: minimal to none

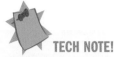

TECH NOTE!

Histamine₁ receptors are located in the lungs, and agents used to treat the effects caused by histamine resulting from allergies are called antihistamines, whereas H₂ receptors are located in the stomach, and agents used to treat the effects of histamine are called H₂ antagonists.

Histamine₂ antagonists. The prescription (Rx) strength is the higher-strength agent indicated next to the trade name and must be filled in the pharmacy. Although most of the prescription agents have normal dosages suggested by their manufacturer, many physicians allow patients to take cimetidine and ranitidine on an as-needed basis for indigestion.

Drug action. H₂ antagonists bind to H₂ receptor sites, lowering acid secretions. Common side effects of histamine antagonists include possible gastrointestinal upset and drowsiness.

H₂ RECEPTOR ANTAGONISTS

GENERIC NAME: cimetidine
TRADE NAME: Tagamet (Rx: 300 mg, 400 mg, 800 mg), Tagamet HB (OTC: 100 mg)
INDICATION: GERD, ulcer, duodenal ulcer prophylaxis (preventive therapy)
ROUTE OF ADMINISTRATION: oral, intravenous
COMMON DOSAGE: oral dosage Rx, 300 mg qid
AUXILIARY LABELS:
- Take with food.
- May cause drowsiness.

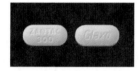

GENERIC NAME: ranitidine
TRADE NAME: Zantac (Rx: 150 mg), Zantac 75 (OTC: 75 mg)
INDICATION: GERD, ulcers, duodenal ulcer prophylaxis
ROUTE OF ADMINISTRATION: oral, intravenous
COMMON DOSAGE: 150 mg bid
AUXILIARY LABELS:
- Take with food.
- May cause drowsiness.

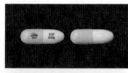
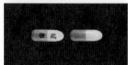

GENERIC NAME: nizatidine
TRADE NAME: Axid Pulvules (Rx: 150 mg, 300 mg), Axid AR (OTC: 75 mg)
INDICATION: GERD, duodenal ulcer
ROUTE OF ADMINISTRATION: oral
COMMON DOSAGE: 150 to 300 mg qhs (once daily at bedtime)
AUXILIARY LABEL:
- May cause dizziness and drowsiness.

GENERIC NAME: famotidine
TRADE NAME: Pepcid (Rx: 20 mg, 40 mg), Pepcid AC (OTC: 10 mg)
INDICATION: GERD, duodenal ulcer (OTC for heartburn and indigestion)
ROUTE OF ADMINISTRATION: oral, intravenous
COMMON DOSAGE: GERD, 20 mg bid up to 6 weeks
AUXILIARY LABELS:
- May cause dizziness and drowsiness.
SPECIAL NOTE: Suspension needs a "shake well" auxiliary label.

Proton pump inhibitors

Proton pump inhibitors have similar indications for use in the treatment of GERD, although at this time they are available only by prescription. All of these agents are available as a delayed-release form so that the patient is able to take them just once daily rather than having to take them at each meal. Drug action for all proton pump inhibitors is to block gastric acid secretions in the stomach.

PROTON PUMP INHIBITORS

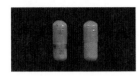

GENERIC NAME: omeprazole
TRADE NAME: Prilosec
INDICATION: peptic ulcer, *H. pylori,* duodenal ulcer; short-term use for esophagitis and GERD
ROUTE OF ADMINISTRATION: oral
COMMON DOSAGE: for GERD, 20 mg qd for 4 to 8 weeks
SIDE EFFECTS: diarrhea
AUXILIARY LABELS:

■ Take before meals.
■ Do not crush or chew capsule.

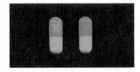

GENERIC NAME: lansoprazole
TRADE NAME: Prevacid
INDICATION: GERD, duodenal ulcer, gastric ulcer disease, erosive esophagitis
ROUTE OF ADMINISTRATION: oral
COMMON DOSAGE: for GERD, 15 mg qd for up to 8 weeks
AUXILIARY LABELS:

■ Take before meals.
■ Do not crush or chew capsules.
■ If capsule is opened and sprinkled onto food: do not chew or crush granules.

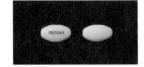

GENERIC NAME: pantoprazole
TRADE NAME: Protonix
INDICATION: GERD
ROUTE OF ADMINISTRATION: oral
COMMON DOSAGE: for GERD, 40 mg qd for 8 to 16 weeks
AUXILIARY LABEL:

■ Do not chew or crush tablet.

GENERIC NAME: esomeprazole magnesium
TRADE NAME: Nexium
INDICATION: GERD
ROUTE OF ADMINISTRATION: oral
COMMON DOSAGE: 20 to 40 mg qd
AUXILIARY LABELS:

■ Take 1 hour before meals.
■ Do not crush or chew tablet.

GENERIC NAME: rabeprazole sodium
TRADE NAME: AcipHex
INDICATION: GERD
ROUTE OF ADMINISTRATION: oral
COMMON DOSAGE: 20 mg qd
AUXILIARY LABELS:

■ Take before meals.
■ Do not crush, chew, or split tablet.

Peptic Ulcer Disease

H. pylori is a gram-negative bacillus. The bacterium can embed itself into the mucosal lining of the stomach, duodenum, and rectum. *H. pylori* is the cause of gastritis and peptic ulcers and is linked to cancer of the stomach. Six laboratory tests can be given to confirm the presence of *H. pylori*. They are listed in Table 20-5.

TABLE 20-5 Diagnostic Tests to Confirm *Helicobacter pylori*

Diagnostic tests	Uses
Blood test	Confirms bacteria by elevated levels of antibody to *H. pylori*
Breath test	Carbon-labeled urea is given to patient. On exhaling, a change in the urea to ammonia detects the presence of bacteria
Tissue biopsy	After obtaining biopsy, four different laboratory tests can be run to confirm *H. pylori*

TABLE 20-6 *Helicobacter pylori* Agents

Regimens	Length of treatment
Amoxicillin (500 mg qid), clarithromycin, omeprazole	1 to 2 weeks
Tetracycline (500 mg qid), metronidazole, bismuth, omeprazole	1 week
Metronidazole (250 mg qid), amoxicillin, bismuth	1 to 2 weeks
Clarithromycin (500 mg tid/qid), omeprazole, metronidazole	1 week
Bismuth (525 mg qid), tetracycline, metronidazole	1 week
Omeprazole (20 mg bid), clarithromycin, amoxicillin, or tetracycline	2 weeks

Medications to treat *H. pylori,* listed in Table 20-6, are the current treatments that have been approved by the FDA for eradication of *H. pylori.* Treatments consist of two, three, or four agents to be given simultaneously. The most effective combination is the four agents (bismuth, metronidazole, tetracycline, and omeprazole).

INTESTINAL CONDITIONS

Two of the most common symptoms affecting the intestinal tract are diarrhea and constipation. These can be caused by various infections of the gastrointestinal system. Infections by bacteria, viruses, and parasites typically result in symptoms of diarrhea. Tumors and other obstructions can cause constipation; although most cases of diarrhea or constipation are isolated symptoms that can be treated with OTC medications. In addition, medications are among one of the most common causes of diarrhea or constipation, and many physicians prescribe stool softeners along with routine medications to alleviate potential problems.

Table 20-7 outlines major illnesses of the upper and lower intestines. Patients who require a bowel resection, such as for the removal of a tumor, may be required to wear a colostomy bag. These bags are attached to the abdominal wall with adhesive strips and allow for the emptying of the intestinal contents. The site of the colostomy varies depending on where the resection has taken place. The location of the colostomy determines the necessary replacement medications that a patient needs to take routinely, such as laxatives or antidiarrheals. Because the intestinal tract is responsible for most of the nutrient absorption, if the colostomy site is close to the stomach, fewer nutrients can be absorbed through the intestine and must be provided to the patient. Other than having to empty the colostomy bag a few times during the day and changing the tubing twice weekly, a person can live a normal life with a colostomy.

Diarrhea

Treatment for diarrhea consists of agents that have an adsorbent and/or protectant quality. Activated attapulgite is used most commonly for its adsorbent

TABLE 20-7 Common Conditions Affecting the Gastrointestinal System

Condition	Definition	Symptoms	Treatment
Diverticular disease	Protrusions of the colon wall resulting from a weakened intestinal wall	Rectal bleeding, inflammation, and bowel obstruction	Surgery
Hemorrhoids	Lesions caused by enlargement and inflammation of veins in the rectum	Rectal bleeding, pain	Suppositories, creams, ointments
Crohn's disease	Congenital or acquired; chronic inflammation of the gastrointestinal tract Commonly occurs within the colon and terminal ileum	Abdominal pain, weight loss, diarrhea	Surgery or medications
Colitis	Congenital or acquired; inflammation of the intestines that commonly occurs in the large intestine	Rectal bleeding, pain	Surgery or medications

TABLE 20-8 Common Over-the-Counter Antidiarrheal Agents

Trade name	Ingredients	Common dosage
Kapectolin	90 g kaolin, 2 g pectin	1 dose following each loose stool
Parepectolin	600 mg attapulgite, sucrose	1 dose following each loose stool up to 7 doses/day
Donnagel	600 mg attapulgite, saccharin, sorbitol	1 dose following each loose stool up to 7 doses/day
Diasorb	750 mg attapulgite, sorbitol	dose following each loose stool up to 3 doses/day
Imodium AD	2 mg loperamide	2 doses stat, then 1 dose following each loose stool up to 4 doses/day

and protectant ability, whereas bismuth has an adsorbent quality along with an antacid effect. These medications can be bought as OTC drugs and are considered safe by the FDA. As with any condition, if the symptoms do not disappear within a few days, it is advisable to visit the doctor to see whether there is another underlying reason for the diarrhea. Diarrhea is also a common side effect caused by medications. Bacteria can be another cause for diarrhea and can be deadly. Symptoms include watery stools, abdominal cramping, and general discomfort. As diarrhea continues, vital fluids and electrolytes are lost through the intestines. If these fluids are not replaced and the diarrhea is brought under control, death can occur within days. Persons who are susceptible to this danger are older adults and children. Several agents, OTC and prescription, can treat this condition (Table 20-8). OTC drugs include Kaopectate, FiberCon, and Pepto-Bismol. More potent drugs or controlled substances require a prescription. Agents such as Lomotil (diphenoxylate/atropine) or paregoric are meant for short-term use because they can become less effective with continued use. In some cases, the lack of normal intestinal bacteria causes diarrhea. In this instance, a bacterial replacement therapy called *Lactobacillus* is used.

Medications Used to Treat Diarrhea
ANTIDIARRHEALS

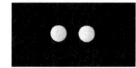

GENERIC NAME: diphenoxylate w/atropine Schedule CV
TRADE NAME: Lomotil
ROUTE OF ADMINISTRATION: oral
INDICATION: acute or chronic diarrhea
DRUG ACTION: slows intestinal motility
COMMON DOSAGE: 2.5 to 5 mg qid, then prn
SIDE EFFECTS: dry mouth, dizziness, drowsiness
AUXILIARY LABELS:
- May cause dizziness and drowsiness.
- Do not drink alcohol.
- Drink plenty of water.

GENERIC NAME: loperamide
TRADE NAME: Imodium (Rx), Imodium AD (OTC)
ROUTE OF ADMINISTRATION: oral
INDICATION: acute or chronic diarrhea
DRUG ACTION: slows gastrointestinal motility and increases viscosity of fecal matter
COMMON DOSAGE: 2 mg following each loose stool (maximum 16 mg/day x 2 days)
SIDE EFFECTS: dizziness, drowsiness, dry mouth
AUXILIARY LABELS:
- May cause dizziness and drowsiness.
- Do not drink alcohol.
- Drink plenty of water.

GENERIC NAME: bismuth subsalicylate
TRADE NAME: Pepto-Bismol (OTC)
ROUTE OF ADMINISTRATION: oral
INDICATION: diarrhea and abdominal cramps
DRUG ACTION: antisecretory and antibacterial effects in gastrointestinal tract
COMMON DOSAGE: two tablets or 30 mL (liquid) prn
SIDE EFFECTS: stools may appear grayish black
AUXILIARY LABELS:
- Drink plenty of water.
- May cause dark stools.
- Chew tablet before swallowing.

Constipation
The lack of defecation or stools that are dry and hard are the symptoms of constipation. This may be caused by a lack of fiber in the diet, a common problem in older adults. Various classes of drugs are used to treat this condition. Laxatives include bulk-forming types, stool softeners, hyperosmotic agents, and powerful stimulants. Bulk-forming agents work by absorbing water from the body to increase the moisture and overall bulk of the stools, allowing for easier elimination. Stool softeners pull water and fatty compounds into the intestine to aid in elimination.

Hyperosmotic agents work by osmosis, increasing pressure within the bowels by drawing in water, similar to bulk-forming agents. For more stubborn bouts of constipation, a stimulant may be used. These agents increase the peristalsis within the intestines (specifically the colon), which forces the contents

TABLE 20-9 Laxatives

Anticonstipation agents	Ingredients	Normal dosage	Route of administration
Over the Counter Laxative			
Phillips' Milk of Magnesia	Magnesium hydroxide	30-60 mL prn	PO (orally)
Sodium phosphates	Sodium phosphate, sodium biphosphate	20-30 mL prn	PO
Stimulants			
Ex-Lax	Senna	1 dose qhs	PO
Bulk-producing laxatives			
FiberCon	500 mg calcium	qd-qid (max 6 g/day)	PO
Enemas			
Fleet Laxative	Bisacodyl	1 dose qd	PR (per rectum)
Fleet mineral oil	Mineral oil	1 dose qd	PR
Prescription Laxative			
Cephulac	Lactulose	15-30 mL qd	PO
Bowel evacuant			
GoLYTELY	Polyethylene glycol, sodium sulfate, sodium bicarbinate, sodium chloride, potassium chloride	1 dose (4 L)	PO

out. Agents listed in Table 20-9 are examples of the many types of laxatives available. Bowel evacuants are used to empty the intestines before a procedure or surgery. Solutions that contain polyethylene glycol and electrolytes are loaded with replacement electrolytes because the intestines are not able to absorb the necessary ions from the expelled fecal material. Typically, the patient must drink approximately 4 L, or 4000 mL, of solution within a relatively short time. Other evacuants consist of a variety of laxatives to attain the same results.

Many gentle laxatives are available OTC, such as psyllium powder; however, there are some available OTC, such as Ex-Lax, that are powerful. Staying at home is recommended while one is taking these agents. Abdominal cramping is also a common occurrence from using more powerful laxatives. Persons who constantly take laxatives eventually may become dependent on them; therefore, it is recommended to take them only as a short-term treatment. Nondrug treatments suggested to avoid constipation include the ingestion of adequate dietary fibers, found in fruits and vegetables, in the daily diet. Roughage also aids in good digestion and elimination. In addition to a well-balanced meal plan, drinking plenty of water also helps prevent constipation.

Bulk-Forming Medications
BULK-FORMING LAXATIVES

GENERIC NAME: psyllium (OTC)
TRADE NAME: Metamucil
INDICATION: constipation

426 Section Two BODY SYSTEMS

ROUTE OF ADMINISTRATION: oral
DRUG ACTION: holds water within the intestine allowing stools to pass
COMMON DOSAGE: prn
SIDE EFFECTS: n/a
SPECIAL NOTES: Psyllium also is used to reduce cholesterol levels in persons with hyperlipidemia. All laxatives should be used only as short-term treatments for constipation.

SURFACTANT

GENERIC NAME: docusate sodium (OTC; also known as DSS)
TRADE NAME: Colace
INDICATION: constipation
ROUTE OF ADMINISTRATION: oral, rectal (enema)
DRUG ACTION: retains fat and water in bowels, allowing stools to pass
COMMON DOSAGE: orally, 50 to 500 mg qd
SIDE EFFECTS: n/a

GENERIC NAME: bisacodyl (OTC)
TRADE NAME: Dulcolax
INDICATION: constipation
ROUTE OF ADMINISTRATION: oral, rectal (suppository or enema)
DRUG ACTION: acts on increasing intestine mucosal lining and softens stools with water
COMMON DOSAGE: one rectally once daily as needed
SIDE EFFECTS: n/a

GENERIC NAME: senna (OTC)
TRADE NAME: Senokot
INDICATION: constipation (also used for constipation from opioid agents)
ROUTE OF ADMINISTRATION: oral
DRUG ACTION: irritates intestinal wall and causes osmotic gradient, softening stools
COMMON DOSAGE: 30 mg 1 to bid
SIDE EFFECTS: n/a

GENERIC NAME: glycerin (OTC)
TRADE NAME: Glycerin
INDICATION: constipation
ROUTE OF ADMINISTRATION: rectal
DRUG ACTION: irritates intestinal wall and causes osmotic gradient, softening stools; rectal lubricant
COMMON DOSAGE: one suppository rectally once daily as needed
SIDE EFFECTS: n/a

OTHER CONDITIONS

Emesis

Although most persons have experienced nausea and vomiting at one time or another, it is usually an isolated event. Persons who are subjected to chemotherapeutic agents as a part of cancer treatment must deal with extreme nausea and vomiting. The chemotherapy agents damage the lining of the stomach and other areas of the body, causing emesis as a common side effect. This violent reaction of the body is controlled from the medulla oblongata located within the brain. Known as the chemoreceptor trigger zone or nausea zone, this small area can be activated by smell, pain, medication, motion sickness (caused by relay from the inner ear), and even emotions. When the chemoreceptor trigger zone is activated, chemical signals are sent via the nervous system to the vomit center, which then relays the message down to the stomach where muscles of the diaphragm, stomach, esophagus, and the salivary glands working together cause the vomiting reflex. Drugs used to treat this condition are referred to as antiemetics.

Most antiemetics require a prescription because of their effects on the chemoreceptor trigger zone, which is located near the respiratory center of the brain. When this area is inhibited, it can cause a decrease in respiration. Agents that do not affect the chemoreceptor trigger zone can be bought OTC and usually are used for motion sickness. All of the following agents are available by prescription. For the following agents, only the normal adult oral dosages are given.

Antiemetic medications
ANTIEMETICS

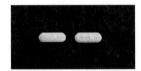

GENERIC NAME: metoclopramide
TRADE NAME: Reglan
INDICATION: for the relief of nausea and vomiting
ROUTE OF ADMINISTRATION: oral, intravenous
DRUG ACTION: blocks dopamine receptors in chemoreceptor trigger zone and increases gastrointestinal motility
COMMON DOSAGE: nonchemotherapy dosing, 10 mg before meals and at bedtime as needed
SIDE EFFECTS: diarrhea, drowsiness, restlessness
AUXILIARY LABELS:
- May cause dizziness and drowsiness.
- Alcohol may intensify this effect.

GENERIC NAME: thiethylperazine maleate
TRADE NAME: Torecan
INDICATION: for the relief of nausea and vomiting
ROUTE OF ADMINISTRATION: oral, intravenous
DRUG ACTION: inhibits chemoreceptor trigger zone and vomit center
COMMON DOSAGE: 10 mg qd to tid as needed
SIDE EFFECTS: dizziness, drowsiness, dry mouth, rash, fever, headache
AUXILIARY LABELS:
- May cause dizziness and drowsiness.
- Alcohol may intensify this effect.
- Drink plenty of water.

GENERIC NAME: trimethobenzamide
TRADE NAME: Tigan
INDICATION: for the relief of nausea and vomiting
ROUTE OF ADMINISTRATION: oral, rectal, intravenous
DRUG ACTION: depresses the chemoreceptor trigger zone
COMMON DOSAGE: 250 mg tid to qid
SIDE EFFECTS: dizziness, drowsiness, diarrhea, headache, blurred vision
AUXILIARY LABELS:
- May cause dizziness and drowsiness.
- Alcohol may intensify this effect.
- Drink plenty of water.

ANTICHOLINERGIC

GENERIC NAME: scopolamine
TRADE NAME: Transderm-scōp
INDICATION: for the relief of nausea and vomiting
ROUTE OF ADMINISTRATION: intramuscular, intravenous, subcutaneous, topical
DRUG ACTION: affects chemoreceptor trigger zone directly by blocking serotonin in brainstem and gastrointestinal tract
COMMON DOSAGE: apply one patch behind ear 4 hours before stimulation every 3 days
SIDE EFFECTS: dizziness, drowsiness, headache
AUXILIARY LABELS:

■ May cause dizziness and drowsiness.
■ Alcohol may intensify this effect.

SEROTONIN RECEPTOR ANTAGONIST

GENERIC NAME: ondansetron
TRADE NAME: Zofran
INDICATION: for the relief of nausea and vomiting, used with chemotherapy
ROUTE OF ADMINISTRATION: oral, injectable
DRUG ACTION: affects chemoreceptor trigger zone directly by blocking serotonin in brainstem and gastrointestinal tract
COMMON DOSAGE: 8 mg 30 minutes before chemotherapy treatment, then 8 mg 8 hours after dose followed by 8 mg every 12 hours for several days
SIDE EFFECTS: fever, headache, constipation, diarrhea
AUXILIARY LABELS:

■ Take as directed.
■ Do not drink alcohol.

ANTICHOLINERGICS

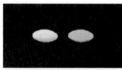
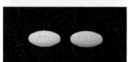

GENERIC NAME: meclizine
TRADE NAME: Antivert, Bonine*, Antivert/50
INDICATION: to relieve nausea and vomiting resulting from motion sickness
ROUTE OF ADMINISTRATION: oral
DRUG ACTION: affects the labyrinth within the inner ear, decreasing stimulation
COMMON DOSAGE: 12.5 to 25 mg 1 hour before exposure to stimulus
SIDE EFFECTS: dizziness, drowsiness, dry mouth
SPECIAL NOTE: Meclizine is also available in 25-mg and 50-mg tablets but requires a prescription.

GENERIC NAME: dimenhydrinate*
TRADE NAME: Dramamine
INDICATION: to relieve nausea and vomiting resulting from motion sickness
ROUTE OF ADMINISTRATION: oral, intramuscular, intravenous
DRUG ACTION: affects the labyrinth within the inner ear decreasing stimulation
COMMON DOSAGE: 50 to 100 mg q4-6h
SIDE EFFECTS: dizziness, drowsiness, dry mouth
*Over-the-counter

Flatulence

More commonly called gas, flatulence can be caused by the by-product of microbial breakdown of food (see Chapter 29). Also, certain foods are known to produce gas, such as broccoli, onions, and garlic. Symptoms are discomfort and pain within the abdominal cavity. The only OTC medication used for the treatment of gas is simethicone. This medication comes in tablets, chewable tablets, and liquid for children.

Antiflatulence medications
ANTIFLATULENT

GENERIC NAME: simethicone
TRADE NAME: Gas-X; Mylicon
INDICATION: for the relief of gas and abdominal distention caused by gas
ROUTE OF ADMINISTRATION: oral
COMMON DOSAGE: 40 to 80 mg up to qid as needed
SIDE EFFECTS: none

Poisoning

If a person should ingest poison accidentally or otherwise, drugs and treatments are available to prevent absorption and possible death. The type of chemical ingested determines what treatment to use. For the removal of a substance before it has been digested, ipecac syrup is sold OTC. Most parents have this medication to use in case their child ingests poison. This agent is made from the roots of the plant *Cephaelis ipecacuanha*. The chemical responsible for causing emesis (vomiting) is cephalenine. In other cases, activated charcoal may be used to absorb the toxins. Syrup of ipecac is derived from a Central American plant and has two active components, the alkaloids cephaline and emetine. Both of these components work locally in the stomach. Cephaline also acts in the area of the brain that triggers vomiting. The onset for vomiting is usually 15 to 30 minutes and can last 1 to 2 hours. Ipecac syrup can remove about one third of the stomach contents if given within the first hour after a substance in swallowed. In November 2003 the American Academy of Pediatrics determined that syrup of ipecac should not be kept in the home, noting that use of syrup of ipecac had not been associated with improvement in patient outcome. Additionally, in June 2003 the Nonprescription Drug Advisory Panel of the FDA recommended that ipecac syrup be removed from OTC status. This is only a recommendation at this time, not an official FDA action. This recommendation is due to studies that have shown that the outcome of a poisoning is not any better if ipecac is used in the home and that there is a high risk of misuse of this agent. Also, in many instances, vomiting is not recommended. If poisoning should occur, one must take the proper steps. This includes calling the poison prevention line (911), bringing the container of ingested substance to the hospital, and acting quickly. A common antidote used in emergency rooms is activated charcoal. This odorless and tasteless agent has the consistency of tar and can adsorb toxins in the stomach to prevent absorption. This medication is given in the emergency room and effectively works on overdoses of acetaminophen (Tylenol), aspirin, barbiturates, digitalis, triyclic antidepressants, and many more drugs.

EMETICS

GENERIC NAME: ipecac
TRADE NAME: Ipecac syrup
INDICATION: to cause emesis to remove poisons that are yet undigested
ROUTE OF ADMINISTRATION: oral
DRUG ACTION: targets the gastric mucosa and the chemoreceptor trigger zone to induce vomiting
COMMON DOSAGE: 30 mL once; may be repeated in 20 minutes if necessary (Each dose should be followed by one to two glasses of water [240 mL each].)

SIDE EFFECTS: Side effects of ipecac syrup may include drowsiness, diarrhea, and prolonged vomiting.

NOTE: Symptoms seen during chronic use, as in persons with eating disorders, include irritability, lowered body temperature, loss of fluids, chemical imbalances, muscle weakness, diarrhea, and *heart problems.* Deaths have been reported from the heart problems caused by chronic abuse. Ipecac syrup also can delay the administration and/or reduce the effectiveness of additional treatments such as activated charcoal.

TECH ALERT!

Remember these soundalike/look-alike drugs:

Hydroxyzine versus hydralazine

Prevacid versus Pravachol or Prinivil

Metoclopramide versus metolazone

Ranitidine versus amantadine

Zantac versus Zofran

General Information

Because the gastrointestinal system can be affected by outside forces—such as bacteria, viruses, parasites, medications, and emotions—this system is a complicated one. Numerous OTC remedies are available to consumers to treat a variety of symptoms. As the median age increases across America and around the world, the amount of routine medication that is taken to help deter illness is increasing. Imbalances that affect the gastrointestinal system can alter the amount of nutrients the body can absorb and the chain reaction that allows for the chemical breakdown of food. If this chain reaction breaks down, side effects may occur. By reducing stress, eating a well-balanced diet, and exercising, the gastrointestinal tract is better able to remain in good working condition. However, those who are diagnosed with a more severe condition have many medications and sometimes surgery available to treat their illness. If at all possible, it is important to take care of the gastrointestinal system before problems occur.

DO YOU REMEMBER THESE KEY POINTS?

- The major parts that make up the digestive system
- The pH of the stomach and its importance
- The function of the stomach and intestines
- The major conditions covered in this chapter that affect the gastrointestinal system
- The agents used to treat common conditions such as indigestion
- The ingredients used in antacids
- The generic names of the medications covered in this chapter
- The difference between GERD and *H. pylori* infection
- The treatment for *H. pylori* infection
- The difference between laxatives such as cathartics and stool softeners

MULTIPLE CHOICE QUESTIONS

1. The primary functions of the gastrointestinal system include all of the following except _____.

A. Digestion

B. Absorption

C. Secretion

D. Metabolism

E. All of the above are functions

2. Auxiliary organs to the gastrointestinal system include all those listed except
_____.

   A. Pancreas
   B. Liver
   C. Gallbladder
   D. Appendix
   E. All of the above are auxiliary organs

3. The function of the epiglottis is to _____.
   A. Break down food particles
   B. Digest food
   C. Block off the tracheal tube
   D. Aid in peristalsis

4. The pH of the stomach is acidic, and its function is to _____.
   A. Help in digestion by breaking down food into chyme
   B. Help move food through the intestines
   C. Help the absorption of food in the stomach
   D. Help in metabolism

5. The pyloric sphincter is located _____ and allows chyme to pass when
_____.

   A. At the top of the stomach; relaxed
   B. At the base of the stomach; tense
   C. At the opening of the small intestine; tense
   D. At the opening of the small intestine; relaxed

6. The duodenum, jejunum, and the ileum make up the _____.
   A. Stomach
   B. Small intestine
   C. Large intestine
   D. Adjacent organs to the gastrointestinal system

7. Bile is made by the _____ and stored by the _____.
   A. Gallbladder; liver   C. Pancreas; gallbladder
   B. Liver; gallbladder   D. Liver; pancreas

8. Excretion takes place mainly in the _____.
   A. Stomach   C. Large intestine
   B. Small intestine   D. Rectum

9. A person diagnosed with gastroesophageal reflux disease may be placed on which of
the following medications?
   A. Antacids
   B. H_2 antagonists
   C. Proton pump inhibitors
   D. All of the above

10. Ulcers that can be attributed to hyperacidity include all those listed except _____.
    A. Peptic
    B. Duodenal
    C. Gastroesophageal reflux disease
    D. *Helicobacter pylori*

TRUE/FALSE   If the statement is false, then change it to make it true.

_____ 1. Chyme is an acidic mixture of small food particles.

_____ 2. Anabolism is the breaking down of molecules, whereas catabolism is the
building of molecules; each represents a part of metabolism.

_____ 3. Proteins are broken into simple sugars by enzymatic actions.

_____ 4. Most antacids should be given twice daily, once in the morning and at bedtime.

_____ **5.** Simethicone is an antacid that is added to many stomach medications.

_____ **6.** H₂ receptors are located in the lungs.

_____ **7.** Carbonates are used to balance pH concentrations.

_____ **8.** The drug action for proton pump inhibitors is that they inhibit gastric secretions and block enzymes.

_____ **9.** Aluminum and magnesium can cause diarrhea as a side effect.

_____ **10.** *H. pylori* is a gram-positive microbe that infects the esophagus.

TECHNICIAN'S CORNER

A. A patient comes in to fill a prescription in your pharmacy. The prescription calls for codeine 30 mg. Take one to two tablets every 4 to 6 hours as needed for pain. The quantity indicates #100.

What over-the-counter medication probably was prescribed by the physician or will be suggested by the pharmacist at the time of consultation and why?

B. A patient who tested positive for *Helicobacter pylori* comes into the pharmacy and gives you a prescription for the following agents:

Clarithromycin
Omeprazole
Metronidazole

Question: What would be the recommended strengths and the dosing of these medications? Also give the length of time the medications should be taken, and how it is determined whether they should be stopped?

BIBLIOGRAPHY

Cincinnati Children's Hospital Medical Center: *Drug and Poison Information Center/DPIC: syrup of ipecac no longer recommended.* Retrieved 10-05 from www.cincinnatichildrens.org/svc/alpha/d/dpic/ipecac

Drug facts and comparisons, ed 60, St Louis, 2005, Wolters Kluwer.

Goodman G, Gillman L: *The pharmacological basis of therapeutics,* ed 11, Elmsford, NY, 2005, McGraw-Hill.

Koda-Kimble M et al: *Applied therapeutics: the clinical use of drugs,* ed 9, Philadelphia, 2004, Lippincott Williams & Wilkins.

McKenry LM, Salerno E: *Mosby's pharmacology in nursing,* ed 21, St Louis, 2001, Mosby.

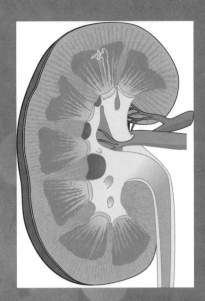

Urinary System

Objectives

UPON COMPLETING THIS CHAPTER, YOU SHOULD BE ABLE TO DO THE FOLLOWING:

- List both trade and generic names covered in this chapter.
- Describe the location and function of the kidneys.
- Explain the functions of the nephrons.
- Describe the location and function of the bladder.
- Differentiate between secretion and reabsorption.
- List the most common conditions that affect the urinary system.
- Describe the drug action of various diuretics discussed in this chapter.
- List the most commonly used diuretics.
- Describe dialysis treatments and the medications that are given with them.
- List the auxiliary labels necessary when filling diuretic prescriptions.
- List the major medications for dialysis.
- Describe the two common types of incontinence and what causes them.
- List the medications and explain the exercises to treat incontinence.

TERMS AND DEFINITIONS

Acidification *The conversion to an acidic environment*

Acidosis *The increase of acid content of the blood resulting from the accumulation of acid or loss of bicarbonate; the pH of blood is lowered*

Alkalosis *The increase of alkalinity of the blood resulting from the accumulation of alkali or reduction of acid content; the pH of blood is raised*

Blood urea nitrogen *A test that measures the nitrogen in the blood in the form of urea*

Congestive heart failure *Accumulation of blood in the circulatory system caused by the inability of the heart to pump efficiently*

Dialysis *The passage of a solute through a semipermeable membrane to remove toxic materials and to maintain fluid, electrolyte, and pH levels of the body system when the kidneys no longer work*

Diuretic *An agent that increases urine output and diuresis*

Dyspepsia *Heartburn, indigestion, epigastric discomfort*

Edema *A local or generalized condition in which body tissues retain an excessive amount of tissue fluid*

Electrolyte *Charged elements called cations (which have positive charges) and anions (which have negative charges)*

Excretion *Elimination of waste products through stools and urine*

Incontinence *Loss of control over excretion of urine or feces*

Micturition *Urination*

Nocturia *Having to urinate excessively at night*

Pyelonephritis *Inflammation of the kidney and renal pelvis*

Urea *The main nitrogenous constituent of urine and final product of protein metabolism; formed in the liver*

Urinary tract infection *Infection of the kidney, bladder, prostate gland, or the urethra*

Urolithiasis *Kidney stones*

COMMONLY USED DRUGS FOR THE URINARY SYSTEM

Trade name	Generic name	Pronunciation	Trade name	Generic name	Pronunciation
Thiazide and Similar Drugs			**Osmotic Diuretics**		
Diuril	chlorothiazide	(klor-oh-**thigh**-ah-zide)	Diamox	acetazolamide	(ah-see-ta-**zoe**-la-myde)
Hygroton	chlorthalidone	(klor-**thal**-ah-doan)	Osmitrol	mannitol	(**man**-ah-tol)
Lozol	indapamide	(in-**dap**-ah-myde)			
Esidrix	hydrochlorothiazide	(high-drow-klor-oh-**thigh**-ah-zide)	**Potassium-Sparing Diuretics**		
			Aldactone	spironolactone	(spear-own-oh-**lak**-tone)
Zaroxolyn	metolazone	(me-**toe**-lah-zone)	Aldactazide	spironolactone with hydrochlorothiazide	
Loop Diuretics			Dyrenium	triamterene	(try-**am**-tur-een)
Bumex	bumetanide	(byew-**met**-ah-nide)	Dyazide, Maxzide	triamterene with hydrochlorothiazide	
Demadex	torsemide	(**tore**-sea-myde)			
Lasix	furosemide	(feur-**oh**-sah-myde)	Midamor	amiloride	(ah-**mill**-or-ide)

Trade name	Generic name	Pronunciation	Trade name	Generic name	Pronunciation
Moduretic	amiloride with hydrochlorothiazide		**Analgesic Agents**		
			Urispas	flavoxate	(fla-**vox**-ate)
Replacement Supplements			Pyridium	phenazopyridine	(fen-az-o-**peer**-i-deen)
K-Dur, Slow-K, K-Lor	potassium chloride	(po-**tass**-ee-um **klor**-ide)	**Urinary Tract Infection Agents**		
			Cinobac	cinoxacin	(sin-**ox**-a-sin)
K-Lyte DS	potassium bicarbonate/ potassium citrate	(po-**tass**-ee-um bi-**kar**-bow-nate/po-**tass**-ee-um **sit**-rait)	Macrobid	nitrofurantoin	(nye-troe-fyoo-**ran**-toyn)
			Monurol	fosfomycin	(fos-fo-**my**-sin)
Feosol	ferrous sulfate	(fair-**us** sul-**fate**)	**Incontinence Agents**		
			Detrol	tolterodine	(tol-**tare**-oh-deen)
Dialysis Agents			Ditropan	oxybutynin	(ox-i-**byoo**-tin-nin)
Epogen, Procrit	epoetin alfa	(eh-**poh**-ee-tin **al**-fah)	Enablex	darifenacin	(dare-ih-**fen**-ah-sin)
			Sanctura	trospium chloride	(trose-**pee**-um)

WHEN THE BODY IS IN BALANCE (EQUILIBRIUM) throughout, this is known as homeostasis. The kidneys are one of two systems that help create and maintain homeostasis. The other system is the lungs (Chapter 18). Homeostasis includes the chemical compositions of the fluids and tissues within the body system. This chapter looks into the location and function of the various parts of the kidneys. This chapter also gives an overview of the conditions that can affect the urinary system along with the medications used to treat these conditions.

Anatomy

The kidneys are located inside the upper abdominal cavity on either side of the vertebra as shown in Figure 21-1. The right kidney is located a little lower than the left because the liver is located directly above it. A fibrous connective tissue called the renal fascia holds the kidneys stationary. The shape of the kidneys is similar to the shape of a kidney bean with a small indentation called the hilus. Blood enters the kidneys at the hilus via the renal artery and is filtered in the kidney. Important ions such as sodium and chloride are reabsorbed into the body and circulatory system. The renal vein and ureter leave the kidney at the hilus. The renal vein returns the blood to the body after it has undergone the filtering process. The ureter carries wastes removed from the blood to the bladder, where the waste is stored for excretion.

The bladder is similar to a holding tank that can expand. When the bladder becomes full, we feel the urge to urinate. The urine is eliminated through the urethra, which is a shorter tube leading from the bladder to the outside of the body (Figure 21-2).

Function of the Kidneys

The kidneys play an important role in our daily lives. All the food and drink that is consumed is metabolized by the liver and ultimately is carried to the kidneys, where filtration is carried out and important nutrients and chemicals are allowed to reenter the body system for cellular use. The remaining waste is eliminated in a process called excretion. Excretion is one of the four major important functions of the body:

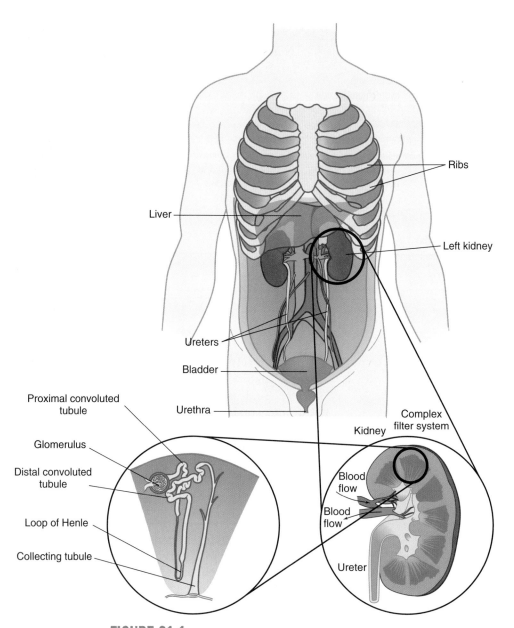

FIGURE 21-1 Anatomy of urinary tract and nephrons.

1. Absorption: the intake of liquids, solids, and gases into the body fluids and tissues
2. Distribution: the way in which chemicals or drug agents are separated throughout the body
3. Metabolism: how chemical changes and all transformations occur within the body system. Metabolism includes anabolism (building up processes) and catabolism (breaking down processes)
4. Excretion: The elimination of chemicals and substances from the body system

The bladder has walls that can expand to hold up to 1000 mL (1 L) of urine if necessary. The body excretes about 960 mL of urine per day. Urine contains urea, which is produced by the liver. Urea is a form of nitrogen that, on standing for a time, changes to ammonia. This gives urine its ammonia odor. The kidneys also have an important function: balancing the fluid content of the body.

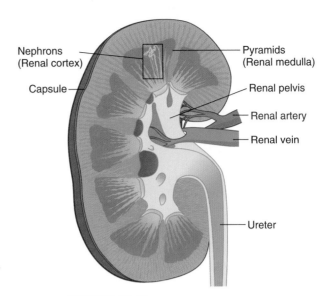

FIGURE 21-2 Anatomy of the kidney.

Most of the body is composed of fluids such as water, blood, and plasma and various ions such as chloride, potassium, and sodium. The kidneys balance ions within the blood and eliminate excess ions in the blood. When excess ions are present in the bloodstream, certain conditions such as acidosis or alkalosis can occur. Acidosis is when too many free hydrogen ions are present, and alkalosis occurs when too many hydroxide ions are present. The blood urea nitrogen test is used to determine the levels of acid in the patient's system. Patients who have kidney conditions or those who are taking medications that may weaken the effectiveness of the kidneys may have this test done. Although the kidneys are only about the size of a fist, they manage to filter about 50 gal of blood products every day. Plasma travels through an amazing 140 miles of tubules contained inside the kidneys.

NEPHRON FUNCTION

The portion of the kidneys that does the work of separation is the nephrons. Each kidney contains millions of microscopic nephrons (Figure 21-3). Each nephron is shaped like an inverted pyramid with many twists and turns of its tubules; the nephrons work 24 hours a day. The following is a step-by-step look into the filtering process by following the blood as it enters the kidney:

1. The renal artery containing blood enters the kidneys where it divides into smaller and smaller vessels until it becomes an afferent arteriole, which in turn enters Bowman's capsule and becomes capillaries. The capillaries are called a glomerulus. Bowman's capsule (which resembles a baseball glove) covers the glomerulus.
2. Blood cells, platelets, and large proteins are not allowed to pass through the capillaries of the glomerulus into Bowman's capsule. Only plasma can pass through the glomerulus. Plasma is composed of all the contents of blood other than the cells and platelets. However, some of the components of plasma are still too large to leave the capillaries, such as albumins and globulins. Other components of plasma include toxins that may build up in the blood. These are so small that they can leave the capillaries easily and enter Bowman's capsule.
3. The filtrate from Bowman's capsule travels down the descending tubule called the proximal convoluted tubule and back up the ascending tubule

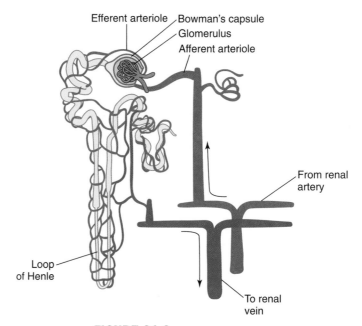

Efferent arteriole
Bowman's capsule
Glomerulus
Afferent arteriole
From renal artery
Loop of Henle
To renal vein

FIGURE 21-3 Nephron anatomy.

called the distal convoluted tubule. The U-turn part of the nephron is called the loop of Henle.

4. As the filtrate passes through the nephron tubules, various nutrients and important chemical ions such as chloride, potassium, and water are pulled out of the filtrate and returned to the plasma to be used for cellular nourishment. At the same time, other ions in the tubules (such as those in excess) are excreted.

5. The filtrate, now called urine, travels to the collecting ducts where it leaves the nephron.

6. The ducts empty directly into the ureter.

7. The ureter goes directly to the bladder.

8. The bladder empties the urine into the urethra and the urine travels out of the body.

Tubular Reabsorption

The first function of the nephrons is tubular reabsorption. This is a process in which important molecules are separated from the filtrate into their individual components. Some of these molecules eventually are excreted in urine, whereas others—such as glucose (sugar), water, sodium, chloride, and amino acids (proteins)—reenter the plasma. This takes place at various points in the proximal convoluted tubule, distal convoluted tubule, and in the loop of Henle (Figure 21-4).

The kidneys balance the acid-base content of the body. Two mechanisms affect the balance of ions. The first is ion exchange. Sodium ions are pulled out of the tubules and are exchanged for hydrogen ions. As sodium builds up on the outside of the proximal convoluted tubules, it creates an osmotic gradient, and water molecules are drawn toward the higher concentration of sodium. This is called osmosis (Figure 21-5). The overall effect is a decrease in excreted water. Ion exchange also can take place in the distal convoluted tubule. As sodium ions exit the nephron tubule, they are exchanged for potassium ions. The loop of Henle has a different mechanism. This mechanism is called active transport. Instead of an exchange of ions, there is a one-way uptake of sodium and chloride from the loop of Henle. These ions return to the circulatory system.

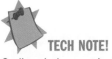

TECH NOTE!

Sodium helps conduct nerve impulses and balance fluid through reabsorption in the kidneys.

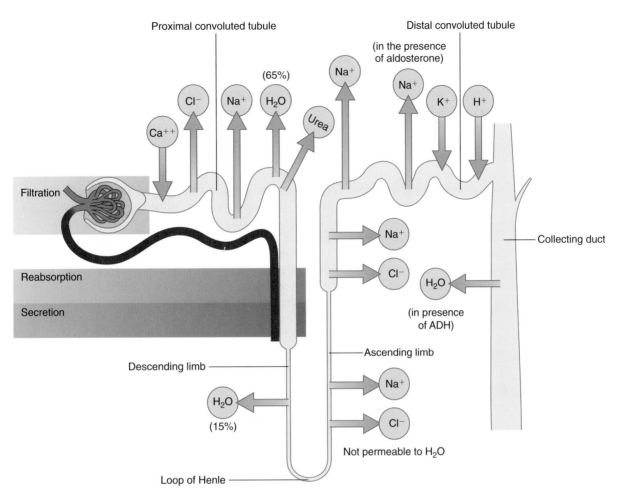

FIGURE 21-4 Tubular reabsorption and secretion.

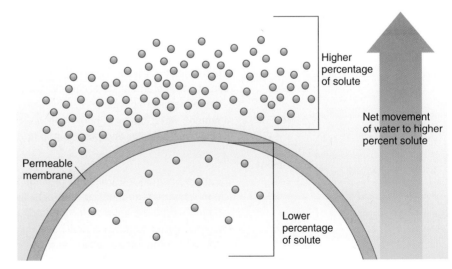

FIGURE 21-5 Also known as an osmotic gradient, the smaller water molecules gravitate toward the highly concentrated sodium ions.

Most of the sodium that enters the renal system is returned to the circulatory system.

Tubular Secretion

Tubular secretion is another major function of the nephrons. This function takes place throughout the nephron. Various ions, toxins, and water are secreted into the collecting duct. First, molecules such as toxins, water-soluble molecules, and excess or unnecessary chemicals are excreted. Weak acids, such as aspirin and penicillin; weak bases, such as narcotic analgesics; and antihistamines are the types of chemicals that are secreted and eliminated. The second function of secretion is to allow the kidneys to regulate the pH of the body through urine acidification. Acidification is the process of eliminating extra hydrogen ions through the urine. This is why urine has an acid content between a pH of 4 and 5, whereas the pH of the blood is maintained at approximately 7.4.

As hydrogen ions are taken into the nephron tubules, they combine with other molecules to produce bicarbonate. This then is released into the bloodstream where it regulates the overall pH of the body, helping to maintain homeostasis. Bicarbonate is a buffer. A buffer has the ability to bind hydrogen (which creates a basic environment) or release hydrogen (which creates an acidic environment by liberating a base) balancing the blood pH. To put it another way, an acid can release hydrogen ions, whereas a base can remove hydrogen by binding the hydrogen to itself. The extra hydrogen ions are taken into the tubules and eventually are excreted.

The Importance of Electrolytes

An important function of the kidneys is to maintain homeostasis through balancing the electrolytes within the body system. To understand the importance of this and other functions of electrolytes we must look at specific cations and anions (see Chapter 30): Na^+ (sodium), K^+ (potassium), Ca^{2+} (calcium), Mg^{2+} (magnesium)/Cl^- (chloride), PO_4^{3-} (phosphate), and HCO_3^- (bicarbonate).

The following is a list of functions of each electrolyte:

Cations

Ca^{2+}	Bone and teeth formation, cell membrane integrity, cardiac conduction nerve impulses, muscle contraction, hormone secretion
K^+	Necessary for glycogen deposits in the liver and skeletal muscles; aids in nerve and cardiac conduction; helps in the contraction within the skeletal and smooth muscle
Mg^{2+}	Aids in cardiac and skeletal muscle excitability, enzyme activities, and neurochemical activities
Na^+	Maintains water balance, nerve impulse transmission, and regulation of acid-base balance and participates in cellular chemical reactions

Anions

Cl^-	The main anion in the transport of chloride following sodium
HCO_3^-	The most important chemical that acts as a buffer; it is essential for the proper acid base balance for the body system
PO_4^{3-}	Aids as a buffer to balance acid-base regulation within the body; promotes normal neuromuscular action and participates in carbohydrate metabolism

Conditions Affecting the Urinary System

It seems as though it would be impossible for individuals to survive long without the constant functioning of both kidneys; however, many persons live with just one kidney. The kidneys are so efficient that as little as 20% of them needs to

TABLE 21-1 Conditions Affecting the Urinary System

Condition	Effect
Anuria	Lack of urine: less than 100 mL over 24 hours
Cystitis	Inflammation of the bladder
Edema	Increase in fluid in cells, tissues, and/or cavities
Hyperkalemia	Excessive increase in potassium in the blood
Hypokalemia	Excessive decrease in potassium in the blood
Incontinence	Lack of control of urination or feces
Oliguria	Little urine output: Between 100 and 400 mL over 24 hours
Polyuria	Excessive or large volume of urine within a certain time
Pyelonephritis	Inflammation of the kidney
Renal failure	Kidney no longer functions
Uremia	Excess urea in the blood
Urethritis	Inflammation of the urethra
Urolithiasis	Kidney stones made of calcium or salts
Urinary tract infection	Infection of the urinary tract caused by microorganisms

be working for survival. This does not mean that a person does not have to watch diet, medications, and activities, but many persons can live normal lives with only one kidney or a partial kidney functioning. In some cases, however, dialysis or even kidney transplants may be necessary. The bladder also can create problems if there is residual urine that does not leave the body. This can lead to infection of the kidneys.

Other conditions that can affect the kidneys and urinary system in general include blockages or infections of the kidney, ureter, bladder, or urethra. Drinking plenty of water is one of the most effective ways of taking care of the urinary system because it helps to cleanse the body of toxins and other unwanted chemicals. Table 21-1 lists other common conditions affecting the urinary system.

RENAL FAILURE

Many possible causes can lead to renal failure, such as accidents, toxic agents, genetic diseases, or certain illnesses. For example, persons who are at high risk of renal failure include those with human immunodeficiency virus, diabetes mellitus, leukemia, and Hodgkin's disease and those with genetic predispositions. A common genetic disease that can cause renal failure is polycystic renal disease. This disease can affect a person in childhood or in adulthood. The kidney becomes enlarged and filled with cysts, and if progression is fast, the kidney eventually fails. In many cases the deterioration of the kidneys at least can be decreased through the use of medications.

Older persons suffer from acute renal failure more often than younger adults. As a kidney ages, it is less able to compensate for fluid imbalances of the body. Cardiovascular disease, diabetes mellitus, and other diseases are the most common causes of renal failure in older persons. As renal failure progresses, every part of the body is affected because of the buildup of waste products and an imbalance of fluids. Table 21-2 lists some of the symptoms of end-stage renal disease.

EDEMA

Millions of persons suffer from edema caused by congestive heart failure (CHF) or hypertension (Figure 21-6). In CHF the heart muscle is weakened by disease.

TABLE 21-2 End-Stage Renal Disease Symptoms*

System	Effect
Cardiovascular	Hypertension, congestive heart failure
Respiratory	Pulmonary edema, dyspnea
Gastrointestinal	Nausea, vomiting, gastrointestinal bleeding
Endocrine	Hyperthyroidism
Ocular	Hypertensive retinopathy
Nervous	Fatigue, confusion, seizures

*Other symptoms include problems with the skin, nerves, blood, and metabolism and psychological problems.

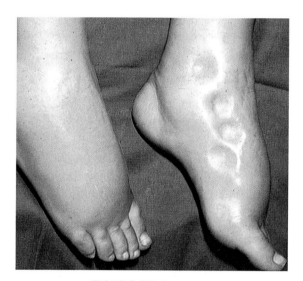

FIGURE 21-6 Edema.

This decreases its efficiency, and as the blood is pumped less and less through the body, the following signs and symptoms may occur:

- Edema in the extremities, such as the legs, ankles, feet, and hands, and edema in the liver, abdominal cavity, lungs, and other areas of the body
- Chest pain resulting from the decreased oxygen to and increased workload of the diseased heart
- Fatigue, dyspnea, and orthopnea from the lack of oxygen in the body

In CHF, when the kidneys get signals that there is a lack of blood content in the body, they try to solve the problem by retaining fluid. This in turn puts more work on the heart, creating the vicious cycle of CHF. Only with the use of medications can a person suffering from CHF extend his or her life. There is no cure. Persons suffering from hypertension must be especially careful because the condition eventually may damage the veins within the heart muscle, which can lead to CHF.

Depending on the disorder of the urinary system, different treatments or medications are prescribed by a physician. In the next section, we discuss the types of treatments and medications used for urinary conditions.

KIDNEY STONES

Hundreds of thousands of Americans experience a condition known as urolithiasis (kidney stones) every year. Although stones most commonly are found in

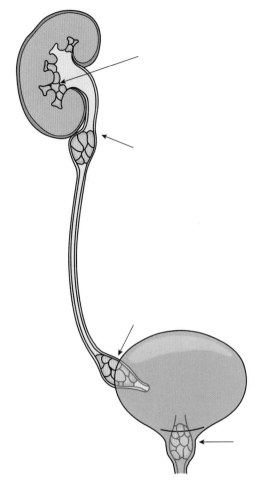

FIGURE 21-7 Common locations of calculus stones.

persons between the ages of 20 and 55, they can affect anyone. They occur at a somewhat higher percentage in whites than blacks, and they tend to run in families. Different types of stones are formed, and each one has a specific treatment. Therefore, it is imperative that a urologist determine which type of stone is causing the problem (Figure 21-7). Table 21-3 lists the different types of stones along with their characteristics and treatments.

URINARY TRACT INFECTIONS

Nosocomial Infection

One of the most common conditions that can affect the urinary system is a urinary tract infection (UTI). Many of the infections are nosocomial. This means the infection was picked up while the patient was in the hospital for a different reason. Most of these types of nosocomial infections are caused by catheterization or cystoscopic examinations. Regardless of the cause, it is important to determine the specific organism in order to prescribe the proper medication. Infections of the kidney are called pyelonephritis, whereas a bladder infection is called cystitis.

INCONTINENCE

A common urinary condition that affects millions of Americans is incontinence. Older adults, especially females, are more prone to this condition; women who

TABLE 21-3 Types of Kidney Stones

Type	Possible cause	Characteristic	Treatment
Cystine	Genetic	Decreased absorption of cystine in gastrointestinal tract causes buildup	Penicillamine, potassium citrate
Uric acid	Gout, genetic	Seen more in men, especially Jewish men	Potassium citrate, diet change
Struvite	Urinary tract infection	Seen more in women	Antimicrobials, surgery
Calcium phosphate	Hyperparathyroidism	Appearance of struvite or oxalate stones	Treat hyperparathyroidism, alkaline urine
Calcium oxalate	Genetic, idiopathic hypercalciuria	Small stones, seen more in men	Increase water intake; decrease oxalate in diet

TABLE 21-4 Types of Incontinence

Type	Possible causes	Possible treatment
Stress	Relaxed pelvic muscles because of lower estrogen levels, multiple pregnancies	Kegel exercises, weight loss, vaginal estrogen creams or rings
Urge	Central nervous system disorders such as Alzheimer's disease, Parkinson's disease, tumors, and bladder disorders	Anticholinergic agents; treat underlying cause or condition; vaginal estrogen creams
Reflex	Central nervous system disorder	Treat underlying cause or condition; surgery; α-adrenergic blockers
Functional	Age: older adults lose mobility and balance	Change in environment, timed voiding, or implement a care plan for person
Overflow	Hyperplasia, bladder neck obstruction following surgery	Catheterization, bethanechol to increase bladder contractions; surgery

have multiple pregnancies tend to develop this condition later in life because of the stretching of the muscles during childbirth. The weakening of these muscles over time can worsen. *Micturition* is the term commonly used to describe urination. Although the bladder can hold up to a liter of fluid, receptors are triggered when the bladder fills about half way. Even after urinating, there is always a small amount (approximately 100 mL) of urine left in the bladder. When coughing or sneezing occurs, there may be enough force placed on the bladder to release a small amount of urine. This is called stress incontinence. Weight gain also can add to this type of condition. In addition, urge incontinence is the involuntary urination when an urgency to urinate happens. Urge incontinence has several causes, such as decreased bladder capacity, infection, or irritation. Also, increased fluid intake, including alcohol or caffeine ingestion, can increase the risk. Table 21-4 lists the types of conditions under this topic along with their treatments. Also examples are given later in the chapter of specific drugs and their dosages.

Treatments for Urinary System Conditions

DIALYSIS: TREATMENT FOR RENAL FAILURE

When a person has lost too much kidney function or has end-stage renal disease and a transplant is not an option, dialysis is the only alternative. Although transplants are relatively common and have a high rate of success, unfortunately there are not enough donors to supply kidneys. Many patients whose names are on transplant waiting lists must wait for years. While they wait, dialysis is the patient's option. Sometimes a transplant may not be an option because the donor's kidneys are not compatible with the recipient's. Also, many times individuals do not want to have surgery to replace their kidneys.

Dialysis is the cleansing of the blood for patients with end-stage renal disease. This treatment replaces the normal kidney function of removing wastes and balancing fluids. Two major methods are in use today: hemodialysis and peritoneal dialysis. A newer, third type—nocturnal dialysis—may be yet another choice. Although each of these types of dialysis has drawbacks, it keeps the person alive. Drawbacks include the additional medications that patients must take to balance pH and fluids further, the inconvenience of having to be stationary for a length of time, and the fact that even sophisticated machinery cannot perform as efficiently as one's own kidneys.

Hemodialysis requires the patient to visit a clinic or hospital for treatment. The patient is hooked up by a vein shunt (needle puncture with a reinforced opening) to a machine that takes a small but steady stream of blood from the body and cleans it of impurities using a mechanical filtration system. Patients undergoing this treatment feel good afterward; however, over time the body builds up toxins again, and they begin to feel ill. Although the length of treatment varies, dialysis normally takes around 5 hours 2 to 3 times weekly.

Peritoneal dialysis is an alternative to hemodialysis. The patient is hooked up to a bag of osmotic solution. A catheter plug is implanted into the abdominal cavity for administration and removal of the solution. The osmotic solution flows into the peritoneal cavity. The peritoneal membrane is a thin lining that encases the organs of the abdomen, including the stomach, liver, spleen, and kidneys. The osmotic solution works in the same fashion as the sodium gradient works in the kidneys. As the solution is allowed to fill the cavity, wastes are pulled into the solution where they can be drained from the cavity into an empty bag attached to the abdominal wall on the outside. This treatment usually is done daily to keep toxins to a minimum. Treatment can be done at home; however, treatment can be done in clinics if the patient cannot afford a home health nurse to assist him or her (Figure 21-8).

Nocturnal dialysis is a newer treatment that is being tested in the United States. Nocturnal dialysis allows the patient to receive treatment while sleeping. Because it can be done slowly over the course of the night, the patient keeps the body system at a steadier state of wellness. Patients do not have to wait between treatments, which is when they begin to feel the effects of toxic buildup, nor do they have to visit clinics or be immobilized for hours at a time. Although this treatment may sound like the best option, the patient must have a full hemodialysis system in the bedroom, which is costly and unwieldy. Also, the patient must be able to troubleshoot problems with the machinery if there is a malfunction. Finally, the patient must have a home health nurse to help with the treatment.

Persons receiving dialysis have to be careful of their fluid and salt intake. With any of these treatments, there is a loss of ions and nutrients that must be replaced with supplements each time dialysis is performed. One of the most common side effects of dialysis is anemia. For this condition iron and erythro-

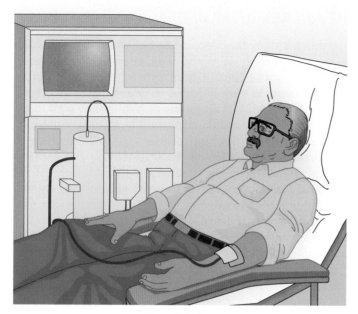

Hemodialysis

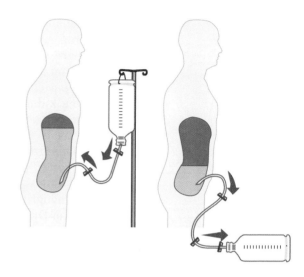

Continuous ambulatory peritoneal dialysis

FIGURE 21-8 Two types of dialysis.

poietin are given to the patient. Iron increases the oxygen-carrying capacity of the hemoglobin. Hemoglobin is a protein within the red blood cells that carries oxygen with the help of iron. Iron and erythropoietin agents are listed in the following.

Replacement Therapy for Dialysis
MINERAL

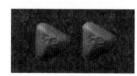

GENERIC NAME: ferrous sulfate
TRADE NAME: Feosol
ROUTE OF ADMINISTRATION: oral
INDICATIONS: dialysis, also for iron deficiency
COMMON DOSAGE: hemodialysis (900 mg); peritoneal dialysis (500 to 900 mg)
SIDE EFFECTS: constipation, black stools
AUXILIARY LABEL:
■ May cause black stools.
SPECIAL NOTE: Iron supplements normally are taken with a stool softener to counteract the side effect of constipation

BLOOD FORMER

GENERIC NAME: epoetin alfa (erythropoietin)
TRADE NAME: Epogen, Procrit
ROUTE OF ADMINISTRATION: subcutaneous or intravenous
INDICATION: dialysis
COMMON DOSAGE: for dialysis patients: 75 units/kg 3 times weekly
SIDE EFFECTS: hypertension, headache, nausea and vomiting
SPECIAL NOTE: Erythropoietin must be kept refrigerated.

TREATMENT OF EDEMA

The main drugs used for the treatment of edema include diuretic thiazides, thiazide-like agents, loop diuretics, potassium-sparing agents, carbonic anhydrase inhibitors, and osmotic diuretics. Each classification is discussed along with its drug action and a listing of each medication.

Thiazides and Thiazide-Like Agents

The drug action of thiazides and thiazide-like agents is the equal increase of urinary excretion of the ions sodium and chloride. These agents do this by inhibiting the normal process of reabsorption within the ascending tubule following the loop of Henle and in the early distal tubules. They also increase the loss of potassium and bicarbonate. Their onset of action is rapid. Because of the loss of potassium, a potassium supplement must be taken concurrently with this type of medication. Common side effects for all thiazides include frequent urination. For this reason, they normally are to be taken early in the day to avoid nocturia.

The normal dosage given is for an adult maintenance dose for edema.

THIAZIDE OR THIAZIDE-LIKE DIURETICS

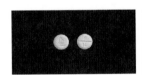

GENERIC NAME: indapamide
TRADE NAME: Lozol
ROUTE OF ADMINISTRATION: oral
COMMON DOSAGE: 2.5 mg qd
SIDE EFFECTS: headache, dizziness, upset stomach
AUXILIARY LABELS:

- Take with food or milk.
- Do not crush tablet.

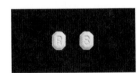

GENERIC NAME: hydrochlorothiazide
TRADE NAME: Esidrix
ROUTE OF ADMINISTRATION: oral
COMMON DOSAGE: 25 to 100 mg daily or intermittently
SIDE EFFECTS: may cause gastrointestinal upset and photosensitivity
AUXILIARY LABELS:

- Take with food or milk.
- May cause photosensitivity.

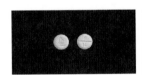

GENERIC NAME: chlorothiazide
TRADE NAME: Diuril
ROUTE OF ADMINISTRATION: oral, intravenous
COMMON DOSAGE: 0.5 to 1 g qd or bid
SIDE EFFECTS: may cause photosensitivity
AUXILIARY LABELS:

- Take with food or milk.
- May cause photosensitivity.

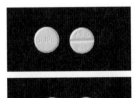

GENERIC NAME: metolazone
TRADE NAME: Zaroxolyn
ROUTE OF ADMINISTRATION: oral
COMMON DOSAGE: 5 to 20 mg qd
SIDE EFFECTS: may cause photosensitivity
AUXILIARY LABELS:

- Take with food or milk.
- May cause photosensitivity.

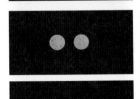

Loop Diuretics

Loop diuretics inhibit reabsorption of sodium and chloride in the proximal convoluted tubule and distal convoluted tubule and within the loop of Henle. Because of the strong action of these agents, a great deal of potassium is lost with urination. They normally are prescribed to be taken early in the day to avoid nocturia.

LOOP DIURETICS

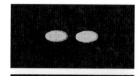

GENERIC NAME: bumetanide
TRADE NAME: Bumex
ROUTE OF ADMINISTRATION: oral
COMMON DOSAGE: 0.5 to 2 mg qd or bid
SIDE EFFECTS: may cause gastrointestinal upset, dizziness, light-headedness
AUXILIARY LABELS:

■ Take with food or milk.
■ May cause dizziness.

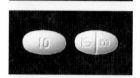

GENERIC NAME: torsemide
TRADE NAME: Demadex
ROUTE OF ADMINISTRATION: oral, intravenous
COMMON DOSAGE: 10 to 20 mg qd
SIDE EFFECTS: may cause dizziness, light-headedness
AUXILIARY LABELS:

■ May cause dizziness.
■ May cause photosensitivity.
SPECIAL NOTE: Torsemide does not need to be taken with food or milk.

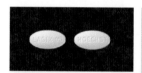

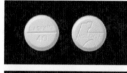

GENERIC NAME: furosemide
TRADE NAME: Lasix
ROUTE OF ADMINISTRATION: oral, intravenous
COMMON DOSAGE: 20 to 80 mg qd
SIDE EFFECTS: may cause gastrointestinal upset
AUXILIARY LABEL:

■ Take with food or milk.

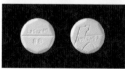

Potassium-Sparing Agents

Because potassium-sparing agents work primarily in the distal convoluted tubule and inhibit sodium reabsorption, which decreases potassium loss, they do not cause large amounts of potassium to be lost in the urine. With these types of agents, it is recommended that patients avoid large quantities of potassium-rich foods.

Table 21-5 gives combination drugs composed of the listed potassium-sparing and thiazide or loop diuretics, along with their indication, dosage form, and auxiliary labels.

POTASSIUM-SPARING DIURETICS

GENERIC NAME: amiloride
TRADE NAME: Midamore
ROUTE OF ADMINISTRATION: oral
COMMON DOSAGE: 5 mg per day

TABLE 21-5 **Combination Diuretics**

Generic name	Trade name	Dosage form	Strength	Normal dosage	Auxiliary label
Amiloride/ hydrochlorothiazide (HCTZ)	Moduretic	Tablet	5 mg/ 50 mg	1-2 tablets daily	Take with food Photosensitivity
Spironolactone/ HCTZ	Aldactazide	Tablet	25 mg/ 25 mg	1-8 tablets daily	Take with food Photosensitivity
	Aldactazide	Tablet	50 mg/ 50 mg	1-4 tablets daily	Take with food Photosensitivity
Triamterene/HCTZ	Dyazide	Capsule	37.5 mg/ 25 mg	1-2 capsules daily	Take with food Photosensitivity
	Maxzide-25	Tablet	37.5 mg/ 25 mg	1-2 tablets daily	Take with food Photosensitivity
	Maxzide	Tablet	75 mg/ 50 mg	1 tablet daily	Take with food Photosensitivity

SIDE EFFECTS: may cause gastrointestinal upset, dizziness, headache, visual disturbances

AUXILIARY LABELS:
- Take with food.
- May cause dizziness.

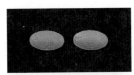
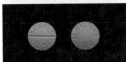

GENERIC NAME: spironolactone
TRADE NAME: Aldactone
ROUTE OF ADMINISTRATION: oral
COMMON DOSAGE: for edema, 25 to 200 mg per day
SIDE EFFECTS: may cause drowsiness, mental confusion
AUXILIARY LABEL:
- May cause dizziness and drowsiness.

GENERIC NAME: triamterene
TRADE NAME: Dyrenium
ROUTE OF ADMINISTRATION: oral
COMMON DOSAGE: 100 mg bid after meals
SIDE EFFECTS: may cause gastrointestinal upset, headache
AUXILIARY LABEL:
- Take after meals.

Carbonic Anhydrase Inhibitors

Carbonic anhydrase inhibitors inhibit the enzyme carbonic anhydrase. Carbonic anhydrase inhibitors include acetazolamide, dichlorphenamide, and methazolamide. They inhibit hydrogen ion secretion by the renal tubule, causing an increase in urination of sodium, potassium bicarbonate, and water. Most of these agents more commonly are used to treat glaucoma (see Chapter 19), although acetazolamide also can be used for the treatment of edema resulting from CHF. Side effects include possible gastrointestinal upset, photosensitivity, and drowsiness.

TABLE 21-6 Osmotic Diuretics

Generic name	Trade name	Dosage form	Strength	Normal dosage
Mannitol	Osmitrol	Injection	5%, 10%, 15%, 20%, 25%	20-200 g over 24 hours
Urea	Ureaphil	Injection	40 g/150 mL	30% solution by slow intravenous infusion not to exceed 4 mL/min
Glycerin	Osmoglyn	Oral solution	50%	1 to 2 g/kg, 1 to 1½ hours before surgery
Isosorbide	Ismotic	Oral solution	45%	1 to 3 g/kg 2 to 4 times a day as needed

CARBONIC ANHYDRASE INHIBITOR

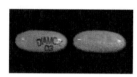

GENERIC NAME: acetazolamide
TRADE NAME: Diamox
ROUTE OF ADMINISTRATION: oral, intravenous, intramuscular
COMMON DOSAGE: 250 to 375 mg qd
AUXILIARY LABELS:

- Take with meals.
- May cause dizziness.

TECH ALERT!

Mannitol is available only in injectable solution. Mannitol must be stored at a temperature between 15° to 30° C (59° to 86° F) because it has a tendency to crystallize at lower temperatures because of its high sugar content. If mannitol does crystallize, it can be placed for short periods of time in 80° C water with periodic vigorous shaking or can be autoclaved at 121° C for 20 minutes at 15 psi. The vials cannot be placed in a microwave or they may explode. Mannitol should not be administered until it is at room temperature or slightly below and requires a filter for infusion. This is a common question on the Pharmacy Technician Certification Board exam.

Osmotic Diuretics

Osmotic diuretics inhibit tubular reabsorption of water by increasing the osmolarity of the glomerular filtrate. They are used for prophylaxis of acute renal failure when the glomerular filtration is reduced. Agents such as urea, glycerin, and isosorbide also are used for glaucoma. Table 21-6 lists osmotic diuretics and their normal dosages.

TREATMENT OF URINARY TRACT INFECTIONS

The most common bacterial infections are those that cause UTIs. Because the urethra is much shorter in women than in men, women are more susceptible to contract infections from bacteria entering the urethra. Another cause of UTIs is catheterization. Infection of the kidney is called glomerulonephritis or pyelonephritis, whereas infection in the bladder is referred to as cystitis. The symptoms of an upper (kidney) UTI include lower back pain, stomach pain, nausea, vomiting, and headache. Symptoms of lower (bladder) UTIs include frequent but small amounts of urine, dysuria, and sometimes incontinence. As discussed before, if the infection is acquired within the hospital, it is referred to as a nosocomial infection. Most of these infections are caused by gram-negative microbes. Table 21-7 lists the most common agents used to treat UTIs. Often a physician will give the patient instructions to take an initial large dose called a loading dose before the normal dosage regimen. This is done to bring the antibiotic quickly up to therapeutic levels within the system so that it can begin to assist the body in fighting off the infection. The drug action for these antibiotics is given in Chapter 24. Depending on the identification of pathogens that are responsible for the UTI, urinary antibiotics can be used for treatment. The following are three examples of medications used specifically for uncomplicated UTIs caused by strains of *E. coli* and *E. faecalis*.

TABLE 21-7 Treatments for Urinary Tract Infections

Generic name	Trade name	Normal dosage
Sulfonamides		
Sulfamethoxazole	Gantanol	2 g loading dose, then 1 g every 8 to 12 hours
Sulfisoxazole	Gantrisin	2-4 g loading dose, then 750 mg-1.5 g every 6 hours
Sulfadiazine	[Generic only]	2-4 g loading dose, then 1 g every 4 to 6 hours
Fluoroquinolones		
Ciprofloxacin	Cipro	250-500 mg every 12 hours
Norfloxacin	Noroxin	400 mg every 12 hours
Ofloxacin	Floxin	200 mg every 12 hours for 3 to 10 days
Enoxacin	Penetrex	200 mg every 12 hours for 7 to 14 days
Miscellaneous Antiinfectives		
Nitrofurantoin	Macrodantin	50-100 mg every 6 hours
Methenamine	Mandelamine	1 g 4 times daily

ANTIINFECTIVE ANTIBIOTIC

GENERIC NAME: fosfomycin
TRADE NAME: Monurol
ROUTE OF ADMINISTRATION: oral granules
COMMON DOSAGE: 3-g packet in 90 to 120 mL cold water 1 time only
SIDE EFFECTS: nausea, diarrhea, abdominal cramps, flatulence
AUXILIARY LABELS:

■ Mix in water.
■ May cause diarrhea.
■ May cause nausea.
■ Do not take if breast-feeding.

UTI ANTIBIOTIC

GENERIC NAME: nitrofurantoin
TRADE NAME: Macrobid, Macrodantin
ROUTE OF ADMINISTRATION: oral
COMMON DOSAGE: Macrobid 100 mg bid or Macrodantin 50 to 100 mg qid
SIDE EFFECTS: Nausea
AUXILIARY LABELS:

■ May cause brownish urine.
■ Do not take if breast-feeding.

QUINOLONE ANTIBIOTIC

GENERIC NAME: cinoxacin
TRADE NAME: Cinobac
ROUTE OF ADMINISTRATION: oral
COMMON DOSAGE: 1 g per day in two to four divided doses
SIDE EFFECTS: edema, dizziness, headache, insomnia, constipation
AUXILIARY LABELS:

■ Take until gone.
■ May cause dizziness.
■ Do not take if breast-feeding.

TREATMENT OF INCONTINENCE

Table 21-4 lists the types of incontinence along with possible treatments. The most common nondrug therapy for most types of incontinence is the Kegel exercise. This is an exercise that involves the pelvic floor muscles. The exercise requires that the patient tighten the muscles around the pelvis in the same fashion as he or she would to hold urine and can be done standing or sitting. The exercise usually is done in sets of 10, 10 times daily over several weeks. Often incontinence can be overcome if the patient seeks help from his or her physician. If incontinence cannot be corrected by exercise or medication, surgery (in some cases) can alleviate the problem. The following are samples of the types of medications commonly used to treat incontinence.

ANTICHOLINERGIC

GENERIC NAME: trospium chloride
TRADE NAME: Sanctura
ROUTE OF ADMINISTRATION: oral
COMMON DOSAGE: 20 mg bid
AUXILIARY LABELS:

- Do not crush or break tablet.
- Take 1 hour before meals or on an empty stomach.
- May cause dry mouth.
- May cause constipation.

ANTISPASMODIC

GENERIC NAME: darifenacin hydrobromide
TRADE NAME: Enablex EX
ROUTE OF ADMINISTRATION: oral
COMMON DOSAGE: 7.5 mg qd; may be increased to 15 mg qd after 2 weeks if needed
AUXILIARY LABELS:

- May cause nausea and vomiting.
- May cause dizziness.
- May cause constipation.

ANTISPASMODIC

GENERIC NAME: tolterodine tartrate
TRADE NAME: Detrol, Detrol LA
ROUTE OF ADMINISTRATION: oral
COMMON DOSAGE: Detrol, 1 to 2 mg qd; Detrol LA, 2 to 4 mg qd (used for cases of severe renal or hepatic impairment)
AUXILIARY LABELS:

- Do not take if breast-feeding.
- May cause dizziness.
- May cause headaches.
- May cause dyspepsia.

TECH ALERT!
Remember the following soundalike/look-alike drugs:
Chlorthalidone versus chlorothiazide
Bumex versus Buprenex
Furosemide versus torsemide
Metolazone versus metoclopramide
Ditropan versus diazepam

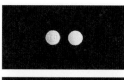
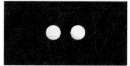
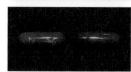
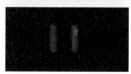

DO YOU REMEMBER THESE KEY POINTS?

- The location of the kidneys
- The function of the kidneys
- The major components of the kidney and urinary system
- The functions of the glomerulus
- What conditions require dialysis and the types available
- The various types of medications that dialysis patients must receive
- The drug action of diuretics
- The major conditions affecting the urinary system and their treatments

MULTIPLE CHOICE QUESTIONS

1. Blood enters the kidneys through the _____.
   A. Renal fascia
   B. Renal artery
   C. Renal vein
   D. Hilus

2. All of the following are components of the nephron except the _____.
   A. Glomerulus
   B. Urethra
   C. Bowman's capsule
   D. Loop of Henle

3. When taking loop diuretics, it should not be necessary to take which of the following supplements?
   A. Potassium
   B. Calcium
   C. Multivitamins
   D. A, B, and C

4. The _____ is where sodium is transported actively along with chloride.
   A. Proximal convoluted tubule
   B. Distal convoluted tubule
   C. Loop of Henle
   D. Glomerulus

5. Edema commonly is associated with all of the following conditions except:
   A. Hypertension
   B. Congestive heart failure
   C. Glaucoma
   D. Nephritis

6. Buffers have the ability to prevent:
   A. Large changes in pH
   B. Edema
   C. Renal failure
   D. Blood loss

7. Plasma is a component of _____.
   A. Buffers
   B. Water
   C. Blood
   D. Dialysis

8. Which of the following classifications of medications include diuretics?
   A. Blood formers
   B. Thiazides
   C. Carbonic anhydrase inhibitors
   D. B and C

9. Active transport is when _____.
   A. Sodium is exchanged for hydrogen
   B. Potassium is exchanged for sodium
   C. Sodium and chloride leave the nephron
   D. Bicarbonate leaves the nephron

10. Loop diuretics and thiazides _____.
    A. Have a slow mechanism of action
    B. Cause a loss of potassium
    C. Cause a loss of sodium
    D. Must be taken with a potassium-sparing agent

TRUE/FALSE **If the statement is false, then change it to make it true.**

_____ 1. The connective tissue that holds the kidneys in place is called the peritoneal membrane.

_____ 2. All food is metabolized and excreted by the kidneys.

_____ 3. When giving thiazide diuretics, a potassium replacement is not necessary.

_____ **4.** A blood urea nitrogen test measures the uric nitrogen content within the liver.

_____ **5.** Urine is collected in the glomerulus and transported to the bladder.

_____ **6.** Weak acids and bases are reabsorbed via the nephron.

_____ **7.** Waste products from the kidneys are called urine.

_____ **8.** Urine pH is between 4 and 6, which is acidic.

_____ **9.** The two mechanisms of reabsorption involve ion exchange and active transport.

_____ **10.** Epoetin is given to dialysis patients to counteract iron deficiency.

TECHNICIAN'S CORNER

Ms. Lewis went to the doctor because of swelling in her legs and shortness of breath. After blood tests and a physical examination, she was diagnosed with congestive heart failure. The doctor prescribed the following medications to be filled in the pharmacy:

Spironolactone 25 mg 1 q am
Furosemide 20 mg 1 tablet q am

Question

What are the classifications of these medications, and what auxiliary labels will you place on the vial? Also, what medication/if any did the doctor omit that you would bring to the attention of the pharmacist?

BIBLIOGRAPHY

Campbell N, Reese J: *Biology,* ed 7, Redwood City, Calif, 2004, Benjamin/Cummings.

Clayton BD, Stock YN: *Basic pharmacology for nurses,* ed 14, St Louis, 2006, Mosby.

Drug facts and comparisons, ed 60, St Louis, 2005, Wolters Kluwer.

Lacy C, Armstrong L, Goldman M, et al: *Lexi Comp's Drug information handbook,* ed 13, Hudson, Ohio, 2005, Lexi-Comp.

Lewis SM, Heitkemper MM, Dirksen SR: *Medical-surgical nursing: assessment and management of clinical problems,* ed 6, St Louis, 2003, Mosby.

Potter PA, Perry AG: *Fundamentals of nursing,* ed 6, St Louis, 2004, Mosby.

Salerno E: *Pharmacology for health professionals,* St Louis, 1999, Mosby.

Stedman's concise medical dictionary for health professionals, ed 3, Baltimore, 1997, Williams & Wilkins.

Wilson BA, et al: *Prentice Hall nurse's drug guide 2006,* Upper Saddle River, NJ, 2006, Prentice Hall.

Cardiovascular System

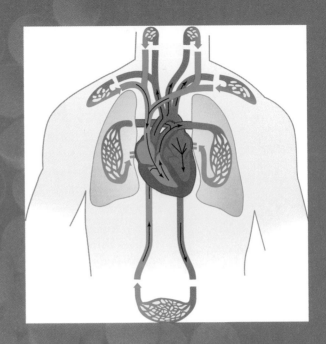

Objectives

UPON COMPLETING THIS CHAPTER, YOU SHOULD BE ABLE TO
DO THE FOLLOWING:

- List both trade and generic names covered in this chapter.

- Describe the location and function of the heart.

- Name the four chambers of the heart.

- Explain how the heart receives nourishment.

- List the major disease states of the heart.

- Explain the possible causes of coronary artery disease, congestive heart failure, and hypertension.

- List the three types of angina.

- Describe how hypertension and hyperlipidemia can contribute to heart conditions.

- List the drugs used for heart conditions.

- List the drugs used for hypertension.

- Describe the indications for and mechanisms of the following classifications of drugs:
    - Angiotensin-converting enzyme inhibitors
    - Anticoagulants
    - β-blockers
    - Calcium channel blockers
    - Nitrates
    - Thrombolytics

455

Angina *A severe, often constricting pain affecting the pectoris, or chest region, caused by lack of oxygen to the heart cells*

Arrhythmia *Irregular rhythm of the heart*

Artery *A vessel that carries oxygenated blood from the heart to the tissues of the body*

Capillary *Extremely small vessel that connects the ends of the smallest arteries (arterioles) to the smallest veins (venules), where exchanges of nutrients and wastes, O_2 and CO_2, occur; blood vessels at cellular level*

Coagulation *To solidify or change from a fluid state to a solid state as in forming a blood clot*

Congestive heart failure (CHF) *Accumulation of blood in the circulatory system caused by the inability of the heart to pump efficiently*

Coronary artery disease (CAD) *A common term used for several diseases that affect the heart*

Diuretic *An agent that increases urine output and diuresis*

Enzyme *A protein that speeds up a reaction by reducing the amount of energy required to initiate a reaction; also called a biological catalyst*

Hyperlipidemia *Abnormally high concentration of lipids in the circulatory system*

Hypertension *High blood pressure*

Hypotension *Low blood pressure*

Myocardial infarction *Death of the heart muscle*

Stroke *Impaired cerebral blood flow caused by thrombosis, hemorrhage, or embolism*

Thrombin *An enzyme that is formed in coagulating blood from prothrombin; this enzyme reacts with fibrinogen, converting it into fibrin, which is essential in the formation of blood clots; tested by performing a prothrombin time or partial thromboplastin time blood test*

Thrombolytic *Medication used to break up a thrombus or blood clot*

Transient ischemic attack *A temporary reduction of oxygen and blood in the brain*

Vein *A vessel that carries deoxygenated blood to or toward the heart*

456

CARDIOVASCULAR DRUGS

Brand name	Generic name	Pronunciation	Brand name	Generic name	Pronunciation
Antihypertensives			Plendil	felodipine	(fe-**low**-de-peen)
Aldomet	methyldopa	(meth-ill-**doe**-pah)	Procardia	nifedipine	(nye-**fed**-ih-peen)
Apresoline	hydralazine	(high-**dral**-ah-zeen)			
Cardura	doxazosin	(dok-**sah**-zo-sin)	**Anticoagulants**		
Catapres	clonidine	(**klon**-ih-deen)	Coumadin	warfarin	(**war**-fair-in)
Diuril	chlorothiazide	(klor-oh-**thigh**-ah-zide)	Liquaemin	heparin	(**hep**-ah-rin)
DynaCirc	isradipine	(is-**rad**-i-peen)			
Hytrin	terazosin	(tur-**ah**-zoh-sin)	**Nitrates/Antianginals**		
Minipress	prazosin	(**pra**-zoe-sin)	Imdur	isosorbide mononitrate	(eye-soe-**sor**-bide mo-no-**ny**-trate)
Reserpine	reserpine	(re-**sir**-peen)	Isordil	isosorbide dinitrate	(eye-soe-**sore**-bide-dye-**ny**trate)
Zaroxolyn	metolazone	(me-**toe**-lah-zone)	Nitrostat, Tridil	nitroglycerin	(nye-troe-**glis**-sir-rin)
Antiarrhythmics			**Antihyperlidemic Agents**		
Lanoxin	digoxin	(di-**jox**-in)	Lipitor	atorvastatin	(a-tore-va-**stat**-in)
Quinidex	quinidine	(**kwin**-ah-deen)	Lopid	gemfibrozil	(gem-**fib**-row-zil)
Norpace	disopyramide	(dye-so-**peer**-a-mide)	Mevacor	lovastatin	(**low**-vah-stat-in)
Pronestyl	procainamide	(pro-**cane**-ah-mide)	Niacor	niacin	(**nye**-a-sin)
			Pravachol	pravastatin	(**prav**-ah-stat-in)
Angiotensin-Converting Enzyme Inhibitors			Questran	cholestyramine	(koe-lee-sty-**rah**-meen)
Accupril	quinapril	(**kwin**-a-pril)	Tricor	fenofibrate	(fee-no-**fye**-brate)
Altace	ramipril	(ray-**mi**-pril)	Zetia	ezetimibe	(eh-**zet**-eh-mi-be)
Capoten	captopril	(**cap**-tow-pril)	Zocor	simvastatin	(sym-vah-**stat**-in)
Lotensin	benazepril	(ben-**ayz**-ah-prill)			
Monopril	fosinopril	(foe-**sin**-oh-pril)	**Bile Acid Sequestrant Agents**		
Prinivil, Zestril	lisinopril	(lih-**sin**-oh-prill)	Colestid	colestipol	(koe-**les**-ti-pole)
Univasc	moexipril	(moe-**ex**-a-prile)	WelChol	colesevelam	(koh-le-**sev**-e-lam)
Vasotec	enalapril	(eh-**nal**-ah-prill)			
			Diuretics		
Angiotensin II Antagonists			Aldactone	spironolactone	(spear-own-oh-**lak**-tone)
Avapro	irbesartan	(erb-ba-**sar**-tan)	Bumex	bumetanide	(byew-**met**-ah-nide)
Cozaar	losartan	(low-**sar**-tan)	Diamox	acetazolamide	(ah-see-ta-**zoe**-la-myde)
Diovan	valsartan	(val-**sar**-tan)	Lasix	furosemide	(feur-**oh**-sah-myde)
Micardis	telmisartan	(tel-meh-**sar**-tan)			
Teveten	eprosartan	(eh-pro-**sar**-tan)	**Vasodilators**		
			Isordil	isosorbide	(eye-soe-**sore**-bide)
β-Blockers			Nitrostat	nitroglycerin	(nye-troe-**glis**-sir-rin)
Brevibloc	esmolol	(**es**-mo-lol)	Transderm Nitro	nitroglycerin patches	(nye-troe-**glis**-sir-rin)
Inderal	propranolol	(pro-**pran**-oh-lol)			
Kerlone	betaxolol	(be-**tax**-oh-lol)	**Coagulants**		
Lopressor	metoprolol	(meh-toe-**pro**-lol)	Mephyton	phytonadione	(fy-toe-na-**dye**-own)
Sectral	acebutolol	(a-se-**byoo**-toe-lole)	Protamine Sulfate	protamine	(**pro**-toe-mean)
Tenormin	atenolol	(ay-**ten**-oh-lol)			
Trandate	labetalol	(lah-**bet**-ah-lol)	**Thrombolytics**		
Visken	pindolol	(**pin**-doe-lole)	Abbokinase	urokinase	(your-oh-**kin**-ase)
			Activase	alteplase	(**al**-tee-plase)
Calcium Channel Blockers			Streptase	streptokinase	(strep-toe-**kye**-nase)
Calan, Isoptin	verapamil	(ver-**ap**-ah-mill)			
Cardene	nicardipine	(nye-**kar**-de-peen)			
Cardizem	diltiazem	(dill-**tie**-ah-zem)			
Nimotop	nimodipine	(nye-**moe**-di-peen)			
Norvasc	amlodipine	(am-**low**-di-peen)			

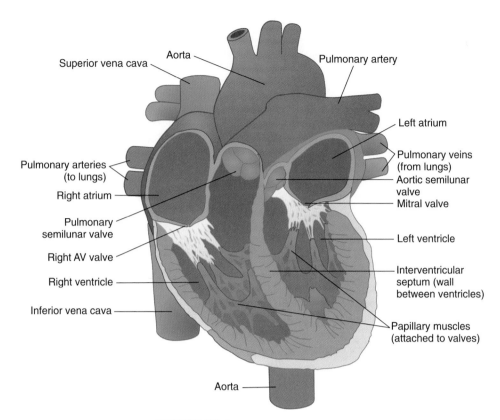

FIGURE 22-1 Anatomy of the heart.

THE CARDIOVASCULAR SYSTEM is a network of many complex interactions. These interactions involve the blood, lungs, arteries, and veins of the body and the heart muscle itself. Millions of persons die each year from heart disease; however, millions are living normal lives because of the advancements made in medicine. In addition, there is an awareness of heart health in the public because of health organizations. Individuals are living longer because of their lifestyle changes and medications and the advancements of new surgical techniques. We begin with an overview of the anatomy of the heart, followed by the most common conditions that affect the heart. The last section is on the treatments available—the focus is on the medications. Technicians fill many prescriptions for heart medications over their careers, and it is important to learn basic information about the classifications to assist the pharmacist.

Location and Anatomy of the Heart

The heart is located in the chest cavity between the lungs. The heart is a large muscle that initiates systemic arterial pulse waves, causing blood to circulate throughout the body and supply it with nutrition and oxygen. Extending from the heart are large transport tubes called arteries. These arteries flow into smaller tubes called arterioles and then ultimately into very small tubes called capillaries. From the capillaries oxygen and nutrients are exchanged throughout the tissues (Figure 22-1).

A normal heart beats anywhere from 60 to 100 times per minute and is about the size of a person's fist. The heart is surrounded by connective tissue called the pericardium, which in turn is anchored by ligaments to the chest wall and diaphragm. The heart is composed of three main layers:

1. *Endocardium* (inside): The endocardium has a smooth accordion pleat–like surface, which allows the heart wall to collapse when it contracts.

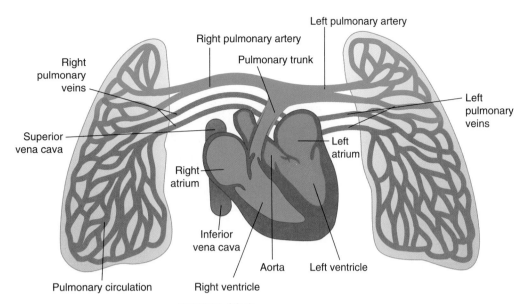

FIGURE 22-2 Blood oxygenation.

2. *Myocardium* (muscle): The myocardium is the heart muscle that contracts.
3. *Epicardium* (outside): The epicardium is the outer layer of the heart. This is also the inner layer of the pericardium. The coronary arteries that supply the heart with oxygenated blood and the coronary veins that return deoxygenated blood to the heart are located in the epicardium.

OXYGENATION

The heart has two pumps, each of which is composed of two chambers (Figure 22-2). The first two chambers are the right atrium and the right ventricle. Blood circulates through the body exchanging oxygen, nutrients, and other substances to tissues and organs. The blood returns to the heart via two large veins called the superior and inferior venae cavae. The superior vena cava brings blood from the upper portion of the body, and the inferior vena cava brings blood into the heart from the lower portion of the body. The blood travels through the right atrium into the right ventricle. The right ventricle contracts, expelling blood into the pulmonary arteries that go to the lungs, where blood is fully oxygenated by the air that we breathe (see Chapter 18). The left atrium of the heart then receives the fully oxygenated blood from the lungs via the pulmonary veins. Blood then is passed into the left ventricle through the mitral valve. The left ventricle then contracts, expelling the blood into the aorta. In the aorta the blood initiates a pulse wave that carries it to all parts of the body (Figure 22-3). Although the heart is an efficient organ, it still must be oxygenated just like other organs. The main arteries that supply blood to the heart are called the coronary arteries.

CARDIAC CONDUCTION SYSTEM

The cardiac conduction system provides the electrical charge that makes the heart pump. This system is a lifetime battery that keeps our heartbeats in rhythm. This cardiac conduction system is run by two nodes: the sinoatrial and atrioventricular. The sinoatrial node is located in the upper right atrium wall (this is where the impulse begins). The signal then is sent down to the atrioventricular node, located in the septum between the right atrium and the right ventricle. As the cardiac impulse is sent from the sinoatrial to the atrioventricular node, it also is sent out to the muscle fibers that run throughout the atria. From the atrioventricular node the impulse goes to the ventricles to initiate a

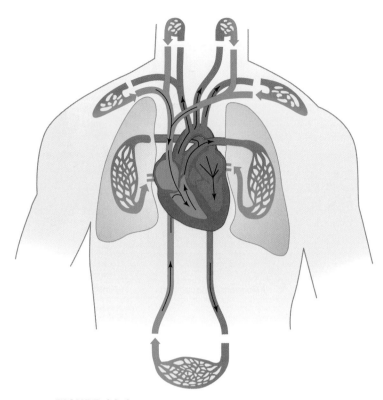

FIGURE 22-3 Circulation of blood through the body.

ventricular beat by stimulation of the bundle branches and Purkinje fibers (Figure 22-4).

The Cardiac Cycle

The series of events that occur for one complete heartbeat is called the cardiac cycle. This cycle is composed of two sequences:

1. Systole: The myocardium squeezes blood from the heart chamber into the pulmonary artery or aorta.
2. Diastole: Blood is allowed to refill the chambers (relaxation). During diastole, the atria contract to pack 20% more blood into the ventricles. Most of your blood supply is cycled every minute through the heart.

Conditions Affecting the Heart

Many heart conditions affect millions of persons each year. Because of the advancements made in the area of health, including the importance of lifestyle choices on our health, new medications, and new surgical techniques available, individuals are living longer lives. Box 22-1 lists some of the most common cardiovascular conditions along with a brief description.

To see how all of these conditions are related to one another is important, so we briefly discuss the differences and similarities between the conditions listed.

CORONARY ARTERY DISEASE

Coronary artery disease is associated with atherosclerosis. This condition can be the result of a lifelong buildup of small plaques mainly composed of lipids (fats) especially cholesterol. Although these lipids can build up anywhere in the large arteries of the body, they also tend to accumulate in the arteries throughout the heart. Atherosclerosis has been linked to high blood pressure. For

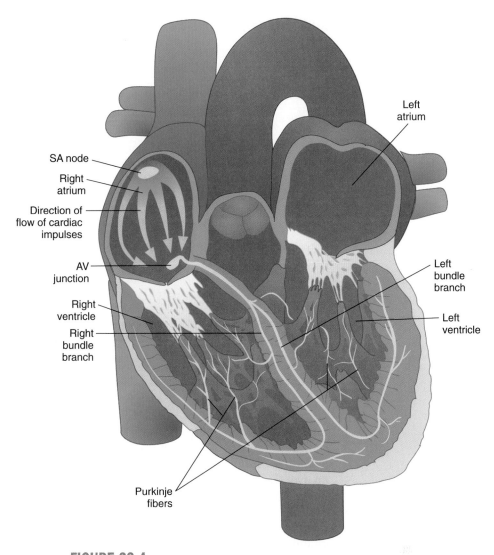

FIGURE 22-4 Conduction system. *SA,* Sinoatrial; *AV,* atrioventricular.

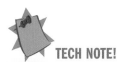

TECH NOTE!

Arteriosclerosis is characterized by hardening and loss of elasticity of the arterial vessels. Three forms of this condition are atherosclerosis, sclerosis of the arterioles, and calcific sclerosis of the medial layer of the arteries. Of these three types, atherosclerosis is the most common type, which causes angina, transient ischemic attacks (TIAs), stroke, or even an MI resulting from the formation of a thrombus (clot).

example, small injuries can occur in the vessel wall. As lipids pass by, they attach and begin to build up along the wall of the artery, eventually blocking the site altogether. Although much of the damage to the heart may be done in adulthood, lipid deposits have been observed in young children as well. Over time, if these fatty deposits build up, a thrombus can be generated that can block the artery. This causes myocardial infarction (MI). Many risk factors can be linked to the development of atherosclerosis and eventual coronary artery disease. These include hypertension, age, gender, race, and genetics. Although these traits cannot be altered, several factors can be altered, such as a fatty diet, no exercise, smoking, and stress.

Hyperlipidemia

Hyperlipidemia is the increase of lipids in the bloodstream and is the precursor to atherosclerosis. When discussing fats (lipids) in the body, the purpose of cholesterol, one type of lipid, is an important aspect. Cholesterol is produced by the body and is vital for making steroid hormones and cell membranes. When persons eat foods that are high in fat, they also are ingesting too much cholesterol and other fatty acids, which our bodies cannot eliminate. Instead, these fatty substances float throughout the bloodstream where they can latch onto large arteries and middle-sized arteries of the heart and brain. Therefore, it is

BOX 22-1 CONDITIONS AND DEFINITIONS

Angina pectoris	Pain and pressure in the chest caused by a lack of proper blood flow and oxygenation to the heart muscle
Arrhythmia	Irregular heartbeats resulting from a malfunction in the conduction system
Arteriosclerosis	A disease of the arterial vessels resulting from thickening, hardening, and loss of elasticity in the arterial walls
Atherosclerosis	A form of arteriosclerosis resulting from cholesterol-lipid calcium deposits in the walls of the arteries
Congestive heart failure	A condition in which the heart is unable to pump the amounts of blood needed to meet the requirements of the body; normally abbreviated CHF
Coronary artery disease	A term used to describe blood vessel disorders that affect the coronary arteries; normally abbreviated CAD
Hyperlipidemia	High or excessive amounts of lipid (fat) in the blood that lead to arteriosclerosis and atherosclerosis
Hypertension	High blood pressure, which is considered a systolic reading of greater than 140 mm Hg or greater than 90 mm Hg diastolic over several readings
Myocardial infarction	An event in which part of the heart muscle dies because of interruption or cessation of blood flow
Prehypertensive state	Blood pressure of 120/80 to 140/90 mm Hg
Thrombosis	The formation of a blood clot within the vascular system

important that regular checkups include a blood test to reveal the amount of cholesterol in the bloodstream. A generic type of test indicating the overall cholesterol levels normally is done; a cholesterol level less than 200 mg/dL indicates an overall low cholesterol, 200 to 239 mg/dL indicates a borderline high reading, and a level at or greater than 240 mg/dL is a high value. In the case of a borderline or above-normal level, a more in-depth look at the low-density lipoprotein (LDL) and high-density lipoprotein (HDL) probably would be indicated. The guidelines for specific cholesterol readings are listed in the following chart. (Values are derived from blood tests or serum of the blood in adults.)

LDL		**HDL**
Less than 130	Good	Greater than 75
130 to 159	Borderline	36 to 44
Greater than 160	High	26 to 35

Another type of cholesterol not normally mentioned in laboratory values is very-low-density lipoproteins (VLDLs). The level of VLDL is an indicator of the amount of LDL because it is a precursor to LDL. Other factors that determine the treatment approach include family history, lifestyle habits, and the patient's personal medical history. The good cholesterol HDL transports fat from tissues. Bad cholesterol LDL carries around lipids (fat) that can attach to artery walls causing atherosclerosis.

Hypertension

Hypertension is defined as persistent high blood pressure. High blood pressure is a prevalent problem in the United States, affecting millions of Americans. This disease also is known as the "silent killer" because there are no obvious signs of its presence.

Why and How Hypertension Occurs. Hypertension is a result of various factors. The heart may be diseased and the blood flow is decreased or another organ,

BOX 22-2 COMMON CONDITIONS THAT CAN LEAD TO HYPERTENSION

Common Conditions for Hypertension
Heart condition
Hyperthyroidism
Kidney conditions

Increased Risk Factors That Can Lead to Hypertension
1. Genetic
   Age
   Gender
   Race
2. Lifestyle
   Diet
   Anxiety
   Alcohol consumption
   Sodium intake

such as the kidney, is not working properly, causing edema (a buildup of watery fluids). When the kidneys are not working properly, the concentration of ions such as sodium can increase throughout the body system. (Remember that water follows salt because of the higher concentration; therefore, when an increase in salt occurs, the patient retains water, resulting in edema.) Whatever the cause of hypertension, the result is that the heart must work much harder to pump blood through the chambers and out into the body. Hypertension also can result from various conditions and risk factors such as those listed in Box 22-2.

The continuous overload on the coronary system also adds to the development of atherosclerosis (hardening of the arteries) and can cause small ruptures of vessels within the heart. Common signs of high blood pressure can be confused with other causes not associated with hypertension, such as blurred vision, headache, and shortness of breath. Another important factor that patients should be made aware of by their physician and pharmacist is that many over-the-counter agents can affect their blood pressure. This includes antihistamines, decongestants, and ingredients in many different cold and allergy remedies.

Blood Pressure Readings. Individuals should have their blood pressure taken regularly throughout their lifetime to evaluate blood pressure for elevations or to seek medical attention if necessary. A person with a systolic blood pressure reading of more than 140 mm Hg is considered to have hypertension. A prehypertensive state is considered when blood pressure reaches 120/80 mm Hg. Four categories of hypertension are based on diastolic readings and three categories are based on systolic readings, as explained in Box 22-3. Blood pressure units are read by mm Hg, which is millimeters of mercury. Even a mild case of hypertension can lead to problems in later life because of the extra work placed on the heart. Blood pressure readings should be taken a few times during each visit to the doctor to obtain an average for each person's blood pressure, because it varies depending on different factors such as emotions and physical activity.

An important note is that hypertension and edema can affect patients concurrently. Edema results from the excessive amount of fluid that is retained in the body tissues (see Chapter 21). This extra fluid must be pumped throughout the body system, which causes vasoconstriction. Drugs such as angiotensin-converting enzyme (ACE) inhibitors can reduce edema by blocking certain hor-

BOX 22-3 CLASSIFICATION OF BLOOD PRESSURE MEASUREMENTS

First or Top Measurement (Systolic Blood Pressure)
Normal: less than or equal to 115 mm Hg
Prehypertensive state: between 120 and 140 mm Hg
High: greater than 160 mm Hg

Second or Bottom Measurement (Diastolic Pressure)
Pre-hypertensive state: between 80 and 90 mm Hg
Mild hypertension: 90 to 100 mm Hg
Moderate hypertension: 105 to 115 mm Hg
Severe hypertension: greater than 115 mm Hg

mones and peptides. This reduces the production of excess fluid and lowers vaso-constriction. Diuretics can lower hypertension by reducing the reabsorption of sodium and water by the kidneys. This results in lowering circulating fluid volume.

Transient Ischemic Attacks and Strokes

TIAs are caused by a short duration of a reduction of oxygen to the brain and are caused by atherosclerotic cerebrovascular disease. The plaque causes narrowing of the blood vessels, which causes a reduction of blood flow. If this plaque increases into a blood clot, a thrombosis is created. This eventually may close off the vessel. TIAs are almost the same as ischemic attacks, except the duration is much shorter. Transient attacks may last only a few minutes or many times over a span of a day. TIAs sometimes are referred to as ministrokes and are thought of as a possible precursor to a stroke.

Two types of strokes are an ischemic (clot) stroke or a hemorrhagic (bleeding) stroke. Hemorrhagic strokes are caused by weakened vessels or aneurysms in the brain that cause a vessel to rupture. When a vessel is ruptured, blood flows into areas of the brain causing damage along with the damage caused by the lack of oxygenated blood for the parts of the brain that are needed. Most of the symptoms of TIAs and strokes may appear rapidly. All of these lead to symptoms such as vision or hearing problems, weakness on one or both sides of the body, dizziness, slurred speech, and sudden severe headache. One of the main chronic causes of TIAs and strokes is high blood pressure (hypertension). Besides hypertension, other contributing factors may lead to the likelihood of a stroke. Persons with diabetes, high cholesterol, heart problems, and obesity run a higher risk. Also certain lifestyle habits such as smoking, lack of exercise, and excessive alcohol intake also can add to the damage of the vessels in the body system.

Angina Pectoris

Angina pectoris results from a decrease in blood flow to the heart, which results in pain in the chest. These pains can vary from minor to severe. Decreased blood flow can be caused by factors such as hardening of the arteries (atherosclerosis), hypertension, cigarette smoking, and diabetes. Environmental and genetic influences also can play a role in acquiring angina (chest pain). Three types of angina are the following:

1. Classic angina
2. Variant angina
3. Unstable angina

In classic angina the patient can experience short ischemic episodes of pain, in which a mild deficiency of oxygen has occurred. Patients may feel as though there is a weight on the chest accompanied with a sharp pain. This pain can occur in the chest, neck, arms, teeth, and jaw. Many times this type of an anginal attack occurs after exercise or excessive activity.

Another type of angina is variant angina. This type may not be related to atherosclerosis; instead the patient experiences spasms of the coronary artery. This is painful and may occur even at rest.

The third type is unstable angina, which may worsen in a person with a known history of anginal attacks. Unstable angina is caused mainly by obstruction of the arteries, which increases over many years.

All three types of anginal pain are treated with medications such as nitrates. In addition to medications, the patient may be required to make certain lifestyle changes that may decrease these attacks. In addition, surgery may be performed to bypass the blockage.

Myocardial Infarction

If coronary blood flow to an area of the heart becomes entirely blocked because of a thrombus or embolism, that area of heart muscle cannot receive the necessary oxygen. This results in the death of that part of the muscle. Depending on the severity of the blockage, the patient may have an MI from which he or she can recover over time or a massive MI that weakens the heart permanently or may even result in death.

Arrhythmias

A person with coronary artery disease can develop arrhythmias (irregular heartbeats), also known as dysrhythmias. As previously discussed in the section on the conduction system, the heart beats in a rhythm. This is done via special fibers that run throughout the heart. The pacemaker is located in the sinoatrial node. Many factors influence the efficient working of the pacemaker, including chemical balance. If an imbalance results from chemicals or oxygen, then irregular heartbeats can occur. Most patients receive short-term treatment in the emergency room. Once stabilized, the patient may be sent home. If so, long-term medications can be given to help keep the heart beating regularly.

Congestive Heart Failure

Congestive heart failure (CHF) is usually a progressive disease. Effective treatments are available to help patients with CHF, but there is no cure. A common heart disease of older persons, CHF occurs when the heart cannot pump as vigorously, thus delivering less blood throughout the body. Edema complicates CHF because the kidneys compensate for the lack of blood flow by retaining more fluid in the body. This fluid adds more work for the heart, further weakening it.

Thrombosis

When bleeding occurs, the body prevents bleeding to death by forming blood clots. Clotting is a normal body function aimed at stopping hemorrhage and starting the healing process. Unfortunately, our bodies also can form unwanted blood clots that can appear in areas such as the heart or brain. This clotting can occur because of an overactive clotting mechanism or narrowing of the arteries, such as those in persons with atherosclerosis. An obstructed blood vessel to the brain can cause a stroke (also known as a brain attack). When it strikes the heart muscle, it can cause an MI, or heart attack.

An embolus is a blood clot that has broken away from the thrombus (main clot) and has traveled through the body to another area where it can become lodged and create a blockage. The body produces chemicals that prevent clotting. Sometimes, however, the body needs additional help in preventing blood clots. This is when prophylactic treatment would be given. A prophylactic is an agent or treatment that is aimed at prevention, in this case preventing a clot.

Hypotension

A person suffering from hypotension has low blood pressure as opposed to high blood pressure. A common problem that persons can experience is orthostatic hypotension. This is caused by standing up quickly from a sitting or lying position. This occurs because a large amount of blood remains in the lower extremities. When one stands quickly, the blood returning to the heart is decreased considerably, and the body responds by raising the heartbeat, compensating for the lack of blood flow. This results in a feeling of lightheadedness. Side effects of hypotension include syncope (fainting) and/or vertigo (dizziness). For persons who suffer often from this condition, physicians may recommend midodrine, which causes vasoconstriction, raising the blood pressure.

Treatments and Medications for the Cardiovascular System

TREATMENT OF HYPERLIPIDEMIA

Because hyperlipidemia is known to lead to atherosclerosis, it is important to obtain an accurate cholesterol level. Factors such as family history and lifestyle are important parts of the assessment as well. These may indicate the likelihood of experiencing further problems. Through diet and exercise, many persons can lower their lipid content. On occasion a physician may suggest niacin, which is available over-the-counter to lower the cholesterol. For persons at high risk because of family history or those who have high levels that do not decrease through diet and exercise, other agents are available (referred to as antihyperlipidemics). In severe cases, bypass surgery may be indicated for those persons who might not be responding to medications and lifestyle changes or those who have had an MI.

Antihyperlipidemics

The classes of drugs that make up the antihyperlipidemics include the bile acid sequestrants and hydroxymethylglutaryl-coenzyme A (HMG-CoA) reductase inhibitors. Bile acid sequestrants, such as cholestyramine, increase the loss of cholesterol, specifically LDL, through *increased* defecation. Many agents effectively help reduce cholesterol in this manner. HMG-CoA reductase agents such as lovastatin, simvastatin, and pravastatin are referred to as the *statins*. They specifically inhibit an enzyme responsible for one of the first steps in the overall conversion of fats into cholesterol. They raise the HDL level and decrease the LDL and VLDL cholesterol levels. Other agents, such as gemfibrozil, work specifically to lower VLDL cholesterol levels by inhibiting the extraction of free fatty acids, which reduces the ability of the liver to produce triglycerides. This agent also increases HDL; however, the specific mechanism of action is not well known. Nicotinic acid (over-the-counter agent) reduces cholesterol, triglyceride, and VLDL levels, which leads to an overall decrease in LDL levels; the exact mechanism is not well known. The recommended maintenance dose for an adult is listed in the following.

BILE ACID SEQUESTRANTS

GENERIC NAME: cholestyramine
TRADE NAME: Questran
ROUTE OF ADMINISTRATION: oral (powder)

COMMON DOSAGE: 4 g qd or bid
SIDE EFFECTS: constipation, flatulence
AUXILIARY LABELS:

- Do not chew or crush tablets.
- Take before meals.

SPECIAL NOTE: Powder form should be mixed into 60 to 180 mL of liquid. Other medications should be taken 4 to 6 hours apart from cholestyramine to avoid interference of absorption.

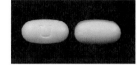

GENERIC NAME: colestipol
TRADE NAME: Colestid
ROUTE OF ADMINISTRATION: oral
COMMON DOSAGE: 5 to 30 g per day (may be given in divided doses)
SIDE EFFECTS: constipation, flatulence
AUXILIARY LABELS:

- Do not chew or crush tablets.
- Take before meals.

SPECIAL NOTE: Powder form should be mixed into at least 90 mL of liquid. Other medications should be taken 4 to 6 hours apart from cholestyramine to avoid interference of absorption.

HMG-COA REDUCTASE INHIBITORS

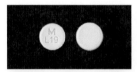

GENERIC NAME: lovastatin
TRADE NAME: Mevacor
ROUTE OF ADMINISTRATION: oral
COMMON DOSAGE: 10 to 80 mg daily in single or divided doses
SIDE EFFECTS: may cause photosensitivity, gastrointestinal upset
AUXILIARY LABELS:

- May cause photosensitivity.
- Take with meals.

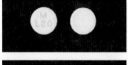
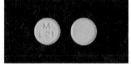

GENERIC NAME: simvastatin
TRADE NAME: Zocor
ROUTE OF ADMINISTRATION: oral
COMMON DOSAGE: 5 to 40 mg qd
SIDE EFFECTS: may cause photosensitivity
AUXILIARY LABEL:

- May cause photosensitivity.

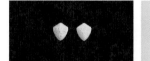
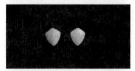
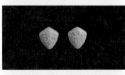
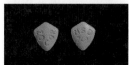
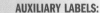
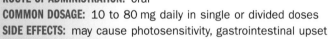

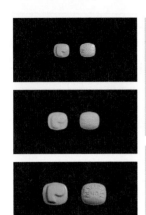

GENERIC NAME: pravastatin
TRADE NAME: Pravachol
ROUTE OF ADMINISTRATION: oral
COMMON DOSAGE: 10 to 40 mg qd at bedtime
SIDE EFFECTS: may cause photosensitivity
AUXILIARY LABEL:
■ May cause photosensitivity.

GENERIC NAME: atorvastatin
TRADE NAME: Lipitor
ROUTE OF ADMINISTRATION: oral
COMMON DOSAGE: 10 to 80 mg qd
SIDE EFFECTS: may cause photosensitivity
AUXILIARY LABEL:
■ May cause photosensitivity.

FIBRIC ACID ANTIHYPERLIPIDEMIC

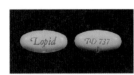

GENERIC NAME: gemfibrozil
TRADE NAME: Lopid
ROUTE OF ADMINISTRATION: oral
COMMON DOSAGE: 600 mg bid, before morning and evening meals
SIDE EFFECTS: may cause dizziness, blurred vision
AUXILIARY LABEL:
■ May cause dizziness.

MISCELLANEOUS ANTIHYPERLIPIDEMIC

GENERIC NAME: nicotinic acid
TRADE NAME: Niaspan RX (niacin over the counter [read package insert for dosage])
ROUTE OF ADMINISTRATION: oral
COMMON DOSAGE: 1 to 2 g tid with or following meals
SIDE EFFECTS: may cause photosensitivity
AUXILIARY LABEL:
■ May cause photosensitivity.

TREATMENT OF ARRHYTHMIAS

The medications used in treating arrhythmias are called antiarrhythmic agents. Quinidine sulfate, procainamide, disopyramide, and verapamil are common agents that may be prescribed. See the following for a complete list of medications and their indications. In severe cases in which medications cannot correct the continuing problem of arrhythmias, a pacemaker implant may be the only alternative.

Drug Action

All of these antiarrhythmic agents work on the conduction system and induce regular heartbeats. Lidocaine is used in an emergency situation to treat arrhythmias resulting from MIs and other conditions. Quinidine sulfate and procainamide slow down the speed of the conduction system and are used for tachycardias (rapid heartbeat) and other arrhythmias. The injectable form of

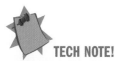

TECH NOTE!

Serious medication errors can occur because of the similar names of quinidine and quinine. Quinine is an antimalarial agent; quinidine is a cardiac agent. These two medications often sit close to one another on a pharmacy shelf and have been mistaken for one another. This can result in a dangerous error.

procainamide normally is used in life-threatening tachycardia episodes in an emergency. Disopyramide slows the heart rate. Again, the injectable form is used in life-threatening tachycardias similar to procainamide. Verapamil slows the conduction system at the atrioventricular node and stabilizes cardiac rhythm.

ANTIARRHYTHMICS

GENERIC NAME: quinidine sulfate, quinidine gluconate
TRADE NAME: Quinidex (oral), Quinalan (intravenous)
ROUTE OF ADMINISTRATION: sulfate, gluconate (injection [intramuscular, intravenous]), and polygalacturonate (oral tablets)
COMMON DOSAGE: 200 to 300 mg tid or qid
SIDE EFFECTS: gastrointestinal upset; do not crush or chew sustained-release tablets
AUXILIARY LABELS:
- Do not break or chew tablet.
- Take with food.
- Take as directed.

GENERIC NAME: procainamide
TRADE NAME: Pronestyl
ROUTE OF ADMINISTRATION: oral, injection (intramuscular, intravenous)
COMMON DOSAGE: to be determined by physician based on weight and age of patient
SIDE EFFECTS: no major effects unless patient does not adhere to dosing schedule
AUXILIARY LABEL:
- Take as directed.

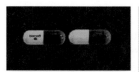
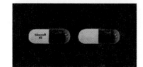

GENERIC NAME: disopyramide
TRADE NAME: Norpace CR (capsules, extended-release)
ROUTE OF ADMINISTRATION: oral
COMMON DOSAGE: 100 to 200 mg q6h or 300 mg CR q12h
SIDE EFFECTS: dry mouth, dizziness, difficulty urinating, constipation, blurred vision
AUXILIARY LABELS:
- Do not break or chew tablet.
- May cause dizziness.
- Take as directed.

GENERIC NAME: Lidocaine
TRADE NAME: Xylocaine
INDICATION: acute management of ventricular arrhythmias
ROUTE OF ADMINISTRATION: injection or intravenous drip
COMMON DOSAGE: for intravenous infusion, 50 to 100 mg at a rate of 25 to 50 mg/min
SPECIAL NOTE: This medication is kept in emergency rooms and other areas where crash carts are located. These carts are used in code blue situations. In the emergency department and intensive care units, a code blue occurs when a patient is having a heart attack or stops breathing.

TREATMENT OF CONGESTIVE HEART FAILURE

The most common treatment for CHF is cardioglycosides. The only one available in the United States is digoxin. Diuretics also commonly are used in addition to glycosides to treat the edema that normally accompanies CHF.

Drug Action
Cardioglycosides increase the forcefulness of the pumping of the heart but not the oxygen requirements. Specifically, it inhibits the sodium-potassium pump,

which works within the heart to increase contractility. In arrhythmias, a suppression of the atrioventricular node increases regularity of the heartbeat and decreases conduction speed and force (velocity); thus (in both cases) the heart works smarter, not harder. Patients must take their medications exactly as directed. Diuretics often are prescribed concurrently. They increase urine output, thus decreasing the overall fluid retention (see Chapter 21) and allowing the heart to work more easily.

CARDIAC GLYCOSIDE

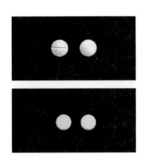

GENERIC NAME: digoxin
TRADE NAME: Lanoxin
INDICATIONS: treatment of CHF and certain arrhythmias
ROUTE OF ADMINISTRATION: oral, injection (intravenous, intramuscular)
COMMON DOSAGE: 0.125 to 0.25 mg (this dosage must be based on body weight and normal renal function for age of patient)
SIDE EFFECTS: nausea and vomiting, diarrhea, dizziness
AUXILIARY LABELS:
- Take as prescribed.
- Do not stop taking medication without consulting physician.

SPECIAL NOTE: The antidote for an overdose of digoxin is Digibind (digoxin immune Fab). This agent binds to the digoxin molecule, and it then is excreted from the body. This treatment must be done in the emergency department and is available in injectable form only.

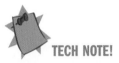

TECH NOTE!
The pharmacy tech should reinforce the fact that the pulse should be taken each day before taking digitalis. If the pulse is less than 60, the patient should call a physician before taking the medicine.

Diuretics Used for Congestive Heart Failure–Related Edema. Different diuretic agents can be used to help reduce edema. With thiazides and loop diuretics, an important consideration is the large amount of potassium lost in the urine. For this reason, both classes of drugs may be supplemented with potassium. Diuretics also are given along with one or more of the listed agents to decrease the effects of sodium retention. Frequent urination leading to a decrease in edema is the main outcome with the use of diuretics. A major side effect of certain diuretics is the loss of potassium along with the urine. An example is the agent hydrochlorothiazide. However, some agents are known as *potassium sparing*. These include agents such as triamterene and hydrochlorothiazide and others listed in Box 22-4. A maximum of two examples of each type of diuretic is given because a more extensive list is provided in Chapter 21.

Thiazides. Thiazide agents are used to increase urinary excretion. They are indicated for use in patients with edema resulting from CHF, hypertension, and other conditions. Their side effects are similar and include frequent urination, gastrointestinal upset, and possible photosensitivity. The auxiliary label of each medication is noted along with the normal dosage for an adult at maintenance.

BOX 22-4 CLASSIFICATION OF DIURETIC AGENTS

Thiazides
Loop diuretics
Potassium-sparing diuretics
Carbonic anhydrase inhibitors
Osmotic diuretics

THAZIDE AND THAZIDE-LIKE DIURETICS

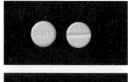
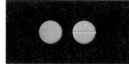

GENERIC NAME: chlorothiazide
TRADE NAME: Diuril
ROUTE OF ADMINISTRATION: oral, injection (intravenous, intramuscular)
COMMON DOSAGE: 0.5 to 1 g qd or bid
AUXILIARY LABELS:

- Take with food or milk.
- May cause photosensitivity.

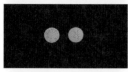
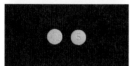

GENERIC NAME: metolazone
TRADE NAME: Zaroxolyn
ROUTE OF ADMINISTRATION: oral
COMMON DOSAGE: 2.5 to 5 mg qd
AUXILIARY LABELS:

- Take with food or milk.
- May cause photosensitivity.

Loop diuretics. Loop diuretics work specifically in the loop of Henle within the renal tubules (see Chapter 21). They work rapidly and cause large amounts of urine to be excreted. They often are prescribed for patients who have edema caused by CHF and hypertension. Their side effects include increase in urination, possible gastrointestinal upset, orthostatic hypotension, and photosensitivity. Because these agents work rapidly, it is advised that the patient take them in the morning or early in the day.

LOOP DIURETICS

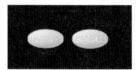
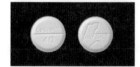
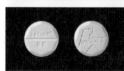

GENERIC NAME: furosemide
TRADE NAME: Lasix
ROUTE OF ADMINISTRATION: oral, injection (intravenous, intramuscular)
COMMON DOSAGE: 20 to 80 mg qd
AUXILIARY LABELS:

- Take with food or milk.
- May cause photosensitivity.

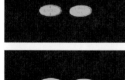
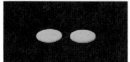

GENERIC NAME: bumetanide
TRADE NAME: Bumex
ROUTE OF ADMINISTRATION: oral, injection (intramuscular, intravenous)
COMMON DOSAGE: 0.5 to 2 mg qd
AUXILIARY LABELS:

- Take with food or milk.
- May cause photosensitivity.

Potassium-sparing diuretics. Potassium-sparing agents work to eliminate urine by way of interrupting the sodium reabsorption within the distal tubules of the kidney. Because of their place of action, they do not cause a large amount of potassium to be excreted along with the urine. Their side effects are similar to other diuretics with possible gastrointestinal upset, but they also may

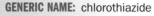

cause dizziness, drowsiness, headache, and diarrhea. Following are a few commonly used agents.

POTASSIUM-SPARING DIURETICS

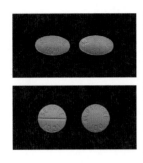

GENERIC NAME: spironolactone
TRADE NAME: Aldactone
ROUTE OF ADMINISTRATION: oral
COMMON DOSAGE: 50 to 100 mg qd
AUXILIARY LABELS:

- Take with food or milk.
- May cause dizziness and drowsiness.

GENERIC NAME: triamterene
TRADE NAME: Dyrenium
ROUTE OF ADMINISTRATION: oral
COMMON DOSAGE: 100 mg bid
AUXILIARY LABEL:

- Take after meals.

Carbonic anhydrase inhibitors. Carbonic anhydrase inhibitors specifically inhibit the enzyme carbonic anhydrase. These agents work to reduce edema by inhibiting the hydrogen ion secretion by the renal tubule, which causes the loss of ions such as sodium and potassium. Acetazolamide also is used to reduce intraocular pressure, which is the cause of glaucoma (see Chapter 19).

CARBONIC ANHYDRASE INHIBITOR

GENERIC NAME: acetazolamide
TRADE NAME: Diamox
ROUTE OF ADMINISTRATION: oral, injection (intramuscular, intravenous), topical (otic)
COMMON DOSAGE: 250 to 375 mg qd
AUXILIARY LABELS:

- Take with food or milk.
- May cause photosensitivity.
- May cause dizziness and drowsiness.

Osmotic diuretics. Osmotic diuretic agents eliminate excess water weight by increasing the osmolarity of the glomerular filtrate, which has the effect of decreasing tubular reabsorption of water. Certain agents such as mannitol are available in injection only and can be used for intraocular pressure and for edema caused by acute renal failure and when the glomerular filtration is dangerously reduced. It is recommended that mannitol be filtered before use to prevent possible crystallization of solution from being injected into patient.

OSMOTIC DIURETIC

GENERIC NAME: mannitol
TRADE NAME: Osmitrol
ROUTE OF ADMINISTRATION: injection (intravenous)
COMMON DOSAGE: usual adult dose ranges from 20 to 200 g over a 24-hour period
AUXILIARY LABEL:

- None: given in the hospital

TREATMENT OF HYPERTENSION

Treatment of hypertension is given by a step care approach. The four steps are based on the severity of the condition. As shown in an example in Table 22-1, diet

TABLE 22-1 Example of Four-Step Approach to Controlling High Blood Pressure

Therapy	Medication
Step 1	
Separate or in combination	
Weight reduction*	None
Step 2	
Angiotensin-converting enzyme inhibitors	captopril
β-blockers	propranolol
Calcium channel blockers	verapamil
Diuretics	furosemide
Step 3: Additional Medication	
Adrenergic blockers	clonidine
Step 4: Additional Medication	
Vasodilators	hydralazine

*A change in diet is indicated regardless of which medications are used. Fat consumption, salty foods, and foods containing tyramine should be decreased. Often fluid restriction also may be recommended.

usually is indicated with or without medication because foods high in fat, sodium, or tyramine are a leading contributor to hypertension. The main agents used for high blood pressure are antihypertensive medications such as methyldopa, doxazosin, clonidine, terazosin, and prazosin. Other agents used to treat high blood pressure include diuretics and vasodilators. Persons who have high blood pressure are not always aware of their condition because of the lack of signs or symptoms. Therefore, compliance in taking medication as directed can be a problem. Because they do not physically feel bad, patients do not take their medications.

Reducing salt intake and alcohol consumption, as well as exercising and abstaining from smoking, has been proved to reduce hypertension, therefore reducing the workload on the heart. However, even with these types of interventions, hypertension still may not be controlled. If medication is required to control hypertension, the initial drug therapy may include diuretics. Along with a diuretic there are many medications available that are effective in controlling hypertension, including ACE inhibitors, β-blockers, and calcium channel blockers. These medications are covered separately, including their drug action, side effects, and commonly used auxiliary labels on prescription vials.

Hypertension and hyperlipidemia go hand in hand in many cases. Several combination drugs are being added constantly to the list of antihypertensive and antilipidemic drugs to treat both conditions at the same time. Combination drugs in general allow for better compliance by the patient. If the patient has fewer medications to take, the patient is more likely to take them. Table 22-2 gives a quick sample of the various combination drugs.

TREATMENT OF TRANSIENT ISCHEMIC ATTACKS AND STROKES

TIAs are treated by improving arterial blood flow to the brain so that a stroke can be avoided. If a patient shows TIA symptoms, certain diagnostic tests can be done to determine the likelihood of more TIAs or even an impending stroke. The use of computed tomography or magnetic resonance imaging scans are common diagnostic tests given. A computed tomography scan shows whether a clot is present and whether it is ischemic or hemorrhagic. Magnetic resonance imaging is used to diagnose brain vessel abnormalities that may be involved in a hemorrhagic stroke. In the case of a TIA, patients may be treated with hypertension medication such as aspirin, to decrease the risk of platelets clumping

TABLE 22-2 **Combination Drugs**

Trade name	Dosage form	Strength
Antihypertensives		
Apresazide	Capsule	Hydralazine 25 mg/hydrochlorothiazide (HCTZ) 25 mg and 50/50 capsules
Hydromox R	Tablet	Quinethazone 50 mg/reserpine 0.125 mg*
Inderide LA	Capsule	Propanolol HCl 160 mg/HCTZ 50 mg
Antihypertensives/Antilipemics		
Caduet	Tablet	Amlodipine 5 mg/atorvastatin 10 mg
Diupres 250	Tablet	Chlorothiazide 500 mg/reserpine 0.125 mg*
Diuretics		
Dyazide	Capsule	Triamterene 37.5 mg/HCTZ 25 mg
Maxzide	Tablet	Triamterene 75 mg/HCTZ 50 mg*
Moduretic	Tablet	Amiloride HCl 5 mg/HCTZ 50 mg
Lipid-Lowering Agent		
Pravigard	Tablet	Pravastatin 20 mg/buffered aspirin 81 mg

*Available in additional strengths.

together that can form a clot, or with anticoagulants such as warfarin. Usually the last resort is surgery to remove the arterial plaque.

The main agents used to treat a stroke in progress would be thrombolytics such as tissue plasminogen activator if indicated because of a clot. Although many medications are used to prevent the onset of a TIA or stroke, there are not many medications to reduce the effects of them once they have occurred. Nonfatal strokes are one of the most common causes of disability, causing possible brain damage and lengthy physical therapy. Through lengthy rehabilitation, sometimes the unaffected portion of the brain can learn to take over the functions that were lost because of the stroke. The following is one agent used specifically to reduce vascular spasms in the cerebral arteries during a stroke. More information on thrombolytics is given later in this chapter.

CALCIUM CHANNEL BLOCKER

GENERIC NAME: nimodipine
TRADE NAME: Nimotop
INDICATION: reduce spasms following TIA or stroke
ROUTE OF ADMINISTRATION: oral, injection (intravenous)
COMMON DOSAGE: oral, 30-mg capsules; or if the patient cannot take it orally, extract the contents in the capsule with an 18-gauge syringe and give intravenously, flushing it with 30 mL of normal saline afterward
AUXILIARY LABEL:
■ Protect from light.

THE ABCS OF HEART MEDICATIONS

Because many different agents are used to treat heart conditions, such as coronary artery disease and hypertension, it is important to learn about the medications and to remember the information. An easy way of remembering the types of medications used to treat the heart conditions discussed in this chapter is to remember "ABCs." This stands for the common classifications of agents used to treat heart conditions. Although more classifications of agents are available, this is a simplified way to begin to remember them.

Angiotensin-Converting Enzyme Agents (ACE Inhibitors)

ACE inhibitors are a set of agents that help reduce blood pressure by causing a decrease of pressure in the arteries. Certain enzymes produced by the kidneys ultimately help produce ACE, which increases sodium content. This allows for further increases of fluid retention. ACE inhibitors stop these enzymes from causing vasoconstriction that normally would result in high blood pressure caused by the sodium imbalance. Side effects for ACE inhibitors may include headache, hypotension, nausea, or vomiting.

ACE AGENTS

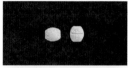
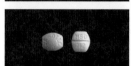
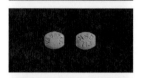
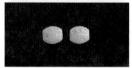

GENERIC NAME: enalapril
TRADE NAME: Vasotec
INDICATION: mild to severe hypertension
ROUTE OF ADMINISTRATION: oral, injection (intravenous)
COMMON DOSAGE: oral, 10 to 40 mg qd or bid (divided doses) for hypertension
AUXILIARY LABEL:
- Take as directed.

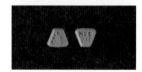

GENERIC NAME: lisinopril
TRADE NAME: Prinivil, Zestril
INDICATION: hypertension
ROUTE OF ADMINISTRATION: oral
COMMON DOSAGE: oral, 40 mg qd
AUXILIARY LABEL:
- Take as directed.

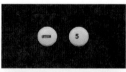
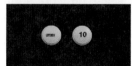

GENERIC NAME: benazepril
TRADE NAME: Lotensin
INDICATION: hypertension
ROUTE OF ADMINISTRATION: oral
COMMON DOSAGE: 20 to 40 mg qd or bid
AUXILIARY LABEL:
- May cause dizziness or drowsiness.

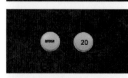
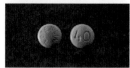

GENERIC NAME: captopril
TRADE NAME: Capoten
INDICATION: hypertension
ROUTE OF ADMINISTRATION: oral
COMMON DOSAGE: 25 mg bid or tid
AUXILIARY LABELS:
- Take before meals.
- May cause dizziness or drowsiness.

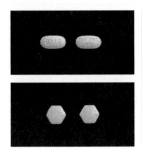

GENERIC NAME: fosinopril
TRADE NAME: Monopril
INDICATION: hypertension
ROUTE OF ADMINISTRATION: oral
COMMON DOSAGE: 20 to 40 mg qd
AUXILIARY LABELS:
- Take before meals.
- May cause dizziness.

Angiotensin II Receptor Antagonists

Angiotensin II receptor antagonists work by inhibiting the effects of angiotensin II receptors located in vascular muscles. This in turn lowers blood pressure via antagonistic effects on vasoconstriction. These agents have no major side effects.

ANGIOTENSIN II RECEPTOR ANTAGONISTS

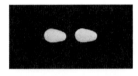

GENERIC NAME: losartan
TRADE NAME: Cozaar
ROUTE OF ADMINISTRATION: oral
COMMON DOSAGE: 50 mg qd
AUXILIARY LABEL:
- Take as directed.

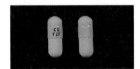

GENERIC NAME: valsartan
TRADE NAME: Diovan
ROUTE OF ADMINISTRATION: oral
COMMON DOSAGE: 80 to 320 mg qd
AUXILIARY LABEL:
- Take as directed.

β-Blocking Agents

β-Blockers are a set of agents that are effective because they block various enzymes, such as epinephrine, that can cause high blood pressure. β-Blockers work at two sites, the β_1 and β_2 receptor sites. β_1 Receptors are located in the heart, whereas β_2 receptors are located in the lungs and deep arteries. The actions of medications can be specific or nonspecific. Nonspecific agents affect β_1 and β_2 sites.

A nonspecific agent would not be recommended if a person were suffering from asthma or another type of respiratory problem. When β_2 sites are inhibited, breathing airways can be restricted; therefore the physician must determine the appropriate agent for the patient. Side effects include dizziness, hypotension, and diarrhea.

β-BLOCKING AGENTS

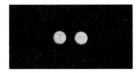

GENERIC NAME: atenolol
TRADE NAME: Tenormin
INDICATIONS: hypertension, angina pectoris, after MI

ROUTE OF ADMINISTRATION: oral, injection (intravenous)
COMMON DOSAGE: 50 mg qd
AUXILIARY LABELS:

■ Take as directed.
■ May cause dizziness.

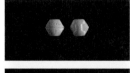
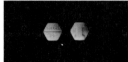

GENERIC NAME: propranolol
TRADE NAME: Inderal
INDICATIONS: hypertension, angina, arrhythmias, and migraines
ROUTE OF ADMINISTRATION: oral, injection (intravenous)
COMMON DOSAGE: for hypertension, 40 mg bid
AUXILIARY LABELS:

■ Take as directed.
■ May cause dizziness.

GENERIC NAME: metoprolol
TRADE NAME: Lopressor
INDICATIONS: hypertension, angina pectoris, arrhythmias
ROUTE OF ADMINISTRATION: oral, injection (intravenous)
COMMON DOSAGE: oral, 100 to 450 mg per day in divided doses, either bid or tid
AUXILIARY LABELS:

■ Take as directed.
■ May cause dizziness.

GENERIC NAME: pindolol
TRADE NAME: Visken
INDICATION: hypertension
ROUTE OF ADMINISTRATION: oral
COMMON DOSAGE: maximum of 60 mg daily
AUXILIARY LABELS:

■ Take as directed.
■ May cause dizziness.

GENERIC NAME: acebutolol
TRADE NAME: Sectral
INDICATIONS: hypertension, ventricular arrhythmias
ROUTE OF ADMINISTRATION: oral
COMMON DOSAGE: 400 to 800 mg qd
AUXILIARY LABEL:

■ Take as directed.

Calcium Channel Blockers

Calcium channel blockers work by decreasing calcium intake by the heart and blood vessels. Calcium is used by the heart to stimulate the conduction system (the electrical pump). When the calcium channel is blocked by these agents, the heart rate slows, which decreases stress on the heart muscle. Common side effects include dizziness, drowsiness, and blurred vision in varying degrees depending on the specific agent.

CALCIUM CHANNEL BLOCKERS

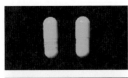
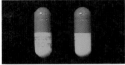
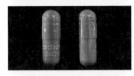

GENERIC NAME: diltiazem
TRADE NAME: Cardizem CD
INDICATIONS: angina pectoris, chronic stable angina, essential hypertension
ROUTE OF ADMINISTRATION: oral, injection (intravenous)
COMMON DOSAGE: oral, for hypertension, 180 to 360 mg daily in divided doses, either 3 or 4 times a day
AUXILIARY LABELS:
- Take as directed.
- Do not crush or chew tablet (for sustained-released tablets).

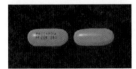
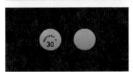
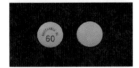

GENERIC NAME: nifedipine
TRADE NAME: Procardia, Adalat
INDICATIONS: chronic stable angina, hypertension
ROUTE OF ADMINISTRATION: oral
COMMON DOSAGE: for hypertension, 30 or 60 mg qd
AUXILIARY LABELS:
- Take as directed.
- Do not chew or break tablet (for sustained-release tablets).

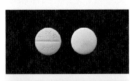
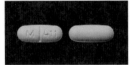

GENERIC NAME: verapamil
TRADE NAME: Calan, Isoptin
INDICATIONS: angina, chronic atrial flutter or fibrillation, essential hypertension
ROUTE OF ADMINISTRATION: oral, injection (intravenous)
COMMON DOSAGE: oral, for hypertension, 80 mg tid; for sustained release, 120 or 240 mg qd
AUXILIARY LABELS:
- Take with food.
- Take as directed.

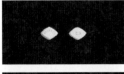
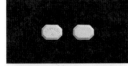

GENERIC NAME: amlodipine
TRADE NAME: Norvasc
INDICATIONS: hypertension, chronic stable angina, variant angina
ROUTE OF ADMINISTRATION: oral
COMMON DOSAGE: for hypertension, 5 to 10 mg qd
AUXILIARY LABEL:
- Take as directed.

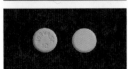

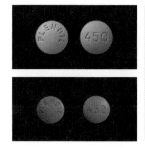

GENERIC NAME: felodipine
TRADE NAME: Plendil
INDICATION: hypertension
ROUTE OF ADMINISTRATION: oral
COMMON DOSAGE: 2.5 to 10 mg qd
AUXILIARY LABELS:

- Take as directed.
- Do not crush or chew tablet.

TREATMENT OF ANGINAL ATTACKS

Nitrates, calcium channel blockers, and β-blockers commonly are used to treat anginal attacks. Probably one of the most prescribed antianginal agents is nitroglycerin. Millions of individuals carry nitroglycerin sublingual tablets in their pockets or purses in the event of an anginal attack. Nitroglycerin has many dosage forms, including capsules, topical patches, paste, and sublingual spray. The sublingual tablets and injectable forms are used for emergencies.

Drug Action

Nitrates are vasodilators that dilate the arteries to permit an increase of blood flow through the heart muscle. They also reduce the workload of the heart. Because more oxygenated blood is allowed to enter the arteries, less blood is returned to the heart, thereby decreasing the workload. Isosorbide and nitroglycerin are the two agents used for the treatment of angina. Both agents are available as sublingual tablets, which are effective because of their rapid absorption; the medication bypasses the gastrointestinal system and enters directly into the bloodstream for a more rapid onset of action. The sublingual route has several benefits. First, the drug is not inactivated by stomach acid (many medications are rendered less active because of the low pH of the stomach). Second, the sublingual route provides faster onset of action (oral medications usually take at least 20 to 30 minutes to work, which is too long for a patient experiencing severe chest pain). Figure 22-5 shows a common prescription order.

Doctor David Gall
1000 Archway
St. Louis, MO
ph: 816-555-5555

Patient name: _B. Jones-Lewis_
Address: _106 Nutree Way_ Date: _1-30-03_

℞: NTG 0.4mg sl #100

Take 1 sl q 5 min x3

if no relief call 911

Dy. Gall
Dr. Signature

Refills: _6_ DEA # _____

FIGURE 22-5 Nitroglycerin sublingual tablet prescription.

TABLE 22-3 Common Nitrate Agents

Trade name	Generic name	Dosage form	Normal usage
Tridil	nitroglycerin	Injectable	Emergency
Ntg in D$_5$W	nitroglycerin	Injection solution	Emergency
Nitrostat	nitroglycerin	Sublingual tablets	Emergency
Nitrogard	nitroglycerin	Buccal tablets	Routine medication
Nitrong	nitroglycerin	Sustained-release tablets	Routine medication
Nitro-Bid	nitroglycerin	Sustained-release capsules	Routine medication
Nitro-Dur, Transderm	nitroglycerin	Nitroglycerin patches	Routine medication
Nitro-Bid	nitroglycerin	Ointment 2% with papers	Routine medication
Monoket, ISMO	isosorbide mononitrate	Tablets, extended-release tablets	Routine medication
Isordil	isosorbide dinitrate	Sublingual tablets, chewable tablets	Emergency
Sorbitrate, Isordil	isosorbide dinitrate	Tablets, capsules, sustained-release tablets	Routine medication

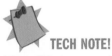

TECH NOTE!

When filling a prescription for nitroglycerin, never take the tablets out of the glass container in which they come. Instead, place the glass container within a larger plastic vial on which the label is attached. Other containers include the box type, which holds four small glass vials each containing 25 tablets and which has a space on the box for the drug label.

Nitroglycerin is good for only 6 months after opening the container. In addition, it must be kept in a dry area and in a light-protected glass container to prevent the active agent from breaking down. Table 22-3 provides a list of the nitrate agents and their dosage forms. Sublingual dosages are kept at the patient's bedside for emergency relief of angina attacks. The nitroglycerin transdermal patches normally are applied once daily in the morning and are taken off at bedtime to decrease the possibility of tolerance to the medication. Ointment tubes are available in 60-g, 30-g, and 1-g unit dose sizes. The ointment also comes with papers premarked in half-inch increments for delivering the proper amount of ointment. The ointment is squeezed onto the paper in increments of $1/2$ inch to 2 inches, similar to toothpaste placed on a toothbrush. The translingual spray is used if an anginal attack occurs. The patient sprays one or two metered doses under the tongue with a maximum of three sprays in a 15-minute period.

TREATMENT OF BLOOD CLOTS

Drug Action of Anticoagulants and Thrombolytics

Clots are formed by fibrin, a type of binding string that holds blood cells together. Heparin converts blood-clotting fibrin into another substance like warfarin does. Each drug works at a different site within the body and blocks the formation of blood clots. However, once a clot is formed, heparin, warfarin (Coumadin), or aspirin cannot be used for treatment. A thrombolytic must be administered as soon as possible.

The medications used for a thrombosis are emergency agents that include streptokinase, urokinase, and tissue plasminogen activator. The dosage forms of these agents are injectable only and are kept in areas within a hospital such as emergency, surgery, and intensive care units. A patient normally does not need more than one dose, and the sooner the drug is administered to the patient, the better the outcome.

To prevent blood from coagulating (binding together), anticoagulants may be prescribed. Two kinds of anticoagulants are heparin and warfarin. Heparin is available in injectable form only. Heparin inhibits thrombosis by inactivating a factor (called Xa) and by preventing the conversion of prothrombin to thrombin. This stops the coagulation mechanism. Heparin is prepackaged by manufacturers in 20,000-unit bags of 500 mL or can be made in various units from a wide variety of vial strengths. Heparin cannot be given orally because stomach acids destroy it. For example, patients who are admitted into the hospital with an MI or stroke may be placed on a heparin intravenous drip to prevent any blood clotting. Heparin is effective and is intended for short-term use in a hospital setting. Some patients are sent home with a low-molecular-weight heparin, such as enoxaparin, which is an subcutaneous injection. The patient may be counseled by a nurse on how to administer this injectable subcutaneous dose. This low-dose heparin normally is given for up to 14 days for prophylactic treatment against embolisms.

Another type of anticoagulant is warfarin. This agent is available in injectable and oral dosage forms. Unlike heparin, orally administered warfarin also is indicated for long-term use and is always taken once a day. Warfarin interferes with the synthesis of vitamin K-dependent coagulation factors (II, VII, IX, and X) in the liver. Prothrombin time tests must be done to monitor how long it takes the blood to form clots while the patient is taking this medication. It is vital that a patient not be overdosed on warfarin or the patient can bleed to death internally. Warfarin has many interactions with other drugs and with certain foods. Any drug that may increase the potency of warfarin must be avoided, as should those that counteract the effectiveness of this medication.

Many over-the-counter agents also are used to prevent thrombosis. One of the best known and popular is aspirin. The advantage of taking aspirin over warfarin is the lower amount of interactions between drugs and food. However, only a doctor can determine which is best for a patient. In addition, the anticoagulant effect of aspirin lasts for 7 days.

ANTICOAGULANTS

GENERIC NAME: heparin
TRADE NAME: Liquaemin
ROUTE OF ADMINISTRATION: injectable forms only (intravenous, subcutaneous)
SIDE EFFECTS: possible hemorrhage (prothrombin time must be monitored closely)
ANTIDOTE: phytonadione injection (vitamin K)

GENERIC NAME: warfarin
TRADE NAME: Coumadin
ROUTE OF ADMINISTRATION: oral, injection (intravenous)
SIDE EFFECTS: possible hemorrhage (prothrombin time must be monitored closely)
ANTIDOTE: phytonadione injection (vitamin K)

Antiplatelet Agents. Antiplatelet drugs work mainly on arterial thrombi, which are made of platelet aggregates (particles). Table 22-4 lists the drugs most commonly used to treat these types of clots.

Drug Action of Thrombolytics

Streptokinase (Streptase) is an enzyme extracted from bacteria that destroys clots after they are formed. Urokinase (Abbokinase) is another type of lytic agent that is retrieved from a human protein that also reduces thrombosis. The newest agent is alteplase (Activase, or t-PA), a natural enzyme that normally is produced by the body to dissolve blood clots. Alteplase binds to fibrin within a

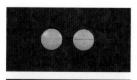
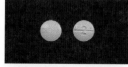
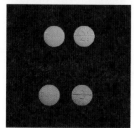

TABLE 22-4 Antiplatelet Agents

Trade name	Generic name	Common prophylaxis dosage
Aspirin	aspirin	81 to 325 mg qd
Persantine	dipyridamole	75 to 100 mg qid
Ticlid	ticlopidine	250 mg bid with food
Plavix	clopidogrel	75 mg qd

thrombus and converts the entrapped plasminogen to plasmin, dissolving the clot. This enzyme is isolated and prepared for parenteral use. Of the three agents, alteplase is the most expensive at well over $1000 per dose. These medications have specific uses and are intended for use as soon as possible after an MI to break up the clot.

NONPHARMACOLOGICAL TREATMENT FOR MYOCARDIAL INFARCTION

The many available medications for patients after MI have been discussed previously in this chapter. With the continued use of a variety of agents and a change in lifestyle, many patients live a normal life span. However, if the patient's MI was severe, an intervention such as bypass surgery may be necessary. Bypass surgery creates new routes for blood flow to the heart muscle. Veins are transplanted from the legs and are rerouted around the damaged vessel within the heart. Newer techniques allow surgeons to conduct bypass surgery without opening the chest wall. This less invasive technique enables the patient to recover more quickly. For more information on new innovative treatments in cardiac surgery, visit the American Heart Association online *(www.heartassociation.org)*.

TECH ALERT!

Remember the following soundalike/look-alike drugs:
Nicobid versus Nitro-Bid
Cardene versus Cardizem
Cardene SR versus Cardizem SR
Nicardipine versus nifedipine
Lotensin versus Lioresal

DO YOU REMEMBER THESE KEY POINTS?

- The location of the heart
- How blood flows through the heart
- The layers of the heart muscle
- Conditions that affect the heart
- Causes for heart problems such as congestive heart failure, coronary artery disease, and hypertension
- Treatments for conditions affecting the heart
- Common side effects for medications mentioned in this chapter
- Types of diuretics and their mechanism of action
- The effects of over-the-counter medications for persons suffering from hypertension
- The types of angina and the medications used to treat them
- The difference between the use of anticoagulants and thrombolytics

MULTIPLE CHOICE QUESTIONS

1. The average adult heart beats _____ times per minute.
   A. 10-50 bpm
   B. 60-100 bpm
   C. 70-90 bpm
   D. 110-120 bpm

2. The artery responsible for supplying the heart muscle with oxygen is called the:
   A. Pulmonary artery
   B. Aorta
   C. Coronary artery
   D. Myocardial passageway

3. The cardiac conduction system is responsible for:
   A. Providing the electrical charge to the heart muscle
   B. Oxygenating the blood
   C. Receiving blood from the body
   D. None of the above

4. A condition in which fluid builds up within tissues is known as:
   A. Myocardial infarction
   B. Angina pectoris
   C. Congestive heart failure
   D. Hypertension

5. Factor(s) that may effect the condition of atherosclerosis is/are:
   A. Lifestyle
   B. Family history
   C. Smoking
   D. All of the above

6. If Mr. Low has a blood pressure of 165/95 mm Hg, he would have:
   A. Low blood pressure
   B. Normal blood pressure
   C. Slightly high blood pressure
   D. High blood pressure

7. ACE inhibitors is an abbreviation for:
   A. Activating coronary electrical site inhibitors
   B. Altering and converting enzyme inhibitors
   C. Angiotensin-converting enzyme inhibitors
   D. Anginal converting enzyme inhibitors

8. β-blockers are effective because they work by:
   A. Blocking receptor sites in the heart
   B. Blocking receptor sites in the heart and kidneys
   C. Activating receptor sites in the heart and lungs
   D. Activating receptor sites in the heart and kidneys

9. Calcium channel blockers are effective because they work by:.
   A. Blocking channel one and two receptors
   B. Reducing cardiac conduction
   C. Speeding up the heart to pump more blood
   D. None of the above

10. Which instruction is NOT patient information necessary about taking oral nitroglycerin medications?
    A. Take with food.
    B. Keep medication within the original container.
    C. Take as needed for chest pain; maximum 3 times in 15 minutes; if no relief, then call 911.
    D. Keep medication out of direct sunlight.

11. Streptase, Abbokinase, and t-PA are classified as _____.
    A. Vasoconstrictors
    B. Vasodilators
    C. Prophylaxis thrombolytics
    D. Thrombolytics

12. The common life span of nitroglycerin (once opened) is _____.
    A. 3 months
    B. 6 months
    C. 12 months
    D. None of the above

13. The four chambers of the heart are _____.
A. Right and left: upper and lower atrium
B. Right and left: atrium and superior and inferior venae cavae
C. Right and left: atrium and ventricle
D. None of the above

14. The medication that dissolves blood clots is called _____.
A. Heparin
B. Aspirin
C. t-PA
D. Warfarin

15. Heparin cannot be given orally because _____.
A. It takes too long to work
B. It is used only for emergencies
C. It is degraded by gastric juices
D. It binds directly to blood products

TRUE/FALSE If the statement is false, then change it to make it true.

_____ **1.** The heart pumps only oxygenated blood.

_____ **2.** Oxygenated blood returns from the lungs via the pulmonary artery.

_____ **3.** The epicardium is the outer layer of the heart muscle, and it protects the heart.

_____ **4.** The vena cava is the large artery that carries blood to the body system.

_____ **5.** Two major types of lipoproteins that should be monitored are HDL and LDL.

_____ **6.** HDL stands for high-density lipoproteins and is considered bad cholesterol.

_____ **7.** Cholesterol has no benefit to the human body.

_____ **8.** The fibers that control the conduction system are called the pacemaker.

_____ **9.** Congestive heart failure can be cured by surgery.

_____ **10.** Hypertension also is known as the silent killer.

_____ **11.** Nitrates are agents that cause vasoconstriction.

_____ **12.** Aspirin is a thrombolytic agent.

_____ **13.** Calcium channel blockers are often the first line of treatment for angina.

_____ **14.** An embolism is a thrombosis or clot that has moved from its origin.

_____ **15.** Aspirin has more side effects than heparin or warfarin.

_____ **16.** β-blockers increase blood pressure, thus helping the heart beat stronger.

_____ **17.** Angiotensin-converting enzyme inhibitors increase blood pressure, thus helping the heart beat faster.

_____ **18.** Nitroglycerin must be kept in a glass container.

_____ **19.** All diuretics cause a loss of potassium through frequent urination.

_____ **20.** Edema is a condition of inflammation of the tissues resulting from hyperlipidemia.

TECHNICIAN'S CORNER

Mrs. Lewis comes into the pharmacy with several prescriptions. Using a comprehensive drug reference, such as *Drug Facts and Comparisons* or *Mosby's Drug Consult,* look up the medications listed and determine what Mrs. Lewis may be suffering from. In addition, for each of the medications, classify each one and transcribe into laymen's terms as though you were preparing a prescription label.

Zocor 5 mg qd, #30
Digoxin 125 mcg qd, #30
Furosemide 40 mg bid, #60
K-Dur 20 mEq bid, #60
Albuterol INH 1 to 2 puffs prn SOB, #17 g
NTG 0.4 mg sl tab prn cp, 1 q 5 min, max 3 tabs over 15 min, then call 911, 4/#25s
Atenolol 25 mg qd, #30

BIBLIOGRAPHY

Clayton BD, et al: *Basic pharmacology for nurses,* ed 14, St Louis, 2006, Mosby.

Drug facts and comparisons, ed 60, St Louis, 2005, Wolters Kluwer.

Lacy C, Armstrong L, Goldman M, et al: Lexis Comp's *Drug information handbook,* ed 13, Hudson, Ohio, 2005, Lexi-Comp.

Lewis SM, Heitkemper MM, Dirksen SR: *Medical-surgical nursing: assessment and management of clinical problems,* ed 6, St Louis, 2003, Mosby.

Mosby's 2006 drug consult for nurses, St Louis, 2006, Mosby.

Potter PA, Perry AG: *Fundamentals of nursing,* ed 6, St Louis, 2004, Mosby.

Filtration Recommendations Summary. http://www.utmb.edu/rxhome/Operations/Filtrations.htm. Retrieved 10/06

Stedman's concise medical dictionary for health professionals, ed 3, Baltimore, 1997, Lippincott, Williams & Wilkins.

Reproductive System

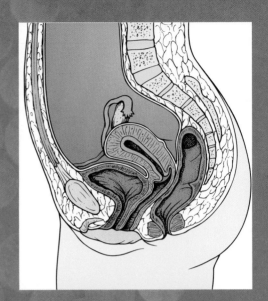

Objectives

UPON COMPLETING THIS CHAPTER, YOU SHOULD BE ABLE TO DO THE FOLLOWING:

- List both trade and generic drug names covered in this chapter.

- Describe the organs of the male and female reproductive tracts and their locations.

- Describe the male and female hormones and their roles in the body.

- List the common conditions affecting the male reproductive system and the medications used to treat these conditions.

- List the common conditions of the female reproductive system and the medications used to treat these conditions.

- Describe hormone replacement therapy in the female, and list the medications used for hormone replacement.

- List the different types of oral contraceptives.

- List other types of contraception and the advantages and disadvantages of each.

- Describe the medications that are used as abortifacients.

- List the types of sexually transmitted diseases and their treatments.

Abortifacient *Any treatment that causes abortion of a fetus*

Amenorrhea *Absence or suppression of menses*

Androgen *Male hormone*

Benign prostatic hypertrophy *Nonmalignant enlargement of prostate gland*

Chloasma *Hyperpigmentation of skin, limited or confined to a certain area*

Depot *An area of the body where a substance can accumulate or be stored for later distribution*

Dysmenorrhea *Painful menstruation*

Endometriosis *Condition in which tissue resembling endometrium is found outside the uterine cavity, usually in the pelvic area*

Endometrium *Mucous membrane lining of the uterus*

Fallopian tube *Narrow passage between the ovary and the uterus*

Fertilization *The process by which a sperm unites with an ovum to create a new life*

Gametes *Sex cells, or ova and sperm*

Inert ingredient *An ingredient that has little or no effect on body functions*

Menopause *Cessation of menstruation; a natural phenomenon in which a woman passes from a reproductive state to a nonreproductive state*

Negative feedback *A self-regulating mechanism in which the output of a system has input or control on the process; a factor within a system that causes a corrective action to return the system to normal range*

Oocyte or ova *The female reproductive germ cell*

Palliative *That which brings relief but does not cure*

Teratogenic *Causing abnormal embryonic development*

REPRODUCTIVE SYSTEM DRUGS

Trade Name	Generic Name	Pronunciation	Trade Name	Generic Name	Pronunciation
Androgens			**Estrogens**		
Androderm	testosterone	(tes-**toss**-ter-one)	Delestrogen	estradiol valerate	(ess-tra-**dye**-ole **val**-er-ate)
Fluoxymesterone	fluoxymesterone	(floo-ox-ee-**mes**-ter-one)	Estrace, Estraderm	estradiol	(ess-tra-**dye**-ole)
Testred, Virilon	methyltestosterone	(meth-ill-tes-**toss**-ter-own)	Estratab, Menest	esterified estrogen	(ess-**ter**-i-fide **ess**-troe-gijen)
Adrenergic Antagonists for Benign Prostatic Hypertrophy			Ogen, Ortho-Est	estropipate	(ess-troe-**pye**-pate)
Cardura	doxazosin	(dokx-**sahy**-zoe-sin)	Premarin	conjugated estrogens	(ckon-juh-**gate**-ed **ess**-troe-gijens)
Flomax	tamsulosin	(tam-**sue**-lo-sin)	Prempro, Premphase	esterified conjugated estrogens/ medroxyprogesterone	(ess-ter-i-**fide kon**-juh-gat-ed **ess**-troe-gijens/me-drockx-see-proe-**jess**-teur-owne)
Hytrin	terazosin	(teur-**ahy**-zohe-sin)			
Androgen Hormone Inhibitor for Benign Prostatic Hypertrophy					
Proscar	finasteride	(fin-**ass**-te-ride)			

REPRODUCTIVE SYSTEM DRUGS—cont'd

Trade Name	Generic Name	Pronunciation	Trade Name	Generic Name	Pronunciation
Progestins			**Long-Acting Contraceptives**		
Crinone	progesterone	(pro-**jess**-tuer-owne)	Depo-Provera	medroxyprogesterone	(me-drock-see-pro-**jess**-tur-own) (me-drock-see-pro-**jess**-tur-own)
Hylutin	hydroxyprogesterone	(highye-drokx-see-proe-**jess**-ture-rowne)			
Micronor	norethindrone	(nor-**eth**-in-drone)	Lunelle	medroxyprogesterone/ estradiol	(me-drock-see-pro-**jess**-tur-own/ess-tra-**dye**-ole)
Ovrette	norgestrel	(nor-**jess**-trel)			
Provera	medroxyprogesterone	(me-drockx-see-proe-**jess**-ture-rowne)	Progestasert	progesterone	(pro-**jess**-tur-own)
			Spermicidals		
Oral Contraceptives			Delfen, Advantage 24, Sheik Elite nonoxynol-9		(non-**ox**-i-nol)
Monophasic combinations					
Alesse, Levlen	esthinyl estradiol/ levonorgestrel	(**eth**ss-tin-ill ess-tra-**dye**-ole/**lev**-o-nor-**jess**-trel)	**Medications for Infertility**		
Demulen	esthinyl estradiol/ ethynodiol diacetate	(**eth**ss-tin-nill ess-tra-**dye**-ole/eh-the-no-**dye**-ol di-**as**-ah-tate)	Clomid	clomiphene	(**kloe**-mi-feen)
			Parlodel	bromocriptine	(bro-mo-**ckrip**-teen)
Desogen, Ortho-Cept	esthinyl estradiol/ desogestrel	(**eth**ss-tin-ill- ess-tra-**dye**-ole/des-o-**ges**-trol)	Pergonal	menotropins	(**men**-o-trop-in)
Lo-Ovral, Ovral	esthinyl estradiol/ norgestrel	(**eth**ss-tin-ill ess-tra-**dye**-ole/nor-**jess**-trel)	**Miscellaneous Medications for the Reproductive System**		
			Emergency contraceptives		
Ortho-Cyclen	esthinyl estradiol/ norgestimate	(**eth**ss-tin-ill ess-tra-**dye**-ole/nor-**jess**-ti-mate)	Plan B	levonorgestrel	(**lev**-o-nor-**jess**-trel)
Ortho-Novum 1/35	ethinyl estradiol/ norethindrone	(**eth**-in-nill ess-tra-**dye**-ole/nor-**eth**-in-drone)	Preven	levonorgestrel/ethinyl estradiol	(**lev**-o-nor-**jess**-trel/ **eth**-in-ill ess-tra-**dye**-ole)
Ortho-Novum 1/50, Genora 1/50	mestranol/ norethindrone	(**mess**-tra-nol/nor-**eth**-in-drone)			
			Drugs for endometriosis		
			Lupron	leuprolide	(loo-**pro**-lide)
Biphasic combination			Synarel	nafarelin	(**naf**-a-rell-in)
Ortho-Novum 10/11	ethinyl estradiol/ norethindrone	(**eth**-in-ill ess-tra-**dye**-ole/nor-**eth**-in-drone)	Zoladex	goserelin	(**goe**-ser-a-lin)
			Drugs for erectile dysfunction		
Triphasic combinations			Caverject	alprostadil	(al-**pros**-ta-dil)
Ortho Tri-Cyclen	ethinyl estradiol/ norgestimate	(**eth**-in-nill ess-tra-**dye**-ole/nor-**jess**-ti-mate)	Cialias	tadalafil	(tah-**dal**-ah-fill)
			Levitra	vardenafil	(var-**den**-ah-fill)
Ortho-Novum 7/7/7	ethinyl estradiol/ norethindrone	(**eth**-in-nill ess-tra-**dye**-ole/nor-**eth**-in-drone)	Viagra	sildenafil	(sil-**den**-a-fil)
Triphasil	ethinyl estradiol/ levonorgestrel	(**eth**-in-nill ess-tra-**jessdye**-treole/ **lev**-o-nor-**jess**-trel)	*Drugs for sexually transmitted diseases*		
			Bicillin C-R benzathine	penicillin	(pen-eyei-**cil**-in)
			Flagyl	metrondiazole	(met-row-**nid**-dah-zole)
Estrophasic combination			Floxin	ofloxacin	(o-**flox**-a-sin)
Estrostep	ethinyl estradiol/ norethindrone	(**eth**-in-ill ess-tra-**dye**-ole/nor-**eth**-in-drone)	Suprax	cefixime	(sef-**ix**-ime)
			Vagistat	tioconazole	(teey-o-**con**-a-zole)
			Zovirax	acyclovir	(a-**sy**-klo-veer)

THE MAJOR FUNCTION of the reproductive system is the production of offspring for the survival of the species. This organ system operates interdependently with other systems such as the endocrine system (for the hormones necessary to function properly) and the urinary system (especially in the male). In men and women, the functions of reproduction are divided between the primary and secondary, or accessory, organs. The primary reproductive organs are the gonads (ovaries or testes), which are necessary to produce the gametes or sex cells (ova or sperm). The gonads are also responsible for the secretion of the hormones that provide gender characteristics of the male or female. The secondary reproductive organs include the structures necessary for transport and sustenance of the gametes and also those organs necessary for the sustenance of the developing fetus in the female. The male and female systems, conditions, and treatments are covered respectively. The coverage of sexually transmitted diseases (STDs) is last because these affect males and females.

Male Reproductive System

In the male the reproductive system is closely tied to the urinary system. The urethra passes through the penis and is surrounded by the prostate gland. The testicles are responsible for the production of sperm after puberty and for the immediate storage of these cells. Once sperm production begins, it continues throughout the lifetime of the male. After formation the sperm pass through the epididymis, where they mature, and into the vas deferens, where peristaltic movements move them into the proximal portion. The sperm then enter the ejaculatory duct.

The prostate is about the size and shape of a walnut. The prostate also encircles part of the urethra, the tube that carries urine out of the bladder and through the penis. The function of the prostate and glands is to secrete fluids to the sperm to enhance their motility and viability and to provide a slightly alkaline environment that will endure the acidic environment of the vagina. Finally, the sperm and fluids pass through the urethra in the penis for ejaculation during sexual intercourse (Figure 23-1).

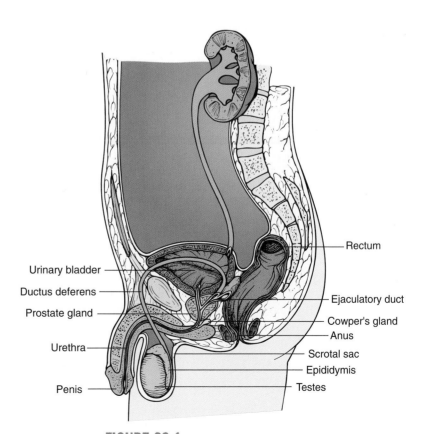

FIGURE 23-1 Male reproductive system.

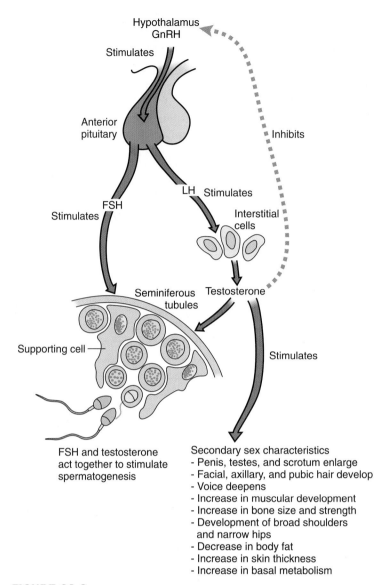

FIGURE 23-2 Function of testes in response to hormone stimulation.

Male sex hormones are stimulated by the gonadotropin-releasing hormone of the anterior pituitary gland that then stimulates the formation of luteinizing hormone (LH), also called interstitial cell–stimulating hormone in the male, and follicle-stimulating hormone (FSH). Interstitial cell–stimulating hormone then promotes the growth of interstitial cells in the testes and stimulates the cells to secrete testosterone. Testosterone and FSH stimulate spermatogenesis in the testicles (Figure 23-2).

Male sex hormones collectively are called androgens, with testosterone being the most abundant androgen. At puberty, the androgens stimulate the formation of secondary male characteristics, such as increased muscle mass, deepening of the voice, and growth of facial hair.

CONDITIONS AFFECTING THE MALE REPRODUCTIVE SYSTEM AND THEIR TREATMENTS

Impotence

Sildenafil (Viagra) was introduced in 1998 for the treatment of impotence. This medication initially was released for use as a cardiovascular agent to lower blood pressure. Today this medication is used for erectile dysfunction by increasing

TABLE 23-1 Two Male Conditions and Their Treatments

Condition	Generic name	Brand name	Dosage forms	Normal dosage
Erectile dysfunction	Alprostadil	Caverject	Urethral suppository	0.125 mg
	Sildenafil	Viagra	Tablet	50 mg
	Tadalafil	Cialas	Tablet	10 mg
	Vardenafil	Levitra	Tablet	10 mg
Prostatitis	Cefazolin	Ancef	Injection	Dosage varies
	Cephalexin	Keflex	Injection	Dosage varies
	Ciprofloxacin	Cipro	Tablet/injection	Dosage varies
	Trovafloxacin	Trovan	Tablet/injection	Dosage varies

blood flow to the penis and causing penile rigidity. The side effects include headaches, flushing of the skin, gastrointestinal symptoms, nasal congestion, and diarrhea. Patients taking nitrates should not take sildenafil because of the dangerous decrease in blood pressure. Table 23-1 lists medications for erectile dysfunction and inflammation of the prostate.

Prostatitis/Prostatism/Prostatocystitis

As men age, there is a higher risk of conditions that can affect the prostate gland. Various conditions include prostatitis (inflammation of the prostate gland); prostatism (enlargement of the gland), which causes nocturia and obstructive symptoms, with symptoms that range from a decrease in stream of urine, dribbling, double voiding, and urinary retention; and prostatocystitis, the inflammation of the prostate gland and the bladder.

Prostate Cancer

Prostate cancer can be treated through the use of surgery, radiological treatment, and hormone therapy. Although prostatic cancer is a serious condition it has become more treatable due to public awareness and new neoplastic agents (see Chapter 28).

Benign Prostatic Hypertrophy

Medications for benign prostatic hypertrophy are used to decrease the mass of an enlarged prostate gland. Benign prostatic hypertrophy occurs in about 73% of men by the age of 70. The goal of treatment for benign prostatic hypertrophy is to relieve the bothersome symptoms such as urinary tract infections, hesitancy on urination, a decrease in the stream of urine, postvoiding dribbling, frequency, and nocturia. Some of the medications, such as finasteride, promote shrinkage of the prostate, whereas the α-adrenergic blockers relax the smooth muscle of the prostatic tissue to reduce obstruction.

Tumors and Other Miscellaneous Conditions

Male hormones also are used as palliative agents in treating male reproductive tumors. In addition to an increased feeling of well-being, the androgens increase bone density and lean body mass. Because of the ability of androgens to reverse tissue wasting, these hormones often are used to reverse the debilitating effects of diseases and the wasting that comes from long-term use of corticosteroids. These medications tend to decrease pain levels, make the male more alert, and increase appetite. These actions lead to an overall feeling of increased well-being.

Testosterone provides a sense of well-being, mental stability, and energy. Testosterone also provides the body with a resistance to fatigue. Natural testosterone that is used for medicinal purposes is obtained from the testes of bulls. Androgens that are produced synthetically are called anabolic steroids—medications that are used to build muscle mass. Because of the misuse and abuse of anabolic steroids, the Drug Enforcement Administration has placed anabolic steroids on the schedule III list of controlled medications.

Androgens are used to produce male secondary sex characteristics and to maintain the male reproductive structures. Therefore, androgens are used to treat hypogonadism or infertility resulting from a low sperm count. The increase in sperm count is achieved through the suppression of negative feedback, causing an increased secretion of testosterone, FSH, and interstitial cell–stimulating hormone.

MEDICATIONS AND THEIR SIDE EFFECTS

The following are samples of medications used to treat conditions of the male reproductive tract. Classifications are given for the various drugs. The strength, indications, routes of administration, and common dosage of each drug also are listed. Patients taking androgens should be informed that weight gain and headaches are common, but a weight gain of more than 2 lb may require medications to rid the body of edema. Taking the medications with food helps decrease undesired gastrointestinal symptoms. Patients taking anticoagulants and hypoglycemics may require smaller doses of these medications when taking androgens. Various side effects may happen when taking testosterone medications, such as nausea, vomiting, and diarrhea. Blood levels of calcium, sodium, phosphorus, potassium, and cholesterol may become elevated. Hypoglycemia, pruritus, jaundice, and alterations in libido also may occur with continued use of testosterone. With men, breast engorgement, impotence, male pattern baldness, and acne are expected.

CLASSIFICATION OF ANDROGENS

Androgens

> **GENERIC NAME:** testosterone
> **TRADE NAME:** Androderm transdermal system
> **INDICATIONS:** androgen replacement therapy, hypogonadism
> **ROUTE OF ADMINISTRATION:** topical patch
> **COMMON DOSAGE:** 5 mg qd (applied at bedtime)

> **GENERIC NAME:** methyltestosterone
> **TRADE NAME:** Testred, Virilon
> **INDICATIONS:** (men) androgen replacement therapy, hypogonadism, delayed puberty; (women) metastatic mammary or breast cancer
> **ROUTE OF ADMINISTRATION:** oral
> **COMMON DOSAGE:** (males) 10 mg to 50 mg daily; (women) 50 mg to 200 mg per day

Synthetic Androgens
Androgen Hormone Inhibitor

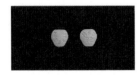

> **GENERIC NAME:** finasteride
> **TRADE NAME:** Proscar
> **INDICATION:** benign prostatic hypertrophy
> **ROUTE OF ADMINISTRATION:** oral
> **COMMON DOSAGE:** 5 mg qd
> **NOTE:** This drug is teratogenic, so a form of contraception should be used, if applicable.

α-Adrenergic Blockers

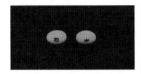

GENERIC NAME: terazosin
TRADE NAME: Hytrin
INDICATION: benign prostatic hypertrophy
ROUTE OF ADMINISTRATION: oral
COMMON DOSAGE: 1 to 10 mg qd

GENERIC NAME: tamsulosin
TRADE NAME: Flomax
INDICATION: benign prostatic hypertrophy
ROUTE OF ADMINISTRATION: oral
COMMON DOSAGE: 0.4 mg qd

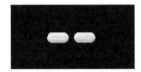

GENERIC NAME: doxazosin
TRADE NAME: Cardura
INDICATIONS: benign prostatic hypertrophy, mild hypertension
ROUTE OF ADMINISTRATION: oral capsule
COMMON DOSAGE: 1 mg qid

Female Reproductive System

The female reproductive system produces and transports ova (or oocytes) from the ovary through the fallopian tube into the uterus, which will house a fertilized ovum. After puberty the female ovary matures an egg each month, although recent science indicates that more than one egg may mature. At birth the female ovary contains all the eggs that the female will ever have. Thus females do not produce ova throughout life but only mature those that are available. When an egg is mature, it is gathered by the fimbriated end of the infundibulum (funnel-shaped structure or passage) of the fallopian tube. The fallopian tubes are in constant motion, but at ovulation their activity increases, and currents in the peritoneal fluid are created to propel the egg into the fallopian tube. During the next 7 days, the ovum is moved down the fallopian tube where it may become fertilized by a sperm. Because an ovum is only viable for 24 to 38 hours, most fertilization occurs in the fallopian tube. At the end of the tube is the uterus that will house the fertilized ovum or slough the ovum and endometrium as menses if fertilization has not occurred. This cycle begins at puberty and continues until menopause, or for a period of about 40 years (Figure 23-3).

As in the male, the gonadotropin-releasing hormone from the anterior pituitary gland begins the secretion of the hormones necessary for ovulation. FSH and LH stimulate the ovaries to secrete estrogen and progesterone. These female hormones found in the endocrine system are controlled by negative feedback and are secreted in cycles, unlike the continuous secretion of sex hormones in males (Figure 23-4). The level of female hormones peaks when a woman is in her 20s and then gradually decreases throughout life.

The accessory organs of the female reproductive tract are the mammary glands or breasts. This tissue also is regulated by hormonal secretions. At puberty the increase in estrogen stimulates the development of glandular tissue, causing an accumulation of adipose tissue, and progesterone stimulates the development of the duct system that is used during milk production.

CONDITIONS AFFECTING THE FEMALE REPRODUCTIVE SYSTEM AND THEIR TREATMENTS

The chief drugs that affect the reproductive system are hormones. Some agents stimulate secretions, whereas others inhibit the action of certain hormones.

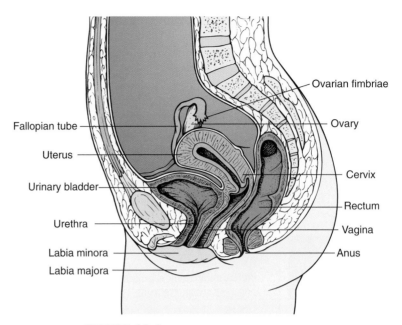

FIGURE 23-3 Female reproductive system.

Medication therapy for conditions of the reproductive tract can be complicated because hormone levels must be considered and must remain fairly constant. Female hormones are used to treat some conditions of the male reproductive tract, such as prostate and testicular cancer, and male hormones are used to treat endometrial or breast cancer, endometriosis, and fibrocystic disease in the female. The inhibition of the natural hormones in either gender is brought about by the use of the hormones of the other gender, much like negative feedback in which the stimulating hormone is inhibited. Remember that the hypothalamus cannot distinguish between hormones naturally produced by the body and those that are administered as medications; therefore the body will react to the medication in the same manner as it reacts to synthetic and naturally occurring hormones.

Estrogens are the dominant form of medical therapy used to treat conditions such as abnormal uterine bleeding resulting from hormone imbalance, abnormal ovulation, and infertility. Estrogens also are used for hormone replacement therapy. One of the main uses of estrogen preparations is for oral contraception. Estrogens also have effects on bone and cardiovascular function and cause reduced levels of low-density lipoproteins, thus raising levels of high-density lipoproteins to lower the risk of cardiac disease. Estrogens support the development and maintenance of the reproductive organs and the secondary sex characteristics and have profound influences on the menstrual cycle. In the male, estrogens are used to treat prostate and breast cancer.

Estradiol is the major natural estrogen that is produced by the ovaries. Estradiol is used for hormone replacement therapy in the naturally postmenopausal woman or in the woman who is experiencing a surgical menopause. Estradiol usually is combined with progestins because of the increased risk of endometrial and breast cancer when combination medications are not used. Estrogen replacement therapy seems to protect the woman against coronary and vascular disease; thus the values of the medications must be weighed against the known risks, such as thromboembolytic diseases and increased risk for neoplasms. Most replacement therapy is in conjugated doses from natural sources such as from the urine of pregnant mares or from placentas, but estrogens also may be formulated synthetically. The naturally occurring estrogens, such as estrone, estradiol, and estriol, are steroids that are converted to estriol by the

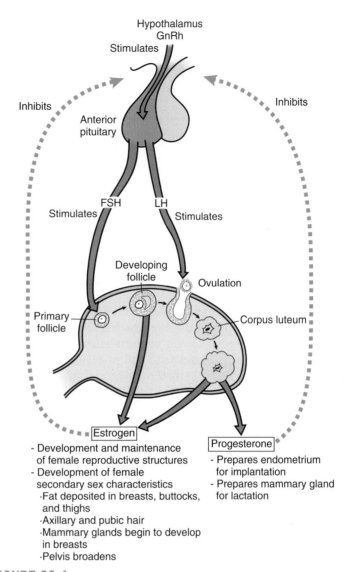

Hypothalamus
GnRh

Stimulates

Inhibits

Anterior
pituitary

Inhibits

FSH   LH
Stimulates   Stimulates

Developing
follicle

Ovulation

Primary
follicle

Corpus luteum

Estrogen
- Development and maintenance
  of female reproductive structures
- Development of female
  secondary sex characteristics
  ·Fat deposited in breasts, buttocks,
   and thighs
  ·Axillary and pubic hair
  ·Mammary glands begin to develop
   in breasts
  ·Pelvis broadens

Progesterone
- Prepares endometrium
  for implantation
- Prepares mammary gland
  for lactation

FIGURE 23-4 Function of ovaries in response to hormone stimulation.

body. Some of the synthetically formulated products are steroidal, whereas others are nonsteroidal.

Estrogens are available in several forms; some forms are unique, such as implants, vaginal inserts, and nasal sprays. The most common forms are oral and injectable (water- or oil-based) preparations. The oil-based medications, called *depot* medications, are prepared to prolong the action by allowing absorption in the fatty tissue for slow distribution. Transdermal preparations are applied to the skin to provide continuous daily release of the medication. Drug-laden vaginal rings are pressed into the vaginal canal for the continuous release of medications into the local tissues. Other locally administered estrogens include vaginal inserts and creams that provide absorption of hormones at the local site. The choice of preparation to be used depends on the reason for use, cost, reliability of the patient to use it correctly, and the convenience of use. Most estrogens are prescribed at the lowest dose needed to provide the desired effect over the shortest time.

The primary actions of estrogens are to maintain reproductive structures such as ova production and to provide secondary sex characteristics. Estrogens also assist with the retention of calcium and phosphorus for bone production in the postmenopausal state. In women, estrogens are used to treat hypogonadism;

for postpartum breast engorgement or lactation; to relieve symptoms of menopause (natural or surgical); and to relieve symptoms of dysmenorrhea, endometriosis, and dysfunctional uterine bleeding. In men, estrogens are used for inoperable prostate and testicular cancer. The increased estrogen in males causes feminization to occur, including voice changes, breast enlargement, loss of body hair, testicular and penile atrophy, and impotence. The feminization and impotence of males usually are reversed on termination of medication.

In the female, adverse effects may include chloasma, photosensitivity, nausea, vomiting, bloating, and risk of gallbladder disease. Infertility, dysmenorrhea, breast tenderness and enlargement, and increased susceptibility to thrombolytic disease are also commonly seen effects. Although estrogens induce a feeling of well-being, high levels tend to cause depression that may progress to psychosis. In addition, estrogens may aggravate asthma, epilepsy, migraines, heart disease, and urinary tract diseases and increase the symptoms of diabetes mellitus.

Male hormones can be used for treating some female breast tumors that grow faster in the presence of estrogen. Androgens suppress the effects of estrogen, thus preventing rapid growth of these tumors. Sometimes the medications may even cause the tumor to atrophy. Other uses of androgens in females are to suppress postpartum breast engorgement and fibrocystic disease by causing atrophy of the breasts. For the woman with endometriosis, androgens cause suppression of the endometrium and thus prevent the excessive uterine bleeding that is found with the disease.

Like testosterone secretion in the male, estrogen and progesterone secretion responds to the secretions of the anterior pituitary gland. Gonadotropin-releasing hormone stimulates FSH and LH to cause the ovaries to secrete estrogen and progesterone. Unlike testosterone in the male, these hormones follow cyclical patterns each month beginning at puberty and continuing until menopause, when hormone secretion decreases. During premenopause, the ovaries gradually decrease estrogen production.

SIDE EFFECTS

Women receiving androgen therapy for prolonged periods may have amenorrhea or menstrual irregularities. Hot flashes, headaches, sleep disorders, increased libido, vaginitis, and masculinization also are found. Changes in the voice (lowering of the voice) are often permanent, whereas other symptoms such as loss of breast mass, increased facial and body hair, and increased muscle mass may reverse when the testosterone therapy is discontinued. Masculinization does not seem to occur with short-term use of androgens by women with conditions such as postpartum engorgement of the breasts.

ESTROGEN PREPARATIONS

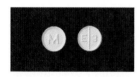

GENERIC NAME: estradiol
TRADE NAME: Estrace (oral), Estraderm (transdermal), Estring (vaginal ring)
INDICATIONS: menopausal symptoms, female hypogonadism
ROUTE OF ADMINISTRATION: oral, topical, vaginal
COMMON DOSAGE: oral, 0.5 to 2 mg qd in cycles; transdermal, 0.05- to 1-mg patch applied once or twice a week; vaginal ring, change ring every 3 months

GENERIC NAME: esterified estrogen
TRADE NAME: Estratab, Menest
INDICATIONS: menopausal symptoms, female hypogonadism, breast cancer
ROUTE OF ADMINISTRATION: oral
COMMON DOSAGE: 0.3 to 1.25 mg qd

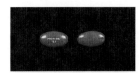
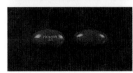

GENERIC NAME: conjugated estrogens
TRADE NAME: Premarin
INDICATIONS: menopausal symptoms, osteoporosis prevention, prostate cancer, breast cancer, hypogonadism, atrophic vaginitis
ROUTE OF ADMINISTRATION: oral, injection, vaginal
COMMON DOSAGE: oral, 0.3 to 2.5 mg qd in cycles; injection, 25 mg IM; vaginal cream, 2 to 4 g vaginally as directed in cycles

GENERIC NAME: conjugated estrogens with medroxyprogesterone
TRADE NAME: Prempro, Premphase
INDICATIONS: menopausal symptoms, osteoporosis prevention, prostate cancer, breast cancer, hypogonadism, atrophic vaginitis
ROUTE OF ADMINISTRATION: oral
COMMON DOSAGE: 0.625 mg/2.5 mg to 0.625 mg/5 mg

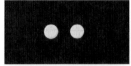
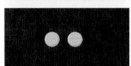
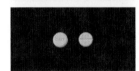

GENERIC NAME: estropipate
TRADE NAME: Ogen, Ortho-Est
ROUTE OF ADMINISTRATION: oral
INDICATIONS: menopausal symptoms, prostate cancer, osteoporosis, hypogonadism
COMMON DOSAGE: 0.75 to 3 mg qd in cycles

PROGESTINS

Progesterone, naturally occurring as progestin, is the female hormone secreted from day 14 through day 28 of the menstrual cycle. This hormone has many functions, including changing the secretions of the cervix, reducing uterine contractility, and maintaining the corpus luteum. Other actions include stimulating the development of ducts and glands of the breasts in preparation of lactation; however, progestin does not cause lactation.

Progestins also may be made synthetically; natural and synthetic forms have similar pharmacological effects on the body. Placentas are one of the natural sources for obtaining progestins. Because the liver rapidly metabolizes progestin preparations, oral administration of natural preparations is not indicated. Injected forms usually are placed in an oil base to delay the absorption and thus prolong effects. Synthetically produced preparations are different from natural progesterone and are called progestins or progestogens. The synthetic form is used most often rather than the natural forms because synthetic forms are more effective. Given by injection and orally, the action of synthetic progestin is prolonged over progesterone, and the oral administration is effective because the synthetically made progestin is not rapidly metabolized by the liver.

Progestins are used for treating amenorrhea, abnormal uterine bleeding from hormone imbalances, for contraception, in combination with estrogen for hormone replacement therapy in menopause, and as therapy for renal and endometrial cancer. When used with estrogen for contraception, the dosage of progestin is measured in milligrams, whereas the estrogen component is measured in micrograms. Used to treat infertility, progesterone and progesterone-like products cause negative feedback and with the gonadotropic hormones stimulate the development of ova and subsequent ovulation.

The side effects of progestins include weight gain, stomach pain and cramping, swelling of the face and legs, headaches, mood swings, anxiety, weakness, rashes, acne, and insomnia. Menstrual changes and breast tenderness may occur, and liver dysfunction and phlebitis are more severe adverse reactions.

Glucose intolerance is seen in women who are prone to diabetes mellitus, and fetal teratogenic effects have occurred.

GENERIC NAME: progesterone
TRADE NAME: Crinone
INDICATIONS: secondary amenorrhea
ROUTE OF ADMINISTRATION: vaginal
COMMON DOSAGE: 45 mg (4% gel) qod × 6 doses

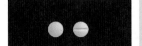
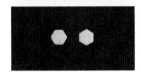

GENERIC NAME: medroxyprogesterone
TRADE NAME: Provera(oral), Depo-Provera (injection)
INDICATIONS: endometrial hyperplasia, secondary amenorrhea, abnormal uterine bleeding; Depo-Provera (contraception)
ROUTE OF ADMINISTRATION: oral, injection
COMMON DOSAGE: 2 to 10 mg qd for 5 to 10 days for amenorrhea and abnormal bleeding; Depo-Provera, 150 mg every 3 months as a contraceptive

GENERIC NAME: hydroxyprogesterone
TRADE NAME: Hylutin
INDICATIONS: amenorrhea, abnormal uterine bleeding
ROUTE OF ADMINISTRATION: injection
COMMON DOSAGE: 375 mg q 4 weeks for amenorrhea and uterine bleeding

GENERIC NAME: norethindrone
TRADE NAME: Micronor, Norlutin
INDICATIONS: amenorrhea, abnormal uterine bleeding, endometriosis, contraception, prevention of endometrial hyperplasia with estrogen therapy
ROUTE OF ADMINISTRATION: oral
COMMON DOSAGE: 2.5 to 10 mg in cycles for amenorrhea; 0.35 mg qd for contraception; 5 mg for prevention of endometrial hyperplasia

CONTRACEPTIVES

Oral contraceptives are used as a means of birth control by preventing fertilization of an ovum and the subsequent pregnancy. Contraception may be accomplished through pharmacological methods such as oral contraceptives or medication-laden devices such as vaginal rings, patches, or intrauterine devices. Nonpharmacological methods such as surgery, the rhythm method, and mechanical devices also may be used. Of the different methods of birth control, the oral contraceptives have the highest incidence of side effects—from nausea and vomiting to menstrual abnormalities to thrombolytic diseases. Barrier methods have the fewest side effects but are not as effective as hormone-based medications (Figure 23-5).

Oral contraceptives are relatively safe when used by nonsmokers who have normal cardiovascular function. Combination oral contraceptives consist of estrogen and progestin to inhibit ovulation. The progestin-only contraceptives are called "minipills." The combination medications are the most often prescribed contraceptives and are almost 100% effective. The combination medications are available in monophasic, biphasic, triphasic, and estrophasic formulas. In the monophasic regimen the daily doses of estrogen and progestin remain constant throughout the menstrual cycle. In the biphasic regimen, the estrogen remains constant but the progestin dose is increased in the second half of the

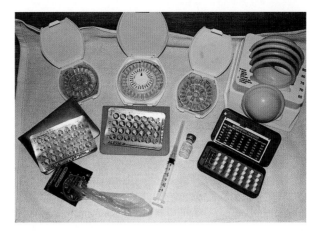

FIGURE 23-5 Common contraceptives, including barrier and medicinal methods: condoms, diaphragm, oral contraceptives, and parenteral contraceptives.

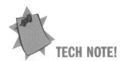

TECH NOTE!

Oral contraceptives should be taken at the same time each day. Oral contraceptives may increase blood glucose levels; thus a person with diabetes mellitus should be monitored closely. Additional methods of contraception should be used during the initial cycle of oral contraceptives. Some oral contraceptives are packaged in 21-tablet packs, whereas others have 21 tablets of the medication and 7 tablets that are an iron preparation or a tablet of an inert ingredient.

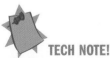

TECH NOTE!

Transdermal patches for contraception should be applied to the upper arms, back, abdomen, or buttocks. The patch should be applied and worn for 1 week; a new patch should be applied on the same day of the week that the first patch was applied. The fourth week should be patch free.

cycle. The triphasic regimen divides the menstrual cycle into three phases, and the amount of progestin changes in each phase. The estrophasic cycle has a constant amount of progestin, and the estrogen component is increased gradually throughout the cycle.

The side effects of oral contraceptives include thromboembolism, increased susceptibility to myocardial infarction, and stroke. These medications can increase blood sugar levels, and gallbladder disease, acne, and hirsutism may develop.

The effectiveness of oral contraceptive use depends on taking the medication as prescribed. The medication is started on the fifth day of the menstrual cycle and should be taken at the same time of the day for 21 days. If a single dose of the contraceptive is missed, the chance of ovulation is small. However, the risk of pregnancy increases with each dose missed. If one dose is missed, it should be taken on the next day. If two doses are missed, two tablets should be taken on each of the next 2 days. If three doses are missed, a new cycle of medications should be started 7 days after the last pill was taken, and additional forms of birth control are needed during the first 2 weeks of the new cycle.

Most oral contraceptives are in tablet form, whereas some are available as transdermal patches. Some contraceptives are given by injection for safety, and each injection is effective for 3 months. These injections, used in persons who may be noncompliant with oral dosage forms, prevent pregnancy in three ways: by suppressing ovulation, by thickening the cervical mucus, and by altering the endometrium to discourage implantation. The adverse reactions are typical of progestins. Oral contraceptives provide no protection against STDs; this is an important factor in patient education.

Contraceptive medications listed are those other than oral cycle packs, which make up most of the contraceptives taken. For drugs separated with a slash, the first drug listed is the estrogen component and second drug is the progestin component.

GENERIC NAME: ethinyl estradiol/norelgestromin
TRADE NAME: Ortho-Evra
ROUTE OF ADMINISTRATION: topical
COMMON DOSAGE: transdermal patch applied weekly for 3 weeks, the 4th week is patch-free

Long-Acting Contraceptive

GENERIC NAME: medroxyprogesterone
TRADE NAME: Depo-Provera
ROUTE OF ADMINISTRATION: injection
COMMON DOSAGE: injection every 3 months

Intrauterine Progesterone Contraception

GENERIC NAME: progesterone
TRADE NAME: Progestasert
ROUTE OF ADMINISTRATION: intrauterine
COMMON DOSAGE: Insert one system into the uterus. Each system is effective for 1 year, at which time a new system is inserted.

Other Contraceptives

Other contraceptives include spermicides that have the active ingredient nonoxynol-9. These contraceptives are available as foam, jelly, gel, cream, suppository, and vaginal film. The correct use of a spermicide is essential for contraceptive efficacy. The spermicide must be applied before coitus but no more than 1 hour in advance of sexual intercourse. Spermicides may be purchased without a prescription and must be applied each time intercourse is anticipated.

Barrier devices are nonpharmacological methods of birth control, although a prescription may be written for cervical caps and diaphragms to ensure proper fitting. These devices include male and female condoms, cervical caps, and diaphragms. The most commonly used is the male condom. Three materials are used in the manufacture of male condoms: latex, polyurethane, and lamb intestine. Lubricants containing mineral oil can decrease the barrier strength of condoms.

Barrier types of contraception for women include the condom, which is a loose-fitting tubular polyurethane pouch with flexible rings at both ends, and the diaphragm, which is a soft rubber cap with a metal spring that fits over the cervix. Before a diaphragm is inserted, it should be filled with spermicide to block the cervix completely from sperm access. The cervical cap, another contraceptive device, is a small cup-shaped barrier that fits directly over the cervical rim and is held in place by suction.

Table 23-2 provides information on the types of contraception and their efficacy.

Postcoital, or emergency, forms of contraceptives may be "morning-after pills" or the "abortion" pill to prevent pregnancy after intercourse. To be effective, the first dose of morning-after medication must be taken within 72 hours of unprotected sexual intercourse. A second dose then is taken 12 hours after the first dose. These medications should not be used as a routine type of contraception because of the potential side effects, but they should be used for sexual attacks, contraception failure, or the like.

The morning-after pill is a high-dose contraceptive formulated of progestin only, estrogen only, or both of these. The combined form of emergency contraception is about 75% effective, but one side effect is nausea and vomiting as if the woman is pregnant. The progestin emergency contraception requires two tablets and is packaged under the name of Plan B. The first tablet is to be taken within 72 hours and the second tablet 12 hours later. Plan B is for women 17 years and older. Plan B is more effective than combined estrogen and progestin forms. Emergency contraception products may lead to infertility, breast tender-

TECH NOTE!
Douching should be postponed for at least 6 hours after intercourse when using spermicides.

TECH NOTE!
Lamb intestine condoms do not provide effective protection against the transmission of viruses and bacteria.

TECH NOTE!
Patches and vaccines for men and women are currently under development. In testing, the male vaccine has been shown to be 99% effective against sperm production. The vaccine for men requires weekly injections of testosterone.

TABLE 23-2 Contraceptive Methods: Risks, Complications, and Failure

Type	Risk/potential complications	Failure rate (%)
Periodic abstinence	Sexual frustration, sexually transmitted diseases (STDs)	20
Calendar abstinence	Sexual frustration, unexpected ovulation, STDs	9-23
Withdrawal (coitus interruptus)	Anxiety, frustration, inability to relax, pregnancy, STDs	19
Vasectomy	Bruising, edema, pain, infection, psychological problems, STDs	0.15
Tubal ligation	Typical abdominal surgical risks, STDs	0.4
Injectible progestogen	Menstrual changes, weight gain, headaches, STDs	0.3-1
Intrauterine devices	Spotting, increased bleeding, uterine cramping, pelvic inflammatory disease, STDs	1-5
Oral contraceptive (estrogen/progesterone tablets)	Nausea, headaches, dizziness, spotting, weight gain, breast disease, ovarian cysts, fluid retention, mood changes, cardiovascular problems, STDs	1-5
Male condom	Allergic reactions, decreased sensitivity, loss of spontaneity, STDs	3-15
Female condom	Visibility, loss of spontaneity	21
Diaphragm	Allergy, toxic shock, vaginal irritation, cervical erosion	4-25
Cervical cap	Allergy, toxic shock, vaginal irritation, cervical erosion	4-25
Sponge	Allergy, toxic shock, vaginal dryness, vaginal irritation	15-30
Spermicides (alone)	Allergy, unpleasant smell or taste	10-25
Douche	Infection, local irritation, STDs	40
None	Pregnancy, STDs	85

ness, chest pain, shortness of breath, blurred vision, and jaundice. If pregnancy is not terminated by the use of this medication, the woman who took the emergency contraception product should consider an abortion because these products are teratogenic to a fetus.

RU-486, or mifepristone, is known as the abortion pill. RU-486 acts as an antiprogestin. Because progesterone is necessary for establishment and maintenance of pregnancy, RU-486 as an antagonist to progesterone prevents the maintenance of the pregnancy. For safety, this medication must be used within the first 9 weeks of pregnancy. Because of the abortifacient effects of the medication, the administration of RU-486 must be performed by a qualified health care professional, and a prescription will not be written for dispensing by a pharmacist.

Infertility

Infertility is the decreased ability to reproduce. Anovulation is a cause of infertility that can be corrected by pharmaceutical means. Agents are given to promote maturation of the graafian follicle and the production of ovulation to release an ovum.

CLASSIFICATION

Ovulation Stimulants

> **GENERIC NAME:** clomiphene
> **TRADE NAME:** Clomid
> **INDICATION:** female infertility
> **ROUTE OF ADMINISTRATION:** oral
> **COMMON DOSAGE:** 1 50-mg tablet qd for 5 days (initial therapy)

Luteinizing Hormone and Follicle-Stimulating Hormone Stimulants

> **GENERIC NAME:** menotropins
> **TRADE NAME:** Pergonal
> **INDICATION:** stimulate follicles to mature in infertility
> **ROUTE OF ADMINISTRATION:** injection
> **COMMON DOSAGE:** 75 to 150 units of FSH/LH

Ergot Alkaloid

> **GENERIC NAME:** bromocriptine
> **TRADE NAME:** Parlodel
> **INDICATION:** stimulates follicle maturity
> **ROUTE OF ADMINISTRATION:** oral
> **COMMON DOSAGE:** 2.5- to 7.5-mg tablet qd with food

TABLE 23-3 Sexually Transmitted Disease Organisms and Various Drug Therapies

Organism	Condition	Generic name	Trade name
Chlamydia trachomatis	Chlamydia	azithromycin	Zithromax
		erythromycin	Erythromycin
		doxycycline	Vibramycin
		ofloxacin	Floxin
Neisseria gonorrhoeae	Gonorrhea	cefixime	Suprax
		ceftriaxone	Rocephin
		ciprofloxacin	Cipro
		ofloxacin	Floxin
Herpes simplex	Genital herpes	acyclovir	Zovirax
		famciclovir	Famvir
		valacyclovir	Valtrex
Treponema pallidum	Syphilis	erythromycin	Erythromycin
		penicillin G benzathine	Bicillin C-R
		tetracycline	Tetracycline
Trichomonas vaginalis	Trichomoniasis vaginalis	metronidazole	Flagyl
Garnerella vaginalis	Bacterial vaginitis	clindamycin	Cleocin
		metronidazole	Flagyl
Candida albicans	Vaginal candidiasis	butoconazole	Femstat, Femstat 3
		clotrimazole	Gyne-Lotrimin, Mycelex-G
		fluconazole	Diflucan
		miconazole	Monistat
		terconazole	Terazol 7, Terazol
		tioconazole	Vagistat

Sexually Transmitted Diseases

TECH ALERT!

Remember these
  soundalike/look-alike
  drugs:
Cardura versus Coumadin
  and Cardene
Clomiphene versus
  clomipramine
Methyltestosterone versus
  methylprednisolone
Parlodel versus pindolol
Provera versus Premarin

STDs have been around for centuries and affect males and females. Any disease that can be transmitted by sexual intercourse is considered to be an STD. This does not mean that these diseases cannot be transmitted in other ways (non-sexually); it is the difference in terminology. Because STDs are embarrassing to the patients, many cases are not reported. Additionally, certain STDs can stay in hiding for long periods, which results in more transferrence between partners until the symptoms occur. Even then, many persons are reluctant to give out names of those who may be infected. STDs are caused by bacterial, viral, fungal, and protozoan organisms (see Chapter 29). If left untreated, STDs can cause irreversible sterility, blindness, and even death. Table 23-3 gives a list of the organisms along with the drug names and dosage forms.

DO YOU REMEMBER THESE KEY POINTS?

- Hormones mimicked by the medications used in reproductive tract therapy
- Conditions that androgens are used to treat
- The danger of synthetically produced androgens
- Uses of testosterone therapy in the male; uses of estrogen therapy in the female
- Action of medications used to treat benign prostatic hypertrophy
- Forms of oral contraceptive preparations
- Packaging of oral contraceptive for ease of compliance
- Uses of progestin therapy
- Method of wearing transdermal contraceptive patches
- Method of taking oral contraceptives; method for taking oral contraceptives after missed doses
- Hormones found in combination oral contraceptives
- Forms of contraception other than oral tablets
- Dangers of sildenafil
- Common sexually transmitted diseases and their treatments

MULTIPLE CHOICE QUESTIONS

1. The primary reproductive organs in the female are _____.
   - A. Uterus
   - B. Ovaries
   - C. Testes
   - D. A and B

2. What are the male sex hormones collectively called?
   - A. Estrogens
   - B. Androgens
   - C. Progestins
   - D. Testosterones

3. What is the major natural hormone produced by women?
   - A. Estradiol
   - B. Androgen
   - C. Progestin
   - D. All of the above

4. Which one of the following is used to obtain progestin naturally?
   - A. Urine of mares
   - B. Testes of bulls
   - C. Placentas
   - D. None of the above

5. Which of the following are classified on the controlled substances list as schedule III drugs?

A. Estrogens

B. Androgens

C. Anabolic steroids

D. All of the above

6. Testosterone is used to treat which of the following?

A. Hypogonadism in females

B. Hypogonadism in males

C. Breast and endometrial cancer in females

D. B and C

7. Estrogens are used to treat which of the following?

A. Menopausal symptoms

B. Hypogonadism in males

C. Hypogonadism in females

D. A and C

8. Medications used to treat benign prostatic hypertrophy include _____.

A. Antiandrogens

B. Estrogens

C. Androgens

D. α-Adrenergic blockers

E. A and D

9. There are four combination forms of oral contraceptives containing estrogen and progestins. In which of the combinations does estrogen gradually increase throughout the cycle?

A. Monophasic

B. Biphasic

C. Triphasic

D. Estrophasic

E. None of the above

10. If two tablets of oral contraceptives are missed and not taken at the correct time, what is the correct procedure?

A. Do not worry about the missed medication, just discard the medication not taken.

B. Take the two extra tablets with the next dose of medication.

C. Take two tablets with the next two doses at the regular time.

D. Take the two extra tablets at the end of the cycle.

TRUE/FALSE If a statement is false, then change it to make it true.

_____ **1.** The female produces ova just as males produce sperm.

_____ **2.** Fertilization of the ovum occurs in the uterus.

_____ **3.** Patients taking androgens should be told that weight gain may occur because of the accumulation of fluids.

_____ **4.** Progestins used with estrogen for contraception are measured in milligrams, and the estrogens are measured in micrograms.

_____ **5.** In biphasic oral contraceptives, the progestin is increased in the first half of the cycle.

_____ **6.** Transdermal estrogen patches should be worn on a hairless area of the body such as the upper arms, back, abdomen, or buttocks.

_____ **7.** Oral contraceptives are effective against sexually transmitted disease.

_____ **8.** A prescription for RU-486 will be brought to the pharmacy for dispensing.

_____ **9.** Sildenafil is safe for use by all men and may be used as often as necessary.

_____ **10.** All types of contraception have approximately the same effectiveness.

TECHNICIAN'S CORNER

A 55-year-old male patient with diabetes mellitus, hypertension, and coronary artery disease presents a prescription to the pharmacy for sildenafil (Viagra). When you, the pharmacy technician, review his medication history, you find that the following medications are taken regularly:

Glucotrol-XL 5 mg daily
metformin 500 mg tid
Tenormin 50 mg daily
Lipitor 20 mg qam
Isordil 10 mg bid

Is the Viagra safe for dispensing with the previously listed medication history? Which of the medications are in a correct dosage? Which medications could be given with sildenafil? Which are contraindicated with sildenafil, if any? What should you as a pharmacy technician do if this prescription is presented for dispensing?

BIBLIOGRAPHY

Applegate EJ: *The anatomy and physiology learning system,* ed 3, Philadelphia, 2006, Saunders.

Clayton BD, Stock YN: *Basic pharmacology for nurses,* ed 14, St Louis, 2006, Mosby.

Drug facts and comparisons, ed 60, St Louis, 2006, Wolters Kluwer.

Fulcher EM, Soto C, Fulcher RM: *Pharmacology: principles and applications,* Philadelphia, 2003, Saunders.

Leifer G: *Introduction to maternity and pediatric nursing,* ed 5, Philadelphia, 2006, Saunders.

Mosby's drug consult 2006, ed 16, St Louis, 2005, Mosby.

Mosby's medical, nursing, & allied health dictionary, ed 6, St Louis, 2002, Mosby.

Stedman's concise medical dictionary for health professionals, ed 3, Baltimore, 1997, Lippincott, Williams & Wilkins.

SECTION
three

Classifications of Drugs

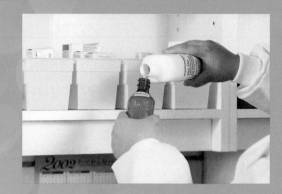

Antiinfectives

Objectives

UPON COMPLETING THIS CHAPTER, YOU SHOULD BE ABLE TO
DO THE FOLLOWING:

- List both trade and generic drug names covered in this chapter.
- Discuss the history of antibiotics and antibacterials.
- Understand the main causes of infections.
- List the various methods of transmission.
- Explain the reasons for antibiotic resistance.
- List the various generations of penicillin and cephalosporin antibiotics.
- Describe the differences in the generations of antibiotics.
- Describe the drug action for the various antibiotics discussed.
- List the common side effects of the antibiotics described in this chapter.
- Describe the types of infections caused by bacterial, fungal, and protozoan microbes.
- Describe the types of conditions caused by viruses.
- Distinguish between different antibiotics used for bacterial, fungal, and protozoan infections and antiviral agents used for viral infections.
- Differentiate between helminthic infestations and typical bacterial, fungal, and other parasitic infections.
- List the products used to treat infestations by helminths.
- Distinguish between gram-negative and gram-positive microbes and agents used to treat them.
- Distinguish between bacteriostatic and bactericidal effects of various agents discussed.

Antibiotic *Chemical agent produced by organisms and used to treat infections*

Antibiotic spectrum *The variety of microbes that a particular antibiotic can treat. Broad spectrum agents can treat many different types of organisms, whereas narrow-spectrum agents treat a lesser amount of organisms*

Antimicrobial *Chemical agent produced by scientists to prevent growth of or kill microorganisms*

Bacteria *Unicellular organisms*

Bactericidal *Agent that kills bacteria*

Bacteriostatic *Agent that prevents the growth of bacteria but does not kill the microbe*

ESBLs *Extended-spectrum beta-lactamases*

Fungicide *Agent that kills fungus*

Gram-negative bacteria *Bacteria that are unable to keep crystal violet stain when washed in acid alcohol*

Gram-positive bacteria *Bacteria that are able to keep crystal violet stain when washed in acid alcohol*

Helminth *Multicellular worm*

Inhibit *To stop or hold back; to keep a reaction from taking place*

Morphology *Appearance, including shape, size, structure, and Gram stain characteristics of organisms; study of organisms without studying the functions of organisms*

MRSA *Methicillin-resistant <u>Staphylococcus aureus</u>*

Mycosis *Fungal disease*

Normal flora *Microorganisms that reside harmlessly in the body and do not cause disease but may aid the host organism*

Nosocomial infection *An infection acquired during hospitalization*

Parasite *Organism that requires a host for nourishment and reproduction*

Pneumonia *Inflammation of the lungs caused by an infection*

Protozoa *Kingdom Protista; unicellular organisms that are parasites*

PRSP *Penicillin-resistant Streptococcus pneumoniae*

Symbiotic *A close relationship between two species*

Synthesis *The formation of chemical components within the body system*

Virus *An organism that replicates by using the host's cell parts, including DNA, ribosomes, and proteins*

VRE *Vancomycin-resistant enterococci*

ANTIINFECTIVES

Trade name	Generic name	Pronunciation
Penicillins		
First Generation		
Pfizerpen	penicillin G	(pen-i-**cil**-in)
Veetids	penicillin V	(pen-i-**cil**-in)
Penicillinase-Resistant Agents		
Dynapen	dicloxacillin	(die-klox-ah-**sil**-lin)
Prostaphlin	oxacillin	(ox-ah-**sil**-lin)
Staphcillin	methicillin	(meth-ah-**sil**-lin)
Tegopen	cloxacillin	(klox-ah-**sil**-lin)
Unipen	nafcillin	(naf-**sil**-lin)
Second Generation		
Amoxil	amoxicillin	(a-mox-ah-**sil**-lin)
Augmentin	amoxicillin/clavulanate	(a-mox-ah-**sil**-lin/**clav**-u-lah-nate)
Omnipen	ampicillin	(amp-ah-**sil**-lin)
Unasyn	ampicillin/sulbactam	(amp-ah-**sil**-lin/sul-**back**-tum)
Third Generation		
Geocillin	carbenicillin	(car-ben-ah-**sil**-lin)
Ticar	ticarcillin	(tie-car-**sil**-lin)
Timentin	ticarcillin/clavulanate	(tie-car-**sil**-lin/**clav**-u-lah-nate)
Fourth Generation		
Mezlin	mezlocillin	(mez-low-**sil**-lin)
Pipracil	piperacillin	(pie-**per**-ah-sil-lin)
Zosyn, Tazocin	piperacillin/tazobactam	(pie-**per**-ah-sil-lin/taz-oh-**back**-tam)
Cephalosporin Agents		
First Generation		
Ancef	cefazolin	(seh-**faz**-oh-lyn)
Keflex	cephalexin	(sef-ah-**lex**-in)
Velosef	cephradine	(**sef**-rah-deen)
Second Generation		
Ceclor	cefaclor	(**sef**-ah-klor)
Cefotan	cefotetan	(**sef**-o-tea-tan)
Cefzil	cefprozil	(cef-**pro**-zil)
Lorabid	loracarbef	(lor-a-**kar**-bef)
Mefoxin	cefoxitin	(ce-**fox**-eye-tin)
Monocid	cefonicid	(seh-**fon**-eye-sid)
Zinacef	cefuroxime	(cef-your-**ox**-zeem)
Third Generation		
Cefizox	ceftizoxime	(cef-tah-**zox**-zeem)
Cefobid	cefoperazone	(cef-o-**pear**-ah-zone)
Fortaz	ceftazidime	(**cef**-taz-eye-deem)
Omnicef	cefdinir	(cef-**deh**-ner)
Rocephin	ceftriaxone	(cef-try-**ax**-zone)
Spectracef	cefditoren pivoxil	(cef-deh-**tor**-en)
Suprax	cefixime	(sef-**ix**-ime)
Vantin	cefpodoxime	(cef-poe-**dox**-zeem)
Zefazone	cefmetazole	(cef-**met**-ah-zole)

Trade name	Generic name	Pronunciation
Fourth Generation		
Maxipime	cefepime	(**cef**-eye-peem)
Aminoglycosides		
Amikin	amikacin	(am-ah-**kay**-sin)
Garamycin	gentamicin	(jent-ah-**my**-sin)
Humatin	paromomycin	(par-oh-mow-**my**-sin)
Kantrex	kanamycin	(cane-ah-**my**-sin)
Nebcin	tobramycin	(tow-bra-**my**-sin)
Streptomycin	streptomycin	(strep-toe-**my**-sin)
Antifungals		
Diflucan	fluconazole	(flew-**kone**-ah-zole)
Fulvicin	griseofulvin	(gri-se-oh-**full**-vin)
Fungizone	amphotericin B	(am-foe-**ter**-i-sin)
Lamisil	terbinafine	(**ter**-bin-a-feen)
Lotrimin	clotrimazole	(kloe-**trim**-ah-zole)
Monistat	miconazole	(my-**kon**e-a-zole)
Nizoral	ketoconazole	(kee-toe-**kone**-ah-zole)
Mycostatin	nystatin	(ny-**stat**-in)
Sporanox	itraconazole	(it-trah-**kone**-ah-zole)
Antiprotozoan Agents		
Aralen	chloroquine	(**klor**-o-kwin)
Biltricide	praziquantel	(pra-ze-**quan**-tell)
Daraprim	pyrimethamine	(pie-rye-**meth**-ah-mean)
Lariam	mefloquine	(**mef**-low-kwin)
Flagyl	metronidazole	(met-row-**nid**-ah-zole)
Primaquine	primaquine	(**prim**-ah-queen)
Vermox	mebendazole	(me-**ben**-dah-zole)
Yodoxin	iodoquinol	(eye-oh-do-**kwin**-ole)
Antituberculin Agents		
INH	isoniazid	(eye-so-**nye**-ah-zid)
Myambutol	ethambutol	(e-**tham**-byoo-tole)
Rifadin	rifampin	(riff-**am**-pin)
Antivirals		
Famvir	famciclovir	(fam-sy-**klo**-veer)
Foscavir	foscarnet	(fos-**car**-net)
Symmetrel	amantidine	(ah-man-**tah**-deen)
Valcyte	valganciclovir	(val-**gan**-sye-kloe-veer)
Zovirax	acyclovir	(aye-sye-**klo**e-veer)
Antiretrovirals		
AZT	zidovudine	(zye-**doe**-vue-deen)
Crixivan	indinavir	(in-**dih**-nah-veer)
Epivir	lamivudine	(la-**miv**-you-deen)
Videx	didanosine	(dye-**dan**-oh-seen)
Viracept	nelfinavir	(nell-**fin**-ah-veer)
β-Lactams		
Azactam	aztreonam	(**az**-tree-oh-nam)
Primaxin	imipenem/cilastatin	(im-eh-**pen**-um/sye-la-**stat**-in)

ANTIINFECTIVES—cont'd

Trade name	Generic name	Pronunciation	Trade name	Generic name	Pronunciation
Carbapenems			**Lipopeptide**		
Invanz	ertapenem	(er-ta-**pen**-um)	Cubicin	daptomycin	(**dap**-toe-mye-sin)
Merrem	meropenem	(mer-o-**pen**-um)			
			Macrolides		
Quinolone			Biaxin	clarithromycin	(clar-ith-**row**-my-sin)
Avelox	moxifloxacin	(mox-i-**floks**-ah-sin)	Dynabac	dirithromycin	(dir-ith-**row**-my-sin)
Cipro	ciprofloxacin	(ci-pro-**flox**-a-sin)	Erythrocin	erythromycin	(er-ith-**row**-my-sin)
Factive	gemifloxacin	(gem-i-**floks**-ah-sin)	Zithromax	azithromycin	(a-zi-**throw**-my-sin)
Levaquin	levofloxacin	(lee-vo-**floks**-ah-sin)			
Maxaquin	lomefloxacin	(low-meh-**floks**-ah-sin)	**Oxalodinones**		
NegGram	nalidixic	(nal-eye-**dix**-ic)	Zyvox	linezolid	(lin-eh-**zo**-lid)
Noroxin	norfloxacin	(nor-**flox**-a-sin)			
Tequin	gatifloxacin	(ga-tee-**floks**-ah-sin)	**Tetracyclines**		
Trovan	trovafloxacin	(troh-vah-**floks**-ah-sin)	Achromycin	tetracycline	(tet-ra-**sye**-kleen)
Zagam	sparfloxacin	(spar-**floks**-ah-sin)	Declomycin	demeclocycline	(deme-**klow**-sye-kleen)
Cinoxacin	cinoxacin	(sin-**ox**-ah-sin)	Terramycin	oxytetracycline	(oxy-**tetra**-sye-kleen)
			Vibramycin	doxycycline	(dox-i-**sye**-kleen)
Ketolides					
Ketek	telithromycin	(tell-lith-row-**mye**-sin)	**Tricyclic Glycopeptide**		
			Vancocin	vancomycin	(van-koe-**mye**-sin)
Lincosamides					
Cleocin	clindamycin	(klin-da-**mye**-sin)			
Lincocin	lincomycin	(lin-koe-**mye**-sin)			

THE BODY HAS A BUILT-IN defense mechanism called the immune system that identifies and kills foreign bodies that have invaded the body. However, if a microorganism cannot be destroyed by our immune systems, then help from antibiotics may be necessary. Infections can occur when the invading microorganisms grow rapidly and the body cannot fight off the invader. This may be because of factors such as a weakened immune system. If the invading organism gets out of hand, antibiotics can help. The word *antibiotic* literally means "against life." Antibiotics are made from natural or synthetic substances that can inhibit or destroy microorganisms. The term *antimicrobial* refers specifically to substances produced by scientists that are used against human infections. However, both terms are used interchangeably in the medical field.

Although it may seem reasonable that bacteria are an unnecessary component for a healthy life, in reality, this is not true. Within the intestines of a normal human body, billions of microbes reside. We refer to these microbes as the normal flora, and their function is a symbiotic one; that is to say, both entities benefit from each other. The human gut provides a warm, nutrient-rich environment for the bacteria to survive, and the bacteria aid in the digestion and absorption of food, from which human beings benefit. Other areas of the human body in which bacteria can be found are in the mouth and throat. However, if the microbial growth does not stay in balance, then even our own normal flora can cause us to become ill. This can occur if our immune system is weakened and cannot keep the bacteria in balance.

Antibiotics have a bacteriostatic or bactericidal effect on microbes. Those agents that arrest the development or stop growth of microbes are considered bacteriostatic. When antibiotics are "static," they do not kill mature cells.

Instead, they inhibit (stop) any new growth, allowing the immune system of the body to kill off the remaining microbes. A bactericidal agent kills the microorganisms.

This chapter discusses a brief history of antibiotics, followed by a description of each body system along with the types of infections that are seen most commonly. Finally, the drugs used to treat various conditions are listed along with their drug action, side effects, auxiliary labels, and any special notes with which pharmacy technicians should be acquainted. More information on microorganisms can be found in Chapter 29.

History of Antibiotics

IMPORTANT "FIRSTS" IN ANTIBIOTIC THERAPY

In the 1930s the first antibiotic, sulfa (sulfanilamide), was discovered. This agent was found to cure staphylococcus infections via bacteriostatic action. With the mass production of sulfa drugs, thousands of military personnel were saved from death from infections during World War II. Sulfa drugs were the first antibiotics produced and were considered a miracle drug; thus they were used often and without knowledge of the possibility of resistance. Resistance allows a microorganism to decrease the action of antibiotics. As patients took their sulfa drugs and began to feel better, they would stop taking their medication. This allowed the remaining microbes to build up a type of immunity to the sulfa drug. The next time the infection appeared, the bacteria were more resistant to the antibiotic. As this trend repeated itself, more bacteria became resistant, eventually making it impossible to kill them with normal antibiotic therapy. Not until decades later did researchers find out that microbes have the ability to alter their genetic makeup. Therefore, because of the overuse and misuse of antibiotics, new strains of bacteria made the antibiotic ineffective. By the 1960s, sulfa drugs were obsolete; however, they have found a limited yet useful place in antibiotic treatment and are used for urinary tract and certain respiratory infections. It is important, however, always to take antibiotics for the full course of treatment, as prescribed.

THE DISCOVERY OF PENICILLIN

Most persons associate penicillin with the mold that forms on bread. Alexander Fleming was an English physician who discovered penicillin by accident. As he worked on his laboratory experiments, he inadvertently contaminated an agar plate with mold called *Penicillium notatum*. As the mold grew within the agar plate, he observed a ring of clearance being formed around the *Penicillium* species. The ring was produced by chemicals emitted from the mold into the agar plate. The chemicals had killed off the surrounding microorganisms (Figure 24-1). This is called the zone of clearance. This substance eventually was isolated and became what we now know as penicillin. Penicillin agents have been around since the 1940s and are effective, having a bactericidal effect toward gram-positive bacteria more than toward gram-negative bacteria.

Advancements in the science world concerning antiinfectives have increased the current treatments to include more than one dozen classifications of antiinfectives and more than 100 individual drugs that are available to combat a range of infections.

GRAM STAIN

A Danish doctor by the name of Hans Christian Gram developed the Gram stain procedure in 1883. The procedure is still in use today to determine the mor-

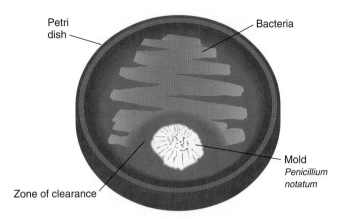

Petri
dish

Bacteria

Mold
*Penicillium
notatum*

Zone of clearance

FIGURE 24-1 A petri dish is prepared with nutrient-rich agar. This nutrient feeds the bacteria that are placed on the plate. The penicillium colony can be seen with an area of clearance where the bacteria cannot grow. This occurs because the penicillium inhibits the bacterial growth.

phology of bacteria. The morphology refers to the shape and appearance of microorganisms. Gram-positive bacteria have a thick outer membrane made of peptidoglycan links. Penicillin molecules enter into these links and break them, which kills the microorganism. Gram-negative organisms have a different type of cell wall and are therefore harder to kill (see Figure 29-2). Several antibiotics, especially newer antibiotics, can kill gram-negative microorganisms.

MODERN ANTIBIOTICS

Because microorganisms have the ability to alter their genetic makeup enough to deter the effects of many antibiotics, stronger antiinfectives had to be developed. A different class or generation of antibiotic is used to overcome these organisms. Antibiotics were altered chemically to be more effective against different microbial infections. Some microbes were able to make penicillin ineffective. These specialized bacteria are referred to as penicillinase-producing microbes. However, there have been advances made in strengthening penicillins by additives such as clavulanate (used with amoxicillin) to make Augmentin and sulbactam (used with ampicillin) to make Unasyn. These agents inhibit the penicillinase enzymes from breaking down the antibiotic. This renders the penicillinase-producing microbes susceptible to the antibiotic. Many antibiotics are available to treat a wide variety of infections; these are covered in the next section.

Types of Infections and Their Treatments

COMMON INFECTIONS

Infections can appear anywhere on or within the body. Some are more common because of exposure to the environment, foods we eat, and contact with others. Box 24-1 outlines the most common types of organisms that attack the major body organs.

The internal body is normally a sterile environment; however, this does not include areas that are open to the outside (air) or those that contain outside substances. Many areas within the body are subject to bacterial, viral, and parasitic infections. Those areas open to the outside are susceptible to infections. The common areas most likely to become infected include the following:

BOX 24-1 TYPES OF MICROORGANISMS

Bacteria
Fungi
Protozoa
Viruses*
Multicellular microscopic parasites

*Not technically an organism.

Male and female genital systems (sexually transmitted diseases)
Gastrointestinal tract
Respiratory system, upper and lower
Urinary tract
Skin
Nose and mouth
Eyes and ears

SEXUALLY TRANSMITTED DISEASES

Sexually transmitted diseases can be caused by various bacteria, protozoan organisms, and viruses. They can do permanent damage to internal organs such as the cervix, kidneys, heart, and brain. They can cause sterility and even death if not treated. Many symptoms of various STDs are different in men than in women. In certain cases the patient is asymptomatic (without symptoms). Proper diagnosis and appropriate treatment with the correct antibiotic or antiviral medication is vital. Table 24-1 lists examples of the most common types of sexually transmitted diseases, their symptoms, and treatments.

GASTROINTESTINAL INFECTIONS

The stomach is subjected to food that normally carries many different bacteria. The highly acidic environment within the stomach usually destroys any bacteria, but if the stomach lining is injured or if the stomach juices are not strong enough to kill microbes, the microbes may settle in the gut, causing infections. One of the major infections of the stomach is from the bacterium *Helicobacter pylori,* also known as *H. pylori.* This bacterium can be eradicated by a triple drug therapy. The primary antibiotics that are used include tetracycline, sulfamethoxazole/trimethoprim (Septra), or metronidazole. These antibiotics have a bactericidal effect on the bacilli. Other areas susceptible to infections include the mouth, throat, and trachea.

Microbes also can infiltrate areas of the body that do not come into contact with air; these microbes are referred to as anaerobic microbes. Microbes that can live in air are aerobic, those that do not live in air are anaerobic, and the types of microbes that can tolerate oxygen to a degree are called facultative anaerobes. The type of antibiotic that is prescribed depends on the type of microbe that is causing the infection.

RESPIRATORY INFECTIONS

Infections of the respiratory system can occur in any part of the respiratory system. When we breathe, small particles and microorganisms can be inhaled on dust. These microorganisms include bacteria, fungi, and viruses. These can settle within the airways and cause infection. Common symptoms of a respiratory infection include wheezing, coughing, and shortness of breath (see Chapter 18).

TABLE 24-1   Common Sexually Transmitted Diseases and Treatments

Sexually transmitted diseases	Species	Symptoms	Drug treatments
Bacterial			
	Chlamydia trachomatis		Gram-negative obligate intracellular microbe
Gonorrhea	*Neisseria gonorrhoeae*	White discharge from penis in men, painful urination, sterility in both sexes	ceftriaxone, cefixime, cefpodoxime, doxycycline, gatifloxacin, oxytetracycline
Syphilis	*Treponema pallidum*	Damages the nervous and circulatory systems	penicillin G, procaine penicillin, tetracycline, doxycycline
Trichomoniasis	*Trichomonas vaginalis*	Causes a thin, malodorous discharge, often asymptomatic	metronidazole

Viral	**Virion**	**Symptoms**	**HIV/AIDS drug treatments may include several agents taken concurrently**
Genital herpes	Enveloped virion or naked viral capsomere	Fever, headaches, genital blisters, mortality in newborns if active	acyclovir or famciclovir or valacyclovir
HIV	Retrovirus	HIV weakens the immune system, when it advances it becomes AIDS	Determined by patient's situation, (i.e., pregnancy onset, blood tests)
AIDS	Retrovirus	AIDS causes severe infections including Kaposi's sarcoma. Other illnesses include dementia, shortness of breath, malnutrition, chronic diarrhea	abacavir, atazanavir, delavirdine, didanosine, efavirenz, indinavir, nelfinavir, lamivudine, nevirapine, ritonavir, saquinavir, zalcitabine, zidovudine

One of the most serious respiratory infections is pneumonia, which affects more than 4 million Americans annually. Pneumonia is an infection of the lungs. Infectious pneumonia can be caused by bacteria, viruses, fungi, parasites, and chemicals. Pneumonia acquired within the hospital or nursing home is referred to as a nosocomial infection. Many elderly persons who are bedridden for long periods are at high risk of acquiring pneumonia, as are persons with chronic conditions such as emphysema, bronchitis, asthma, and immunosuppressive disorders.

Unlike pneumonia, tuberculosis is a highly contagious respiratory infection that is caused by the bacterium *Mycobacterium tuberculosis*. Tuberculosis causes inflammation, abscesses, necrosis, and fibrosis of the respiratory system and can spread to other parts of the body. Because of the increase in immunodeficiency from human immunodeficiency virus (HIV) and acquired immunodeficiency syndrome (AIDS), tuberculosis has been increasing. An estimated 10 million to 15 million Americans have tuberculosis, and more than 1.7 billion persons are infected worldwide. Symptoms include chronic coughing, fever, sweating, and weight loss. Tuberculosis is diagnosed in the United States by a tuberculin skin test, but this must be confirmed by a sputum test that isolates the bacteria.

Fungal infections are more prone to infect persons with other major illnesses such as cystic fibrosis and those whose immune systems are compromised, such as persons with AIDS, cancer patients receiving chemotherapy, or patients taking multiple antibiotics. Fungal infections normally are acquired while persons are in the hospital or nursing home. The two most common fungal infections of this type are *Candida albicans* and *Aspergillus fumigatus*.

Bacterial infections resulting from chemical exposure include those toxins that are inhaled in fumes. For example, if inhaled, asbestosis causes scarring of the lungs, decreasing the capacity of the lungs to take in oxygen. This eventually can cause emphysema, pulmonary edema, and even cancer. These conditions in turn can lead to infections within the respiratory system.

NOSOCOMIAL INFECTIONS

Most hospitalizations are a result of illness, trauma, or surgery or to conduct tests to determine the cause of a problem. Nursing homes are necessary for long-term care of older adults and severely ill persons. Infections that are acquired within hospitals or nursing homes are known as nosocomial infections, and they can be deadly. Hand sanitization and hand washing are the major steps for the prevention of nosocomial infections. See Appendix F. Patients who have conditions that weaken their immune system and who are bedridden are more susceptible to infection. Whether these nosocomial infections are bacterial, fungal, or viral, they are hard to fight. With more antibiotics being used to fight infections, more multidrug-resistant organisms in the hospital and in nonhospital health care settings are emerging.

MULTIDRUG-RESISTANT ORGANISMS

Multidrug-resistant organisms are increasing as more persons are living longer. More infections may affect older citizens who are in hospitals, nursing homes, long-term care, and even doctor's offices. Any area that may harbor bacteria can infect several types of persons. These include the young, those with weakened immune systems, and those with major trauma or preexisting diseases. Also those persons who have poor nutrition or receive kidney dialysis are at risk. In the hospital setting, two of the most common antibiotic-resistant organisms are methicillin-resistant *Staphylococcus aureus* (MRSA) and vancomycin-resistant enterococci (VRE). Two additional types of resistant organisms that are emerging in doctor's offices, clinics, and pediatric settings include extended-spectrum beta-lactamases (ESBLs), which are resistant to cephalosporins and monobactams, and penicillin-resistant *Streptococcus pneumoniae* (PRSP).

INFECTIONS OF THE SKIN

Skin abrasions, cuts, and scrapes are a common occurrence with growing children and should be cleaned and kept free of bacteria that can infect the area and cause disease. Diabetic persons are at high risk for infections of the skin. Because of the lack of blood flow to the extremities in some diabetic persons, minor injuries to the feet can get infected and cause septic infections that can cause gangrene. For these types of infections, hospitalization and treatment with strong antibiotics may be necessary.

Fungal infections are common on the skin surface because fungi need a high concentration of oxygen to live. A common fungal infection is *tinea pedis,* or athlete's foot. For this condition there are several over-the-counter (OTC) medications available.

INFECTIONS OF THE NOSE AND MOUTH

The nose and mouth come in constant contact with airborne microbes. Colds and the yearly flu (influenza) are common conditions experienced by most persons at one time or another. For minor colds and flulike symptoms, OTC products can bring some relief of the symptoms experienced. Unfortunately, because viruses cause colds and flu, antibiotics are useless against them. If the normal (bacterial) flora within the mouth, nose, or throat should grow out of control, antibiotics may be prescribed. In addition to bacteria, some antivirals and antifungals are used to treat a variety of infections.

INFECTIONS OF THE EYES AND EARS

The eyes and the ears are susceptible to infections because they are exposed to the environment. The eyes most often are infected by bacteria or viruses. The most common eye infection is conjunctivitis. Conjunctivitis is an inflammation of the lining of the eyelids and cornea called the conjunctiva. Within the eyelids, styes may appear, as well as a discharge of pus. The eye may swell and close. Seasonal allergies also can cause conjunctivitis. If an infection of the underlying cornea develops, it is called keratitis.

Otitis media is a common ear infection that many babies and young children experience. Two types of otitis media, or middle ear infection, are acute and chronic. The acute form normally is caused by a bacterial infection that begins as an upper respiratory tract infection and proceeds to infect the ear. The chronic form is caused by repeated infections. Both forms cause inflammation of the tympanic membrane and are painful. Chronic otitis media also may result from rupture of the tympanic membrane. Table 24-2 gives a list of ophthalmic and otic antiinfectives.

Antibiotic Treatments

Many types of microorganisms can cause infections. Antibiotics often are referred to as wide-spectrum or narrow-spectrum agents. This refers to the variety of microorganisms that they can stop or kill. An antibiotic narrow-spectrum agent typically covers mostly gram-positive microbes, whereas wide-spectrum agents cover many gram-positive and gram-negative microorganisms. Another important morphologic characteristic is whether the organism shape is a rod, coccus, spiral, or other type. Once the microorganism is identified, a physician can determine the best antibiotic to use for the infection. Several classifications of antibiotics are known. In addition to those agents listed at the beginning of the chapter are several more that cover specific gram-negative and/or gram-positive microorganisms.

Table 24-3 lists some of the most common types of infections based on their bacterial morphology and their treatments. This includes the outcome of a Gram stain, the shape of the microbe, and where the microbe is located.

PENICILLIN

Penicillin antibiotics are taken from two different molds, *Penicillium notatum* and *P. chrysogenum*. These molds are grown in laboratories and are altered synthetically to fight off many microorganisms. The drug action of penicillin is bactericidal toward microbes that are currently reproducing. They disrupt the formation of the cell wall so that the bacteria cannot keep a constant osmotic gradient and lyse (break open). Penicillin-type agents cover mostly gram-positive organisms. Because penicillins are susceptible to degradation from stomach acids, it is important that they be taken 1 to 2 hours before or after meals.

For some infections, such as those that can affect the gastrointestinal system, more potent antibiotics are required. In this case, broader-spectrum "cillins" such as ampicillin and carbenicillin can kill gram-positive and some gram-negative organisms.

Mild side effects make these agents a good choice. However, if someone has a penicillin allergy, other agents must be used. If penicillin is to be given to a person suspected of having an allergy, a skin test can be performed to see

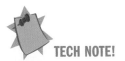

TECH NOTE!

Gram-positive microbes have a different cell wall than gram-negative microbes. Antibiotics can kill microbes by breaking down their cell walls. The reason they do not kill human cells is because human cells do not have a cell wall.

TABLE 24-2 Otic and Ophthalmic Antiinfectives

Classification	Generic name	Trade name	Indication	Dosage forms	Auxiliary label
Otic Agents					
Antiinfective	chloramphenicol	Chloromycetin	External ear infections	Solution, ointment	For the ear
Fluoroquinolone	ciprofloxacin	Cipro-NC	External ear infections	Solution	For the ear
Cephalosporin	cefaclor	Ceclor	Otitis media	Tablets, suspension	For the ear
Ophthalmic Agents					
Fluoroquinolone	ciprofloxacin	Ciloxan	A broad spectrum of Gram microorganisms	Solution, ointment	For the eye
Macrolide	erythromycin	Ilotycin	Neonatal prophylaxis of *Neisseria gonorrhoeae* or *Chlamydia trachomatis* ocular infections	Ointment	For the eye
Aminoglycoside	gentamicin	Garamycin	A broad spectrum of Gram microorganisms	Solution, ointment	For the eye
Antiviral	idoxuridine	Herplex	Herpes simplex virus keratitis	Solution, ointment	For the eye
Antifungal	natamycin	Natacyn	Conjunctivitis, keratitis, blepharitis from fungal infection	Solution	For the eye
Triple antibiotic	neomycin, polymyxin B sulfate, bacitracin	Neosporin	Superficial ocular infections	Solution, ointment	For the eye
Fluoroquinolone	norfloxacin	Chibroxin	A broad spectrum of Gram microorganisms	Solution	For the eye
Fluoroquinolone	ofloxacin	Ocuflox	Conjunctivitis, corneal ulcers that are caused by susceptible organisms	Solution	For the eye
Antibiotic	polymyxin B sulfate	Aerosporin	Susceptible gram-negative organisms	Solution	For the eye
Sulfonamide	sulfacetamide	Bleph-10, Sulamyd	Susceptible Gram organisms	Solution, ointment	For the eye
Sulfonamide	sulfisoxazole	Gantrisin	Acute otitis media and susceptible Gram organisms	Solution	For the eye
Antiviral	tifluridine	Viroptic	Herpes simplex virus keratoconjunctivitis	Solution	For the eye
Aminoglycoside	tobramycin	Tobrex	A broad spectrum of Gram microorganisms	Solution, ointment	For the eye
Antiviral	vidarabine	Vira-A	Herpes simplex virus keratoconjunctivitis	Ointment	For the eye

TABLE 24-3 **Antibiotic Reference Table 1: Bacterial Morphology, Areas Affected, Conditions, and Treatment**

Affected area	Treatment	Conditions
Gram-Positive Cocci (Spherical-Shaped Microbe): Aerobic and Anaerobic		
Skin, systemic	penicillin G	Throat infections, cuts, sepsis
Systemic, respiratory	penicillin G, penicillin VK	Strep throat, pneumonia, sepsis
Sepsis	penicillin G, ampicillin	Urinary tract infections
Gram-Negative Cocci (Spherical-Shaped Microbe): Aerobic and Anaerobic		
Sexually transmitted disease	ceftriaxone, spectinomycin	Gonorrhea
Brain	penicillin G	Meningitis
Respiratory	ampicillin/sulbactam amoxicillin/clavulanate	Pneumonia
Gram-Positive Bacilli (Rod-Shaped Microbe): Aerobic and Anaerobic		
Respiratory	penicillin G	Pneumonia
Systemic	vancomycin	Sepsis of the blood
Peripheral	penicillin G	Necrosis, gangrene
Gram-Negative Bacilli (Rod-Shaped Microbe): Aerobic and Anaerobic		
	cefazolin, cephradine, cefotetan, cefoxitin, cefonicid, lomefloxacin, gatifloxacin, cinoxacin, nalidixic, doxycycline, sulfa ampicillin, piperacillin, gentamicin	Urinary tract infections
Sepsis	ampicillin, glycosides, cephalosporins	Sepsis, bacteremia, stomach infections
Respiratory	Fourth-generation penicillin, aminoglycosides	Pneumonia

whether there is any sensitivity. Nausea, vomiting, and diarrhea; headache; sore mouth or rashes; pain; and fever may be signs of allergic reaction. One of each generation of penicillins is listed along with its individual information. The normal dosage of each drug is the recommended oral adult dosage.

ANTIBACTERIAL, PENICILLINS

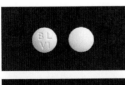
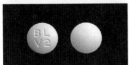

GENERIC NAME: penicillin V potassium
TRADE NAME: Veetids
GENERATION: first-generation penicillin
ROUTE OF ADMINISTRATION: oral
INDICATIONS: pneumonococcal pneumonia, streptococcal pharyngitis, syphilis, gonorrhea
DOSAGE FORMS: tablet, oral solution
COMMON DOSAGE: 125 to 500 mg PO q6-8h
AUXILIARY LABELS:
- Take on an empty stomach.
- Take until gone.

SPECIAL NOTE: Liquid should have a "shake well and refrigerate" auxiliary label and 14-day expiration date after reconstitution if stored in a refrigerator.

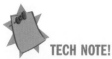

TECH NOTE!

Normal practice is for a physician to write for a loading dose of an antibiotic followed by a lower routine dose. The reason for a loading dose is to bring the antibiotic up to its therapeutic level as quickly as possible.

GENERIC NAME: ampicillin
TRADE NAME: Omnipen, Polycillin
GENERATION: second-generation penicillin
ROUTE OF ADMINISTRATION: oral
INDICATIONS: skin/soft tissue infections, otitis media, sinusitis, respiratory, gastrointestinal, meningitis, and septicemia
DOSAGE FORMS: capsules, suspension, injection
COMMON DOSAGE: 250 to 500 mg PO q6h
AUXILIARY LABELS:
- Take on an empty stomach.
- Take until gone.
SPECIAL NOTE: Suspension should have a "shake well and refrigerate" auxiliary label and 14-day expiration date after reconstitution if stored in a refrigerator.

GENERIC NAME: ticarcillin
TRADE NAME: Ticar
GENERATION: third-generation penicillin
ROUTE OF ADMINISTRATION: injection (intramuscular, intravenous)
INDICATIONS: drug-resistant or severe skin infections, bone/joint infections, septicemia, respiratory infections, urinary tract infections (UTIs)
DOSAGE FORM: injection only
COMMON DOSAGE: 3 g IV q4-6h; 200 mg/kg qd or 15 to 40 g q4h
SPECIAL NOTE: After reconstitution, drug is good for 72 hours if kept in the refrigerator.

CEPHALOSPORINS

Cephalosporins are less affected by stomach acids; therefore, they can be taken with meals. Although cephalosporins are not exactly like penicillins, there is a 10% chance of an allergic reaction for those who have penicillin allergies.

An example of one cephalosporin from each generation is listed. In addition, the common dosage forms and dosages are listed, as well as any special notes of which technicians should be aware.

CEPHALOSPORINS

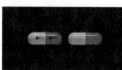

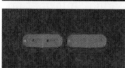

GENERIC NAME: cephalexin
TRADE NAME: Keflex
GENERATION: first-generation cephalosporin
ROUTE OF ADMINISTRATION: oral
INDICATIONS: most infections, cystitis, skin/soft tissue infections, streptococcal pharyngitis
DOSAGE FORMS: tablet, capsules, suspension
COMMON DOSAGE: 250 mg to 1 g PO q6h
AUXILIARY LABEL:
- Take until gone.
SPECIAL NOTE: Suspension should have a "shake well and refrigerate" auxiliary label and 14-day expiration date after reconstitution if stored in a refrigerator.

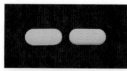

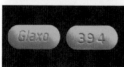

GENERIC NAME: cefuroxime
TRADE NAME: Ceftin (tablet), ? (suspension), Zinacef (injection)
GENERATION: second-generation cephalosporin
ROUTE OF ADMINISTRATION: oral, intramuscular
INDICATIONS: most infections, UTI, gonorrhea
DOSAGE FORMS: tablet, suspension, injection
COMMON DOSAGE: 250 to 500 mg PO bid
AUXILIARY LABEL:
- Take until gone.
SPECIAL NOTE: Suspension should have a "shake well and refrigerate" auxiliary label.

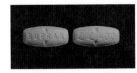

GENERIC NAME: cefixime
TRADE NAME: Suprax
GENERATION: third-generation cephalosporin
ROUTE OF ADMINISTRATION: oral
INDICATIONS: most infections, gonorrhea
DOSAGE FORMS: tablet, suspension
COMMON DOSAGE: 400 mg PO qd or divided every 12 hours
AUXILIARY LABEL:
■ Take as directed.
SPECIAL NOTE: Suspension should have "shake well" auxiliary label. Storage and
stability: May be kept at room temperature for up to 14 days.

GENERIC NAME: cefepime
TRADE NAME: Maxipime
GENERATION: fourth-generation cephalosporin
ROUTE OF ADMINISTRATION: intravenous
INDICATIONS: skin infections, UTI, moderate to severe pneumonia; wide range of gram-
negative bacilli and other microorganisms
DOSAGE FORMS: injection
COMMON DOSAGE: most infections: 1 to 2 g IV q12h for 5 to 10 days
SPECIAL NOTE: Drug is stable 7 days if refrigerated.

Penicillin and cephalosporins are popular agents used to fight off bacterial infections caused by gram-negative and gram-positive microbes. However, other classes of antibiotics are available, such as those listed in Table 24-4. These medications are used depending on the specific microbe that has been isolated. A culture is taken of the area infected, and by using various laboratory methods, the specific microbe in most cases can be identified (see Chapter 29). In addition, the organism is tested for its sensitivity to various antibiotics; thus the right drug can be used. If the microbe cannot be isolated or the infection is severe, doctors may give a broad-spectrum antibiotic in hopes that it will cover the microbe in question. In addition to this alternative type of treatment, a combination of agents can be used to cover many different species of bacterial infections.

MYCOBACTERIUM AND MYCOBACTERIAL TREATMENT

Two main infections in human beings caused by a mycobacterium are tuberculosis and leprosy. (*Mycobacterium* is related closely to bacteria but is considered a different species than those that fit into the general class of bacteria.) Both of these conditions are chronic. Leprosy (Hansen's disease) is an infectious disease that is caused by *Mycobacterium leprae.* In the past, it affected millions of persons across the world, with most cases in Asia and Africa. Recently, the disease has decreased progressively. Noticeable skin lesions appear. Ulceration of the feet and loss of hand function may occur, and corneal abrasions may cause blindness. This condition can be treated with dapsone (bacteriostatic) and clofazimine (bactericidal).

Tuberculosis is a disease that was known as the wasting disease because it robs a person of breath and strength. Eventually, death occurred. Tuberculosis has been responsible for millions of deaths throughout history, but in the 1960s tuberculosis was disappearing as new drugs were invented to eradicate the disease. Unfortunately, many individuals quit taking their medication once they felt better; thus the microbe was able to withstand low doses of antibiotics until it became resistant. Now, entering the new millennium, tuberculosis is once again occurring in staggering numbers. Two thirds of prisoners are

TABLE 24-4 Antibiotic Reference Table 2: Antibiotics Other Than Penicillins and Cephalosporins

Antibiotic	Trade name	Generic name	Effects	Normal adult dosage
Aminoglycosides	Garamycin	gentamicin	Mostly gram-negative microbes: bactericidal	Normally based on peak/trough levels: see *Drug Facts and Comparisons*
	Kantrex	kanamycin	Mostly gram-negative microbes: bactericidal	1 g q6h, max 3-4 days
	Amikin	amikacin	Mostly gram-negative microbes: bactericidal	15 g/kg per day IV/IM q6-8h
	Nebcin	tobramycin	Mostly gram-negative microbes: bactericidal	3 g/kg per day IV/IM q8h
Carbapenems	Merrem	meropenem	Broad spectrum: bactericidal	1 g IV q8h
	Primaxin	imipenem-cilastatin	Broad spectrum: bactericidal	250 mg IV q6-8h; 500 mg IV q6-8h
Monobactams	Azactam	aztreonam	Broad spectrum: bactericidal	500 mg-1 g IV q8-12h: 2 g IV q6-8h
Quinolones	Cipro	ciprofloxacin	Broad spectrum: bactericidal	250-750 g PO q12h; 200-400 g IV q12h
	Noroxin	norfloxacin	Broad spectrum: bactericidal	200-400 g PO/IV q12h
	Trovan	trovafloxacin mesylate/ alatrofloxacin mesylate	Broad spectrum: bactericidal	100-200 g PO q24h; 200-300 g IV q24h
	Levaquin	levofloxacin	Broad spectrum: bactericidal	500 g IV/PO q24h
Lincosamides	Cleocin	clindamycin	Gram-positive microbes; anaerobes: bacteriostatic	150-300 g PO q6h; 300-600 g IV q6-12h
	Lincocin	lincomycin	Gram-positive microbes; anaerobes: bacteriostatic	500 g PO q6-8h; 600 g IV q12h to qd
Macrolides	Biaxin	clarithromycin	Broad spectrum: bactericidal/ bacteriostatic	250-500 g PO q12h
	E-Mycin	erythromycin	Broad spectrum: bactericidal/ bacteriostatic	Dosage varies depending on what type of erythromycin is given: see *Drug Facts and Comparisons*
	Zithromax	azithromycin	Broad spectrum: bactericidal/ bacteriostatic	250-500 mg PO qd
Ketolides	Ketek	telithromycin	Broad spectrum: pneumonia	800 mg PO 7 to 10 days
Tetracyclines	Achromycin	tetracycline	Broad spectrum: bacteriostatic	250-500 g PO q6-12h
	Vibramycin	doxycycline	Broad spectrum: bacteriostatic	100 g PO qd to bid
Vancomycin	Vancocin	vancomycin	Active against gram-positive microbes: bactericidal/ bacteriostatic	125-500 g PO q6-8h; 500 mg IV q12h

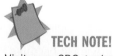

TECH NOTE!

Visit *www.CDC.gov/mmwr (Mortality and Morbidity Weekly Report)* to see what type of outbreaks occur in the United States and the world.

estimated to have tuberculosis. Millions of persons are dying each year, and for those persons who acquire the resistant strain, there is no medication available to combat this deadly disease. Tuberculosis is prevalent in the United States and around the world. For positive results on a TB test refer to Figure 18-4.

A few antituberculin-type medications are used to treat tuberculosis, but they must be taken for the full course of treatment. This can last from 6 months to years depending on test results and must not be stopped regardless of how well the person feels. As the microbes are decreased, the person begins to feel

TABLE 24-5 Antituberculin Agents

Generic name	Trade name	Dosing regimen	Common length of time
isoniazid	INH	5 mg/kg/day	6-24 months
rifampin	Rifadin	600 mg qd	6-9 months
ethambutol	Myambutol	15 mg/kg/day	6-9 months
pyrazinamide	Pyrazinamide	15-35 mg/kg/day	6-9 months
cycloserine	Seromycin	750 mg to 1 g qd	Up to 18 to 24 months
streptomycin	Streptomycin	15 mg/kg/day (IM)	Up to 12 months
kanamycin	Kantrex	500 mg to 1 g qd	Up to 12 months

better, but if the medication is stopped, the microbe reoccurs and it is stronger and much harder to kill (Table 24-5).

AMINOGLYCOSIDES

Aminoglycosides are among the strongest antibiotic agents in use today. They are bactericidal to many varieties of gram-negative microorganisms. The drug action for parenterally administered aminoglycosides is their ability to bind to ribosomes of the microorganism, stopping the protein synthesis, which ultimately causes the death of the organism. Many of these medications come in parenteral (intravenous) form only and are used mainly in hospitals for severe infections. Often, they are given with other antibiotics to further their microbial coverage. A serious side effect of high doses of aminoglycosides is possible nephrotoxicity or ototoxicity. Because aminoglycosides have a narrow range between therapeutic and toxic serum levels, careful calculations must be made to determine the appropriate dosage. This is done by evaluation of the patient's blood levels of antibiotic, drawn at specific times (called peak and trough levels). In this way the patient's clearance of the aminoglycoside drug can be seen, and changes can be made in the dosage or dosing time if necessary. Patients with renal disease and older adults are more susceptible to toxic levels of these agents because of decreased excretion. A sample of the types of agents most commonly seen by technicians is listed next, along with their specifics.

AMINOGLYCOSIDES

GENERIC NAME: amikacin
TRADE NAME: Amikin
INDICATIONS: serious infections such as *Pseudomonas, Proteus, Serratia,* and various gram-positive bacilli that cause bone and respiratory infections, endocarditis, and septicemia
DOSAGE FORMS: injection, 50 mg/mL in 2-mL and 4-mL vials; 250 mg/mL in 2-mL and 4-mL vials
COMMON DOSAGE: based on weight of patient: normally 5 to 7.5 mg/kg per dose every 8 hours
SPECIAL NOTE: stable for 2 days if refrigerated after mixing into appropriate solution

GENERIC NAME: gentamicin
TRADE NAME: Garamycin (intravenous), Genoptic (ophthalmic), G-Myticin (topical)
INDICATIONS: for gram-negative organisms such as *Pseudomonas, Proteus,* and *Serratia* and gram-positive staphylococcus; bone and respiratory tract infections, skin and soft tissue infections, UTI and abdominal infections, and eye infections caused by susceptible bacteria
DOSAGE FORMS: infusion, ophthalmic ointment, solution, topical cream

COMMON DOSAGE: based on weight of patient: for UTI, 1.5 mg/kg per dose IV; ophthalmic, instill $\frac{1}{2}$ inch of ointment 2 to 3 times daily every 3 to 4 hours or drops in infected eye tid to qid; topical, apply 3 to 4 times per day to affected area(s)

AUXILIARY LABELS:

■ For ophthalmic: For the eye.

■ For topical cream: Topical use only.

SPECIAL NOTE: Intravenous solution does not need to be refrigerated before or after mixing into solution. Stability is 24 hours only after mixing.

GENERIC NAME: tobramycin

TRADE NAME: Nebcin (intravenous), Tobrex (ophthalmic), Tobi (inhalant)

INDICATIONS: for susceptible gram-negative bacilli including *Pseudomonas aeruginosa;* ophthalmic use for superficial infections to the eye from susceptible bacteria

DOSAGE FORMS: infusion, ophthalmic ointment, solution, inhalation solution

COMMON DOSAGE: based on weight of patient; for UTI, 1.5 mg/kg per dose IV; ophthalmic, instill ointment 2 to 3 times daily every 3 to 4 hours; for inhalation, 60 to 80 mg tid

AUXILIARY LABEL:

■ For ophthalmics: For the eye.

SPECIAL NOTE: After reconstitution of powder, intravenous solution is stable for 96 hours if refrigerated.

DRUG-RESISTANT AND MISCELLANEOUS ANTIBIOTICS

The following agents are commonly used antibiotics for a variety of infections. Their classification, drug action, indications, and generic and trade names are listed in Table 24-6. Only certain antibiotics can be used on the resistant microorganisms. These agents are listed next:

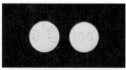
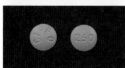

GENERIC NAME: ciprofloxacin

TRADE NAME: Cipro

INDICATION: Complicated severe UTIs

DOSAGE FORMS: tablet, suspension, infusion

COMMON DOSAGE: 500 mg q12h

SPECIAL NOTE: Ciprofloxacin has bactericidal action against a wide range of gram-positive organisms such as *Staphylococcus epidermidis,* methicillin-resistant strains of *S. aureus,* and gram-negative organisms such as *Escherichia coli*

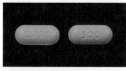
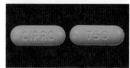

GENERIC NAME: vancomycin

TRADE NAME: Vancocin

INDICATION: staphylococcal infections

DOSAGE FORMS: tablet infusion used for serious staphylococcal infections

COMMON DOSAGE: IV 500 mg (7.5 mg/kg) q6-8h or 1 g (15 mg/kg) q12h

SPECIAL NOTE: bactericidal for staphylococci and streptococci; also used for resistant staphylococcal infections

TABLE 24-6 Antibiotic Reference Table 3: Antibiotics for Resistant Microorganisms

Class	Generic name	Trade name	Indication	Drug action
Tetracyclines*	doxycycline tetracycline minocycline	Vibramycin Achromycin Minocin	Severe infections such as respiratory, gastrointestinal, and integumentary	Inhibits protein synthesis
Quinolones†	ciprofloxacin levofloxacin ofloxacin norfloxacin	Cipro Levaquin Floxin Noroxin	Tuberculosis and respiratory and urinary tract infections	Interferes with bacterial DNA synthesis
Macrolides	azithromycin clarithromycin erythromycin erythro ethylsuccinate erythromycin state	Zithromax Biaxin Emycin, Ery-Tab E.E.S. Erythrocin	Respiratory, genital, gastrointestinal, and skin infections	Inhibits protein synthesis
Carbapenems	imipenem/ cilastatin	Primaxin	Serious infections	Inhibits bacterial cell wall synthesis
Monobactam	aztreonam	Azactam	Wide-spectrum gram-negative aerobic organisms	Inhibits bacterial cell wall synthesis
Vancomycin	vancomycin	Vancocin	Serious/severe infections	Inhibits bacterial cell wall synthesis

*Auxiliary labels: Take on an empty stomach. Take with plenty of water. Avoid dairy products. Avoid antacids. Avoid direct sunlight.
†Auxiliary labels: Do not take antacids. Avoid iron/zinc supplements 4 hours before or 2 hours after taking.

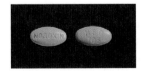

GENERIC NAME: norfloxacin
TRADE NAME: Noroxin
INDICATION: Complicated UTIs and infections
DOSAGE FORMS: oral, ophthalmic
COMMON DOSAGE: 400 mg bid for 10 to 21 days
SPECIAL NOTE: bactericidal action against methicillin-resistant strains of *S. aureus* infections

ANTIFUNGALS

Fungi are plantlike organisms that can grow on cloth, food, showers, people, or in any warm, moist environment. They absorb nutrients from the environment or hosts such as animals and human beings. Most conditions caused by fungi tend to affect the outside of the body and are not life threatening but do cause great annoyance. A systemic infection is much more serious. This is when the fungus invades inside the body. For these types of infections, more potent agents called fungicides are used (Table 24-7).

TABLE 24-7 Antifungal Infections and Their Treatments

Type of infection	Generic name	Trade name	Drug action	Indications
Candidiasis, fungal septicemia, cryptococcal meningitis	amphotericin B	Fungizone	Affects fungus cell membrane, causing lysing to occur; bactericidal and bacteriostatic	Systemic mycosis
Candidiasis, tinea	clotrimazole	Lotrimin, Gyne-Lotrimin	Alters cell membrane permeability	Vaginal, oral, and topical fungal infections
Cryptococcal meningitis	fluconazole	Diflucan	Affects biosynthesis, inhibiting growth; bactericidal and bacteriostatic	Esophageal, urinary tract infection, and vaginal mycosis
Candida spp., fungal pneumonia, septicemia	flucytosine	Ancobon	Inhibits DNA synthesis and metabolism of pyrimidine; bactericidal	Serious mycosis
Tinea infections	griseofulvin	Fulvicin U/F, Grisovin F/P	Inhibits cell mitosis; bactericidal	Ringworm, toe/fingernail mycosis
Histoplasmosis, blastomycosis	itraconazole	Sporanox	Affects biosynthesis, inhibiting growth; bactericidal	Lung infections
Tinea infections	ketoconazole	Nizoral	Affects biosynthesis, inhibiting growth; bactericidal	Systemic mycosis
Candidiasis	miconazole	Monistat, Monistat IV, Monistat-Derm	Affects biosynthesis, inhibiting growth; bactericidal	Skin, vaginal mycosis
Candida albicans	nystatin	Mycostatin	Affects fungus cell membrane, causing lysing to occur; bactericidal	Vaginal, intestinal mycosis
Onychomycosis, tinea infections	terbinafine	Lamisil	Inhibits cell wall synthesis; bactericidal	Skin, toe, and fingernail mycosis

Candida Infections

A common fungal species that resides inside the human body is *Candida albicans*. Although this fungal species is found within a human being's normal flora, if it gets out of control because of a weakened immune system or because of use of potent antibiotics, it can cause serious effects.

There are different species of *Candida*. Depending on the specific species, the organism is responsible for infections of the mouth or vagina or under the fingernails and toenails. When fungal infections occur on the skin surface, they are referred to as dermatophytic infections. The agents used are applied directly

TABLE 24-8 Protozoan Infections and Their Treatments

Species	Disease name	Transmission	Treatment
Toxoplasma gondii	Toxoplasmosis	Contaminated food, water, feces of a bug or cat; sand flies; tsetse flies also carry the disease	primethamine/sulfadiazine trimethoprim/sulfamethoxazole pentamidine (intravenous) azithromycin
Plasmodium vivax	Malaria	Female mosquitoes	chloroquine quinine mefloquine primaquine

to the skin unless the infection has advanced into the bloodstream, and then parenterally administered antifungals must be used. Topical agents are available in different dosage forms: lotions, creams, ointment, powders, and sprays. A person can use what works best for him or her. Many antifungal agents are available OTC to treat mild cases of mycosis (fungus infections). Some of the agents listed are fungicidal (killing fungi) or fungistatic (inhibiting further growth) depending on the organism for which they are used.

Tinea Infections

One of the most common conditions caused by a fungus is dermatophytosis, caused by fungi from the genera *Trichophyton, Microsporum,* or *Epidermophyton.* Tinea pedis (foot) is also known as athlete's foot. If it appears on the scalp, it is known as tinea capitis or ringworm. If it appears on babies in the groin area, it is called tinea cruris or diaper rash.

Parasites

Parasites are organisms that benefit at the expense of another. The host is the organism that is being used by the parasite. Under the kingdom Protista, the phylum Sporozoa consists of parasitic organisms. The morphology (characteristics) of an organism depends on whether it is multicellular or unicellular and how it is transmitted. How these organisms are distinguished from one another depends on several factors, such as morphology and locomotion (movement), as listed in Box 24-2. The life cycles of many of the organisms that affect human beings are explained in Chapter 29. Some major conditions that can occur from protozoa are listed in Table 24-8.

Parasitic Conditions **Protozoa.** Many protozoa are human parasites. Amebiasis is an infection caused by the protozoan species *Entamoeba histolytica.* The cyst form is transferred via fecal-oral routes. Symptoms can include abdominal pain, nausea, flatulence, and fatigue. Treatments include iodoquinol, which rids the body of the infestation. Another protozoan disease that is more dangerous to human beings is toxoplasmosis. The species *Toxoplasma gondii* is transferred via uncooked meat or cysts that may be present in cat feces. Although the symptoms may be mild in most adults, it can be deadly to infants and the unborn fetus. Treatment includes pyrimethamine and sulfadiazine. Trichomoniasis is caused by the species *Trichomonas vaginalis.* This disease affects the vaginal area; the cervical area becomes red and inflamed. These protozoa also can infect the female and male urethra. Metronidazole is the drug of choice and must be used by both sexual partners.

BOX 24-2 PARASITIC ORGANISMS AND THEIR DESCRIPTION

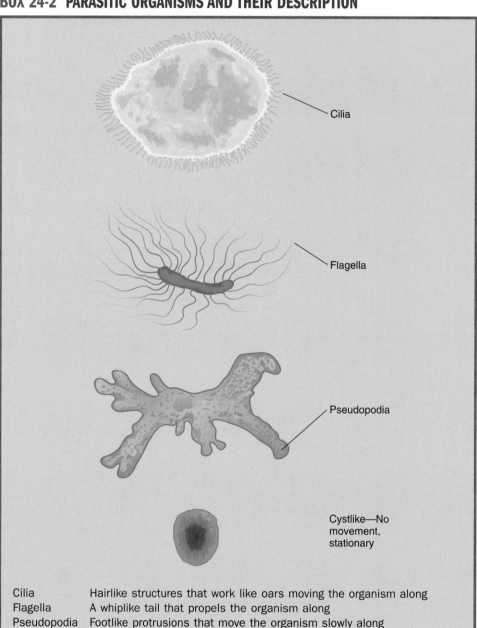

Cilia	Hairlike structures that work like oars moving the organism along
Flagella	A whiplike tail that propels the organism along
Pseudopodia	Footlike protrusions that move the organism slowly along
Stationary	A cyst form that waits for an opportunistic environment before regenerating

Helminths (worms). Helminths are parasitic worms. They are not microscopic organisms, but the procedures used to diagnose infections are done in a clinical laboratory. These parasites are multicellular. The two major worms that affect Americans are roundworms (nematodes) and flatworms (platyhelminthes). Fifty species of roundworms can infect human beings. Many can be transferred in undercooked meat. Some species can lodge in the intestine or lymph nodes, causing harm to the host. Hookworms are another type of roundworm and are transferred via feces infected with the worm through skin contact. For example, if someone walks on soil that has been contaminated with human feces that contains hookworms, the hookworms will enter through the skin of the foot.

TABLE 24-9 Helminthic Infestations and Their Treatments

	Species or disease name	Symptoms	Treatment
Class Nematoda			
Roundworms	*Trichinella spiralis* (trichinosis)	Inflammation	diethylcarbamazine, ivermectin
Hookworms	*Ankylostoma duodenale, Necator americanus*	Anemia, weakness, fatigue	mebendazole, albendazole, pyrantel
Pinworms	*Enterobius vermicularis*	Anal itching	mebendazole, albendazole, pyrantel
Bladder worm	*Cysticercus*	Forms a cyst that can be as large as an orange; symptoms vary depending on area infected	praziquantel
Phylum Platyhelminthes			
Tapeworms	*Taenia saginata, Taenia solium*	Diarrhea, weight loss, perforation of intestine	praziquantel, niclosamide, paromomycin
Flukes	Schistosomiasis	Loss of blood in feces	praziquantel

Flatworms are divided further into tapeworms and flukes. Many flatworms live by feeding off dead matter or small organisms and are not harmful to human beings. Tapeworms reside in the intestines of most vertebrates, where they absorb digested food from the host. Eating undercooked meat can transfer them to human beings. Flukes have an interesting life cycle that involves freshwater snails and human beings. Persons who drink water from feces-contaminated water can acquire flukes. Many helminthic diseases are caused by undercooked meat or contaminated water and soil. Most helminthic infections occur in persons who live in areas where sanitation is nonexistent or in persons who are not aware of the problem with eating raw meat. Table 24-9 lists the species, symptoms, and treatments.

Parasitic Treatments. Parasites can be dealt with in only a few ways: kill them and wash them away, rid them from the body alive or dead, or surgically remove them. Whichever mechanism is used, the main goal is to remove them from the body. All agents used to rid the parasites from the body are oral dosage forms; therefore, hospitalization is rarely necessary. In addition, the dosage regimen is normally short term, and treatment can be done in just a few oral doses.

All parasites can cause damage to the tissues or organs that they invade. Although parasites may weaken the host, most parasites do not kill their host because this would cut off their food and shelter. Table 24-10 lists the main anthelmintic agents and their drug action.

Malaria
Malaria is a sporozoan infection with symptoms consisting of fever, chills, sweating, headache, and nausea. The cycle of chills, fever, and sweating varies depend-

TABLE 24-10 Antihelmintic Drug Actions and Common Dosage

Generic name	Trade name	Drug action	Common dosage
diethylcarbamazine	Hetrazan	Vermicidal: increases the loss of filariae, decreases ability to produce more	2-3 mg/kg PO tid
mebendazole	Vermox	Vermicidal: stops glucose uptake in worm	100 mg PO bid × 3 days
niclosamide	Niclocide	Vermicidal: affects mitochondria, decreases metabolism	8 g × 1 dose or 2 g PO qd × 1 week (depends on type of worm infestation)
oxamniquine	Vansil	Vermicidal: causes worms to move to liver where they are killed	12-15 mg/kg PO × 1 (dose may vary depending on type of worm infestation)
praziquantel	Biltricide	Paralysis: causes loss of calcium and eventual paralysis of worm, which then is flushed out	25 mg/kg PO tid × 1 day
pyrantel	Antiminth	Paralysis: causes depolarization and eventual paralysis of worm, which is then flushed out	11 mg/kg PO × 1 dose; may be repeated in 2-3 weeks if necessary
thiabendazole	Mintezol	Vermicidal: inhibits essential enzymes, causing death	25 mg/kg PO bid × 2 days

ing on the particular pathogen. The genus *Plasmodium* has four different species that are responsible for malaria. Some cause severe side effects, such as the species *P. falciparum,* which can cause death. The human body, the site of sporozoan reproduction, is called the reservoir. Transmission is usually via an infected mosquito, but the sporozoa also can be transmitted by infected needles or syringes or by blood transfusion. The incubation period ranges from 1 week to 1 month depending on the species.

Malaria is a major health problem in more than 100 countries. Reported cases of malaria are responsible for more than 1 million deaths annually. Approximately 1200 cases are diagnosed in the United States annually. The prevention and control of malaria consists of controlling mosquitoes by using insect repellents, filling in water holes where mosquitoes breed, and using insecticides.

The diagnosis of malaria is made based on blood smears. Chloroquine phosphate is used as treatment when possible. However, if the strain is resistant to chloroquine, other agents such as mefloquine, doxycycline, or primaquine can be used.

ANTIVIRALS

Viruses are organisms that cannot live outside their host. They are unlike bacteria or any other organisms because of their structure and design. Viruses are classified by the following criteria:

1. Nucleic acid makeup (single- or double-stranded DNA or RNA)
2. Size
3. Host it infects
4. Enveloped or naked

Debate continues within the scientific community as to whether viruses should be classified as a living organism because they differ in most criteria that are used to classify living organisms. All living organisms replicate or reproduce themselves with their own set of blueprints or DNA; however, viruses do not. They require a host's DNA to replicate. Unlike parasites, viruses kill the host's cell on leaving or bud off, allowing further reinfections. Another major difference between the kingdom Protista and viruses is that they do not have the ability to reproduce themselves in the same way that other organisms do. Most organisms reproduce sexually or asexually; however, viruses cannot reproduce by themselves. They must use their host's components to replicate. The makeup of the virus is related closely to a human being's DNA. Therefore, when agents are used to destroy a virus, they inadvertently can destroy human cells along with the virions. Plants and animals can contract many types of viral diseases. For animals, these include chickenpox, colds, influenza, polio, rabies, warts, HIV, AIDS, and some types of cancer.

The following analogy will help explain viral replication. Let's say you have been given the key to an automobile manufacturing plant, but instead of making one of the cars normally made in the plant, you want a truck specialized to fit your needs. You have all the necessary components within the auto shop, but the outcome will be different from what normally is manufactured in the plant. This is the same type of action that a virion (one virus particle) has on your body. The virus invades your cells and uses your components to assemble its own blueprints. The invasion and spread of virions has five steps:

1. Attachment: This is a lock-and-key mechanism that allows virions to attach to specific host cells.
2. Injection of nucleic acids: the whole virion enters the cell or it injects its nucleic acids to begin the replication process.
3. Synthesis: The virion takes over the controls of the cell and begins to use them to make its own necessary enzymes and proteins to replicate its RNA or DNA and component parts.
4. Assembly: Once all the parts are made, then the parts are assembled to create a new virion. Millions of new virions are assembled and readied for transport.
5. Spread via lyse or budding: When the assembly is completed, the virions leave the manufacturing plant (host cell) and continue to reinfect other cells.

Agents that can slow down and, in some cases, kill viruses. To interrupt the process outlined previously in the manufacturing plant analogy, an antiviral agent can affect the virus by the processes listed in Box 24-3. In addition Table 24-11 lists both antiviral and antiretroviral agents and examples of the types of viruses in which they are indicated.

ANTIVIRAL

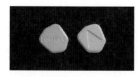

GENERIC NAME: acyclovir
TRADE NAME: Zovirax (Glaxo Wellcome)
DOSAGE FORMS: tablet, capsules, injection, suspension, ointment
DRUG ACTION: interferes with DNA synthesis of the virion by inhibiting viral replication
SIDE EFFECTS: headache, dizziness, rash, nausea
AUXILIARY LABELS:
■ Suspension: Shake well.
■ Ointment: Topical use only.
SPECIAL NOTE: Suspension is banana flavored.

TABLE 24-11 Antiviral and Antiretroviral Agents

Classification	Generic name	Trade name	Indications
Antivirals	acyclovir	Zovirax	Herpes simplex, herpes zoster
	amantidine	Symmetrel	Influenza A strains, Parkinson's disease
	famciclovir	Famvir	Herpes zoster, recurrent genital herpes
	foscarnet	Foscavir	Herpes simplex, CMV retinitis, Acyclovir-resistant HSV in immunocompromised patients
Antiretrovirals	didanosine	Videx	HIV infection
	indinavir	Crixivan	HIV infection
	lamivudine	Epivir	HIV infection, chronic hepatitis B
	nelfinavir	Viracept	HIV infection
	zidovudine	AZT	HIV infection, prevention of maternal-fetal transmission

ANTI-RETROVIRAL

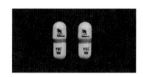

GENERIC NAME: zidovudine
TRADE NAME: Retrovir (also known as AZT)
DOSAGE FORMS: tablet, capsule, injection, syrup
DRUG ACTION: zidovudine is an analog of thymidine that interferes with the HIV viral RNA-dependent DNA polymerase (enzyme), which results in the inhibition of viral replication
SIDE EFFECTS: headache, weakness, abdominal pain, diarrhea, nausea, anemia
AUXILIARY LABEL:

■ Take as directed.

SPECIAL NOTE: Syrup is strawberry flavored.

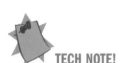

TECH NOTE!
Did you know that there are even smaller virus-type particles called viroids? They have only a single strand of RNA. Fortunately, they do not affect human beings but have been found in plant species. They are responsible for the destruction of many plants and important food crops.

Colds/Flu

Everyone gets a cold now and then without much concern, and it is common knowledge that there is no cure for the common cold. The reason is that colds are caused by viruses. Viruses, as you may have learned, mutate very well; therefore, they change each year. New products claim to decrease the chance or severity of colds, but the cold still rules. The good news is that although it is inconvenient, in a healthy person, it is not deadly. Influenza is another type of virus that affects millions of persons each year. This condition, unlike the common cold, causes death in many older adults and immunocompromised persons every year. For this reason, vaccines, which contain the viruses that are most likely to cause influenza that year, are given each year (in late fall or early winter) to persons who are at higher risk. These include older adults, health care workers, and immunocompromised persons such as those who are receiving chemotherapy or those with HIV or AIDS.

Viral Sexually Transmitted Diseases
HIV/AIDS

Since the 1970s, HIV (the resulting disease is called AIDS) infections have been increasing. HIV is a blood-borne, sexually transmitted virus. Although there are many agents now available to treat AIDS, there is no cure for this disease. The virion does not cause death, but instead it renders the host too weak to fight off any infection; thus a person with AIDS will succumb to common illnesses. The HIV virus attacks the immune system of human beings. HIV can be transmitted by bodily fluids containing the virus. Simple sexual safety steps, which include having both partners tested for HIV before sexual activities, or wearing

BOX 24-3 ANTIVIRAL MECHANISMS OF ACTION

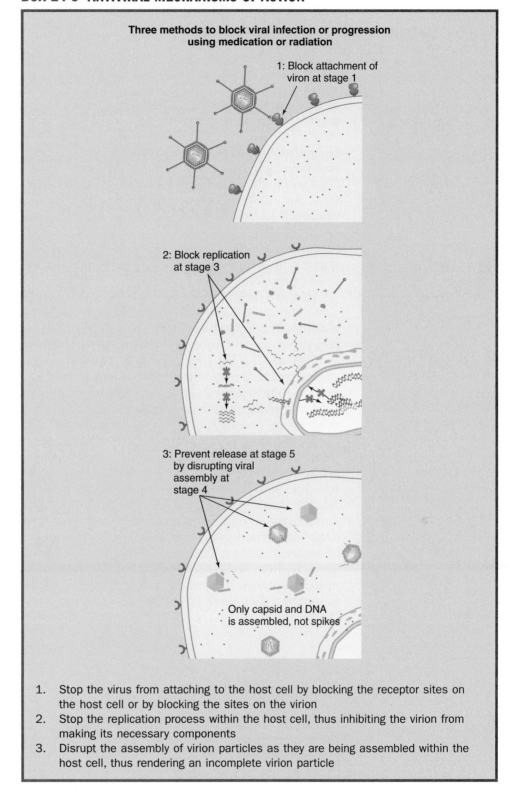

Three methods to block viral infection or progression using medication or radiation

1: Block attachment of viron at stage 1

2: Block replication at stage 3

3: Prevent release at stage 5 by disrupting viral assembly at stage 4

Only capsid and DNA is assembled, not spikes

1. Stop the virus from attaching to the host cell by blocking the receptor sites on the host cell or by blocking the sites on the virion
2. Stop the replication process within the host cell, thus inhibiting the virion from making its necessary components
3. Disrupt the assembly of virion particles as they are being assembled within the host cell, thus rendering an incomplete virion particle

condoms, reduce the chances of acquiring HIV. In medical settings, protective wear such as gloves and face shields is used to decrease the risk of contamination. HIV could be transmitted to a nurse or doctor via fluids such as blood or even vaginal secretions. New syringes are also now in use to decrease the possibility of needle sticks.

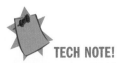

In the beginning stages of HIV, the body weakens because of the virus replication process within the immune system. Specifically, the number of T4 lymphocytes decreases; the infected person is diagnosed as having AIDS when the T-cell count is less than 200.

The onset of AIDS is estimated to be able to occur up to 20 years after one acquires HIV. However, the virus is always contagious. All agents that are available to treat HIV and AIDS are aimed at controlling the progression of the disease but cannot cure it. Therefore the only way to avoid this disease is to prevent contracting it.

Miscellaneous Viral Conditions

Papillomavirus. The papillomavirus is a virus that causes the common wart. Most warts disappear on their own within 6 months. Many agents are available OTC, such as Wart-Off, to treat warts if they do not go away on their own (see Chapter 9 for additional information about OTC drugs).

Herpes Viruses. The three main types of herpes are herpes simplex type 1 and type 2 and herpes zoster. Their activities within the human body vary, as outlined in Box 24-4.

Herpes type 1 causes blisters on the surface of the skin. This virus also can cause blindness if left untreated. Herpes type 2 causes infections in adults and neonates. If a mother has an active case of herpes type 2 when the baby is being born, the neonate can acquire the virus. Herpes zoster affects the nerves endings, and results in severe pain. The virus also causes lesions on the skin surface, referred to as shingles. This form of the virus tends to have cyclical reinfections. Chickenpox also is caused by herpes zoster, although after infection the body may build up an immunity (see Chapter 27) so that the virus cannot cause reinfection.

Two types of immunity are active or passive. Active immunity occurs if the immunity is from antibodies produced by the body. This can be natural or artificial. An example of active natural immunity is when children are exposed to a child with the measles; those who then acquire the virus from the child who has the measles have contracted measles in a natural way. Artificial natural immunity is when the dead or attenuated (weakened) virus is given as an injection. The second type of immunity, passive, can be natural or artificial. An example of passive natural immunity is when antibodies are passed, for example, from mother to the newly born child, providing immunity for up to 3 months. Passive artificial immunity is when an injection of the antibodies or immune globulin is given. These antibodies and globulins are prepared in a laboratory.

BOX 24-4 TYPES OF HUMAN HERPES VIRUSES

Herpes Simplex	
Type 1	Causes disease of the mouth, face, skin, esophagus, or brain
Type 2	Causes disease of the rectum, genitals, and meninges
Herpes Zoster	
Shingles	Lesions on the skin surface appearing on torso, arms, and legs
Chickenpox	Childhood disease: the body normally will produce immunity against reinfection

DO YOU REMEMBER THESE KEY POINTS?

- The generations of penicillins and cephalosporins
- The drug actions of the drugs discussed in this chapter
- What types of bacteria are good and where they reside
- How the Gram stain is done and what it indicates
- What causes tuberculosis and the treatment
- What are some of the most common fungal infections
- How viruses proliferate
- The three mechanisms of destroying or stopping viruses

MULTIPLE CHOICE QUESTIONS

1. Penicillin agents are most effective against which type of microbes?
   A. Gram positive
   B. Gram negative
   C. Gram positive and fungus
   D. Gram positive and viruses

2. The difference in the "generations" of penicillin and cephalosporin agents is that _____.
   A. Generations determine the spectrum of gram-negative and gram-positive microbes against which they work
   B. Generations determine the types of microbes against which they work
   C. Generations determine the length and course of treatment
   D. Generations are determined by when they were discovered

3. The following diseases are caused by sexually transmitted diseases except _____.
   A. Chlamydia
   B. Syphilis
   C. Trichomoniasis
   D. Trichinosis

4. The following conditions are *always* caused by viruses except _____.
   A. Colds
   B. Warts
   C. Acquired immunodeficiency syndrome
   D. Pneumonia

5. A person with an allergy to penicillin who has a urinary tract infection most likely would be treated with which of the following agents?
   A. Second-generation penicillin
   B. Third-generation penicillin
   C. Cephalosporin
   D. Aminoglycoside

6. All of the following agents are third-generation cephalosporins except _____.
   A. Vantin
   B. Cefixime
   C. Ceftizoxime
   D. Cefprozil

7. Corneal abrasions and skin lesions that are progressive are symptoms of _____.
   A. Sexually transmitted diseases
   B. Tuberculosis
   C. Human immunodefiency virus
   D. Hansen's disease

8. The most common treatment for tuberculosis is the combination regimen of _____.
   A. Penicillin G and gentamicin
   B. Isoniazid, rifampin, and ethambutol
   C. Kanamycin, cycloserine, and isoniazid
   D. Amikacin, kanamycin, and rifampin

9. Fungus grows best in or on _____.
   A. Shower floors
   B. In very dry environments
   C. On clothes
   D. On cooked food

10. Antiparasitic agents work by all of the methods listed except _____.
   A. Killing the parasite
   B. Killing the host
   C. Ridding the body of the live parasite
   D. Paralyzing the parasites and then flushing them out of the body

11. One way to avoid a parasitic infestation is to _____.
   A. Cook all meat thoroughly
   B. Do not drink from rivers or streams
   C. Wash your hands before eating food
   D. All of the above

12. The following anthelmintic agents are vermicidal except _____.
   A. Thiabendazole
   B. Oxamniquine
   C. Praziquantel
   D. Mebendazole

13. Malaria is a disease that is caused by _____.
   A. Mosquitoes
   B. Blood transfusions
   C. Tropical climates
   D. Sporozoan species

14. The actions of antiviral agents include all of the following except _____.
   A. They can interrupt the attachment of the virion to the host cell
   B. They can affect the replication phase of the virion within the host cell
   C. They can affect the assembly of the viral parts within the host cell
   D. They can lyse open the viral particles before they reach the host cell

15. Influenza is most dangerous to all of the following groups of persons except _____.
   A. Babies
   B. Older adults
   C. Immunosuppressed
   D. Adults aged 18 to 25 years

16. The type of herpes that is related closely to chickenpox is _____.
   A. Herpes type 1
   B. Herpes type 2
   C. Herpes simplex
   D. Shingles

TRUE/FALSE   If the statement is false, then change it to make it true.

_____ **1.** All microbes cause disease.

_____ **2.** Bacteriostatic agents kill microbes, whereas bactericidal agents only stop the growth.

_____ **3.** Anaerobic organisms need oxygen to survive, whereas aerobic organisms do not.

_____ **4.** A nosocomial infection is an infection within the nose such as a cold.

_____ **5.** Tinea pedis is a viral infection affecting the feet.

_____ **6.** Terbinafine normally is used to treat fungal infections such as onychomycosis.

_____ **7.** The most common form of fungus found as part of the normal flora is the species *Candida albicans*.

_____ **8.** All parasites cause problems for the host because they benefit at the expense of another.

_____ **9.** The sexually transmitted disease *Trichomonas vaginalis* is a parasitic infection.

_____ **10.** AIDS causes similar conditions such as HIV.

_____ **11.** Not all herpes viruses are contagious.

_____ **12.** Chickenpox is a childhood disease that will bring about passive immunity.

TECHNICIAN'S CORNER

Use a reference book to determine the following information about the listed antiinfective agents:

Use
> Necessary auxiliary label
> Dosage forms
> Routes of administration

Agents
> Zidovudine
> Ethambutol
> Miconazole
> Ticarcillin/clavulanate
> Maxipime

BIBLIOGRAPHY

Center for Disease Control and Prevention: Retrieved January 30, 2002, from www.cdc.gov/travel/., Travelers Health. National Center for Infectious Diseases, Division of Global Migration and Quarantine. 10-24-2006

Drug facts and comparisons, ed 60, St Louis, 2006, Wolters Kluwer.

Goodman G, Gillman L: *The pharmacological basis of therapeutics,* ed 10, Elmsford, NY, 2001, McGraw-Hill.

McKenry LM, Salerno E: *Mosby's pharmacology in nursing,* ed 22, St Louis, 2005, Mosby.

Wilson BA, Shannon M, Stang C: *Nurse's Drug Guide 2006, ed 1,* Upper Saddle River, NJ, Pearson Education, Inc.

Skidmore-Roth L: *Mosby's drug guide for nurses,* ed 6, St Louis, 2005, Mosby.

Thibodeau GA, Patton KT: *Structure & function of the body,* ed 12, St Louis, 2004, Mosby.

25

Antiinflammatories and Antihistamines

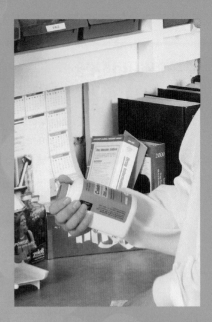

Objectives

UPON COMPLETING THIS CHAPTER, YOU SHOULD BE ABLE TO DO THE FOLLOWING:

- List both trade and generic names covered in this chapter.

- Describe the symptoms of inflammation.

- Differentiate between steroidal and nonsteroidal antiinflammatories.

- List the major side effects of the agents discussed.

- List the major cells that are activated from the immune system to repair damaged cells.

- List the major inflammatory conditions.

- List the drug action of pain receptors.

- List the major medications used in the treatment of arthritis, rheumatoid arthritis, osteoarthritis, and other major conditions.

- Describe the symptoms of asthma and the classifications of drugs used to treat asthma.

- Explain the use of inhalers as opposed to nebulizers and when they are used.

TERMS AND DEFINITIONS

Analgesic *A drug that relieves pain by reducing the perception of pain*

Anaphylactic shock *A severe allergic reaction that causes blood pressure to decrease rapidly, the heart to go into ventricular tachycardia, and the airways to close; a medical emergency that will cause death if not treated immediately*

Antigen *The marker on cell surfaces that marks the cell as a "self-cell"; it stimulates the production of antibodies*

Antipyretic *Medication that reduces fever*

Bradykinins *Chemicals produced by the body and responsible for inflammation and pain*

Corticosteroid *A steroid produced by the adrenal cortex*

Débride *To remove dead or damaged tissue*

Histamine *A substance that interacts with tissues, producing an allergic reaction*

NSAIDs *Nonsteroidal antiinflammatory drugs*

Osteoarthritis *Also known as degenerative joint disease*

OTC (Over-the-counter) *Medication that can be purchased without a prescription; nonlegend medications*

Rheumatoid arthritis *A progressive degenerative and crippling immune disease*

Rhinitis *Inflammation of the lining of the nose; runny nose*

Steroid *Messenger chemical produced by the body that helps fight inflammation and pain*

Systemic *Pertaining to the entire body rather than to individual body parts*

Urticaria *A skin eruption of itching wheals*

Vasodilation *Widening of the blood vessels that allows for increased blood flow*

ANTIINFLAMMATORY AGENTS

Trade Name	Generic Name	Pronunciation	Trade Name	Generic Name	Pronunciation
Salicylates/Nonsteroidal Antiinflammatory Drugs			Mobic	meloxicam	(mel-**ox**-i-cam)
Arthropan	choline salicylate	(**coe**-leen sall-**ih**-sa-late)	Motrin	ibuprofen	(eye-bu-**pro**-fen)
Bayer	aspirin	(**ass**-pur-in)	Nalfon	fenoprofen	(fen-oh-**pro**-fen)
Trilisate	choline magnesium trisalicylate	(**coe**-leen mag-**knee**-see-um try-sall-**ih**-sa-late)	Orudis	ketoprofen	(key-toe-**pro**-fin)
			Relafen	nabumetone	(na-**byoo**-me-tone)
			Tolectin	tolmetin	(**tole**-met-in)
Nonsteroidal Antiinflammatory Drugs			Toradol	ketorolac	(key-toh-**row**-lack)
Aleve	naproxen	(nah-**prox**-sin)			
Ansaid	flurbiprofen	(flur-**bip**-row-fin)	**Cyclooxygenase Inhibitors (COX-2 Inhibitors)**		
Clinoril	sulindac	(suh-**lin**-dack)	Celebrex	celecoxib	(ce-lee-**cox**-ib)
Daypro	oxaprozin	(ox-ah-**pro**-sin)			
Feldene	piroxicam	(peer-**ox**-i-kam)	**Corticosteroids: Oral and Nasal Inhalants**		
Indocin	indomethacin	(in-doe-**meth**-ah-sin)	AeroBid	flunisolide	(floo-**nis**-oh-lide)
Lodine	etodolac	(ee-toe-**doe**-lak)	Aeroseb-Dex	dexamethasone	(dex-ah-**meth**-ah-sown)
Meclomen	meclofenamate	(mea-kloe-**fen**-ah-mate)	Azmacort	triamcinolone	(try-am-**sin**-oh-lone)

539

ANTIINFLAMMATORY AGENTS—cont'd

Trade Name	Generic Name	Pronunciation
Beclovent	beclomethasone	(beck-low-**meth**-the-sewn)
Beconase*	beclomethasone	(beck-low-**meth**-the-sewn)
Decaspray*	dexamethasone	(dex-ah-**meth**-ah-sown)
Flonase*	fluticasone	(flu-**tick**-ah-sone)
Flovent	fluticasone	(flu-**tick**-ah-sone)
Nasalide*	flunisolide	(floo-**nis**-oh-lide)
Nasonex*	mometasone furoate	(mo-**met**-a-sone)
Pulmicort	budesonide	(bu-**des**-oh-nide)
Rhinocort*	budesonide	(bu-**des**-oh-nide)
Tri-Nasal*	triamcinolone	(trye-am-**sin**-oh-lone)

Corticosteroids: Oral/Injectable

Trade Name	Generic Name	Pronunciation
Deltasone	prednisone	(**pred**-ni-sone)
Solu-Cortef	hydrocortisone sodium succinate	(hye-droe-**kor**-ti-sone **so**-dee-um **suck**-seh-nate)
Solu-Medrol	methylprednisolone sodium succinate	(meth-il-pred-**nis**-oh-lone **so**-dee-um **suck**-seh-nate)

Bronchodilators (β-Adrenergic Agonists)

Trade Name	Generic Name	Pronunciation
Alupent	metaproterenol	(met-a-pro-**tear**-in-all)
Foradil Aerolizer	formoterol fumarate	(for-**mot**-er-ol **fu**-mah-rate)
Serevent	salmeterol	(sal-**met**-er-ol)

Bronchodilators (Leukotriene Receptor Antagonists)

Trade Name	Generic Name	Pronunciation
Accolate	zafirlukast	(zay-**fur**-lu-cast)
Singulair	montelukast	(mon-tea-**lu**-cast)
Zyflo	zileuton	(zi-**leu**-ton)

Bronchodilators (Xanthines)

Trade Name	Generic Name	Pronunciation
Phyllocontin	aminophylline	(am-in-**off**-eh-lin)
Theo-Dur	theophylline	(thee-**off**-ah-lin)

Bronchodilators (Anticholinergics)

Trade Name	Generic Name	Pronunciation
Atrovent	ipratropium	(ih-prah-**trow**-pea-um)
Combivent	ipratropium/albuterol	(ih-prah-**trow**-pea-um/al-**byoo**-tur-ol)

Analgesic Medications

Trade Name	Generic Name	Pronunciation
Lortab ASA	hydrocodone/ aspirin	(hye-droe-**koe**-done/ **ass**-pur-in)
Percocet	oxycodone/ acetaminophen	(ox-e-**koe**-done/ a-sea-tah-**men**-oh-phen)
Percodan	oxycodone/aspirin	(ox-e-**koe**-done/**ass**-pur-in)
Tylenol w/ Codeine	acetaminophen/ codeine	(as-sea-tah-**men**-oh-phen/**koe**-deen)
Vicodin	hydrocodone/ acetaminophen	(hye-droe-**koe**-done/a-sea-tah-**men**-oh-phen)

Antihistamine Drugs

Trade Name	Generic Name	Pronunciation
Atarax, Vistaril	hydroxyzine	(high-**drok**-seh-zeen)
Benadryl	diphenhydramine	(dye-fen-**hi**-dra-meen)
Chlor-Trimeton	chlorpheniramine	(klor-fen-**air**-ah-meen)
Dimetane	brompheniramine	(brom-fen-**ir**-a-meen)
PBZ	tripelennamine	(tri-pel-**en**-na-meen)
Periactin	cyproheptadine	(sye-pro-**hep**-tah-deen)
Tavist	clemastine	(**klee**-mas-teen)
Trinalin	azatadine	(a-**za**-ta-deen)

Antihistamine Drugs (Nonsedative)

Trade Name	Generic Name	Pronunciation
Allegra	fexofenadine	(fex-oh-**fen**-ah-deen)
Claritin	loratadine	(lo-**rat**-ah-dean)
Zyrtec	cetirizine	(sea-**tur**-eye-zeen)

*Nasal

U NLIKE FOR MANY OTHER CONDITIONS, several over-the-counter medications are available to treat inflammation. Aside from the common cold, muscle pain resulting from inflammation is one of the leading causes for self-medication. Most pharmacies sell more over-the-counter (OTC) nonsteroidal antiinflammatory drugs (NSAIDs) and analgesics than any other type of agent. This is partially because of the hectic lifestyle many persons live and the accessibility of OTC drugs. Although many OTC drugs are considered safe and effective, they can cause adverse side effects if taken inappropriately, especially when the patient may be taking other medications concurrently or if he or she has a preexisting condition. In addition, many legend drugs can make a person feel better; however, these too can have serious side effects if not taken correctly.

In this chapter we explore the conditions with which inflammation is associated and the use of steroidal and nonsteroidal medications to treat inflammation. We cover causes of allergies and asthma, as well as agents used to treat them. An overview is given of the types of associated conditions, such as pain, and the most common agents used to treat them. We look at the structures of

TABLE 25-1 **Immune Cell Responses in Injury**

Name of cell or molecule	Type of cell involved	Effects
Antibodies	Produced by B lymphocytes in response to an antigen; memory cells previously produced increase in population to fight off infection; found in the blood	Can neutralize or destroy antigens in different ways such as by coating or lysing the antigen; they can stimulate phagocytosis and prevent the antigen from adhering to host cells
Fibrinogen	A globulin found in blood plasma	Helps in coagulating blood
Granulocytes	Mature leukocyte cells that contain granules, including neutrophils and other types of immune response cells	Fight off infection
Leukocytes	White blood cells formed in bone marrow, including granulocytes and nongranulocytes	Fight off infection and tissue damage; they destroy foreign organisms and also clean up damaged cells by phagocytosis
Lymphocytes	White blood cells formed in the spleen and bone marrow	Adhere to endothelial cells: intensify inflammation by causing direct cell injury and promoting formation of antibodies that increase the inflammatory response
Monocytes	Large type of leukocyte	Eventually become macrophages; macrophages are one of the first line of defenses in the inflammatory process
Neutrophils	Mature white blood cells in the granulocytic series; make up more than 50% of the leukocytes present in the body	Adhere to damaged site to protect against infection by destroying infectious microbes; also destroy antigens
Macrophages	Large cells called phagocytes that secrete cytokines	Ingest dead tissue, bacterial cells, or dying cells

antiinflammatory agents and their derivatives to understand the differences between them.

Inflammation

Inflammation can be caused by infection, allergic reactions, or injury. Inflammation is a necessary response if the body is to heal itself.

Along with the obvious swelling effects of inflammation, other effects are felt rather than seen. Thousands of years ago the Romans described the symptoms of inflammation as redness, swelling, heat, pain, and the eventual loss of function of the affected area. The body tries to repair the damages with the help of blood and cells and natural chemicals. Some chemicals send messages to the smooth muscles causing vasodilation, allowing more blood to reach the affected area. Because the blood rushes in, the area is warmer. Areas surrounding the damaged area may not be able to adapt to the increase in blood, resulting in edema (buildup of fluids) within the surrounding tissues. Specialized cells are sent to the area, and the repair process begins. Table 25-1 lists some of the major

TABLE 25-2 Types of Inflammation

Condition	Location of inflammation	Notes
Pneumonia	Lungs	Alveolar spaces swell
Pericarditis	Heart	Lining of the heart swells
Strep throat	Throat lining	Caused by bacterial infection
Abscess	Organs or tissues	Pus- or liquid-filled spaces
Colitis	Colon (large intestine)	Bacterial or ulcerous
Ulcer	Epithelial lining such as in the stomach or duodenum	Peptic ulcers and duodenal ulcers

types of cells that make up our immune system and their effects on the body system.

The cells of the body contain many different chemicals that have a role in inflammation. Each chemical has a specific job to perform. One such chemical found in many cells is an enzyme called cyclooxygenase. This enzyme produces various hormones called prostaglandins, which are responsible for other chemical reactions that cause inflammation, pain, and increased temperature. Aspirin is one agent that inhibits cyclooxygenase pathways and thereby stops the production of prostaglandin.

Inflammation can occur only in living tissue; therefore, if an area undergoes necrosis (death of the tissue), such as necrosis of the hands or feet from frostbite, there will be no apparent swelling of the tissue. Instead, as blood flow diminishes, the skin turns black, and because the tissue has no blood supply, the area needs débriding to prevent the infection from spreading further.

The two different types of inflammation are acute and chronic. Acute inflammation only lasts a few days, and the body usually can recover without any help from medication. Chronic inflammation can arise from an acute case of inflammation or from an injury. Chronic inflammation can occur locally, such as at a cut on the surface of the skin, or systemically within areas of the body. When inflammation becomes chronic, the site of injury may swell again, and a low-grade fever can result. Table 25-2 describes types of inflammation.

Chronic inflammation can cause damage to the affected sites or internal organs. As the body heals, it leaves behind scar tissue. This scar tissue can alter the normal workings of the body system. For instance, if the heart becomes scarred, it may not work as well in pumping or circulating the blood. If the fallopian tubes are scarred by pelvic inflammatory disease, the woman may become sterile. Inflammation also can damage the kidneys to the extent that the person needs dialysis. Along with inflammation there can be varying degrees of pain associated with the swelling.

GLUCOCORTICOIDS (STEROIDS)

Different types of steroids are produced by the body. They are secreted from the endocrine glands and are chemical messengers of the body. The main gland that produces steroids is the adrenal gland. The adrenal cortex makes glucocorticoids and mineralocorticoids (both are referred to as corticosteroids). Another steroid, corticotropin, which is secreted by the anterior pituitary gland, is a regulator of the adrenal gland. Steroids have an important role in the maintenance of the body system. The imbalance of normal steroid levels can cause various diseases. Because of the common use of high doses of glucocorticoids, we focus on these agents in this chapter.

The glucocorticoids have two major effects on the body—physiologic and pharmacological. When low doses are given, a physiologic effect is seen (for treatment of adrenocortical insufficiency). When high doses are given, pharmacological effects are seen. This involves the ability of these agents to decrease inflammatory conditions caused by various types of arthritis, such as rheumatoid arthritis and osteoarthritis. Other uses include treatment of asthma and certain types of cancer and suppression of the immune response in organ transplant recipients.

Because of their strong effects on the immune system, corticosteroids can cause many serious side effects if they are taken over long periods, are taken inappropriately, or are stopped abruptly. To understand why this can happen, we first must review the mechanism of action of high doses of steroids.

Glucocorticoid therapy has the same effects as naturally produced glucocorticoids. Glucocorticoid affects protein, fat, and glucose metabolism within the body by raising the blood glucose levels. One way in which this is accomplished is by decreasing the metabolism of proteins by converting them into glucose. The overall effect reduces muscle mass and bone density and causes thinning of the skin. Glucocorticoid therapy also causes fat redistribution by alteration of fat metabolism. This can lead to the appearance of a "moon face," a symptom of Cushing's disease.

Normally the release of glucocorticoids in the body is regulated by a negative feedback system. For example, when a physiologically stressful event occurs, the brain sends signals to the adrenal glands. Glucocorticoids and other chemicals, such as prostaglandins and leukotrienes, are released into the body system and reduce inflammation.

Although glucocorticoids are effective in reducing inflammation, they can have adverse effects if their secretion is prolonged. Stressful events, such as surgery, high doses, or prolonged use of glucocorticoid medications, may cause a suppression of lymphocytes, which may in turn lower resistance to infections. Other side effects may include increased appetite, increased bruising, insomnia, restlessness, anxiety, hypotension, and headache.

OSTEOARTHRITIS (DEGENERATIVE JOINT DISEASE)

Osteoarthritis is also known as degenerative joint disease and is a common type of arthritis seen in persons over the age of 45 years. Although osteoarthritis is not as severe as rheumatoid arthritis, it is painful. Because of the degradation of the cartilage between the joints, an overgrowth of bone (such as bone spurs) may occur (Figure 25-1). Because of the wear and tear on the bone itself from constant movement, it can cause extreme pain. Eventually, when the bone is smooth from long-term use, the pain may decrease. Treatment of osteoarthritis

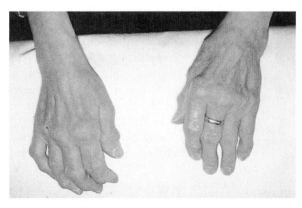

FIGURE 25-1 Severe osteoarthritis.

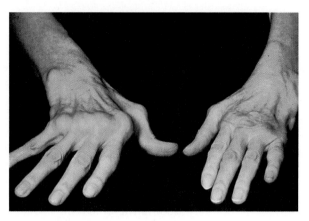

FIGURE 25-2 Severe rheumatoid arthritis.

consists of medication, the removal of the synovial membrane (synovectomy), or even total joint replacement (arthroplasty). Medications such as NSAIDs are listed later in the treatment section.

RHEUMATOID ARTHRITIS

Unlike osteoarthritis, rheumatoid arthritis (RA) not only is painful but also can be bone deforming (Figure 25-2). More women are struck by RA than men. Whether this condition is genetic is not known, although it can run in families. RA also affects young adults between the ages of 20 and 30 years old. RA is believed possibly to be viral. The cause of RA is within the immune system. As more synovial fluid is produced than normal, the area swells, causing painful inflammation; and the cartilage within the joint area degrades. Bones and cartilage eventually are eroded away, making movement extremely painful. If the joint freezes through calcification, it is impossible for the person to move the joint any longer. This deformity of the joints is irreversible. Treatment for RA includes physical therapy, medications (antiinflammatories and/or analgesics), or diet. The removal of excess synovial fluid may be an option for the patient to relieve pain and joint damage.

Pain

Inflammation and pain run hand in hand because of the various hormones that the body secretes when damaged; therefore, most patients treated for inflammation may receive analgesics as well for a short time until the swelling has subsided. Each person's perception of pain is specific to him or her and cannot be measured by scientific methods. Most pain lasts only a short time. This is referred to as acute pain; however, if the pain is persistent (lasts for 3 months or longer), it is called chronic pain.

When consulting a health care provider, a patient may be asked to rate the severity of pain using a numerical scale from 1 to 10. The number 1 indicates very little pain, and 10 indicates severe pain. If pain is severe, it may be called acute pain. Most muscle or tendon sprains result in acute pain and last only a few weeks. Several types of medications, mostly combination drugs, can be prescribed to treat pain, inflammation, and even fever that may be associated with injury or chronic pain that affects joints and other areas of the body.

Asthma

Millions of Americans suffer from asthma, a chronic inflammatory disorder of the airways that can occur in childhood or adulthood. Because of many envi-

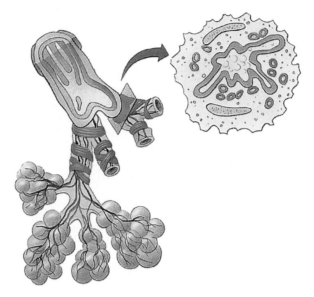

FIGURE 25-3 Asthma: Airways become obstructed by mucus and edema, causing dyspnea.

ronmental factors, the incidence of asthma is increasing. Smoking, sickness such as cold or flu, animal dander, environmental contaminants, and even stressful situations can cause the onset of an asthmatic attack. Because of the inflammation of the lining and constriction of the bronchioles that occurs during an attack, a person can die if not treated quickly (Figure 25-3).

After the airway is exposed to an irritant, different cells within the body (mast cells, T lymphocytes, neutrophils, and epithelial cells) are altered. Various chemicals that are released from these cells cause the smooth muscle in the airway to become inflamed. Epithelial layers become damaged, and mucous membranes secrete large amounts of mucus. All of these events contribute to the overall decrease in normal breathing. An acute attack of asthma has been known to cause anaphylaxis if not treated quickly. Anaphylaxis is a severe allergic condition in which the smooth muscles of the body, including the airways, constrict and the capillaries dilate. Death may occur if the condition goes untreated. Fortunately, many medications are available to treat asthma. Most commonly, corticosteroids are used to treat asthma. Other medications help prevent asthma attacks from occurring. Even with the wide variety of asthma treatments available, there is currently no cure for this common disease.

Allergies

When the body first comes into contact with any antigens, the body produces immunoglobulin E antibodies that attach to mast cells. These sensitized mast cells are found in tissues of the gastrointestinal tract, skin, and the respiratory tract. They attach to the mast cells throughout the body, waiting for the next stimulation from antigens. Histamine$_1$ receptors are found in the lower respiratory tract and skin, whereas histamine$_2$ receptors are located in the gastrointestinal tract. With the second exposure to an antigen, the antigen binds to the immunoglobulin E antibodies on the mast cells (Figure 25-4). This binding causes a release of the contents of the mast cells. Histamine is released and binds to histamine receptor sites in tissues, causing an allergic response that commonly includes coughing, sneezing, wheezing, and urticaria (rash). More severe reactions can include decreased blood pressure, migraine headache, bronchiolar constriction, increased heart rhythm, and anaphylactic shock (Figure 25-5).

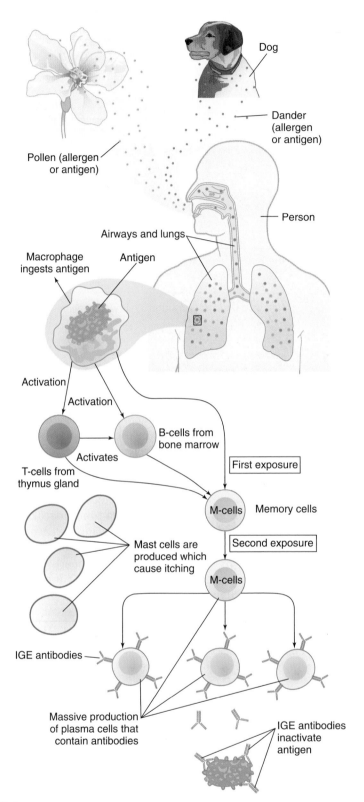

FIGURE 25-4 Events that take place in an allergic reaction, from the first exposure to an antigen then to the allergic reaction.

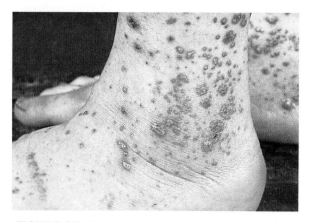

FIGURE 25-5 Allergic vasculitis caused by allergens.

Histamine can produce a drop in blood pressure because it can dilate small blood vessels and capillaries. This dilation then can stimulate pain receptors in the head, causing severe headaches or migraines. Histamine also causes bronchoconstriction, making it difficult to breathe. In extremely severe reactions, the airways of a person can become swollen and close; this is called anaphylactic shock. This systemic affect can result in death if not treated immediately.

When an allergic reaction takes place, antihistamines decrease the release of histamines by binding the antigen to the mast cells. Allergic reactions can be blocked in two ways:

1. Mast cells are prevented from releasing histamine.
2. Histamine$_1$ receptors are blocked from interacting with histamine.

Antihistamine drugs specifically block histamine$_1$ receptors. These agents commonly are found in cold and cough medications because of their ability to dry secretions (some antihistamines work against cholinergic responses of the nervous system). These agents are classified as anticholinergics (see Chapter 17).

Histamine$_2$ receptors are located in the gastrointestinal tract—the stomach and intestines. Foods that cause an allergic reaction can result in vomiting, diarrhea, and cramps. A different class of drugs is used to treat this type of allergic reaction. The histamine$_2$ blockers, called H$_2$ antagonists, block the receptor sites within the gastrointestinal tract. (See Chapter 20.)

Antihistamines are of two generations. The first-generation drugs are considered nonspecific antihistamines. They were found to bind to histamine$_1$ and histamine$_2$ receptors. Many can cause sedation because of their effect on the central nervous system if used in higher concentrations. Some of the first-generation agents also decrease nausea, vomiting, and motion sickness by their actions on the central nervous system. Second-generation antihistamines became available more recently. These agents can affect histamine$_1$ receptors specifically, thus they do not cause the same amount of sedation. Table 25-3 gives examples of the two generations of antihistamines, along with their common uses.

Treatment of Inflammation

THE HISTORY OF ASPIRIN

In England in the early 1800s, it was reported that the bark from the willow tree was effective as a pain, fever, and inflammation reducer. Many cultures had known this for centuries, but it was not until the early 1800s that the medical

TABLE 25-3 Antihistamine Agents

Trade name	Generic name	Dosage form	Uses
Benadryl*	Diphenhydramine	Capsule, tablet, solution(s), injection	Allergies, sedation
Chlor-Trimeton*	Chlorpheniramine	Tablet, syrup, injection	Allergies
Tavist 1.25*; 2.68[†]	Clemastine	Tablet, syrup	Allergies
Phenergan[†]	Promethazine	Tablet, syrup, suppository, injection	Allergies, sedation, antiemetic, motion sickness
Atarax, Vistaril[†]	Hydroxyzine	Tablet, capsule, syrup, injection	Allergies, sedation (oral), antiemetic (intravenous)
Claritin*	Loratadine	Tablet, syrup	Allergies
Second-Generation Drugs			
Zyrtec[†]	Cetirizine	Tablet, syrup	Allergies

*Over the counter.
[†]Prescription.

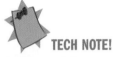

TECH NOTE!

Aspirin contains a chemical called acetylsalicylic acid. This chemical inhibits prostaglandins. This inhibition decreases inflammation and helps decrease pain and fever.

community began to isolate the active ingredients. A French chemist by the name of Henri Leroux found that a bitter glycoside was responsible for the medicinal properties of the bark. This chemical was referred to as salicin. When this chemical breaks apart, it creates glucose (sugar) and salicylic alcohol. The salicylic alcohol ultimately can be broken down into acetylsalicylic acid.

Scientists were aware of the effects of salicin and wanted to know exactly how it produced these effects. For the effects of decreasing pain, they discovered that it inhibits prostaglandins. Prostaglandins, produced naturally by the body, are a group of hormonal chemicals that are responsible for pain, inflammation, and the elevated temperature associated with injury. Although salicin helps decrease inflammation, pain, and the heat associated with injury, it will not lower body temperature caused from normal activities, such as exercising.

As this new information became available, salicin was considered a miracle drug and was used to treat illnesses such as gout, inflammation from injury, and pain and to reduce high fever, which could cause death. The first company to market this miracle agent was the Bayer Company in 1899. They called their new wonder drug aspirin. Since then there have been many new drugs introduced into the marketplace that work similarly; aspirin is still a popular drug because of how well it works and is the most inexpensive treatment.

WHAT IS ASPIRIN USED FOR?

Aspirin is an inexpensive and effective agent against fever, pain, and inflammation, although it should not be given to children, especially those with flulike symptoms because of Reye's syndrome, which may occur following chickenpox or upper respiratory infection. Reye's syndrome is a childhood disease that causes vomiting, lethargy, and encephalopathy, which can lead to coma and death. For children suffering from chickenpox or flulike symptoms, acetaminophen (Tylenol) can be given without fear of Reye's syndrome.

Aspirin has a maximum dosing range for adults that should not exceed 4 g per day. A common side effect is upset stomach. Therefore, an auxiliary label "take with food" should be affixed to any aspirin prescription. In addition, persons taking anticoagulation agents normally should not take aspirin because

TABLE 25-4 Various Strengths of Aspirin Available

Trade name	Strength	Dosage form
1/2 Halfprin	165 mg	Enteric-coated* tablet
Arthritis Foundation Pain Reliever	500 mg	Tablets
Aspergum	227.5 mg	Gum tablet
Bayer Low Adult Strength	81 mg	Tablet
Ecotrin Adult Low Strength	81 mg	Tablet
Ecotrin	325 mg	Enteric-coated tablet, caplet
Extra Strength Bayer EC	500 mg	Enteric-coated tablet, caplet
Halfprin	81 mg	Tablet
Heartline	81 mg	Tablet
Maximum Bayer	500 mg	Tablet, caplet
St. Joseph Adult Chewable Aspirin	81 mg	Chewable tablet

*Enteric coated: a film coating protects the stomach from irritation.

it increases the anticoagulation effects of the prescribed agent, which may result in internal bleeding. Pharmacists should counsel patients any time an anticoagulant is prescribed. One of the most common uses of aspirin is for the prevention of strokes or heart attacks. Aspirin decreases platelet aggregation (blood clotting). If a clot occurs in the brain, it can cause a stroke. If the clot occurs in the blood vessels of the heart, it can cause a heart attack. If it occurs in the lungs, it can cause a pulmonary embolism. All of these conditions are life threatening. Many physicians prescribe 81 to 325 mg per day to decrease blood clotting (Table 25-4). Anticoagulation medication often is called a "blood thinner."

NONSTEROIDAL ANTIINFLAMMATORY AGENTS

Aspirin is a salicylate drug and the prototype agent for the newer NSAIDs. Although NSAIDs have a different chemical structure than aspirin, they have the same basic benzene ring attached to a (acid) carboxyl group. A close similarity exists between the structure of aspirin and aspirin-like drugs and NSAIDs. All of these agents have analgesic, antipyretic, and antiinflammatory properties that make them popular in the retail marketplace. Other chemicals in the body are able to help with the reduction of inflammation, such as corticosteroids. In contrast, NSAIDs suppress inflammation by inhibiting prostaglandin production. The glucocorticoids not only inhibit prostaglandin synthesis but also suppress inflammation.

More than a dozen NSAIDs are available in prescription form, and about four different types of medications are available OTC. In contrast, most aspirin is sold OTC by dozens of different manufacturers in various strengths and dosage forms and in combinations with other drugs. NSAIDs can be used for mild to moderate pain. They have several positive effects on the body, such as the following:

1. They are not addictive, unlike controlled substances.
2. They decrease pain (analgesic).
3. They decrease fever (antipyretic).
4. They decrease inflammation (antiinflammatory).
5. Many can be purchased OTC.

Their method of action includes inhibition of cyclooxygenase, which is the enzyme responsible for the formation of prostaglandins and bradykinins. These chemicals are responsible for pain and inflammation. NSAIDs also have an

TABLE 25-5 Nonsteroidal Antiinflammatory Drugs, Cyclooxygenase-2, and Similar Agents

Generic name	Brand name	Adult dosage	Note
Nonsteroidal Antiinflammatory Drugs			
Etodolac	Lodine*	200 to 400 mg q6-12h	Max 1.2 g qd
Fenoprofen	Nalfon*	200 mg q4-6h	Max 3.2 g qd
Flurbiprofen	Ansaid*	50 to 100 mg q6-12h	Max 300 mg qd
Ibuprofen	Motrin†	300 to 800 mg q6-8h	Max 1.2 g qd
Indomethacin	Indocin*	25 to 50 mg q8-12h	Max 200 mg qd
Ketoprofen	Orudis*	12.5 to 75 mg q6-8h	Max 300 mg qd
	Orudis SR*	100 to 200 mg qd	Max 200 qd sustained release
Ketorolac	Toradol*	15 to 60 mg q6h	Max 60 mg (IM or IV)
		10 mg q4-6h	Max 40 mg qd (PO)
Meclofenamate	Meclomen*	50 to 100 mg q4-6h	Max 400 mg qd
Meloxicam	Mobic	7.5 to 15 mg qd	Max 15 mg qd
Nabumetone	Relafen*	1 g q12-24h	Max 2 g qd†
Naproxen	Naprosyn*	275 to 500 mg q12h	Max 1.25 g qd
Piroxicam	Feldene*	20 mg q24h	Max 20 mg qd
Sulindac	Clinoril*	150 to 200 mg q12h	Max 400 mg qd
Tolmetin	Tolectin*	200 to 600 mg q6-8h	Max 1.8 g qd
	Tolectin DS*	400 mg tid	Max 2 g qd
Cyclooxygenase-2			
Celecoxib	Celebrex*	100 to 200 mg q12-24h	Max 400 mg qd†
Salicylate Agents			
Aspirin	Bayer†	325 mg to 1 g q 4-6h	Max 4 g qd
Choline magnesium trisalicylates	Trilisate*	2-3 g bid-tid	Max 3 g qd
Choline salicylate	Arthropan*	1 to 1.5 g q12h	Max 4 g qd

*Prescription only.
†Over the counter only.

antipyretic effect by acting on the hypothalamus (the body thermostat). Wide variations have been documented among different NSAIDs, even if they are related and in the same chemical family. Because each type of NSAID tends to work differently, if one brand does not work, another one might.

NSAIDs are used to treat many different types of conditions and chronic illnesses such as the following:

1. Muscle pain
2. RA
3. Bone pain such as in osteoarthritis
4. Premenstrual syndrome

Millions of persons use OTC and legend NSAIDs to treat various inflammatory conditions. However, overuse of these agents can cause major problems. NSAIDs can worsen stomach problems such as gastroesophageal reflux disease. They also can cause ulcers if used for a long time. All NSAIDs should be taken with food to prevent stomach problems. In addition, they can increase bleeding and should not be used by those taking warfarin or other anticoagulants. Table 25-5 lists some of the common NSAIDs, COX-2 inhibitors and aspirin-like agents. Lower dosages of some of these agents are available OTC (see Chapter 9). The following are three prescription NSAIDs used to relieve inflammation and the associated pain associated.

GENERIC NAME: Etodolac
TRADE NAME: Lodine, Lodine XL
ROUTE OF ADMINISTRATION: oral
INDICATIONS: inflammation, pain, osteoarthritis
DOSAGE FORMS: tablet, sustained-release tablets, capsules
COMMON DOSAGE: 200-400 mg q6-8h prn for acute pain; 800 to 1200 mg/day q6-8h
AUXILIARY LABELS:

- May cause dizziness or drowsiness.
- Take with food or milk.
- Do not take aspirin while taking this medication.
- Do not crush or chew sustained-release tablets.

GENERIC NAME: ibuprofen
TRADE NAME: Motrin, Advil
ROUTE OF ADMINISTRATION: oral
INDICATIONS: inflammation, pain, osteoarthritis
DOSAGE FORMS: tablet, capsule, liquid-gel, oral suspension, liquid, chewable tablet, drops
COMMON DOSAGE: 200-400 mg q6-8h prn for acute pain; 800 to 1200 mg/day q6-8h
AUXILIARY LABELS:

- May cause dizziness or drowsiness.
- Take with food or milk.
- Do not take aspirin while taking this medication.
- Do not crush or chew sustained-release tablets.

GENERIC NAME: ketorolac
TRADE NAME: Toradol
ROUTE OF ADMINISTRATION: oral, intravenous
INDICATIONS: Short-term mild to moderate pain, inflammation
DOSAGE FORMS: tablet, single-dose vial, multiple-dose vial for injection, prefilled syringes
COMMON DOSAGE: oral, 10 mg q4-6h prn max 5 days
AUXILIARY LABELS:

- May cause dizziness or drowsiness.
- Take with food or milk.
- Avoid alcohol.

CYCLOOXYGENASE-2 INHIBITORS

Cyclooxygenase (COX) is an enzyme that works along a pathway that synthesizes prostaglandins and other compounds. Cyclooxygenase is a substance found in all tissues where it helps regulate many processes. Cyclooxygenase has two forms, COX-1 and COX-2. COX-1 is present in most tissues and helps to take care of many normal functions, including protecting gastric mucosa and promoting platelet aggregation. COX-2 is found mainly at sites of tissue injury, where it helps sensitize receptors to pain and mediates inflammation. COX-2 also is located within the brain, where it affects fever and pain perception. Therefore, COX-1 can be thought of as taking care of the more normal processes, whereas COX-2 takes care of the processes when pain and discomfort are present.

First-generation NSAIDs inhibit COX-1 and COX-2 enzymes, which results in a decrease in inflammation, pain, and fever. Unfortunately, inhibiting COX-1 enzymes have serious side effects such as gastric erosion, ulceration, bleeding, and renal damage. The previous use of COX-1 inhibitors has been shown to be

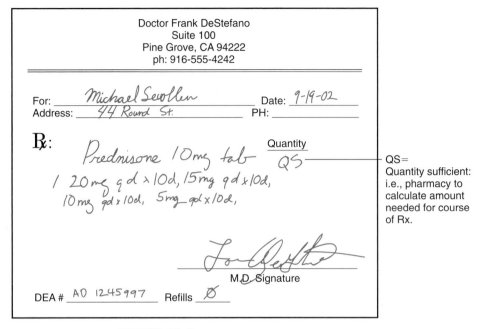

FIGURE 25-6 Prednisone tapered prescription.

more dangerous than useful; therefore, drugs such as rofecoxib (Vioxx) and valdecoxib (Bextra), both of which are COX-1 inhibitors, were withdrawn from the market. Most of the antiinflammatories are NSAIDs. The following is a COX-2 inhibitor that is approved for use.

COX-2 INHIBITOR

GENERIC NAME: celecoxib
TRADE NAME: Celebrex
ROUTE OF ADMINISTRATION: oral
INDICATIONS: acute or chronic pain, RA, or degenerative joint disease
DOSAGE FORMS: Capsules
COMMON DOSAGE: RA, 100-200 mg bid; degenerative joint disease, 200 mg qd or 100 mg bid
AUXILIARY LABELS:

- May cause dizziness or drowsiness.
- Take with food or milk.
- Do not crush or chew capsules.

Adrenal Effects of Steroid Agents

Glucocorticoids are essential to the wellness of the body. One problem of long-term use of steroids is that the ability of the body to produce glucocorticoids on its own is decreased and eventually may stop altogether. Depending on the length of time that steroids are used, the body can take from days to a year to begin production of glucocorticoids. When it is determined that it is time to discontinue a steroid, it must be done slowly to allow the body to begin production of glucocorticoids by tapering the dose over a month or more. An example of a tapered order is given in Figure 25-6.

Several routes of administration for steroids are oral, parenteral (intravenous, intramuscular, subcutaneous), topical, and inhalation. Prescriptions normally are written for the smallest effective amount of steroids and for the least amount of time necessary to treat the condition. Side effects of oral dosages include gastrointestinal upset; therefore, all steroids should have the auxiliary label "take with food." Because dosages are varied based on the severity of the condition and patient's health, we have not included them in the drug monographs in this chapter. The following are examples of oral, topical, and injectable agents used to treat inflammation and pain.

CORTICOSTEROIDS

GENERIC NAME: prednisone
TRADE NAME: Deltasone
INDICATIONS: for the treatment of a wide variety of diseases such as adrenocortical insufficiency and respiratory, gastrointestinal, and neoplastic diseases; also used for allergic, inflammatory, and autoimmune conditions
DOSAGE FORMS: tablets, solution, syrup

GENERIC NAME: hydrocortisone (available in many different forms, such as hydrocortisone acetate, butyrate, cypionate, sodium phosphate, valerate, and sodium succinate)
TRADE NAME: Cortef (oral), Hytone (topical), Procort (spray), Anusol-HC (suppository), Cortenema (enema), Solu-Cortef (injection)
INDICATIONS: oral—management of adrenocortical insufficiency, relief of inflammation of dermatosis, and adjunctive treatment of ulcerative colitis; suppositories—for hemorrhoids
DOSAGE FORMS: injection; aerosol; topical forms—ointment, cream, lotion; oral forms—tablet, solution, syrup, suspension

GENERIC NAME: methylprednisolone
TRADE NAME: Medrol (oral), Depo-Medrol (injection)
INDICATIONS: antiinflammatory or immunosuppressive agents used to treat a variety of diseases; also used after bone marrow transplants
DOSAGE FORMS: injection as methylprednisolone acetate or methylprednisolone sodium succinate; tablet, tablet dose pack (tapered dose)

AGENTS USED TO TREAT DEGENERATIVE JOINT DISEASE AND RHEUMATOID ARTHRITIS

Various salicylate chemical combinations can be prescribed for pain resulting from degenerative joint disease or RA. Table 25-6 lists salicylate agents. The following are medications used in addition to previously described NSAIDs.

GENERIC NAME: ketoprofen
TRADE NAME: Orudis
ROUTE OF ADMINISTRATION: oral
INDICATIONS: mild to moderate pain, osteoarthritis, RA
DOSAGE FORMS: tablets, capsules, extended-release capsules
COMMON DOSAGE: 150-300 mg tid to qid
AUXILIARY LABELS:
- May cause dizziness or drowsiness.
- Take with food.
- Do not crush or chew extended-release capsules.

GENERIC NAME: meloxicam
TRADE NAME: Mobic
ROUTE OF ADMINISTRATION: oral
INDICATION: osteoarthritis
DOSAGE FORM: tablet

TABLE 25-6 Conditions Treated and Common Dosing of Aspirin or Aspirin-Like Agents

Availability	Type of salicylate agent	Condition/symptoms	Dosing
Over the counter/ prescription	Aspirin	Antipyretic/analgesic	325 mg up to 650 mg q4h prn, 975 mg (prescription)
Prescription	Salsalate (Disalcid)	Antipyretic/analgesic	3 g/day in divided doses
Over the counter	Sodium salicylate	Antipyretic/analgesic	325 to 650 mg q4h
Prescription	Sodium thiosalicylate (Rexolate)	Gout	100 mg q3-4h × 2 days, and then 100 mg qd until symptoms disappear
		Muscle pain	50 to 100 mg qd
		Rheumatic fever	100 to 150 mg q4-8h × 3 days, and then 100 mg bid until symptoms disappear
Over the counter	Choline salicylate	Antipyretic/analgesic	870 mg q3-4h
		Rheumatoid arthritis	870 mg to 1.74 g qid
Prescription	Diflunisal (Dolobid)	Mild to moderate pain	500 mg q8-12h
		Osteoarthritis/ rheumatoid arthritis	250 to 500 mg bid

COMMON DOSAGE: 1 tab qd
AUXILIARY LABELS:

- May cause dizziness or drowsiness.
- Avoid aspirin, acetaminophen, and NSAIDs while taking this medication.
- Do not drink alcohol.
- Take with water.

GENERIC NAME: nambumetone
TRADE NAME: Relafen
ROUTE OF ADMINISTRATION: oral
INDICATIONS: osteoarthritis, RA, acute or chronic treatment
DOSAGE FORMS: tablet
COMMON DOSAGE: 1 g qd; may increase if necessary up to 2 g qd in divided doses
AUXILIARY LABELS:

- May cause dizziness or drowsiness.
- Take with water.
- Avoid aspirin, NSAIDS.
- Avoid prolonged or excessive exposure to sunlight.

AGENTS USED TO TREAT PAIN

For pain caused by inflammation, a variety of medications can be used to relieve it, including NSAIDs. These medications can play an important part in the reduction of pain through their mechanism of action. The following sections include a brief overview of the types of medications used with antiinflammatories. These agents specifically treat pain and are scheduled CII to CIII.

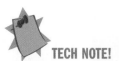

TECH NOTE!

Acetaminophen (Tylenol) is not an antiinflammatory agent. Although it does affect cyclooxygenase enzymes in an inhibitory way by relieving pain and fever, it does not alleviate inflammation.

ANALGESIC AGENTS

GENERIC NAME: acetaminophen and hydrocodone
TRADE NAME: Vicodin, Lortab (CIII)
ROUTE OF ADMINISTRATION: oral
INDICATION: moderate to severe pain
DOSAGE FORMS: tablets, capsules, elixir
COMMON DOSAGE: Tablet: 1 to 2 q 4 to 6 hrs prn pain (Maximum dose 8 tablets/day)
AUXILIARY LABELS:
- May cause dizziness or drowsiness.
- Do not drink alcohol while taking this medication.

GENERIC NAME: acetaminophen and oxycodone
TRADE NAME: Percocet, Tylox, Roxicet, (CII)
ROUTE OF ADMINISTRATION: oral
INDICATION: Moderate to severe pain
DOSAGE FORMS: tablets, capsules, solution
COMMON DOSAGE: Tablet: 1 q 6 hrs prn pain (Maximum dose 8 tablets/day)
AUXILIARY LABELS:
- May cause dizziness or drowsiness.
- Do not drink alcohol while taking this medication.

GENERIC NAME: acetaminophen and codeine (CIII)
TRADE NAME: Tylenol w/Codeine #3 (300 mg APAP/30 mg codeine) and #4 (300 mg APAP/60 mg codeine)
ROUTE OF ADMINISTRATION: oral
INDICATION: Moderate to severe pain
DOSAGE FORMS: tablet. Solution, suspension and elixir contain 120 mg APAP/12 mg codeine.
COMMON DOSAGE: Tablets: 1 to 2 tabs q 4 to 6 hrs prn pain (Maximum dose of! APAP is 4 gm/day)
AUXILIARY LABELS:
- May cause dizziness or drowsiness.
- Do not drink alcohol while taking this medication.

AGENTS USED TO TREAT ASTHMA

The most common medications used to treat acute asthma are β-adrenergic agonists. These can be used along with bronchodilators such as corticosteroids. The effect of β-adrenergics is to dilate the bronchial airways. Short- and long-acting agents work effectively. In addition to β-adrenergic agents, corticosteroids also commonly are used. These agents are available in inhalant or parenteral (injectable) forms. Corticosteroids can be short term and long term. Other agents that can be used to treat asthma are anticholinergics. Anticholinergics may be administered parenterally (by injection); however, the most common route is inhalation. Two methods of inhalation are by a nebulizer (Figure 25-7) or a metered dose inhaler. Table 25-7 presents examples of inhalants used for asthma prophylaxis and attacks.

Sympathomimetics not only reduce inflammation of the bronchi but also relieve spasms within the smooth muscle of the airway. Because these agents mimic the sympathetic system, they affect α-adrenergic receptors and β-adrenergic receptors. α-Adrenergic receptors are located in the smooth muscles of the lungs, whereas β-adrenergic receptors are located in the heart. These agents can be used to treat bronchitis and emphysema, as well as asthma. Side effects of these agents can range from lightheadedness to increased heart rate.

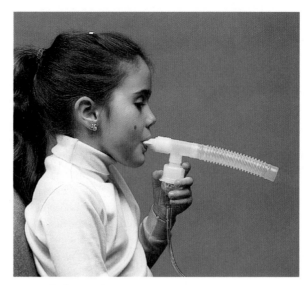

FIGURE 25-7 Proper use of a nebulizer.

Xanthine agents also work on the smooth muscle of the bronchioles. The main difference between sympathomimetics and xanthine agents is their route of administration. Xanthine agents such as aminophylline and theophylline are given in oral and parenteral form, not as inhalants as the sympathomimetics are. Parenterally administered theophylline can worsen heart conditions such as arrhythmias. Indications include symptomatic relief or prevention of bronchial asthma and other associated bronchial disorders. Auxiliary labels include "take with food," "do not chew or crush tablets," "take as directed."

β-ADRENERGIC AGONISTS (BRONCHODILATORS)

GENERIC NAME: metaproterenol
TRADE NAME: Alupent
ROUTE OF ADMINISTRATION: oral
INDICATIONS: bronchial asthma, bronchospasms
DOSAGE FORMS: inhalant solution,
COMMON DOSAGE: Inhalant: two to three puffs; may repeat every 3 to 4 hours; do not exceed 12 puffs per day
AUXILIARY LABELS:
- Shake well before using.
- Take as directed.

GENERIC NAME: salmeterol xinafoate
TRADE NAME: Serevent
ROUTE OF ADMINISTRATION: oral
INDICATIONS: prevention of exercise-induced asthma, bronchospasms, chronic obstructive pulmonary disease
DOSAGE FORMS: inhalant
COMMON DOSAGE: two puffs bid (morning and evening)
AUXILIARY LABELS:
- Shake well before using.
- Take as directed.

TABLE 25-7 **Inhalants in Asthma Agents**

Trade name	Generic name	Adult dose of inhalant	Route of administration	Specific targets
Short-Acting β₂-Agonists (Sympathomimetics)				Relax bronchial smooth muscle. Specifically affect β₂ sites.
Proventil, Ventolin	albuterol	1-2 puffs q4-6h	PO, Inh	
Bronkosol[check]	isoetharine	1-2 puffs q4h	Inh	
Maxair	pirbuterol	1-2 puffs q6h	Inh	
Adrenalin	epinephrine	1-2 puffs qid	SC, Inh	
Alupent	metaproterenol	1 puff q4h	PO, Inh	
Isuprel	isoproterenol	2-3 puffs q3-4h	Inh, IV	
Brethine	terbutaline	Max 12/day	PO, Inh, IV	
Serevent	salmeterol	2 puffs qid		
Corticosteroid Agents				Inhibit certain enzymes that are responsible for inflammation. Stabilize lysosomal membranes.
Vanceril, Beclovent	beclomethasone	2 puffs q6-8h	Inh	
Pulmicort	budesonide	1-2 puffs bid	Inh	
Azmacort	triamcinolone	2 puffs qid	Inh	
AeroBid	flunisolide	2 sprays each nostril bid	Nasal	
Flovent	fluticasone	1 puff bid	Inh	
Anticholinergic				
Atrovent	ipratropium bromide	1-2 puffs qid	Nebulizer	
Leukotriene Agonists				Block leukotriene receptors, stop anaphylaxis
Singulair	montelukast	10 mg daily (4 mg and 5 mg pediatric)	PO, chew tab	
Accolate	zafirlukast	20 mg bid	PO	
Prophylactic				Used in the prevention of asthma attacks. It inhibits the release of histamine, leukotrienes, and other inflammatory producing cells.
Intal	cromolyn sodium	1 spray or capsule qid	Nebulizer, Inh, Nasal	

BRONCHODILATORS (XANTHINES)

GENERIC NAME: aminophylline
TRADE NAME: Phyllocontin
ROUTE OF ADMINISTRATION: oral
DOSAGE FORMS: tablet, enteric-coated tablet, liquid, rectal suppository, injection
INDICATIONS: bronchial asthma, chronic bronchitis, emphysema, bradycardia
COMMON DOSAGE: Oral: 3 mg/kg q8h

AUXILIARY LABELS:

■ Take on an empty stomach.

■ Do not crush or chew enteric-coated tablets.

GENERIC NAME: theophylline
TRADE NAME: Theo-Dur, Slobid
ROUTE OF ADMINISTRATION: oral
INDICATIONS: bronchial asthma, bronchospasms of chronic obstructive pulmonary disease, acute bronchitis
DOSAGE FORMS: tablets, sustained release, LA (long-acting), capsules, elixir, liquid, suspension; injection
COMMON DOSAGE: Oral; 100 to 200 mg q6h
AUXILIARY LABELS:

■ Take as directed.

■ Do not crush or chew slow-release tablets or capsules.

Leukotrienes

Leukotrienes are substances that cause the smooth muscle of the bronchi to contract, causing labored breathing. Zafirlukast, montelukast, and zileuton work to decrease bronchoconstriction of the airways. These drugs also can be given to prevent asthma attacks caused by pollen, dander, cold air, or other antigens if taken before contact is made. The auxiliary label is "take as directed."

GENERIC NAME: zileuton
TRADE NAME: Zyflo
ROUTE OF ADMINISTRATION: oral
INDICATION: asthma
DOSAGE FORMS: 600-mg tablet
COMMON DOSAGE: 600 mg qid with meals and at bedtime
AUXILIARY LABEL:

■ Take with food.

GENERIC NAME: montelukast
TRADE NAME: Singulair
ROUTE OF ADMINISTRATION: oral
INDICATION: chronic asthma
DOSAGE FORMS: tablets and chewable tablets (pediatric 4 mg to 5 mg chewable)
COMMON DOSAGE: 10 mg qd in the evening
AUXILIARY LABEL:

■ Chewable tablet.

GENERIC NAME: zafirlukast
TRADE NAME: Accolate
ROUTE OF ADMINISTRATION: oral
INDICATION: prophylaxis and chronic treatment of asthma
DOSAGE FORMS: 10-mg and 20-mg tablets
COMMON DOSAGE: 20 mg bid
AUXILIARY LABELS:

■ Do not stop taking this medication unless otherwise prescribed by doctor.

■ Do not take this medication while breast-feeding.

Corticosteroids

Corticosteroids, unlike the agents mentioned previously, are not to be used over a long time but normally are used short-term to treat asthma. They help the other agents stop the asthmatic response of bronchiole constriction. Because administered corticosteroids replace the steroid production of the body, they have special dosing requirements. Commonly used inhalers along with normal dosages are listed for the treatment of asthma in adults. Always remember that all metered dose inhalers require a "shake well" auxiliary label.

CORTICOSTEROIDS

GENERIC NAME: beclomethasone
TRADE NAME: Beclovent, Vanceril
INDICATION: chronic asthma
DOSAGE FORMS: aerosol
COMMON DOSAGE: Beclovent—two inhalations tid to qid; Vanceril—two puffs bid
AUXILIARY LABELS:
- Inhalant.
- Shake well before using.

GENERIC NAME: flunisolide
TRADE NAME: AeroBid
INDICATION: chronic asthma
DOSAGE FORMS: aerosol
COMMON DOSAGE: two puffs bid
AUXILIARY LABELS:
- Inhalant.
- Shake well before using.

GENERIC NAME: triamcinolone acetonide
TRADE NAME: Azmacort
INDICATION: chronic asthma
DOSAGE FORMS: aerosol
COMMON DOSAGE: two puffs tid to qid or four puffs bid
AUXILIARY LABELS:
- Inhalant.
- Shake well before using.

Antiasthmatics

Antiasthmatics such as cromolyn sodium are considered antiasthmatic and antiallergic agents. They prevent mast cells from releasing histamine, which is one cause of asthmatic symptoms. Cromolyn is inhaled via a metered dose inhaler, nebulizer, or a nasal inhaler. The use of cromolyn can prevent allergic reactions from occurring if taken before contact with the allergen. The nasal inhaler is available OTC.

GENERIC NAME: cromolyn sodium
TRADE NAME: Intal
INDICATIONS: severe bronchial asthma, prevention of exercise-induced bronchospasm, allergic rhinitis
DOSAGE FORMS: inhalation solution, aerosol spray, nasal solution, capsules for inhalation
AUXILIARY LABEL:
- Inhalant.
- Shake well before using.

Most patients with asthma are given a prescription for an inhaler, and they keep it close by for emergencies. The specific administration method takes

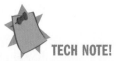

TECH NOTE!
To find out if an inhaler is empty, simply place it into a bowl of water. The empty container will float; a partial container will have only one end floating; and a full container will drop to the bottom of the bowl.

practice and usually is explained by the doctor or pharmacist. The inhaler must be shaken before use.

Because it is difficult for many patients to dose themselves correctly, devices called an Aerochamber or spacers fit over the end of the mouthpiece of the inhaler to aid administration. As the dose of medicine is released from the inhaler, it fills the spacer, and the patient slowly and more accurately can inhale more of the drug.

ASTHMA TREATMENT DOSAGE FORMS

A wide range of agents can be used with multiple routes of administration. The more common route for adults is by inhalation. In young children, oral liquid is used more commonly. A metered dose inhaler is convenient and can be kept easily in a purse or pocket for emergency use. For a more thorough treatment, nebulizers can be used at home or may be given in a clinic or hospital by respiratory therapy. Finally, in severe cases, there are parenteral medications, such as xanthines, that can be used. Spin inhalers or aerochambers are used to increase the dose of medication ejected from the metered dose inhaler.

Nebulizer treatments are given by a respiratory therapist in a hospital if ordered by the physician, or they can be used at home with proper training. Many of the agents, such as metaproterenol and albuterol, are available in unit dose containers that deliver only one dose. The exact number of drops can be placed into the nebulizer reservoir. The machine creates a steam that is filled with the medication. The drug is inhaled via a nose and mouth mask, allowing for deep, thorough inhalation treatments.

PREVENTION OF ANAPHYLAXIS

For the most severe reactions that cause swelling of the airways, epinephrine is given either by inhalation or, if necessary, by injection to open the airways

Allergy Agents (Antihistamines)

Antihistamine agents are used to decrease inflammation and irritation from allergens. Allergens are also known as antigens. They are substances that are capable of stimulating an immune response. Millions of Americans suffer from seasonal allergies, as well as allergies from other common substances. Box 25-1 lists the most common allergenic substances. The three types of nondrowsy antihistamines are listed next, followed by three nasal antihistamines. Medica-

BOX 25-1 TYPES OF ANTIGENS

Synthetic Chemicals
Detergents, cleaners
Drugs
Topical agents such as soaps, lotions, and creams

Naturally Occurring Chemicals
Heavy-molecular-weight compounds such as blood or dextran
Pollen
Venom from snake bites or bee stings

Miscellaneous
Animal dander
Dust
Large lacerations

tions that can be taken to prevent an allergic response by stabilization of the mast cell membranes include cromolyn, cetirizine (Zyrtec), and fexofenadine (Allegra). The main side effects experienced when taking antihistamines include drowsiness, dry mouth, constipation, urinary retention, sedation, and increase in intraocular pressure.

ANTIHISTAMINES

GENERIC NAME: loratadine
TRADE NAME: Claritin
ROUTE OF ADMINISTRATION: oral
INDICATION: seasonal rhinitis
DOSAGE FORMS: oral tablet, syrup
AUXILIARY LABELS:
- Do not take with food.
- Do not use if breast-feeding.
- Take as prescribed.

GENERIC NAME: fexofenadine
TRADE NAME: Allegra
ROUTE OF ADMINISTRATION: oral
INDICATIONS: rhinitis and allergies
DOSAGE FORMS: oral tablet, syrup
AUXILIARY LABELS:
- Do not take with food.
- Do not use if breast-feeding.
- Take as prescribed.

GENERIC NAME: cetirizine
TRADE NAME: Zyrtec
ROUTE OF ADMINISTRATION: oral
INDICATIONS: rhinitis and allergies
DOSAGE FORMS: oral tablet, syrup
AUXILIARY LABELS:
- Do not take with food.
- Do not use if breast-feeding.
- Take as prescribed.
- Avoid prolonged or excessive exposure to direct sunlight.

Nasal agents are used for seasonal allergies or chronic rhinitis. The oral dosage forms are not listed because those are used for asthma or prophylaxis treatment.

CORTICOSTEROIDS (NASAL)

GENERIC NAME: budesonide
TRADE NAME: Rhinocort
ROUTE OF ADMINISTRATION: nasal
INDICATION: seasonal and perennial allergic rhinitis
DOSAGE FORMS: nasal spray, 32 mcg per spray
NORMAL DOSAGE: either two sprays into each nostril in the morning and evening or as four sprays in each nostril once daily in the morning
AUXILIARY LABELS:
- For the nose.
- Shake well before using.

TECH ALERT!

Many generic drug names are similar. Do not confuse drugs such as flunisolide with fluticasone and dexamethasone with beclomethasone. Also make sure you double-check the route of administration because these agents have several different dosage forms!

TECH ALERT!

Many generic drug names are similar. Do not confuse drugs such as fluticasone, dexamethasone, or beclomethasone with one another. Also make sure you double check the route of administration as these agents are available in several different dosage forms.

GENERIC NAME: flunisolide
TRADE NAME: Nasalide
ROUTE OF ADMINISTRATION: nasal
INDICATION: rhinitis
DOSAGE FORMS: nasal spray, 25 mcg per actuation
NORMAL DOSAGE: two sprays into each nostril twice daily in the morning and evening
AUXILIARY LABELS:
- For the nose.
- Shake well before using.

GENERIC NAME: fluticasone
TRADE NAME: Flonase
ROUTE OF ADMINISTRATION: nasal
INDICATION: seasonal and perennial allergic rhinitis in patient 12 years or older
DOSAGE FORMS: 50 mcg per spray
NORMAL DOSAGE: one spray into each nostril daily
AUXILIARY LABELS:
- For the nose.
- Shake well before using.

DRUG INTERACTIONS

The effects of drugs that suppress the central nervous system will increase if used with first-generation antihistamines. Alcohol should not be consumed if one is taking antihistamines because it can intensify drowsiness. Some antibiotics such as macrolides, ketoconazole, and itraconazole can intensify the effects of second-generation antihistamines. All first-generation antihistamines should be given an auxiliary label that states "may cause drowsiness." All OTC antihistamines have labeling that cautions consumers of their ability to cause drowsiness. The only OTC nondrowsy antihistamine is Claritin, and this can cause drowsiness if taken more than recommended.

DO YOU REMEMBER THESE KEY POINTS?

- The commonly used agents for each of the conditions discussed in this chapter
- What chemicals produced by the body cause inflammation
- What chemicals can be used to reduce inflammation
- What are the risks of taking steroids
- How should steroids be discontinued
- What are the symptoms associated with asthma
- Why asthma is considered an inflammatory condition
- What types of agents are used to treat asthma
- What causes the symptoms of seasonal allergies
- What over-the-counter remedies are available to treat allergies
- What are the side effects of most agents used to treat allergies

1. Inflammation is caused by all of the following except _____.
   A. Infection
   B. Temperature
   C. Allergic reactions
   D. Injury

2. All of the following symptoms accompany inflammation except _____.
   A. Swelling
   B. Pain
   C. Redness
   D. Dizziness

3. Nonspecific antihistamines are used for all of the following symptoms except

   _____.
   A. Sleepiness
   B. Motion sickness
   C. Allergies
   D. All of the above

4. The enzyme that is responsible for pain, inflammation, and fever is _____.
   A. Prostaglandin
   B. Acetylsalicylic acid
   C. Cyclooxygenase
   D. Inflammatory disease

5. Histamine$_1$ receptors are located in the _____.
   A. Gastrointestinal system
   B. Skin
   C. Bronchioles
   D. Both B and C

6. Aspirin should not be given to children because _____.
   A. It can cause Reye's syndrome in children with flulike symptoms
   B. It can cause vomiting
   C. It can cause lethargy
   D. All of the above

7. Aspirin often is given to patients who have had a TIA because _____.
   A. It stops inflammation and infection
   B. It lowers body temperature
   C. It decreases chances of blood clotting
   D. It speeds up the flow of blood

8. Common side effects of steroidal use include _____.
   A. Ability to bruise easier
   B. Easier to get an infection
   C. Increase in heart rate
   D. All of the above

9. Those cells that contain histamine are called _____.
   A. Immunoglobulin E antibodies
   B. Antihistamines
   C. Mast cells
   D. Immune cells

10. Corticosteroids are available in all dosage forms except _____.
    A. Injection
    B. Inhalant
    C. Liquid
    D. Tablet
    E. All of the above

If the statement is false, then change it to make it true.

_____ 1. All antiinflammatory agents are legend drugs.

_____ 2. Edema is a result of blood rushing to the damaged tissue or organ.

_____ 3. Promethazine suppositories are used commonly for allergies.

_____ 4. Acetylsalicylic acid increases inflammation.

_____ 5. All aspirin strengths are available over-the-counter.

_____ 6. All nonsteroidal antiinflammatory drugs work the same; therefore, if one does not work, none of them will.

_____ 7. Corticosteroids are used solely for asthma patients.

_____ 8. α-Adrenergic agents affect the bronchiole tubes by causing dilation.

_____ 9. Asthma is genetically inherited, or only affects persons who smoke.

_____ 10. Antihistamine agents bind to mast cells and stop all allergic reactions.

TECHNICIAN'S CORNER

Transcribe the following order into layperson terms and answer the following questions. Prednisone order as follows:

Give orally 30 mg bid ¥ 2 days, 25 mg bid ¥ 2 days, 20 mg bid ¥ 2 days, 15 mg bid ¥ 2 days, 10 mg qd ¥ 2 days, 5 mg bid ¥ 2 days, 5 mg qd ¥ 2 days, stop.

How many tablets and of which strength will you use to fill this order?
What auxiliary label(s) will you need to apply, if any?
What side effects will the pharmacist probably inform the patient about?

BIBLIOGRAPHY

Clayton BD, Stock YN: *Basic pharmacology for nurses,* ed 14, St Louis, 2006, Mosby.

Drug facts and comparisons, ed 60, St Louis, 2005, Wolters Kluwer.

Hardman JG, Gilman AG, Limbird LE, editors: *Goodman & Gilman's the pharmaceutical basis of therapeutics,* ed 10, New York, 2001, McGraw-Hill.

Koda-Kimble MA, Young LY: *Applied therapeutics: the clinical use of drugs,* ed 9, Baltimore, 2004, Lippincott, Williams & Wilkins.

Potter PA, Perry AG: *Fundamentals of nursing,* ed 6, St Louis, 2004, Mosby.

Rang HP, Dale MM, Ritter JM et al: *Pharmacology,* ed 5, Philadelphia, 2003, Churchill Livingstone.

Rosdahl CB: *Textbook of basic nursing,* ed 8, Philadelphia, 2003, Lippincott, Williams & Wilkins.

Shargel L, Mutnick A, Souney P et al: *Comprehensive pharmacy review,* ed 6, Baltimore, 2006, Lippincott, Williams & Wilkins.

Stedman's concise medical dictionary of the health professions, ed 3, Baltimore, 1997, Lippincott, Williams & Wilkins.

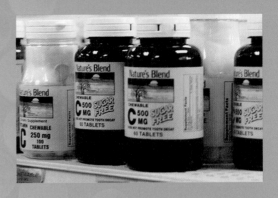

CHAPTER
26

Vitamins and Minerals

Objectives

UPON COMPLETING THIS CHAPTER, YOU SHOULD BE ABLE TO
DO THE FOLLOWING:

- List the conditions that can occur from a deficiency of the vitamins covered in this chapter.

- Explain the functions of vitamins and minerals.

- Describe the difference between water-soluble and fat-soluble vitamins.

- List the recommended daily allowance of each vitamin.

- List the trace elements and the importance of each.

- List the most common minerals.

- Write the chemical symbol for the most commonly used minerals.

- Describe the adverse effects if vitamins and minerals are overused.

- List the foods in which these common elements can be found.

565

Anemia *A deficiency of circulating red blood cells; a symptom of disease, not a disease*

Avitaminosis *Vitamin deficiency*

Coenzyme *A compound that activates an enzyme*

Cofactor *A factor that must be present for other factors to be active*

Fat-soluble vitamin *Vitamin that is soluble in fat and therefore is stored in body fat; vitamins A, D, E, and K are fat-soluble*

Hemoglobin *The iron-containing pigment on red blood cells that carries oxygen to the tissues*

Hypervitaminosis *A disorder caused by the intake of too many vitamins; more common with fat-soluble vitamins.*

Intrinsic factor *A naturally produced protein that is necessary for the absorption of vitamin B_{12}*

Vitamins

A	Retinol	B_{12}	Cyanocobalamin
B_1	Thiamine	C	Ascorbic acid
B_2	Riboflavin	D_2	Ergocalciferol
B_3	Nicotinic acid, niacin	D_3	Cholecalciferol
B_5	Pantothenic acid	E	α-Tocopherol
B_6	Pyridoxine	K	Phytonadione
B_9	Folic acid		

MINERALS

Name	Chemical Symbol (Example of Form Found in Drug Preparations)
Major Minerals	
Calcium	Ca (calcium carbonate, calcium acetate, many others)
Chlorine	Cl (available as a mineral chloride)
Magnesium	Mg (magnesium sulfate, magnesium chloride)
Phosphorus	P (dibasic calcium phosphate, tricalcium phosphate, others)
Potassium	K (potassium chloride, salt substitute, others)
Sodium	Na (NaCl, table salt)
Sulfur	S (available as a mineral sulfate)
Trace Mineral Elements (10 Currently Known to Be Essential in Human Beings)	
Chromium	Cr
Cobalt	Co
Copper	Cu (cupric sulfate)
Fluorine	F
Iodine	I (iodized table salt)
Iron	Fe (ferrous sulfate, ferrous fumarate, ferrous gluconate, iron dextran, and iron sucrose)
Manganese	Mn
Molybdenum	Mo (not currently available as a separate supplement because of its toxicity)
Selenium	Se
Zinc	Zn (zinc sulfate, zinc acetate)

LIKE HERBALS, MOST VITAMINS and minerals in small quantities are considered supplements and do not require a prescription. They are sold over the counter in pharmacies, grocery markets, and in herbal stores across America. The Food and Drug Administration (FDA) regulates all drugs that are sold over the counter to ensure proper manufacturing and labeling. Vitamins and minerals are termed "essential" if disorders occur when they are not present in large enough amounts. Many vitamins are essential, such as vitamins A, B, C, D, and E. Examples of the important essential minerals found in the body are calcium, chlorine, magnesium, potassium, phosphorus, and sodium. Trace elements are agents that the body requires to run various enzymatic reactions; however, they are needed only in extremely small amounts. Examples of trace elements are cobalt, copper, iodine, selenium, manganese, and zinc.

Vitamins and minerals are necessary for proper growth and development. Most of these supplements are contained in everyday foods. If one has a well-balanced diet, then all the daily nutritional requirements normally are met. These include the larger quantities of various vitamins and the necessary mineral elements and trace mineral elements. When one suffers from a depletion of necessary vitamins caused by either a deficiency or lack of absorption results in a condition called avitaminosis. This chapter covers three main types of supplements: vitamins, mineral elements, and trace mineral elements. Each type differs in its function in the body. All water-soluble vitamins function as coenzymes causing important reactions to occur in the body.

Fat-soluble vitamins act in several ways. Vitamin D acts on the nucleus of the cell to cause a normal physiological change in the cell. Vitamin K acts as a coenzyme to produce four factors that enable the blood to clot. Vitamin A becomes incorporated in the rod cells of the eyes, enabling us to see at night. Vitamin E (and other vitamins) bind to free radicals that would otherwise damage cells.

The mineral elements usually are called "minerals" and in the body are found in very large or extremely small quantities. Most minerals found in the body in large quantities usually form structures in the body, such as the calcium and phosphate in bone, or make up a large portion of essential ions in body fluids, such as sodium, chloride, and calcium.

When a major or trace mineral element combines with another molecule to enable that molecule to do something, the element is called a cofactor. For example, calcium also combines with several separate clotting factors that, when activated, enable the blood to clot. Many of the trace elements are cofactors for different enzymes.

Certain elements are needed by the body in only trace or very small amounts. Although vitamins and minerals are essential in keeping the body healthy, they should never be taken in excess. If this happens, toxicity called hypervitaminosis may occur.

In addition to hypervitaminosis, potential toxic problems can be caused if a person supplements his or her diet with various vitamins or minerals but neglects to ask the doctor or pharmacist about possible interactions between the prescription drugs taken and the vitamin or mineral supplement. Many of these vitamin and mineral supplements have interactions with medications and could affect the patient's health. Therefore, it is important for the pharmacy technician to know the interactions of supplements. As always, if the pharmacy technician suspects a patient may be taking a vitamin or mineral supplement that might interact with the patient's prescription, he or she should alert the pharmacist.

TECH ALERT!

Fat-soluble vitamins and minerals such as vitamin E and iron, respectively, can build up in the body system and cause great illness and even death. This must be taken into consideration especially when a technician prepares intravenous preparations that contain these types of additives.

Vitamins

When supplementing a diet with vitamins, one must make an important distinction between the fat-soluble and water-soluble types. Vitamin B (including all of the B complex) and vitamin C are water-soluble. Any excess B or C vitamins usually can be excreted in the urine. In contrast, fat-soluble vitamins such as vitamins A, D, E, and K may be stored by the body in the lipids of a cell. These vitamins accumulate instead of being excreted. As these vitamins accumulate in a cell, they may reach such a high level that they interfere with the function of the cell. This makes fat-soluble vitamins a greater source of potential toxic effects when they are taken in excess.

The FDA considers all vitamins, minerals, herbs, amino acids, and extracts as dietary supplements. Manufacturers must meet the guidelines that are listed in Box 26-1.

Although the FDA has limited control over supplements, these supplements are classified as a food ingredient. Therefore the FDA Center for Food Safety and Applied Nutrition is responsible for the safety of any food including these food supplements. When an illness or accident concerning a supplement is reported to the FDA, an inspection of the manufacturing plant, formulation, or processing method may be done. This is the only time that a supplement may be inspected. All of this information obtained by the FDA is available to consumers.

In addition to ensuring that all regulatory requirements are met, the FDA also regulates the recommended daily allowance (RDA) of vitamins and

BOX 26-1 FOOD AND DRUG ADMINISTRATION REGULATORY REQUIREMENTS FOR DIETARY SUPPLEMENTS AND NONREGULATED ITEMS

Regulatory Requirements

Manufacturers must notify the Food and Drug Administration (FDA) of any "new" dietary ingredient that is not already present in a food substance.

Label Information

The agent that is a food supplement

The name and address of the manufacturer (packer or distributor)

A complete list of all ingredients

The net contents of the package

A "supplement facts" panel listing each ingredient within the package, or ingredients may be listed in the "other ingredient" area below the panel

The statement "This statement has not been evaluated by the FDA. This product is not intended to diagnose, treat, cure, or prevent any disease." This is to ensure that consumers do not believe it is a medication approved by the FDA.

Not Regulated by the FDA

The safety of the ingredients within the container (FDA only regulates the safety of prescription medications)

Specific quantity of supplement in a tablet or capsule

Disclosure of proprietary information pertaining to the supplement (such as the formulation used to make a vitamin tablet). Proprietary information would include, for example, the filler used in making a tablet or capsule and the chemical coating on a tablet.

minerals. This regulatory guideline is used to inform consumers of the necessary requirements of average healthy adults and to make certain that overdosing resulting from lack of supplement information does not occur. The FDA has a MedWatch hotline (1-800-FDA-1088, or e-mail at *www.fda.gov/medwatch/ report/consumer/consumer.htm*) to which all health care providers or consumers can report problems concerning supplements, medical foods, devices, and drugs. All information regarding who reported the information is kept confidential.

Table 26-1 lists examples of the most common vitamins, along with their RDA and possible toxic side effects.

FAT-SOLUBLE VITAMINS (A, D, E, AND K)

Vitamin A

Vitamin A is also called β-carotene or retinol. Vitamin A has four primary functions. First, vitamin A is an important part of the visual pigment for rods in the retina of the eye. Rods enable us to see in dim light. Because rods have no color pigment, there is no color perception in dim light. Without an adequate intake of vitamin A, individuals have night blindness and cannot see well or at all in dim light. Severe deficiency of vitamin A over a long period can result in blindness. The second function of vitamin A is to protect against cancer in the skin and other epithelial (surface) cell types in the respiratory and digestive tracts, urinary bladder, and breast. Patients who are deficient in vitamin A may be more susceptible to these types of cancer. A third major function is to stimulate the immune system so that bacterial, viral, and parasitic infections are dealt with efficiently and the organisms eventually are destroyed. The final, most important, function is that vitamin A acts as an antioxidant, soaking up free radicals that could be dangerous to cells. The full extent of damage that free radicals can cause is unknown, but they have been implicated in cancer, Alzheimer's disease, and aging.

Vitamin A also has several functions that are not as important. Vitamin A is necessary for proper bone growth, renal function, and digestive activity, and it is associated with normal reproductive function in both sexes.

Sources of Vitamin A. Vitamin A sources include dairy products (whole milk, butter, cheese, and egg yolks), liver, and fish. Vitamin A is also present in yellow and green fruits and vegetables. Many dairy products, such as butter substitutes and all forms of milk, are fortified with vitamin A.

Hypervitaminosis A. Symptoms of hypervitaminosis A include headaches, vomiting, skin peeling, loss of appetite, irritability, and a wasting away of bone mass and, in fatal cases, destruction of the liver. Birth defects also can occur in children whose mothers ingested large amounts of vitamin A during the first 3 months of pregnancy.

Vitamin D

The two precursors of vitamin D are cholecalciferol and ergocalciferol. Cholecalciferol (vitamin D_3) is produced by the skin in the presence of ultraviolet light. The ultraviolet light changes modified cholesterol present in the skin to vitamin D_3. Ergocalciferol (vitamin D_2) is the result of ultraviolet radiation on a yeast product called ergosterol found in bread and milk. This is the form of vitamin D that is added to dairy products and bread. Ingested ergocalciferol or cholecalciferol absorbed through the skin is transported to the liver where the

TABLE 26-1 Drug Interactions of Fat- and Water-Soluble Vitamins

Vitamin	Solubility	Chemical name	Overdose	Drug interactions
A	Fat	Retinol, β-carotene	Nausea, vomiting, diarrhea	Mineral oil (interferes with vitamin A absorption)
B vitamins	Water	See Table 26-2	B_1: none B_2: none B_3: liver damage, heartburn, nausea, vomiting, diarrhea B_5: none B_6: ataxia, neuropathy B_{12}: none	B_1: none B_2: none B_3: inhibits the effects of sulfinpyrazone B_5: none B_6: none B_{12}: none
C	Water	Ascorbic acid	Damage to heart and kidneys, fatigue, nausea	Warfarin (decreases effects); iron (increases absorption)
D	Fat	Ergocalciferol (vitamin D_2); cholecalciferol (vitamin D_3)	Weakness, nausea, vomiting, headache, dry mouth	Digoxin (increases vitamin D_2 toxicity); mineral oil (decreases oral absorption)
E	Fat	α-Tocopherol	Anemia	May decrease iron intake in children; may increase bleeding if patient is taking anticoagulants or vitamin K
K	Fat	Phytonadione		Mineral oil (interferes with vitamin A and K absorption) Decreases warfarin effectiveness

hormone calciferol is formed. Calciferol then is transported to the kidney where the final product, a hormone called calcitriol (also called vitamin D hormone), is produced.

Calcitriol increases phosphorus absorption and calcium intake. Calcitriol is also necessary for providing adequate calcium and phosphate to mother and child during pregnancy and during breast-feeding.

Sources of Vitamin D. Dairy foods such as milk and cheeses and eggs contain vitamin D in the form of ergocalciferol. Natural and artificial sunlight provide ultraviolet radiation that makes vitamin D in the skin.

Deficiency of Vitamin D. A deficiency of vitamin D can cause bone weakness and deformities called rickets in children, and in adults it can cause a similar weakened bone structure called osteomalacia. In osteomalacia there is also a reduction in bone mass called osteoporosis. Osteoporosis also can occur in postmenopausal women and in older men if vitamin D and calcium intake is not sufficiently high.

Hypervitaminosis D. Vitamin D excess may cause hypercalcemia (higher than normal calcium blood levels). Toxic effects of vitamin D can cause calcium deposits in various areas, such as in soft tissue and joints, causing muscle weakness or pain. In severe cases, convulsions or even death can occur.

Drug Interactions. Interactions between vitamin D and digitalis may cause arrhythmias. Thiazide diuretics and vitamin D can cause hypercalcemia, and mineral oil may antagonize the absorption of vitamin D.

Vitamin E

Vitamin E has been promoted extensively over the past decade as a potent antioxidant. Vitamin E is essential for normal metabolism and protection of the skin, eyes, tissues, and muscles. Vitamin E also seems to protect red blood cells from damage.

Source of Vitamin E. Vitamin E can be found in whole grains such as wheat and rice germ, nuts, corn, vegetables, and dairy products (eggs and butter).

Deficiency of Vitamin E. A vitamin E deficiency may cause anemia and cardiovascular disease.

Hypervitaminosis E. Fully documented cases of hypervitaminosis E have not been reported in the literature.

Drug Interactions. The use of mineral oil may decrease the absorption of vitamin E.

Vitamin K (Phytonadione)

Vitamin K is responsible for the formation of blood coagulation factors.

Source of Vitamin K. Vitamin K can be found in wheat, legumes, egg yolks, milk, and vegetables such as broccoli and spinach. Certain bacteria in the intestine also produce vitamin K as a by-product of their metabolism.

Deficiency of Vitamin K. Deficiency of vitamin K can cause an increased tendency to bleed. The bleeding may be manifested as repeated nosebleeds, blood in the sputum without coughing, spontaneous bruising (i.e., bruising not caused by injury) in several parts of the body, or blood in the urine. Excess bleeding also may be a sign that the patient is taking an excess of drugs that prevent the clotting of blood: for example, if a patient misses a dose or doses of warfarin (an oral anticoagulant) and takes double or triple the normal dose to make up for it, or if a patient takes lots of aspirin for a headache or cold and also is taking warfarin (because aspirin behaves similarly to an anticoagulant).

Hypervitaminosis K. Hypervitaminosis K has not been reported.

WATER-SOLUBLE VITAMINS (B AND C)

All of the B complex vitamins are water-soluble. This includes B_1 (thiamine), B_2 (riboflavin), B_3 (nicotinic acid [niacin]), B_5 (pantothenic acid), B_6 (pyridoxine), B_9 (folic acid), and B_{12} (cyanocobalamin).

TABLE 26-2 B Vitamins: Sources, Function, and Deficiency States

Vitamin	Chemical name	Food sources	Function	Deficiency
B_1	Thiamine	Grains, cereals, beans, pork, liver	Metabolism	Beriberi (wet and/or dry forms)
B_2	Riboflavin	Cereals, eggs, dark green vegetables, milk, liver	Maintains mucous membranes, metabolic energy pathways	Discolored tongue and dry scaling and fissuring of the lips
B_3	Nicotinic acid	Nuts, beans, peas, wheat, rice, grains	Fat synthesis, protein metabolism and electron transport	Diarrhea, dementia, depression, skin discoloration
B_5	Pantothenic acid	Vegetables, cereals, yeast, liver	Coenzyme	Fatigue, headaches, nausea, muscle spasms
B_6	Pyridoxine	Meat, liver, chicken, salmon, trout, beans, rice, whole grains	Amino acid and fatty acid metabolism	Skin disorders, depression, nausea, impaired vision and nerve function
B_9	Folic acid	Green vegetables and liver	Production of red blood cells	Nerve damage
B_{12}	Cyanocobalamin	Meats, liver, chicken, dairy products	Formation of red blood cells	Pernicious anemia, megaloblastic anemia

Sources of B Vitamins

B vitamins can be found in foods such as peas, beans, red meats, flour, and yeasts. Table 26-2 lists common B vitamins and their sources. Depending on which B vitamin is deficient, different side effects can occur. These effects are discussed in the following section.

Deficiencies of B Vitamins

Persons at high risk of vitamin B deficiencies include older adults, if they have poor diets, and pregnant or lactating (breast-feeding) women, because of the additional requirements of the fetus. Table 26-3 lists the four major B deficiencies. Anyone who suffers from a poor diet is prone to be deficient in many other vitamins and minerals.

Persons who may be more susceptible to vitamin B deficiencies, as well as a wide variety of other vitamin deficiencies, include alcoholics, smokers, and those persons with any disease that may affect intake or processing of necessary vitamins and/or minerals. Deficiencies may go unnoticed for several years until illness occurs. Fortunately, there are many medications that can be taken to replace the necessary amounts of the B vitamins.

B vitamins enable proper cellular functioning of the body system. They do this by acting as coenzymes that combine with the protein portions of enzymes

TABLE 26-3 Four Major Deficiency Diseases Resulting from a Lack of B Vitamins

Disorder	Vitamin deficiency
Pernicious anemia	Cyanocobalamin (B_{12})
Megaloblastic anemia	Folic acid (B_9)
Pellagra	Nicotinic acid (niacin), nicotinamide
Beriberi	Thiamine (B_1)

TABLE 26-4 Recommended Daily Allowances (RDA) of Vitamins for Men and Women

Vitamin (common name)	RDA* (women/men)	Solubility
Vitamin A	800 mcg/1000 mcg	Fat
Vitamin B_1 (thiamine)	1000 mcg/1200 mcg	Water
Vitamin B_2 (riboflavin)	1200 mcg/1500 mcg	Water
Vitamin B_3 (nicotinic acid)	14 mg/15 mg	Water
Vitamin B_5 (pantothenic acid)	No RDA, but 5 mg/day is the accepted amount	Water
Vitamin B_6 (pyridoxine)	1.5 mg/1.7 mg	Water
Vitamin B_9 (folic acid)	150 mcg/150 mcg	Water
Vitamin B_{12} (cyanocobalamin)	2 mcg/2 mcg	Water
Vitamin C (ascorbic acid)	50 mg/50 mg	Water
Vitamin D	5 mcg/5 mcg	Fat
Vitamin E	8 mcg/10 mcg	Fat
Vitamin K	50 mcg/45 mcg	Fat

*In some cases these amounts are based on the lowest end of the range. For information regarding the full range, refer to the Food and Drug Administration website at www.fda.gov/medwatch/report/consumer.htm

to form the complete enzymes. The enzymes cause important reactions to occur within the cell. If the body becomes vitamin B deficient, the enzymes will not work and the cells will not function properly. Some of the important enzymatic reactions that fail to occur include those involved in the immune system, carbohydrate metabolism, protein synthesis, neurotransmission, and blood formation. For the current RDA of all B vitamins and other vitamins covered in this chapter, see Table 26-4.

The B Vitamins in Greater Detail

Vitamin B_1 (Coenzyme). Thiamine has three major functions that help maintain the body system. Thiamine is important for proper carbohydrate metabolism so that energy can be produced from ingested carbohydrates. In this process the carbohydrates are broken down and energy in the form of adenosine triphosphate is produced; this energy is transferred by carrier molecules to the mitochondria of the cell. Water is a by-product of this process, and some of this water is excreted as urine or perspiration. Another role thiamine plays is in the wellbeing of the nervous and cardiovascular system.

Deficiency of vitamin B_1. A deficiency in vitamin B_1 can cause a condition known as beriberi. The symptoms include wasting of the muscles and the malfunctioning of the nervous system. Other signs of a deficiency include anorexia, constipation, nausea, mental confusion, and depression.

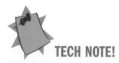

Vitamin B_2 (Coenzyme). Riboflavin is another important component for proper enzymatic activity in the metabolism of carbohydrates and its production of energy for the body system. Riboflavin is necessary for proper growth and maintenance of the body.

Deficiency of vitamin B_2. A deficiency of vitamin B_2 can cause anemia and affect the nervous system and cause depression. In addition, because of the part of vitamin B_2 in the maintenance of healthy mucous membranes, the tongue, mouth, eyes, and skin may be affected adversely by drying out or soreness. Headaches, burning sensations of the skin (especially the feet), cracking of the corners of the mouth, and seborrheic dermatitis are other symptoms of vitamin B deficiency.

Vitamin B_3 (Coenzyme). Nicotinic acid is also known as niacin. This vitamin is used in tissue respiration and metabolism. Although there are two related compounds, nicotinic acid and nicotinamide, they are used in much the same way in the body because nicotinic acid eventually is converted to nicotinamide. However, when nicotinic acid and nicotinamide are taken orally, they do behave differently shortly after ingestion. Nicotinic acid has been found to reduce low-density lipoprotein (the bad cholesterol). Nicotinic acid also releases histamine and causes peripheral vasodilation. Its counterpart, nicotinamide, does not have these effects. However, nicotinamide may help prevent insulin-dependent diabetes mellitus in high-risk patients. Nicotinic acid and nicotinamide are also necessary for lipid metabolism, proper nerve functioning, and overall maintenance of cells.

Deficiency of vitamin B_3. A deficiency of niacin can cause a condition known as pellagra. The symptoms include diarrhea, weakness, lethargy, dermatitis, dementia, sores in the mouth, and gastrointestinal problems.

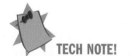

Vitamin B_5 (Coenzyme). Pantothenic acid is another compound that is a coenzyme and thus affects body metabolism. Pantothenic acid is incorporated into a coenzyme or into the enzyme itself, where it is used to synthesize important compounds in the body such as fatty acids, steroid hormones, and other molecules necessary for protein and carbohydrate metabolic processes. Pantothenic acid is produced by bacteria within the gastrointestinal tract of many animals and also can be found in plant cells.

Deficiency of vitamin B_5. Symptoms of vitamin B_5 deficiency include headache, sleep disturbances, muscle cramps, and fatigue. The medication used to replace pantothenic acid is calcium pantothenate.

Vitamin B_6 (Coenzyme). Pyridoxine functions in the metabolism of carbohydrates, proteins, and fats in the diet. The increased metabolism that is an effect of vitamin B_6 is the main reason this vitamin is added to diet preparation. Increased metabolism reduces the breakdown of carbohydrates so that they are not absorbed by the body. Pyridoxine also helps in the absorption of vitamin B_{12} and is a component needed for the production of many different amino acids, including a major amino acid neurotransmitter found in the brain and spinal cord.

Deficiency of vitamin B_6. A vitamin B_6 deficiency causes skin problems such as seborrheic-type lesions, stomatitis, and even seizures, depending on the severity. A deficiency can cause dwarfism, blindness, dementia, depression, and osteoporosis.

Drug interactions with vitamin B_6. Pyridoxine may antagonize the effect of a medication called levodopa used to treat Parkinson's disease.

Vitamin B_9 (Coenzyme). Folic acid is an essential vitamin for DNA synthesis and the creation of cells in areas that have high growth turnover. These areas include the bone marrow where red and white blood cells are formed and the gastrointestinal tract. Folic acid can be found in green vegetables such as broccoli, avocado, and beets. Other sources include orange juice and meats such as liver. Folic acid is metabolized in the liver and then goes to the bone marrow cells where it can be used.

Deficiency of vitamin B$_9$. Vitamin B$_9$ deficiencies include diarrhea, weight loss, weakness, sore mouth, irritability, and behavior disorders. Interactions may occur with phenytoin, estrogen, or nitrofurantoin.

Vitamin B$_{12}$ (Coenzyme). Cyanocobalamin is obtained mainly from dietary intake. Cyanocobalamin is required by the body for red blood cell production, myelin sheath production (myelin speeds the conduction of nerve impulses in the nervous system), and the synthesis of nucleic acids. Smokers have an increased need for vitamin B$_{12}$.

Deficiency of vitamin B$_{12}$. Persons deficient in Vitamin B$_{12}$ may experience anemia, dementia, depression, hair loss, poor growth rate in children, and loss of appetite. The specific type of red cell anemia that is seen in pernicious anemia is called megaloblastic anemia. The term *pernicious* means "serious" or "severe" and does not relate to a particular cell type. *Megaloblastic* means that the red cells are formed abnormally. Pernicious anemia results from the loss of intrinsic factor, a protein produced by the same stomach cells that produce hydrochloric acid. Normally, vitamin B$_{12}$ is bound to intrinsic factor, enabling vitamin B$_{12}$ to be absorbed into the blood. If there is no intrinsic factor produced, vitamin B$_{12}$ is not absorbed. Persons suffering from disorders of the stomach or those who have had gastric surgery such as gastrectomies (removal of the stomach) may develop vitamin B$_{12}$ deficiency. Most cases of pernicious anemia are autoimmune, in which the body develops antibodies against the cells that produce intrinsic factor. As a result, the cells are destroyed and not replaced. After a time, there are too few cells left to produce intrinsic factor, and pernicious anemia develops. Persons who have no vitamin B$_{12}$ absorption at all require vitamin B$_{12}$ injections for the rest of their lives. If there are some stomach cells left that produce intrinsic factor, there may be limited absorption; in those cases, a larger than normal oral dose would be required to ensure that some of the vitamin is absorbed. Vitamin B$_{12}$ is available over the counter in an oral form and by prescription for the injectable form.

Vitamin C
Vitamin C also is known as ascorbic acid and is also well known as another antioxidant. The main function of vitamin C is the formation of the connective tissue that is found in bones, teeth, and gums. It also aids in healing wounds.

Deficiency of Vitamin C. Vitamin C cannot be synthesized by the body, so this vitamin must be consumed daily. Vitamin C deficiency results in the disease known as scurvy. This condition causes excessive bleeding in the skin and gums and causes the teeth to become loose. Vitamin C is important for the proper nutrition of cells and their permeability (how easily molecules can penetrate the membrane). A deficiency can decrease the ability of the immune system to produce T cells. These cells aid in fighting infection. Vitamin C is found in citrus fruits and a wide variety of vegetables. The RDA of vitamin C for adults is listed in Table 26-4.

ANTIOXIDANTS

Many of the vitamins that are popular are advertised as being antioxidants. Although there has been much research on antioxidants, there are still many

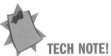

TECH NOTE!
Before the 1900s pernicious anemia was a fatal disease often affecting older adults. By the early 1900s patients were being treated by feeding them large amounts of liver to build up red blood cells. Not until 1948 was vitamin B$_{12}$ isolated, and not until the 1950s were supplements available.

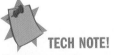

TECH NOTE!
If you overcook vegetables, the vitamin C can be lost. Cooking vegetables as little as possible is recommended to reduce the destruction of vitamin C and all other vitamins.

debates regarding whether antioxidants actually can increase the lifespan. Nevertheless, antioxidants do bind to free radicals that are responsible for damage to the cells and tissues inside the body. The main antioxidant vitamins are vitamins A, C, and E.

Minerals

Minerals are inorganic elements (i.e., they do not contain carbon) and are the ingredients of the earth's crust. Only small amounts are necessary for proper functioning of many metabolic steps within the body. For instance, zinc sulfate is important for normal growth, for the sense of smell and taste, and for skin hydration. Zinc sulfate also helps heal wounds. The normal recommended dose for an adult is 15 mg per day. Table 26-5 lists common minerals and trace elements.

ZINC EXCESS

If zinc is taken in excess, side effects can range from nausea, vomiting, and diarrhea to pulmonary edema, hypotension, and tachycardia.

Drug Interactions

Penicillamine, a chelator, is a drug that binds to metals and is used to treat metal toxicity. Penicillamine binds to zinc and increases its renal excretion.

IRON

Iron (ferrous sulfate, ferrous fumarate, ferrous gluconate) is also an important mineral that plays a role in the transport of oxygen within the blood. Within the red blood cell, iron in hemoglobin binds tightly to the oxygen molecule, thus allowing oxygen to be transported throughout the body. Iron gives blood its red color. Much of the iron within the body is found in hemoglobin. Iron is used in other metabolic body functions, and iron also is found in all muscles (it gives muscles their red color). Iron also is stored in the liver, giving that organ its color.

Iron Deficiency

Iron deficiency anemia is one of the most common types of anemia, and it affects more than 30% of the world population. Iron deficiency can occur for many reasons:

- Lack of iron in the diet
- Pregnancy: typically, pregnant women require 12 mg more per day than non-pregnant women
- Inadequate intestinal absorption
- Excessive blood loss
- Certain forms of kidney failure in which the kidneys fail to produce erythropoietin*
- Alcoholism
- Blood loss in women during menstruation

Symptoms of iron deficiency include hair loss, shortness of breath, lethargy, and even heart palpitations. The toxic effects of an overdose are severe and include acidosis, liver and kidney impairment, and coma. Table 26-6 gives the recommended daily allowance for iron.

---

*Erythropoietin is a hormone necessary to make red blood cells. Epoetin is available in injectable form and normally is given to dialysis patients but also can be given to patients with severe anemia.

TABLE 26-5 Common Minerals and Trace Elements, Their Actions, and Deficiencies

Mineral/trace element	Indication	Deficiency	Overdosage
Calcium	Bone formation, cell transport, nerve and muscle functions	Osteoporosis, rickets	Kidney stones or damage
Copper	Iron utilization, skin pigmentation, nervous system functions	Poor bone growth, nausea, nervous system disorders, poor response of immune system	Jaundice
Magnesium	Normal muscle and heart function; necessary for vitamin C and calcium metabolism	High blood pressure, kidney and heart problems, mental confusion	
Phosphorus	Necessary for healthy bones and teeth; component of phospholipids*	Muscle weakness, defective bone function, arthritis	
Potassium	Cellular transport, normal muscle, heart, kidney, and nervous system functions	Muscle weakness, lethargy, poor growth, and cardiac disturbance	Cardiac arrhythmias; cardiac arrest
Iron	Hemoglobin/oxygen transport	Anemia, poor growth, confusion, loss of appetite	Gastrointestinal disturbance, black stools
Selenium	Proper immune functioning and growth	Heart and bone disease	Gastrointestinal disturbance, liver damage
Manganese	Necessary for bone formation and for metabolism of amino acids, lipids, and cholesterol	Poor hair growth, nails, and osteoporosis	None known
Zinc	Proper growth and reproduction; helps heal wounds	Decreased vitamin D absorption, nausea, hair loss, birth defects, decreased immune response, decreased sperm count	Blurred vision, decreased consciousness, tachycardia

*Phospholipids are required for the formation of cell membranes.

TABLE 26-6 Recommended Daily Allowance for Iron

Age	Amount
7-12 months	11 mg
1-3 years	7 mg
4-8 years	10 mg
9-13 years	8 mg
14-18 years	11-15 mg
19-50 years	8-18 mg
>50 years	8 mg

**DO YOU
REMEMBER THESE
KEY POINTS?**

- The main vitamins required by the body and their functions
- Water-soluble vitamins
- Fat-soluble vitamins
- The main minerals required by the body and their functions
- The cause of pernicious anemia
- The RDA for vitamins
- How iron is used in the body
- Causes of iron deficiencies
- The supposed effects of free radicals and how antioxidants are used to limit the damage from them

**MULTIPLE
CHOICE
QUESTIONS**

1. All of the following vitamins are water-soluble except _____.
   A. Vitamin C
   B. Vitamin E
   C. Vitamin B
   D. Ascorbic acid

2. Cyanocobalamin is the chemical term for _____ and is important in avoiding _____.
   A. Vitamin B_{12}, pernicious anemia
   B. Vitamin K, anemia
   C. Vitamin C, free radicals
   D. Vitamin E, immunity problems

3. Two important minerals that human beings require are _____.
   A. Ascorbic acid and pyridoxine
   B. Zinc sulfate and phytonadione
   C. Folic acid and calcitriol
   D. Ferrous and zinc sulfate

4. All of the following vitamins have antioxidant properties except _____.
   A. Vitamin A
   B. Vitamin C
   C. Vitamin E
   D. Vitamin D

5. The FDA considers all the following substances as food ingredients except _____.
   A. Amino acids
   B. Vitamins
   C. Minerals
   D. Aspirin

6. All of the following statements are true concerning retinol except _____.
   A. It also is called vitamin A
   B. It is an antioxidant
   C. It aids in the absorption of vitamin D
   D. It can be found in several dairy products, fruits, and vegetables

7. The vitamin most associated with proper blood clotting is _____.
   A. Phytonadione
   B. Niacin
   C. Thiamine
   D. Vitamin A

8. Of the statements listed, which is not true concerning the condition pernicious anemia?
   A. It can be caused by a lack of vitamin B.
   B. It commonly is experienced by individuals with a deficiency of intrinsic factor.
   C. Intrinsic factor is caused by hydrochloric acid.
   D. It is a fatal disease.

9. Iron deficiency can be caused by the following reasons except _____.
   A. Alcoholism
   B. Pregnancy
   C. Coffee
   D. Kidney failure

10. Calcium deficiency can cause which of the following condition(s)?
   A. Rickets
   B. Osteoporosis
   C. Osteomalacia
   D. All of the above

TRUE/FALSE

If the statement is false, then change it to make it true.

_____ **1.** All minerals are natural and do not have to be taken through supplements if a proper diet is eaten.

_____ **2.** All vitamins are water-soluble; therefore, all can be taken as often as needed or wanted.

_____ **3.** The initials "FDA" stand for the "Federal Department of Agriculture."

_____ **4.** The FDA considers all over-the-counter vitamins and minerals as food supplements.

_____ **5.** Iron is a main component of hemoglobin and is responsible for oxygen content.

_____ **6.** A deficiency of vitamin D can cause rickets.

_____ **7.** Goiter can be caused by too much iodine.

_____ **8.** Antioxidants are agents that combine with and reduce free radicals.

_____ **9.** Vitamin A is responsible for normal metabolism.

_____ **10.** Nicotinic acid is believed to be active in lowering cholesterol.

TECHNICIAN'S CORNER

An elderly female patient presents herself at the pharmacy window with the following questions: She is currently taking vitamins A, B, C, D, and E. She would like to know if that is okay.

1. What do you know about these vitamins?
2. What would you tell her?

BIBLIOGRAPHY

Bryant B, Knights K, Salerno E: *Pharmacology for health professionals,* St Louis, 2003, Mosby.

Food and Drug Administration: www.fda.gov

Hillman RS: Hematopoietic agents: growth factors, minerals, and vitamins. In Hardman JG, Gilman AG, Limbird LE, editors: *Goodman and Gilman's the pharmacological basis of therapeutics,* ed 10, New York, 2001, McGraw-Hill.

Marcus R: Agents affecting calcification and bone turnover: calcium, phosphate, parathyroid hormone, vitamin D, calcitonin, and other compounds. In Hardman JG, Gilman AG, Limbird LE, editors: *Goodman and Gilman's the pharmacological basis of therapeutics,* ed 10, New York, 2001, McGraw-Hill.

Marcus R, Coulston AM: The fat-soluble vitamins: vitamins A, K, and E. In Hardman JG, Gilman AG, Limbird LE, editors: *Goodman and Gilman's the pharmacological basis of therapeutics,* ed 10, New York, 2001, McGraw-Hill.

Marcus R, Coulston AM: The vitamins: introduction. In Hardman JG, Gilman AG, Limbird LE, editors: *Goodman and Gilman's the pharmacological basis of therapeutics,* ed 10, New York, 2001, McGraw-Hill.

Marcus R, Coulston AM: The water-soluble vitamins: the vitamin B complex and ascorbic acid. In Hardman JG, Gilman AG, Limbird LE, editors: *Goodman and Gilman's the pharmacological basis of therapeutics,* ed 10, New York, 2001, McGraw-Hill.

Mason JB: Consequences of altered micronutrient status. In Goldman L, Bennett JC, editors: *Cecil textbook of medicine,* ed 21, Philadelphia, 2000, Saunders.

McKenry LM, Salerno E: *Mosby's pharmacology in nursing,* ed 22, St Louis, 2005, Mosby.

Schlenker E, Long S: *Williams' Essentials of nutrition and diet therapy,* ed 9, St Louis, 2006, Mosby.

Vaccines

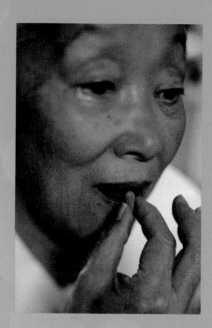

Objectives

UPON COMPLETING THIS CHAPTER, YOU SHOULD BE ABLE TO
DO THE FOLLOWING:

- Describe the importance of vaccines.

- Explain how vaccines are produced.

- List the most common vaccines.

- Explain how the body builds up immunity against diseases.

- Describe where immune cells are produced and what their function is.

- Differentiate between active and passive immunity.

- List the schedule for administering vaccines.

- Explain why some vaccines need boosters, whereas others do not.

- Explain under which circumstances adults should receive vaccines.

Acquired immunity *Immunity that has been acquired through exposure to an antigen or infectious agent*

Antibodies *Proteins contained within plasma cells that neutralize or destroy antigens; also known as immunoglobulins*

Antigen *The marker on cell surfaces that marks the cell as a "self-cell"; it stimulates the production of antibodies*

Attenuated *An altered or weakened live vaccine made from the disease organism against which the vaccine protects*

Globulin *Protein that is insoluble in water; immune globulins protect against disease*

Immunity *A type of resistance to infection resulting from an immune response from the body or from agents such as vaccinations*

Immunosuppresive agent *The immunosuppressive drugs used frequently to prevent rejection. Also used to treat certain autoimmune diseases.*

Lymph node *Composed of many small oval structures that filter the lymph and fight infection. Also where lymphocytes, monocytes, and plasma cells are formed.*

Passive immunity *Resistance that has been acquired through a transfer of antibodies from another person or animal or from mother to child*

Toxoid *A toxin that has been rendered harmless but still invokes an antigenic response*

Vaccine *Toxoids or attenuated viral components that are given to create a response from the body that results in immunity*

TYPES OF VACCINES

Immune Globulins
Cytomegalovirus immune globulin
γ-Globulin
Hepatitis B immune globulin
Tetanus immune globulin
Varicella-zoster immune globulin

Antitoxins/Antivenins
Black widow spider
Diphtheria
Rabies

Toxoids
Diphtheria
Tetanus

Viral Vaccines
Hepatitis A
Hepatitis B
Influenza virus
Measles, mumps, rubella
Poliovirus
Varicella (chickenpox)
Yellow fever

Immunosuppressive Agents					
Trade name	Generic name	Pronunciation	Trade name	Generic name	Pronunciation
Enbrel	etanercept	(e-**tan**-er-cept)	**Immunosuppressants**		
Intron A	interferon alfa-2b	(in-ter-**fear**-on **al**-fa)	Prograf, Protopic	tacrolimus	(tac-ro-**li**-mus)
Iressa	gefitinib	(gee-**fi**-ti-nib)	Ridaura	auranofin	(au-**rane**-eh-fin)
Kineret	anakinra	(an-na-**kin**-rah)	Sandimmune	cyclosporine	(sye-kloe-**spoor**-en)
Remicade	infliximab	(in-**flix**-i-mab)			
Tarceva	erlotinib	(er-**low**-ti-nib)			

HUMAN BEINGS HAVE ALWAYS BEEN plagued by bacterial and viral microbes that have caused disease and even death. In addition to outside invaders, the body may need to deal with cancer cells or a misdirected attack from the immune system (autoimmune disease). Fortunately, highly organized defense mechanisms work specifically on eliminating unwanted entities.

Several factors contribute to the overall wellness of a person. The development of vaccines to prevent infections has contributed directly to the current longevity of human beings. However, specific regions of the earth, such as Third World countries, still face a higher risk of contracting bacterial and viral infections.

This chapter describes the major functions of the immune system and then focuses on the various types of bacteria and viruses that can affect the body. This chapter also explains the timetable for immunizations. In addition, the immunological malfunctions of the body and the agents given to treat them are discussed.

Lymphatic System

The body has a built-in defense mechanism that helps protect it from invading organisms. From birth, one of the most important functions of the body is to defend against invasion. The lymphatic system is a primary source of immune cell production and commonly is referred to as the immune system. The lymph nodes produce our natural arsenal of weapons. The many lymph nodes serve the body by destroying bacteria and cancer cells, using various methods to stop them from entering the bloodstream. Although many lymphoid tissues and small vessels are located throughout the body, a few main production centers are responsible for much of the immune arsenal. The thymus, tonsils, and spleen are larger organs of the lymphatic system, each having specific functions.

THYMUS

The thymus is an important organ located in the upper chest and in the middle of the neck region as shown in Figure 27-1. The primary function of the thymus is to produce lymphocytes, which ultimately circulate through lymph nodes and lymphatic tissues and help provide immunity. The thymus begins producing these lymphocytes before birth, and the organ is much larger in childhood than in adulthood.

TONSILS

Other important lymphoid tissues are the tonsils and the adenoids, located in the throat and nose, respectively. The tonsils help fight off infection by filtering bacteria and other infective material.

SPLEEN

The spleen is located in the left side of the upper abdomen (Figure 27-1). The spleen is also the largest lymphatic organ in the body. The function of the spleen is to filter large amounts of blood cells as they reach the end of their life cycle. Macrophages within the spleen help in the removal of cellular debris. The result is the destruction of old blood cells, bacteria, and any foreign bodies.

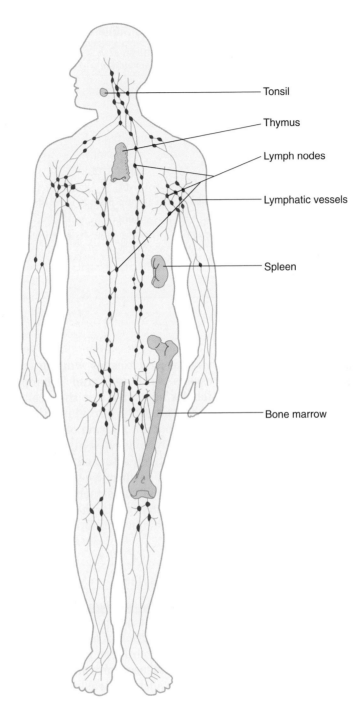

FIGURE 27-1 Overview of the major lymphatic organs within the body.

TYPES OF IMMUNE CELLS

The many nodes and tissues located throughout the body produce some of the fighting cells of the immune system. When first contact is made with a foreign body (antigen), antibodies are formed. Then, certain immune system cells remember that specific antigen until the next time contact is made and more antibodies can be formed quickly. The body, having built up its arsenal, has the necessary forces then to fight off that antigen invader.

Lymphocytes make up a major portion of the fighting cells of the body. They patrol the body, circulating through the bloodstream. Many lymphocytes reside

TABLE 27-1 Major Immune Response Cells

Major cell types	Origin of production	Location in body	Function
T lymphocytes	Lymph nodes	Lymph nodes	Produce more T lymphocytes that are sensitized to specific antigens
B lymphocytes	Bone marrow (prenatal, produced in liver)	Lymph nodes	Produce specific antibodies
Plasma cells	Lymph from B cells	Bloodstream	Antibodies
Memory cells	Lymph from B cells	Lymph nodes	Create a memory antibody
T cells	Thymus gland	Bloodstream, lymph nodes	Bind to a specific antigen

in lymph nodes and tissues waiting to attack foreign bodies. The two types of lymphocytes are B cells and T lymphocytes. B cells are smaller cells that have antibodies imbedded into their cell walls. They mainly reside in the lymph nodes and can multiply into many thousands of the same type of cells. When activated, they become plasma cells that initiate an antibody response to invading antigens. T lymphocytes also are located in the lymph nodes and remain there until an antigen attaches to their surface protein at specific receptor sites. These T cells then perform a cell-mediated immune response. This response can be a direct killing of the attached cell and antigen, or the T cells can release a chemical signal that calls in macrophages that destroy the invading cells. Table 27-1 lists major immune cells along with their location and primary function.

Immunizations

For diseases such as whooping cough, tetanus, and polio, a weakened form of the agent (which acts as an antigen in the body) is given as an immunization to stimulate the production of antibodies, which protect the body from the disease. It is important that children receive the course of vaccinations recommended by the Centers for Disease Control and Prevention because they are at risk for contracting diseases such as measles, mumps, rubella, chickenpox, whooping cough, and polio. Without the benefit of immunizations, many children may contract these childhood diseases. Historically, thousands of children have died from diseases such as measles and mumps or have been physically scarred by the effects of polio. Although children still can contract these diseases today, they are seen less commonly, and death is rare because of the widespread use of immunizations.

By immunizing children and adults, society is better protected against diseases such as chickenpox, measles, and influenza. Those persons with weakened immune systems, such as older adults, chemotherapy patients, transplant recipients, and persons with acquired immunodeficiency syndrome, are also at higher risk than most to catch and succumb to these diseases. Another high-risk group is persons from countries where immunizations are not given. In addition, many diseases can be transmitted through blood or other body fluids. Therefore, anyone sharing needles or having unprotected sex with an infected person is at risk. Unfortunately, not all conditions may be detected. Many newly infected persons do not know that they are infected or how they contracted the disease.

TYPES OF IMMUNITY

The two types of immunity are active and passive.

Active Immunity

Active natural immunity occurs when the body is exposed to a disease and actively produces antibodies to respond to the disease the next time that the body comes in contact with it.

Active acquired immunity occurs when a vaccine is administered. Vaccines are of two types: live or inactive. Live vaccines must be attenuated or weakened. With these vaccines, there is a small risk of developing a full-blown infection. However, once the body builds antibodies against the injected antigen, the body has a long-lasting immunity. For vaccines that are made from killed or inactive antigens, the risk of infection is lower. The disadvantage is that booster shots are needed to keep the antibodies at a high enough level.

Passive Immunity

Passive immunity does not require any work on the part of the body. The body receives protection from outside sources, such as by administration of immune globulin in passive acquired immunity, or from mother to child in passive natural immunity.

HOW VACCINES ARE PREPARED

Viral Vaccines

Live virus vaccines must be attenuated before they are given to patients. The virions taken are weakened or defused so that they do not cause the full-blown disease. This is achieved by treating the virions with various chemicals that destroy the interior components—the disease-causing portion of the virus. A virus, or any foreign substance that causes a disease or allergy, can be referred to as an antigen. When a vaccine is injected into the body, the immune system responds by making antibodies. Millions of antibodies overcome the small number of antigens injected in the vaccine. Table 27-2 gives examples of major types of viral vaccines.

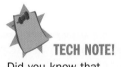

TECH NOTE!

Did you know that vaccines are always kept in the refrigerator at the pharmacy?

TABLE 27-2 Common Viral Vaccines, Diseases Treated, and Route of Administration

Vaccine agents	Disease treated	Route of administration
Havrix	Hepatitis A	Intramuscular (IM)
Recombivax HB	Hepatitis B	IM
Fluzone	Influenza	IM
MMR II	Measles, mumps, and rubella	Subcutaneous (SC)
Attenuvax	Measles	SC
Mumpsvax	Mumps	SC
Meruvax II	Rubella	SC
Orimune	Polio	IM/SC
Varivax	Chickenpox	SC
YF-Vax	Yellow fever	SC

TABLE 27-3 Common Toxoids and Route of Administration

Toxoid agents	Disease treated	Route of administration
Tetanus toxoid	Tetanus	Subcutaneous Intramuscular
Diphtheria and tetanus	Diphtheria, tetanus	Intramuscular
DPT	Diphtheria, pertussis, tetanus	Intramuscular

For those vaccines that need to be given in a series or as boosters, the outer shell of the virus is used as an antigen. Because the capsule or outer shell of the antigen may not invoke the response needed for the body to fight off further attacks, boosters must be given to remind the body and build up antibodies within the immune system. Some bacterial antigens, such as those from cholera and typhoid, may require boosters.

Bacterial Vaccines

Toxoids. Some vaccines are referred to as toxoids. These are inactivated bacterial toxins. Although the bacterial cell has been altered so that it cannot cause disease, it still can induce an antibody response within the body. Table 27-3 lists major toxoids.

Many persons believe that after they are 18 years old, they never need immunizations again. However, there are vaccines, such as the tetanus vaccine, that also should be given to adults. Although tetanus immunizations are given to children combined with diphtheria and pertussis, tetanus immunizations should be given every 10 years throughout one's life. Tetanus is a disease caused by a bacterium that can be contracted through scrapes and cuts from dirty objects.

Miscellaneous Vaccines. Although the two most common vaccines are inactivated (killed) or attenuated (weakened), there are other less common types of vaccines available, as shown in Box 27-1. These vaccines are slightly different in their composition from the usual types.

Unfortunately, the only two types of vaccines that are available are those that protect against viruses and bacterial microbes. Immunizations for other diseases such as malaria (caused by a parasite) and fungal infections have not been developed.

DEVELOPMENT OF VACCINES

To develop a vaccine, researchers must collect a large number of contagious cells. Most vaccine development has come about through the use of laboratory animals. For instance, the rabies vaccine was first grown in the nervous systems of rabbits. Most vaccines, however, were created to protect against bacterial microbes or those viruses that could be grown in or on animal tissue. In the beginning of vaccine research, this was difficult to accomplish if the diseases only occurred in human beings. Since then, scientists have discovered how to retrieve culture cells from human beings. This paved the way for the development of vaccines against polio, mumps, and measles.

Currently, research is being done on a vaccine for the human immunodeficiency virus, the virus that causes acquired immunodeficiency syndrome. Although the viral particles can be grown in monkey tissue, monkeys do not develop the disease. Even if researchers succeed in developing a vaccine, there is a danger with vaccine administration. If even a few virions are not killed

TABLE 27-4 Childhood Immunization Schedule

Vaccine	1 month	2 months	4 months	6 months	12 months	15 months	1½ years	2 years	4-6 years	11-12 years	13-18 years
Hepatitis B	X	X	X	X	X	X	X				
DPT		X	X	X		X	X		X		
HiB		X	X	X	X	X					
Polio		X	X	X	X	X	X		X		
MMR					X	X			X	X	X
Varicella					X	X	X	X	X	X	X

DPT, Diphtheria, pertussis, tetanus; *HiB, Haemophilus influenzae; MMR,* measles, mumps, rubella.

BOX 27-1 THREE TYPES OF LESS COMMON VACCINES AND THEIR SPECIFIC CHARACTERISTICS

Antiidiotypic Vaccines

A newer type of vaccine based on using an antibody that is shaped like the antigen. When the antibody is administered to a person, the body will react as though it were the antigen. The immune system will create antibodies to fight off the disease. In effect, the body is making an antibody against the injected antibody. This second antibody then can be injected to act as the vaccine and will create a third antibody. In the future, this method may make it possible to kill deadly viruses such as human immunodeficiency virus.

Subunit Vaccines

Subunit vaccines are small pieces of the genetic code that come from the disease microbe. These pieces are injected into a bacterium or yeast and are grown. They then are harvested and used as a vaccine to stimulate the body to produce an immune response. Because there are only pieces of the original virion or antigen, they do not carry the coverage of immunity that a complete antigen would. Hepatitis B is a subunit vaccine that is grown in yeast cells and then is given as a vaccine.

Acellular and Conjugated Vaccines

When a vaccine is disassembled or fragmented to isolate specific antigens from entire cells, it is referred to as an acellular vaccine. Pertussis is one type of vaccine made in this manner. Bacterial cells that have been altered and mixed with toxoids to increase their overall effectiveness are called conjugated vaccines. Such is the case with tetanus or diphtheria.

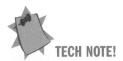

TECH NOTE!

Many hospitals require proof of childhood immunizations before hiring technicians. Keeping your records available for proof will help you avoid having to get a blood test to check for previous immunizations.

before being used in a vaccine (i.e., the vaccine contains live virus particles), an epidemic could spread across the country. This scenario occurred in the 1950s when the first polio vaccine was produced and given to millions of persons. A few batches containing live viruses were injected accidentally into well persons who then contracted polio.

CHILDHOOD IMMUNIZATION

Because children are at a high risk for catching many airborne diseases, a series of immunizations has been recommended. In the United States, children cannot register for school unless they have proof of their immunizations. Table 27-4 gives a recommended schedule for immunizations for children through 18 years of age.

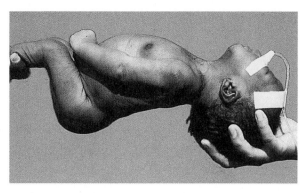

FIGURE 27-2 Tetanus. Caused by a bacillus toxin that causes a wide range of symptoms, which may include tonic spasms as shown.

Hepatitis Vaccine

Hepatitis B can cause many serious side effects including diarrhea, vomiting, jaundice, and lack of energy. Infection can lead to liver damage or even death if left untreated. This virus is contagious via blood and body fluids. Hepatitis B can be contracted through having unprotected sex, sharing syringes, or being stuck with an infected needle. The virus also can be transferred from the mother to the newborn at birth. The vaccine for hepatitis B is given in a series of three to four doses depending on age at the initial dose. Newborns receive their first immunization soon after birth. The second dose is given about 1 month after the first. The third is given at 4 months, followed by the last dose when the child is approximately 6 months old.

Side Effects. Usual side effects of the hepatitis B vaccine include soreness at the injection site and sometimes a slight fever.

Diphtheria, Pertussis, and Tetanus Vaccine

Diphtheria is a disease that causes breathing problems resulting from thick mucus covering the back of the throat.

Pertussis is also known as whooping cough because of the traumatic coughing spasms it can cause. Coughing can be so severe that it is hard to eat, drink, or even breathe. Pertussis may lead to pneumonia and possibly death.

Tetanus is known commonly as lockjaw because the victim's jaw locks in place; the person cannot eat or swallow food. Tetanus also causes painful muscle spasms all over the body (Figure 27-2).

Vaccines for diphtheria, pertussis, and tetanus can be given together in five separate doses. These doses are spread out over several years. The doses are given at 2 months of age, at 4 months, 6 months, 15 to 18 months, and at 4 to 6 years.

Side Effects. Side effects include fever and soreness at the injection site. Children older than the age of 7 years should not receive the combination diphtheria, pertussis, and tetanus; they should receive the diphtheria and tetanus vaccine. Pertussis vaccine is given only to those younger than the age of 7 because pertussis is not seen in children after age 7.

Haemophilus influenzae Type B Vaccine

The *Haemophilus influenzae* type B vaccine is given to prevent the bacterial infection *Haemophilus influenzae* type B. Children younger than 5 years can contract this bacterial infection from other children or adults. The symptoms can be mild if the infection remains in the nose or throat. However, the infection may spread into the lungs. Pneumonia, meningitis, brain damage, and entire body infections known as systemic infections can occur, and death can result. A series of four shots is given to children at 2, 4, and 6 months and between 12 to 15 months of age.

Side Effects. Common side effects include redness and swelling at the injection site and sometimes a fever.

Influenza Vaccines

Flu vaccines are popular because of their effectiveness to protect various groups of persons who are at higher risk of becoming ill with influenza. The common months of transmittance of influenza are between October and April each year. Persons should get their immunization in the month of October or November for best coverage. In 2003 the Food and Drug Administration approved a new intranasal spray vaccine. This vaccine is an attenuated live virus called FluMist. This vaccine allows the virus to grow in the temperature of the nasal mucosa but not the warmer temperature of the body. Side effects such as runny nose, nasal congestion, headache, sore throat, chills, and cough may occur.

The intranasal live influenza vaccine can be used only on healthy children over 5 years and adults up to age 49 years. Others who should not receive the live vaccine are those who are immunosuppressed, pregnant women, and those with a chronic condition such as asthma, diabetes, or cardiovascular disorders. In addition to these individuals, the nasal spray vaccine should be avoided in health care workers and other persons who may come into contact with immuno-compromised individuals.

Another type of influenza vaccine is the inactivated products Fluvin and Fluzone, which can be given intramuscularly. Side effects found with this vaccine are soreness at the injection site, fever, myalgia, and malaise.

The intramuscular inactivated influenza vaccine Fluzone can be given to children 6 to 23 months of age. The vaccine is also safe for ages from 2 years to those up to 49 years of age. Other persons who can receive this injectable vaccine safely include health care workers, caregivers, nursing mothers, and pregnant women after the first trimester. Neither type of influenza vaccine can be given to children less than 6 months old or those with a history of egg allergy.

According to the Centers for Disease Control and Prevention, the only influenza vaccine that can be given to persons 50 years or older is the killed trivalent influenza vaccine (TIV). This vaccine is given annually and provides between 70% and 90% protection for healthy persons 65 years or younger. The percentage decreases as persons age because of the reduction of the immune system functioning.

HPV Vaccine

Human papillomavirus is common around the world and affects both genders. There are 100 types of HPV. It is estimated that approximately 50% of sexually active persons will contract HPV at some time. The CDC reports that nearly 2.6 million persons are diagnosed yearly with HPV. The most vulnerable age category are teens up to the early twenties. This virus can cause cervical cancer and genital warts. A new vaccine has been tested for safety in individuals between the ages of 9 to 26 years. The best time to receive the vaccine is before any sexual activity occurs. The vaccine is given in three injections over a 6-month period–the second injection is given at 2 months, and the final one at 6 months. This provides protection against four types of HPV, which are responsible for 70% of cervical cancer and 90% of genital warts. The only side effect is brief soreness at the injection site. The vaccine is not safe in pregnant women. Research on a vaccine for older women (over 26 years) as well as boys and men is being explored at this time.

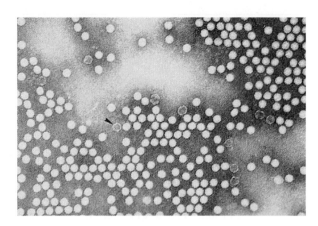

FIGURE 27-3 Poliovirus. Electron micrograph of virus, which is a ribonucleic acid. There are three forms of this viron. Immunization against one form does not provide protection against another.

Polio Vaccine

Polio was once a common disease affecting many persons in America. The main symptom of polio is paralysis of the muscles of the legs and respiratory system (Figure 27-3). Many children and adults who contracted this disease died. Some who survived had to wear leg braces to help them walk. The polio vaccine was developed in the mid-1950s and soon was given to all persons free of charge in a sugar tablet. Persons went to nearby schools where the vaccine was given to all adults and children. Because of this effective vaccine, polio was eradicated totally from the United States. Unfortunately, we still must immunize against this disease because some countries have not had the same success in eradicating the disease as the United States has.

Until recently, oral polio vaccines were an option, but an oral dose can cause polio in 1 in 2.4 million persons, so today only the injectable form is used because it has not caused any infection. Children should receive the series of four immunizations at 2 and 4 months, then between 6 and 18 months, and a booster between 4 to 6 years of age. Because all children have been given this vaccine since the mid-1950s, most adults do not need to receive it because they already are immunized.

Side Effects. Some soreness at the injection site is not uncommon.

Measles, Mumps, and Rubella Vaccine

Measles is a serious disease that begins with flulike symptoms and fever (Figure 27-4, *A*). If the symptoms are ignored, the disease can progress to a major infection, causing pneumonia, brain damage, or even death. Throughout history this disease has been responsible for thousands of deaths among children and adults alike.

Mumps is a disease that affects the parotid glands of the body (Figure 27-4, *B*). These glands become visibly enlarged, and the disease is accompanied by a fever. Mumps also may cause meningitis and deafness.

Rubella also is known as German measles (Figure 27-4, *C*). In pregnant women, this contagious disease can cause birth defects in the unborn child or even a miscarriage. For this reason, women should be given this vaccine 3 months before becoming pregnant if they have never had rubella. In children the main symptoms include rash and fever.

Immunization against measles, mumps, and rubella are given together as one vaccination. This is normally done twice; once between 12 and 15 months old and again between 4 to 6 years of age.

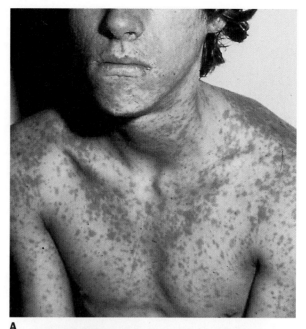

A

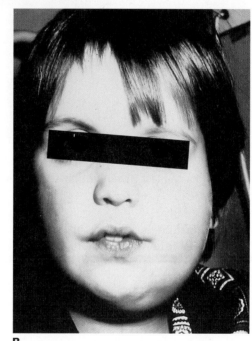

B

FIGURE 27-4 **A,** Measles. Symptoms include rash, composed of both papules and macules, which spread over the body and lasts 3 to 5 days. **B,** Mumps. Glands become swollen, causing pain when chewing or drinking liquids. Symptoms last approximately 24 hours.

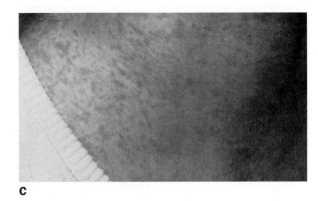

c

FIGURE 27-4, cont'd **c,** Rubella. Lymph nodes enlarge, and a fine red rash occurs. Symptoms last approximately 2 to 3 days.

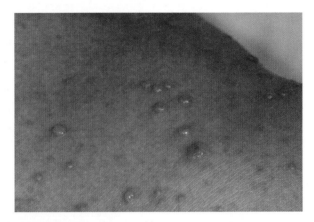

FIGURE 27-5 Chickenpox. Rash begins with macules, which turn into severe papules. Symptoms can last from a few days to 2 weeks.

Side Effects. The most common side effects include fever and rash. In some cases, allergic reactions can cause more serious problems; however, these are rare.

Chickenpox Vaccine

Varicella vaccine is known more commonly as the chickenpox vaccine (Figure 27-5). This vaccine is relatively new. Most children have contracted this disease from other children via air or by touching the fluid within the skin blisters of infected children. Although this is a contagious disease, it rarely causes death. Symptoms include skin blisters, fever, and an itchy rash. Some persons can experience more severe effects, such as brain damage, infection, or (rarely) even death.

Another disorder caused by the same virus that causes chickenpox (herpes zoster) is shingles, which may appear in adulthood in a person who had childhood chickenpox. After lying dormant for several years, the virus may become activated and cause acute inflammation of the dorsal root ganglia. Symptoms include painful lesions along the nerves. Treatment for shingles includes medications such as valacyclovir (Valtrex), which can be given orally or intravenously. Acyclovir (Zovirax) also may be used over a 7-day period to reduce pain and promote healing. In 2006 a single dose vaccine was introduced for adults over the age of 60. The vaccine prevented shingles in about half the subjects tested and can reduce the pain associated with this condition.

Side Effects. If the disease is contracted through immunization, only a mild form of disease results. After the injection there can be soreness at the injection site and mild fever.

Considerations. Although the vaccine is recommended between 12 and 18 months of age, anyone can be given this vaccine. Persons who should not get this vaccine include pregnant mothers or those who are immunocompromised.

Storage Note. This vaccine must be continuously frozen at $-15°C$ ($5°F$) or colder.

Pneumonia Vaccine

Pneumococcal conjugate vaccine is given for *Streptococcus pneumoniae,* which causes meningitis. This is a serious disease that still affects children, causing pneumonia, brain damage, and death. Children younger than the age of 5 years are at the highest risk for this bacterial infection. The vaccine results in immunity for 3 years, and it is given in three doses spaced at 2, 4, and 6 months and then between 12 and 15 months of age. Older children who might be at high risk of infection also can be given the vaccine. The total number of doses may vary. Older children and adults can be given another type of vaccine to protect them from meningitis and pneumonia. This vaccine is called pneumococcal polysaccharide.

Side Effects. Side effects include redness or tenderness at the injection site, and some children have a slight fever. In rare cases, all vaccines may cause an allergic reaction. Therefore, it is important to watch for any severe reactions after the vaccine is given.

National Childhood Vaccine Injury Act of 1986

In 1986 the U.S. Congress passed the National Childhood Vaccine Injury Act. This act provided a National Vaccine Injury Compensation Program for those persons who may have been injured after receiving a routine vaccine. These vaccines include measles, mumps, rubella or a combination thereof and tetanus toxoid, pertussis, polio, influenza, varicella, rotavirus vaccine and/or pneumococcal vaccines. Studies have shown the possibility that a low number of patients who were given vaccines had severe side effects. More information can be found on the website *www.vaccineinjury.org.*

ADULT VACCINES

If a pregnant mother should contract hepatitis, there is a high risk of transmitting the disease to the fetus. Therefore, doctors weigh the potential risk of the mother contracting the disease from the vaccine and causing damage to the fetus against the possibility of catching the disease if the vaccine is not given. Vaccines such as diphtheria and tetanus, hepatitis B, and influenza may be given to high-risk women. If a mother has not been given the rubella vaccine previously, she must wait until the child is born before receiving the vaccine because of the risk of getting a mild case of rubella, which could be harmful to the fetus.

Immune globulins are different from vaccines because they are not prepared in a laboratory, but must be obtained from a human or animal donor. γ-Globulins contain antibodies that can be passed to the recipient, giving them passive immunity. Immune globulins are given for immediate protection against a specific virus. Because the immunity is passive, the protection does not last long. Examples of common globulins are the following:

TABLE 27-5 Types of Vaccines

Vaccine	Disease or organism	Recommendation
Cholera	*Vibrio cholerae*	Persons living or traveling to endemic areas where the disease occurs; military
Plague	*Yersinia pestis*	Persons protecting against wild rodents in endemic areas; military
Yellow fever	Flavivirus	Persons living in or traveling to endemic areas; military
Anthrax	Anthrax	Military only at this time

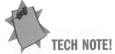

TECH NOTE!

Tuberculosis vaccine is given routinely by many countries such as the Philippines. As health care workers, pharmacy technicians get a yearly tuberculosis test to test for exposure to tuberculosis. Although there is a vaccine for tuberculosis, we do not use it in the United States. A tuberculosis vaccine does not guarantee immunity, which is why the United States does not use it. If a vaccine is given, antibodies are developed against the antigen; therefore, all tuberculosis tests would show positive results and a chest x-ray film would be necessary to rule out tuberculosis. Chapter 18 discusses the microbe that causes tuberculosis.

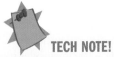

TECH NOTE!

Remember that in all cases it is far worse to contract the disease than to risk the chance of adverse reactions from a vaccine.

- Cytomegalovirus immune globulin
- γ-Globulin
- Hepatitis B immune globulin
- Tetanus immune globulin
- Varicella-zoster immune globulin

Adults primarily receive immunizations when they are planning to travel outside of the United States. The U.S. military immunizes all troops against 12 top contagions that exist across the world. On a smaller scale, persons who are traveling to foreign countries often get specific vaccines to guard against contagions. Other persons who may need a specific vaccine are scientists; researchers; or those who work in close contact with a disease, such as those caring for laboratory animals; or those who live in regions that have an epidemic outbreak. Table 27-5 lists the types of vaccines available and when they should be administered.

Antitoxins and antivenins are yet another type of passive immunity system that can give short-term immediate protection from serious symptoms. These agents contain antibodies that can neutralize dangerous toxins. For example, stepping on a rusty nail may allow the pathogen *Clostridium tetani* to enter through the wound and into the bloodstream where it may cause poisoning. The tetanus antitoxin can be given to the victim against this life-threatening condition. Antivenins are given to counteract poison from creatures such as snakes and spiders. Common antitoxins include those for diphtheria, rabies, and botulism. Common antivenins include antivenin for black widow spider (*Latrodectus mactans*) venom, and Crotalidae polyvalent for rattlesnake venom.

STORAGE OF VACCINES

The Centers for Disease Control and Prevention have guidelines on the storage of vaccines in order to preserve their effectiveness. Most vaccines should be kept at temperatures between 2° and 8°C (36° to 46°F). The cold-adaptive FluMist (an intranasal live influenza vaccine) can be frozen if kept in a specially made freeze box (32°F) issued by the manufacturer.

IMMUNE THERAPIES

Immune therapy, also known as biological therapy or biotherapy, can be used on persons with specific conditions. Depending on the type of condition affecting the patient, certain biological response modifiers (BRMs) may be able to suppress or stimulate the immune system.

The body normally produces small amounts of BRMs that respond to infections and/or a disease. Scientists have been able to produce BRMs in large amounts in the laboratory. These then can be used in the treatment, for example, of cancer, rheumatoid arthritis, and Crohn's disease.

TABLE 27-6 Immune Therapies

Generic name	Trade name	Indication
Immunostimulants		
Etanercept	Enbrel	Crohn's disease
Interferon alfa-2b	Intron A	Hairy cell leukemia, hepatitis, Kaposi's sarcoma related to acquired immunodeficiency syndrome
Anakinra	Kineret	Rheumatoid arthritis
Infliximab	Remicade	Crohn's disease, rheumatoid arthritis
Erlotinib	Tarceva	Metastatic non–small cell lung cancer
Gefitinib	Iressa	Head and neck cancers, non–small cell lung cancer
Immunosuppressives		
Cyclosporine	Sandimmune	Transplant rejections, rheumatoid arthritis, severe psoriasis
Tacrolimus	Prograf, Protopic	Organ rejections, severe plaque-type psoriasis, atopic dermatitis (ointment)
Auranofin	Ridaura	Rheumatoid arthritis, psoriatic arthritis

TECH ALERT!

Remember these soundalike/look-alike drugs:

Cyclosporine versus cycloserine or cyclophosphamide
Interleukin-2 versus interferon-2
Erlotinib versus gefitinib
Ridaura versus Cardura
Protopic versus Protonix, Protopam, or Protropin

This type of therapy is not without side effects such as loss of appetite, nausea, vomiting, and diarrhea. Other effects include fever, chills, and muscle aches. If side effects are severe enough, the patient may be admitted into the hospital for the course of the treatment. The good news is that these side effects usually last only for the duration of the treatment.

Table 27-6 gives a brief list of the two types of BRM medications used, along with their indications.

DO YOU REMEMBER THESE KEY POINTS?

- The various types of immunity
- How vaccines work
- The common childhood diseases
- Which diseases each immunization covers
- The major types of adult immunizations that are given and why
- Where most vaccines are kept in the pharmacy

MULTIPLE CHOICE QUESTIONS

1. The most common side effects from vaccinations are _____.
   A. Fever
   B. Soreness at the injection site
   C. Vomiting
   D. Both A and B

2. The vaccine given to protect against *Streptococcus pneumoniae* is _____.
   A. *Haemophilus Influenzae* type B vaccine
   B. Varicella-zoster
   C. Pneumococcal conjugate vaccine
   D. None of the above

3. Shingles is related to the childhood disease _____.
   A. Measles
   B. Mumps
   C. Rubella
   D. Chickenpox

4. Vaccines can protect human beings against all of the following organisms except _____.
   A. Viruses
   B. Fungus
   C. Bacteria
   D. All of the above

5. The two basic types of immunity are _____.
   A. Bacterial and viral
   B. Live and inactive
   C. Active and inactive
   D. Active and passive

6. Vaccines can be altered by which of the following ways?
   A. Attenuated or weakened
   B. Inactivated or killed
   C. Attenuated or activated
   D. A and B

7. When the body comes into contact with a contagious disease, it causes _____.
   A. Antibodies to be produced
   B. Antigens to be produced
   C. A body rash
   D. No reaction

8. Which of the statements is true concerning toxoids?
   A. Toxoids are bacterial toxins that have been inactivated
   B. All bacterial vaccines are toxoids
   C. Both A and B
   D. None of the above

9. Vaccines that are composed of small pieces of genetic code harvested from bacterium or yeast are _____.
   A. Acellular vaccines
   B. Conjugated vaccines
   C. Subunit vaccines
   D. Toxoid vaccines

10. Most adults need vaccines for all of these reasons, except _____.
   A. They never got them as children.
   B. They are in the military.
   C. They are health care workers.
   D. Adults need vaccines for all of the above.

TRUE/FALSE — If the statement is false, then change it to make it true.

_____ **1.** The thymus helps provide immunity.

_____ **2.** Most vaccinations have no side effects.

_____ **3.** Hospital technicians must have an annual tuberculosis test.

_____ **4.** Polio vaccine is given routinely in an oral form rather than by injection.

_____ **5.** Hepatitis B is a serious condition affecting the kidneys.

_____ **6.** Pertussis vaccine normally is combined with diphtheria and tetanus vaccines.

_____ **7.** Attenuated vaccines often can give protection for a lifetime.

_____ **8.** Tetanus vaccine should be given every 5 years.

_____ **9.** When vaccines are injected, antibodies are produced by the body to fight off antigens injected.

_____ **10.** Many Third World countries do not immunize children.

TECHNICIAN'S CORNER Visit the website of the Centers for Disease Control and Prevention at *www.cdc.gov*, and print out the most recent list of suggested immunizations for children.

BIBLIOGRAPHY

Centers for Disease Control and Prevention: www.cdc.gov

Gardner P, Pabbatireddy S: Vaccines for Women Age 50 and Older. Emerging Infectious Diseases 10(11). Retrieved 11/05, from www.cdc.ogv/nicdod/EID/wol10no11/04-0469.htm.

McKenry LM, Salerno E: *Mosby's pharmacology in nursing,* ed 22, St Louis, 2005, Mosby.

Nathan JP, Rosenberg JM: Who should get the flu vaccine and who shouldn't? *Drug Topics* 147:28, 2003.

National Immunization Program. HPV Vaccine. 8/02/06. Retrieved 11/06 from www.cdc.gov/nip/vaccine/hpv/hpv-facts.htm.

Tortora GJ, Funke BR, Case CL: *Microbiology: an introduction,* ed 8, Redwood City, Calif, 2003, Benjamin Cummings.

WEBSITES

www.ncbi.nlm.nih.gov
www.vaccineinjury.org
www.webmd.com

CHAPTER 28

Oncology Agents

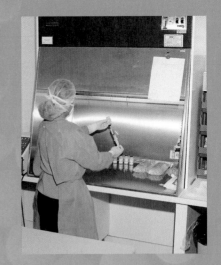

Objectives

UPON COMPLETING THIS CHAPTER, YOU SHOULD BE ABLE TO
DO THE FOLLOWING:

- List both trade and generic drug names covered in this chapter.
- List common types of cancer.
- List four causes of cancer.
- Describe how cancer spreads.
- Describe the methods used to diagnose cancer.
- Explain the method of action for the classification of drugs listed in this chapter.
- Define oncology terms.
- Describe the stages of normal cell reproduction.
- List the types of agents that are vesicants and the precautions technicians need to take when preparing them.
- Describe the most common side effects of chemotherapy.
- List the treatments used in fighting cancer.
- Differentiate between acute lymphocytic and myelogenous leukemia.
- Describe how nuclear medicine is used in oncology.

Antineoplastic *An agent used to prevent the development, proliferation, or growth of neoplastic cells; a medication used in treatment of abnormal cells*

Benign *A nonmalignant neoplasm*

Biopsy *A procedure in which a piece of tissue is removed from a patient for examination and diagnosis; the tissue is a sample of the whole*

Bolus *A single dose of drug*

Cancer *A general term used to describe malignant neoplasms*

Carcinogen *A substance or chemical that can increase the risk of developing cancer*

Chemotherapy *The treatment of a disease with toxic chemical substances to slow the disease process or to kill cells*

Deoxyribonucleic acid (DNA) *The complex nucleic acids that are bases for genetic continuance*

Invasive *The tendency for a tumor or mass to move into tissues and/or organs in proximity*

Leukemia *A progressive disease marked by malignancy of the blood-forming cells found in the hemopoietic tissues, organs, and bloodstream, causing the circulation of abnormal blood cells*

Lymphoma *A term used to describe a malignant disorder of lymphoid tissue*

Malignant *An invasive and destructive pattern of rapid, abnormal cell growth; often fatal*

Melanoma *A malignant neoplasm of the pigmented cells of skin; it may metastasize to other organs*

Metastasis *The movement or spread of cancerous cells through the body to organs in distant areas*

Mitosis *Cellular reproduction that creates two identical daughter cells from the DNA of the parent cell*

Mutation *An unexpected change in the molecular structure within the DNA, causing a permanant change in cells*

Neoplasm *An abnormal tissue growth*

Oncogene *A previously normal gene that may be affected adversely by an infection such as a retrovirus, which causes a mutation and may produce cancer*

PCA *Patient-controlled analgesia*

Remission *The span of time during which a disease, such as cancer, is not spreading; this may be permanent or temporary*

Sarcoma *A malignant neoplastic growth arising from the connective tissue*

CHEMOTHERAPEUTIC AGENTS

Trade Name	Generic Name	Pronunciation	Trade Name	Generic Name	Pronunciation
Adriamycin	doxorubicin	(dox-oh-**ru**-bi-sin)	Matulane	procarbazine	(proe-**kar**-ba-zeen)
Adrucil	fluorouracil	(flure-oh-**your**-a-sil)	Methotrex	methotrexate	(meth-oh-**trex**-ate)
Alkeran	melphalan	(**mel**-fa-lan)	Mithracin	plicamycin	(plick-a-**my**-sin)
BiCNU	carmustine	(kar-**mus**-teen)	Mustargen	mechlorethamine	(me-klor-**eth**-ah-meen)
Blenoxane	bleomycin	(blee-oh-**my**-sin)	Mutamycin	mitomycin	(mye-toe-**my**-sin)
CCNU	lomustine	(low-**mus**-ten)	Myleran	busulfan	(byoo-**sul**-fan)
Cerubidine	daunorubicin	(daw-**now**-roo-bi-sin)	Navelbine	vinorelbine	(vin-**nor**-ell-been)
Cosmegen	dactinomycin	(dak-tin-oh-**my**-sin)	Nipent	pentostatin	(pen-toe-**sta**-tin)
Cytosar-U	cytarabine	(sye-**tare**-ah-been)	Novantrone	mitoxantrone	(mi-to-**zan**-trone)
Cytoxan	cyclophosphamide	(sye-kloe-**fos**-fa-mide)	Oncovin	vincristine	(vin-**kris**-teen)
DTIC-Dome	dacarbazine	(da-kar-ba-zeen)	Paraplatin	carboplatin	(**car**-bow-pla-tin)
Fludara	fludarabine	(flew-**dare**-ah-been)	Platinol	cisplatin	(**sis**-pla-tin)
FUDR	floxuridine	(flox-**yoor**-eye-deen)	Purinethol	mercaptopurine	(mer-kap-toe-**pur**-een)
Gemzar	gemcitabine	(gem-**sit**-ah-been)	Taxol	paclitaxel	(pack-li-**tax**-el)
Hycamtin	topotecan	(toe-po-**tee**-can)	Taxotere	docetaxel	(doc-e-**tax**-el)
Hydrea	hydroxyurea	(high-drok-see-you-**re**-ah)	Tabloid	thioguanine	(thye-oh-**gwah**-neen)
Idamycin	idarubicin	(eye-da-**roo**-bi-sin)	Velban	vinblastine	(vin-**blas**-teen)
Ifex	ifosfamide	(i-**fos**-fa-myde)	VePesid	etoposide	(e-teh-**poh**-side)
Iressa	gefitinib	(gee-**fi**-ti-nib)	Vumon	teniposide	(ten-nye-**poe**-side)
Leukeran	chlorambucil	(klor-**am**-byoo-sil)	Zanosar	streptozocin	(strep-toe-**zoe**-sin)

PAIN AGENTS

Trade Name	Generic Name	Pronunciation	Trade Name	Generic Name	Pronunciation
Codeine	codeine	(**koe**-deen)	OxyContin	oxycodone	(ox-e-**koe**-done)
Demerol	meperidine	(me-**pear**-eye-deen)	Percocet	oxycodone/ acetaminophen	(ox-e-**koe**-done/a-sea-tah-**men**-oh-phen)
Dilaudid	hydromorphone	(hye-droe-**mor**-fone)			
Duragesic	fentanyl	(**phen**-tah-nill)	Percodan	oxycodone/aspirin	(ox-e-**koe**-done/**ass**-peh-rin)
Duramorph	morphine sulfate	(**mor**-feen **sul**-fate)	Vicodin	hydrocodone/ acetaminophen	(hye-droe-**koe**-done/a-sea-tah-**men**-oh-phen)
Hycodan	hydrocodone	(hye-droe-**koe**-done)			
Lorcet	hydrocodone/ acetaminophen	(hye-droe-**koe**-done/a-sea-tah-**men**-oh-phen)	Vicoprofen	hydrocodone/ ibuprofen	(hye-droe-**koe**-done/eye-bu-**pro**-fen)

NOT LONG AGO, THE DIAGNOSIS OF cancer meant certain death. The lack of knowledge pertaining to this life-changing disease led most persons to feel hopelessness. As the scientific community began to attain more knowledge about the causes of cancer (etiology is the study of causes of disease), its early diagnosis, and various treatments, the diagnosis of cancer resulted in less invasive changes in everyday life. Today, the chances of getting cancer can be decreased, and many cancers can be cured. Because of early detection and more advanced treatments, more persons are cancer survivors today than ever before.

This chapter covers the process by which cancer arises, how it metastasizes, and the medications used to treat some of the most common cancers. Many different types of cancer can strike different areas of the body. The incidence of some cancers, such as skin cancer, may be decreased. The chances of acquiring skin cancer increase the longer the skin is exposed to direct sunlight. If precautionary measures are taken, such as wearing sunscreen, the chances of skin cancer may decrease. Unfortunately, the prevention of cancer is not an exact science.

One of the frustrating aspects of headline news stories regarding cancer is the continuous inference that every conceivable food product or eating habit may lead to cancer. In reality, everything in life should be done in moderation. Even then, there is the genetic factor that none of us can alter. Although much research and testing are being done by geneticists to alter genes, it is not a treatment for cancer at this time. In the meantime, the most effective way to fight cancer is to lessen the risk by treating the body in a responsible manner and by making routine visits to the doctor.

In this chapter we define cancer and its nature and introduce some of the more common medications used in its treatment. Common side effects from antineoplastics also are covered. Much of the information pertaining to the preparation of chemotherapeutic agents is in Chapter 13.

What Is Cancer?

Under normal circumstances, cells within the body proliferate, especially in the intestinal epithelium and within the bone marrow. Our body constantly replicates cells to replace old cells or damaged cells or to increase the cell population. The normal cycle of life for cells is required if the body is to remain in homeostasis. Cells normally follow a set of steps. An important step, in addition to replication of new cells, is their eventual death. If the cell controls malfunction and the cells grow much faster than normal and do not stop proliferating, tumors may form. Benign tumors are noncancerous and may include moles, warts, and other lesions. Melanomas and other cancers continuously produce cells that can metastasize and colonize at new sites within the body. However, malignant or cancerous tumors also can begin as moles, warts, or lesions. Only proper diagnosis can determine the nature of the growth.

Four main types of cancer are based on their location and on four possible outcomes, as covered in Box 28-1. The outcome of cancer treatments is determined by early diagnosis, type of treatment, genetics, and finally the attitude of the patient.

BOX 28-1 TYPES OF CANCER AND THEIR POSSIBLE OUTCOMES

Types of Cancer

Carcinomas	These originate in the epithelial tissues of organs such as the lungs and intestines.
Leukemias	These originate in the bone marrow and the spleen. These are areas that produce a large number of blood cells. Leukemia often strikes children.
Lymphoma	This general term is used for malignant tumors within the lymphatic tissues.
Sarcomas	This term is used to describe cancers of the muscle and bone. They stem from the connective tissue within these areas.

Possible Outcomes of Tumor Growth

A possibility exists that the growth of benign cells will be limited to a specific location and may cause no problems for the individual.

The benign cell growth may get large enough to affect the normal functioning of an organ or tissue.

Cancerous cells may break off and travel to other parts of the body, where they grow in an uncontrolled manner.

Cancerous cells may become invasive, moving into adjoining tissue and/or organs and becoming life-threatening.

What Causes Cancer?

The three different causes of cancer (in addition to genetics) are environmental contaminants, radiation, and viruses. Many different environmental contaminants, known as carcinogens, can cause cancer. For example, cigarette smoking may cause cancer because of the many additives contained in tobacco that have been isolated, tested, and proved to cause cancer in laboratory animals. Another causative agent of cancer is radiation. Any type of radiation that breaks the bonds of the deoxyribonucleic acid (DNA) can lead to mutations in the DNA that can result in cancer. For example, radiation in the form of the sun rays or x-rays may lead to mutations if the body is exposed long enough. Other types of cancer-causing agents include radioactive materials, coal, soot, and certain dyes. Viruses also can cause certain types of cancers. Viruses replicate by using their host's components. The host is the person who has contracted the virus. The virus inserts itself into human DNA and creates proteins from the host's DNA to build new virions. The normal genes are affected by the virus, and the newly mutated genes are referred to as oncogenes. Oncogenes are small bits of genes that are normally present in cells but are not dangerous unless they are not "turned off" through normal reactions. Another possible cause of cancer under investigation is genetics. Although no clear evidence indicates for certain that cancer-causing genes are inherited, this possible cause remains a theory.

Diagnosis of Cancer

Although cancer can strike any area of the body, this chapter covers the most common types of cancers and their progression. Through the use of x-ray examinations, magnetic resonance imaging, sonograms, biopsies, and radiopharmaceuticals, many cancers can be identified and treated. A pathologist determines the level or grade of the tumor based on its appearance when observed under a microscope. As the diagnosis is being made, several aspects of the cancer must be considered, such as the morphology, growth pattern, karyotype, and response to chemotherapy agents. Box 28-2 gives an explanation of each consideration.

BOX 28-2 CHARACTERISTICS OF CANCER GROWTH AND TREATMENT

Morphology: The morphology of a cell or organism is its shape characteristics. Most cancerous cells have rigid edges or edges that are not smooth, unlike noncancerous cells that tend to be smooth and round. Cells also can form large masses or may remain as small cells. Normal cells tend to have an appearance of flattened cells, whereas cancer cells tend to be more round.

Growth pattern: Cell types have different characteristics. Whether they grow quickly or slowly and how fast they travel to different parts of the body are some of the patterns that identify types of cancer. When cancer cells are grown in a culture dish, they tend to form multiple layers because they do not follow the same growth pattern as normal cells. Normal cells form a single layer.

Karyotype: The actual mutation that a cancer cell has is contained in the karyotype (see Figure 28-1). Within the DNA of the cell is the mutation or cancer gene that initiates uncontrollable growth. Included in the DNA are also various components that can help speed up the growth. Normal cells have the capability to divide between 20 to 60 times before they are too old to continue; however, cancer cells have been observed to divide thousands of times, furthering their out-of-control nature. This rate of reproduction may decrease the effectiveness of the medication or treatment given to kill the cancer cells.

Response to therapy: Because different cancers have different morphologies, growth patterns, and karyotype, they may or may not be responsive to treatment. Many times, multiple agents are used to treat the growth of cancer cells.

Ordinarily, if a cancer is diagnosed in the early stages, it may be removed surgically. If there is no recurrence within 5 years, the cancer normally is considered cured. With new advancements in the treatment of cancers, some cancers can be cured even if they are discovered in later stages. For example, many leukemias are curable—especially in children. Other cancers such as skin melanomas are being detected in the early stages because of new types of diagnosis and early detection. This can be attributed to public education. For example, breast cancer and prostate cancer are cured more often because persons are having checkups that detect cancerous masses in time.

Types of Cancer

More than 100 known cancers affect the human body. The following cancers have multiple agents that can be used to treat them. They are a sample of the types of diseases that can strike most age groups.

Hodgkin's lymphoma, or Hodgkin's disease, is a cancer of the lymphatic cells that are located in the lymph nodes. This disease was named after Thomas Hodgkin, who was the doctor who first described its features.

Non-Hodgkin's lymphoma is not Hodgkin's disease but is named after Hodgkin because it also affects the lymphatic system. This cancer may have a nodular or diffuse pattern that spreads; non-Hodgkin's lymphoma may have a low, moderate, or high rate of malignancy. Its morphology is different from that of Hodgkin's disease.

Kaposi sarcoma is a type of cancer that affects the skin and is marked by brownish-purplish skin lesions that can spread to internal organs. Persons who are most likely to acquire this type of cancer are those who suffer from acquired immunodeficiency syndrome. Because the immune system is compromised, the body is more susceptible to a variety of diseases.

Leukemia arises in the bone marrow and lymphatic system. A malfunctioning bone marrow produces abnormal leukocytes (white blood cells [WBCs]). These leukocytes can crowd out normal blood cell production; the disease is often fatal. Two major groups of leukemias are lymphocytic leukemia and myelogenous leukemia. Each group is subdivided into many different types of cancer:

- Acute lymphocytic leukemia: The cure rate of this type of leukemia is more than 90%. This type of leukemia usually affects children, although adults also can get it. Approximately 75% of those with the disease will go into remission.
- Acute myelogenous leukemia: This type of leukemia is the most common among adults, with 10% to 20% of those affected being children. The increase of WBCs, in addition to a decreased production of red blood cells, makes the body more susceptible to infection. In fact, the cause of death is usually an invading microorganism rather than the disease itself. The disease progresses rapidly, and a person can succumb to it in less than 6 months.

Most treatments for cancer include more than one agent and also may be followed by or preceded by radiation therapy.

Treatments for Cancer

The four standard types of treatments used to treat cancer are surgery, radiation therapy, implanted radioactive isotopes, and chemotherapy. Nuclear medicine is another advancing treatment that is discussed later in the chapter. New advancements in each type of treatment have lessened the risk of recurrence and side effects. Age is an important factor that must be considered in patients who have been diagnosed with cancer. The risk of cancer increases in individuals older than 65 years. Age can make treatment difficult because older adults

TABLE 28-1 Sample of Combination Therapies

Disease	Drug set	Agents
Ovarian cancer	CC	Carboplatin, cyclophosphamide
Breast cancer	CFM	Cyclophosphamide, fluorouracil, mitoxantrone
Lung cancer	CAV	Cyclophosphamide, doxorubicin, vincristine
Testicular cancer	BEP	Bleomycin, etoposide, cisplatin
Hodgkin's lymphoma (pediatric)	COMP	Cyclophosphamide, vincristine, methotrexate, prednisone
Sarcoma	DI	Doxorubicin, ifosfamide, mesna
Non-Hodgkin's lymphoma	MIV	Mitoxantrone, ifosfamide, etoposide

usually have other illnesses that can make treatment more dangerous. In children, cancer can grow quickly because they are growing rapidly. However, children tend to respond to chemotherapy and recuperate more quickly than older patients.

For many types of cancer, oncologists (doctors who specialize in the treatment of cancer) refer to a protocol (a set of guidelines) that recommends multiple agents used simultaneously to treat cancer. Table 28-1 lists examples of combination therapy.

SURGERY

Surgery, usually one of the first courses of treatments, can eliminate tumors quickly and effectively. When a mass or tissue is removed, a large area of surrounding normal tissue also is taken to ensure that all cancer cells have been removed. Although the procedure may be a success, an oncologist normally follows up with radiation or chemotherapy to ensure that all the cancerous cells are gone.

RADIATION

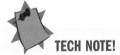

TECH NOTE!

A bone marrow transplant has a much greater chance of curing adults and children with leukemia who do not respond to traditional treatments. The bone marrow is transplanted by intravenous infusion. The new bone marrow naturally attaches to the patient's bones and alters the defective bone marrow by making healthy red blood cells and WBCs.

Radiation can be used to diagnose or treat certain diseases. For example, x-ray imaging, computed tomography scans, and radioisotope scans use electromagnetic waves to project images as the waves pass through the body. Although radiation also is known to be a carcinogen, if used correctly, it can kill cancer cells. In cancer treatment, radiation is categorized by the intensity of the rays. These are α-, β-, and γ-rays. Both α- and β-rays normally are used to treat superficial lesions, whereas γ-rays are stronger and can treat deeper lesions.

RADIOACTIVE ISOTOPES

Certain cancers may require alternative types of treatment because of their location or nature. In this case, implants can be placed directly into the cancer site. This may be effective in cancers of the tongue or the cervix. The implants may be left in from hours to a few days.

CHEMOTHERAPY

Many different types of medications are used to treat cancers. Table 28-2 lists some of these agents. Often, these agents are effective at eradicating cancer cells. The disruption caused by interfering with the normal metabolism of cancer

TABLE 28-2 Common Types of Chemotherapeutic Agents

Generic name	Trade name	Classification	Indication	Route of administration
bleomycin	Blenoxane	Antibiotic	Lymphomas, squamous cell carcinomas	IV
busulfan	Myleran	Alkylating agent	Leukemia	PO, IV
carboplatin	Paraplatin	Alkylating agent	Ovarian cancer and tumors	IV
carmustine	BiCNU	Alkylating agent	Brain tumors, Hodgkin's and non-Hodgkin's lymphomas	IV, wafer
chlorambucil	Leukeran	Alkylating agent	Leukemia, lymphomas	PO
cisplatin	Platinol	Alkylating agent	Ovarian/testicular tumor	IV
cyclophosphamide	Cytoxan	Alkylating agent	Leukemias, Hodgkin's disease, lymphomas	PO, IV
cytarabine	Cytosar-U	Antimetabolite	Myelocytic leukemias	IV
dacarbazine	DTIC-Dome	Alkylating agent	Melanoma, Hodgkin's disease	IV
dactinomycin	Cosmegen	Antibiotic	Wilms' tumor	IV
doxorubicin	Adriamycin	Antibiotic	Leukemias, tumors	IV
etoposide	VePesid	Plant extract	Lung and testicular cancer	PO, IV
fludarabine phosphate	Fludara	Antimetabolite	Leukemia	IV
fluorouracil	Adrucil	Antimetabolite	Cancer of the colon, rectum, breast, stomach, pancreas	IV
gefitinib	Iressa	Antineoplastic	Non–small cell lung cancer	PO
gemcitabine	Gemzar	Miscellaneous antineoplastic	Adenocarcinoma of the pancreas; antimetabolite	IV
hydroxyurea	Hydrea	Miscellaneous antineoplastic	Leukemia, recurrent cancer of the ovary	PO
idarubicin	Idamycin	Antibiotic	Adult leukemias	IV
ifosfamide	Ifex	Alkylating agent	Sarcoma, cancer of testes	IV
mechlorethamine	Mustargen	Alkylating agent	Hodgkin's disease, lymphomas	IV
melphalan	Alkeran	Alkylating agent	Multiple myelomas	PO, IV
methotrexate	Methotrex	Antimetabolite	Leukemia, psoriasis, rheumatoid arthritis	PO, IV
paclitaxel	Taxol	Antimitotic	Ovarian/breast cancer	PO, IV
streptozocin	Zanosar	Alkylating agent	Cancer of the pancreas	IV
teniposide	Vumon	Plant extract	Childhood leukemia	IV
topotecan	Hycamtin	Hormone	Ovarian cancer	IV
vinblastine	Velban	Antimitotic	Hodgkin's disease, tumors	IV
vincristine	Oncovin	Antimitotic	Leukemia, tumors	IV
vinorelbine	Navelbine	Antimitotic	Lung cancer	IV

IV, Intravenous; *PO,* oral.

cells causes them to die. Table 28-3 lists the different routes of administration of chemotherapeutic agents. Other agents commonly given during the treatment of cancer are those that relieve symptoms of cancer or the side effects of chemotherapeutic agents, such as the loss of hair, emesis, loss of energy, loss of weight, and pain.

TABLE 28-3 Routes of Administration of Chemotherapeutic Agents

Abbreviation	Definition	Specifics of use
Traditional		
PO	By mouth	Tablets, capsules taken orally
IM	Intramuscular	Into the muscle
IT	Intrathecal	Into a sheath
IV	Intravenous	Into the vein
Newer Routes		
Infusion pumps	Syringe pump	A portable pump worn by the patient that administers a preset amount of drug through a catheter inserted into the tumor
Implants	Tablet/capsules	Implanted into the cancerous area where the medication can be dispersed over a set time

Agents Used in the Treatment of Neoplastic Diseases

Antimetabolite Agents. The building blocks of DNA are formed by nucleic acids often referred to as bases. These bases form the fundamental configuration of DNA. The structure of antimetabolites is similar to the bases that form the DNA strands, but because they are not identical, they do not allow the process of mitosis to finish. Therefore the cells into which these substances are introduced are not able to replicate. Antimetabolites often are used to treat leukemia. The most common side effects include nausea, vomiting, fever, anorexia, bone marrow depression, and jaundice. Antimetabolites include the following:

Cytarabine
Floxuridine
Fludarabine
Fluorouracil
Mercaptopurine
Methotrexate
Thioguanine

Antibiotics. The antibiotics used to treat certain types of cancers are not in the same category as those used to treat infections. They are specific to tumors that cause cancer. These antibiotics bind directly to the DNA of the cancer cells and prevent the synthesis of any new cells. These agents are not used to treat infections because of their toxic effects. Instead, they are used to destroy newly forming cancer cells. Because they also destroy normal cells along with the cancer cells, they produce side effects that include severe emesis (vomiting), nausea, diarrhea, red urine, and a loss of hair. Agents of this type include the following:

Bleomycin
Dactinomycin
Daunorubicin
Doxorubicin
Idarubicin
Mitomycin
Mitoxantrone
Pentostatin
Plicamycin

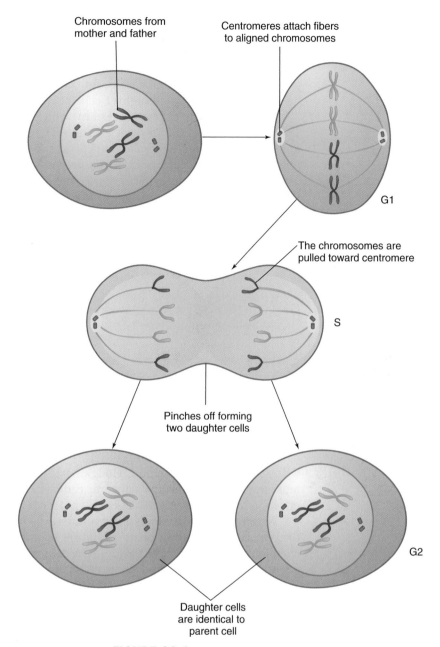

Chromosomes from mother and father

Centromeres attach fibers to aligned chromosomes

G1

The chromosomes are pulled toward centromere

S

Pinches off forming two daughter cells

G2

Daughter cells are identical to parent cell

FIGURE 28-1 Cell reproduction: mitosis.

Mitotic Inhibitors. Mitotic inhibitors prevent mitosis at the metaphase stage. Mitosis is the process of cell division that all cells must perform (Figure 28-1). The agents used to prevent this synthesis are a group of alkaloids derived from plants. Diseases such as Hodgkin's disease and various cancers that may not respond to other treatment often are treated with these types of agents. Side effects of these agents are common side effects of chemotherapy. These agents include the following:

Etoposide
Teniposide
Vinblastine
Vincristine
Vinorelbine

Each cell that produces the next generation of cells leaves a part its genetic makeup behind. Genes are contained within the chromosomes of the DNA, located in the nucleus of the cell. The process of producing new cells is referred to as replication. When a cell replicates, it copies all the chromosomes (all of the genes of the cell are replicated). As the chromosomes are duplicated, they are divided evenly into two daughter cells or new cells and are contained within the new nuclei. Mitosis is the process by which the nucleus of the cell is divided. The entire process of mitosis starts with prophase, followed by metaphase, anaphase, and then telophase. This process sometimes is abbreviated as the "M" phase for mitosis. Each part of the process is specific and lasts a certain time. The last stage, called cytokinesis, is the separation of the daughter cells. The mitotic phase and cytokinesis are the end processes of the life span of the cell. After cytokinesis takes place, the new cell enters a much longer phase referred to as interphase. Interphase process has three parts, the first of which is called G1 (see Figure 28-1). The replication process begins in this stage as the centrioles pull apart chromosomes preparing for mitosis once again. Centrioles anchor to the chromosomes at opposite ends of the cell and separate them. The second part of interphase is the S phase in which DNA replication starts. Lastly, the G2 phase of interphase prepares the cells for the mitotic phase, and the process begins over again.

Alkylating Agents. The two major types of alkylating agents are the nitrogen mustards and nitrosoureas. Although their structures are similar, their methods of action and side effects are different. Because alkylation is a normal reaction that takes place in the DNA between chemical compounds, these agents are able to bind to certain bases of the DNA. New bonds (created by alkylation) are made between components; when this happens, the rapidly dividing cancer cells are damaged and are unable to proliferate any further. Diseases most often treated with these agents include Hodgkin's disease, retinoblastoma, lymphocytic leukemia, and inoperable cancers. Side effects are the same as the common effects of chemotherapeutic agents.

Nitrogen mustards. Nitrogen mustards were some of the first agents used to treat cancer in addition to radiation or surgery. These agents were used in chemical warfare in World War I. On examination of soldiers exposed to these agents, it was discovered that nitrogen mustards decreased the number of WBCs. Because of this effect on WBCs, they were used to treat leukemia, which is marked by a high WBC count. Although effective, the first nitrogen mustards had severe side effects and since have been replaced with agents that are derived from the same chemical structure but are better tolerated. These agents are the following:

Chlorambucil
Cyclophosphamide
Ifosfamide
Mechlorethamine
Melphalan

Nitrosoureas. These agents cross the blood-brain barrier that surrounds the central nervous system. Because of this ability, they can be used to treat cancers within the brain. The following drugs are nitrosoureas:

Carmustine
Lomustine
Streptozocin

Miscellaneous Agents. Various other agents commonly are used to treat cancer. One group, hormones, includes the corticosteroids, androgens, and antiandro-

TABLE 28-4 Miscellaneous Cancer Treatment Agents

Agent	Mode of administration	Types of cancer
Asparaginase	Depletes asparagine (necessary for cell survival)	Lymphocytic leukemia
Dacarbazine	Inhibits synthesis in the G2 phase	Hodgkin's disease
Docetaxel	Inhibits activity of microtubules in the G1 phase	Breast cancer
Gemcitabine	Inhibits synthesis in S phase	Adenocarcinoma of pancreas
Hydroxyurea	Inhibits specific DNA synthesis	Head, neck, and ovarian cancer; melanomas
Paclitaxel	Antimicrotubule agent in the G2 phase	Metastatic ovarian cancer
Procarbazine	Inhibitor in the S phase	Hodgkin's disease

gens. Most hormone agents are indicated for cancers that are influenced by hormonal control. Corticosteroids can be useful in treating leukemia and lymphomas. They also work to decrease inflammation and edema in vital areas. Estrogen and androgens can be used to treat breast cancer. Antiandrogens are used to treat prostate cancer.

Other agents do not fall neatly into the categories previously discussed. One such agent is interferon, a natural protein found in the body. When used in treatment, it boosts immune cells, which are then better able to attack cancerous cells. Interferon also changes the structure of the cells, making them less "cancerlike" and more normal in their behavior. Interferon is used for a special form of leukemia known as hairy cell leukemia. Table 28-4 lists the specific actions of other miscellaneous agents used to treat cancer, along with the types of cancers for which they are used.

Side Effects of Chemotherapy

Because cancer is caused by a malfunction of our own cells, it is difficult to differentiate between defective cells and normal cells. The components are the same in both. This is not the problem for antibiotics used to treat infections caused by microbes because the cells of microbes are not the same as human cells. Therefore, medications can be made that will attack microbial cells and not our own. When fighting off cancerous cells, the only way to ensure a full remission is to kill off the cells. Unfortunately, good cells are killed off along with them, especially fast-growing cells such as those responsible for hair growth. As the cancer cells are killed off, the cells of the hair are too. Fortunately, hair will grow back in time.

Besides hair loss, another common side effect of chemotherapy is emesis (vomiting). Although many patients experience emesis, many antiemetic agents can be given to offset this side effect. For further information on antiemetics, refer to Chapter 20.

PAIN CONTROL

For cancer patients who are in pain there are many medications that can be used to control acute and chronic pain. These medications range from schedule III up to schedule II controlled substances that can be given in a variety of dosage strengths and forms. This enables patients to manage their pain at

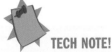

TECH NOTE!

Various agents are classified as vesicants. These agents must be handled carefully because any contact with exposed skin can cause irritation and sloughing of the skin. When preparing chemotherapeutic agents, special chemotherapy gloves must be worn or the technician must double glove to protect the skin. If a chemotherapeutic agent spills on the gloves, the top glove can be removed and discarded into an appropriate container, and a new pair of gloves can be worn. All agents that are vesicant have special auxiliary labels adhered to the container. The auxiliary label alerts the nurse who will be handling and administering the agent.

home or outside the hospital. Dosage forms may be oral liquids, tablets, capsules, patches, or suppositories. In the hospital, injectable analgesics may be given intramuscularly or intravenously. A patient-controlled analgesic (or PCA) pump also may be ordered that dispenses a predetermined amount of drug at set times from a preloaded syringe. The patient also has the ability to push a button for an additional amount of medication for maximum pain relief. The patient-controlled analgesia is preset for bolus doses so that regardless of how many times the patient may push the button, the pump will release only the preset dose. In this way the patient cannot overdose. The amount of medication must be monitored closely by the physician based on the severity of the pain of the patient. The following is a sample of the medications and their dosage forms that the pharmacy commonly stocks. They are intended to be used for moderate to severe pain.

Analgesic/Narcotic Agents	Dosage Forms
Codeine	Tablet, solution, injection
Fentanyl	Lozenge, injection, transdermal
Hydrocodone and acetaminophen	Capsule, elixir, solution, tablet
Hydrocodone and aspirin	Tablet
Hydrocodone and ibuprofen	Tablet
Hydromorphone	Tablet, liquid, suppository, injection
Oxycodone	Capsule, tablet, liquid, solution
Oxycodone and acetaminophen	Caplet, capsule, solution, tablet
Oxycodone and aspirin	Tablet
Meperidine	Oral solution, tablet, injection
Morphine sulfate*	Oral tablet, capsule, solution, injection

Biological Response Modifiers

Chemotherapeutic agents may destroy not only cancer cells but also the cells of the immune system. Patients treated with chemotherapeutic agents often become anemic or, because of a reduction of WBCs, they develop leukopenia. Because WBCs are essential in protecting the body from various infections, special medications are used to boost the immune cells. Two main agents used to treat chemotherapy side effects are erythropoietin and filgrastim. Both agents are used to stimulate specific bone marrow production of blood cells; erythropoietin stimulates red blood cell production, and filgrastim stimulates WBC production. The patient's blood serum must be monitored to dose these medications properly. The manufacturer's storage instructions require them to be stored in the refrigerator between 2° and 8°C. They must not be shaken or frozen.

Erythropoietin. Erythropoietin is used primarily to treat anemia in patients with malignant neoplasms who acquire anemia during chemotherapy. Erythropoietin also may be used to treat persons with human immunodeficiency virus infection or end-stage renal disease. Normal doses of erythropoietin range from 2000 to 10,000 units/mL. A normal dosing regimen is 150 units/kg 3 times a week.

Filgrastim. Filgrastim binds to bone marrow cells and stimulates growth of neutrophils. Neutrophils are key players in the immune system. They are part of the WBC defense mechanisms and often are destroyed by the chemotherapy treatment. When this happens, a condition known as leukopenia may occur, increasing the risk of infection to the patient.

---

*Used in patient-controlled analgesia pumps

BOX 28-3 EXAMPLES OF RADIOPHARMACEUTICALS AND THEIR USE

Chromium-51 sodium chromate	For labeling red blood cells for examination
Indium-111 capromab	For prostate cancer imaging
Iodine-131 sodium iodide	For thyroid imaging
Strontium-89	Treatment of pain from bone cancer
Technetium-99m	Used as a diagnostic tool to determine coronary artery disease (see Chapter 22.)
Gallium scan	To evaluate infections of the kidney and certain tumors; used in brain, gastrointestinal bleeding, bone, liver, gallbladder, thyroid gland, lung, and heart scans

Normal dosage of filgrastim is 5 mcg/kg per day. The dosage is given when WBCs decrease below a certain level and may be given daily until the WBC levels increase to a normal level. Dosage strength is 300 mcg/mL.

Cytoprotective Agents

Mesna is a cytoprotective agent used to treat the side effect of hemorrhagic cystitis caused by ifosfamide. Mesna is given intravenously at a concentration of no more than 20% of the ifosfamide dose. Another agent used to lessen side effects is amifostine. This agent is given along with the chemotherapy agent cisplatin to prevent its toxic effects.

Nuclear Pharmacy Technician

Nuclear pharmacy is a new area of pharmacy to which technicians may be exposed and about which they therefore must be educated. The agents used in nuclear pharmacy are referred to as radiopharmaceuticals. These agents are used as diagnostic tools and for treatments and may be administered to the patient in oral, intravenous, or inhaled forms. Just as chemotherapy agents must be handled carefully when being prepared in the pharmacy, so must nuclear medications. Radiopharmaceuticals are isotopes that can be seen on radiographs as small specks as they participate in the cell activity within the body system. Box 28-3 lists the types of nuclear medicine scans.

A nuclear pharmacy technician is expected to help prepare the medications, label them, and perform quality control testing under the direction of a licensed pharmacist. For safety purposes, each person in the nuclear pharmacy must wear a meter that gives a reading of the radioactive levels to which he or she is exposed. In addition, each medication package is labeled with a monitor that gives a reading of radioactive level. If the contents are damaged somehow, the meter will reflect the level of exposure. Compliance with the proper handling of the radioisotopes during preparation and disposal is imperative for all personnel. All medications are prepared in a vertical flow hood (see Chapter 13) and are disposed of in a special lead container. The half-life of the radioisotope determines how long it takes for the isotope to decay.

TECH ALERT!

Remember the following soundalike/look-alike drugs:

Cyclophosphamide versus cyclosporine
Cytoxan versus Cytosar
Cisplatin versus carboplatin
VePesid versus Versed
Leukeran versus leucovorin

- What types of elements may cause cancer
- How to decrease the possibility of acquiring certain cancers
- What are the diagnostic tools used to determine the type and stage of cancer
- What is leukemia, and what are the various types
- How cancer grows
- What are the types of treatments available to cancer patients
- What are the main types of chemotherapy treatments
- Why side effects of chemotherapy are similar
- How is nuclear pharmacy used in the diagnosis and treatment of cancer
- The method of action for each of the chemotherapeutic agents covered
- Terminology used to describe cancer and its treatments

MULTIPLE CHOICE QUESTIONS

1. Which of the following cell processes are not normally seen in cells?
   A. Replication
   B. Mitosis
   C. Death
   D. Metastasis

2. The term used to define the spread of cancer cells into other areas of the body is _____.
   A. Melanoma
   B. Cancerous
   C. Malignant
   D. Metastasis

3. Factors that are taken into account when diagnosing cancer include _____.
   A. Etiology
   B. Karyotype
   C. Morphology
   D. All of the above

4. The small sections of a gene that usually perform normally within a cell but when altered by a retrovirus can produce cancerous cells are referred to as _____.
   A. Oncogenes
   B. Tumors
   C. Neoplasms
   D. None of the above

5. A type of cancer that affects the lymphatic system and may or may not have a high grade of malignancy is referred to as _____.
   A. Leukemia
   B. Hodgkin's disease
   C. Non-Hodgkin's disease
   D. Kaposi sarcoma

6. Which of the following chemotherapeutic agents is NOT used to treat cancer?
   A. Antimetabolites
   B. Mitotic inhibitors
   C. Nitrogen mustards
   D. Filgrastim

7. The process of mitosis is a set of stages that begins with _____.
   A. G2 phase
   B. Cytokinesis
   C. S phase
   D. G1 phase

8. When preparing radiopharmaceuticals, guidelines require _____.
   A. The use of radioactive meter
   B. Specialized containers for disposal
   C. Preparation within a vertical flow hood
   D. All of the above

9. Which of the following person(s) may be at higher risk for acquiring cancer?
   A. Persons older than 65 years
   B. Children
   C. Smokers
   D. All of the above

10. Which of the following side effects are seen most commonly after chemotherapy treatment?
    A. Nausea and vomiting
    B. Diarrhea
    C. Immunosuppression or anemia
    D. All of the above

TRUE/FALSE **If the statement is false, then change it to make it true.**

_____ **1.** Cancer can be caused by a virus.

_____ **2.** Preventive measures can eliminate any chance of acquiring cancer.

_____ **3.** Only pharmacists can prepare radiopharmaceuticals.

_____ **4.** Surgery does not necessarily eliminate cancers and normally is followed with radiological therapy and/or chemotherapy.

_____ **5.** Radioactive isotopes often are implanted directly into the cancer site for treatment.

_____ **6.** Anticancer agents that alter normal hormone levels include corticosteroids.

_____ **7.** Vesicant agents must be prepared by a pharmacist.

_____ **8.** Chemotherapy drugs are administered intravenously or intramuscularly only.

_____ **9.** Erythropoietin is used to promote growth of neutrophils.

_____ **10.** Traditional antibiotics can be used to treat cancer.

TECHNICIAN'S CORNER

Using a comprehensive drug textbook, such as *Drug Facts and Comparisons* or *Mosby's Drug Consult,* look up the following chemotherapy agents and list their brand name, route of administration, and preparation guidelines:

Idarubicin

Doxorubicin

Mitomycin

BIBLIOGRAPHY

Drug facts and comparisons, ed 60, St Louis, 2005, Wolters Kluwer.

Fremgen B, Frucht S: *Medical terminology,* ed 2, Upper Saddle River, NJ, 2002, Prentice Hall.

Harman JG, Gilman AG, Limbird LE, editors: *Goodman and Gilman's the pharmacological basis of therapeutics,* New York, 2001, McGraw-Hill.

Malarkey LM, McMorrow ME: *Nurse's manual of laboratory tests and diagnostic procedures,* ed 2, Philadelphia, 2000, Saunders.

Stedman's concise medical dictionary for health professionals, ed 3, Baltimore, 1997, Williams & Wilkins.

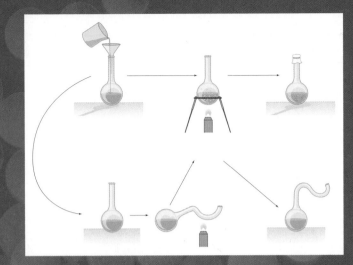

Microbiology

Objectives

UPON COMPLETING THIS CHAPTER, YOU SHOULD BE ABLE TO
DO THE FOLLOWING:

- Describe the Golden Age of Microbiology and its importance in the medical field.

- List the five kingdoms.

- List at least two different types of organisms within each kingdom.

- Differentiate between prokaryotic and eukaryotic cells.

- List the major components of the eukaryotic cell.

- Describe the functions of the major components of eukaryotic cells.

- List the steps required to perform a Gram stain.

- Describe the characteristics of bacterial cell walls of gram-positive and gram-negative microbes.

- Differentiate between gram-positive and gram-negative results.

- Describe the differences between microbes and viruses.

- List some of the most common conditions caused by species within each kingdom.

- Explain how and why bacteriophages are used to protect against viruses.

Aerobic *A term that describes organisms that need oxygen to survive*

Anaerobic *A term that describes organisms that live in the absence of oxygen*

Binary fission *The method of reproduction by which a single cell divides into two separate cells*

Biology *The study of life*

Enzyme *A protein that speeds up a reaction by reducing the amount of energy required to initiate a reaction; also called a biological catalyst*

Facultative anaerobe *A microorganism that can live with or without oxygen*

Heterotrophic *The ability to reproduce asexually*

Microbial *Refers to microorganisms (very small organisms) not visible without a microscope*

Microbiology *The study of microscopic organisms*

Morphology *Appearance, including shape, size, structure, and Gram stain characteristics of organisms; study of organisms without studying the function of organisms*

Peptidoglycan *The substance that comprises bacterial cell walls, specifically of gram-negative and gram-positive microbes*

Species *Of Latin origin meaning "kind"*

Taxonomy *The science of classification and nomenclature of organisms*

Vector *An entity by which infections are transferred, but the entity of transference does not have the disease and does not need to be living. For example, a mosquito bite transfers malaria. In this case, the mosquito is the vector.*

Virology *The study of viruses*

Virus *An organism that replicates by using the host's cell parts, including DNA, ribosomes, and proteins*

ORGANISMS AND DISEASES THEY CAUSE

Organisms	Species	Condition/s	Organisms	Species	Condition/s
Protozoa	*Plasmodium falciparum*	Malaria	Helminths	Helminths	
Fungi	*Candida albicans*	Candidiasis		Roundworms	
	Epidermophyton	Skin and nail infections		Flatworms	
	Microsporum	Hair and skin infections		Flukes	
	Trichophyton	Hair, skin, and nail infections		Tapeworms	
			Viruses	Human immunodeficiency virus	Acquired immunodeficiency syndrome
Bacteria	*Borrelia burgdorferi*	Lyme disease			
	Clostridium botulinum	Botulism		Herpesvirus	Herpes
	Clostridium tetani	Tetanus		Poliovirus	Polio
	Helicobacter pylori	Stomach ulcers		Poxvirus	Chickenpox
	Haemophilus influenzae	Meningitis		Rabies virus	Rabies
	Mycobacterium leprae	Leprosy		Rhinovirus	Common cold
	Mycobacterium tuberculosis	Tuberculosis			
	Neisseria gonorrhoeae	Gonorrhea			
	Staphylococcus aureus	Meningitis			
	Streptococcus pneumoniae	Meningitis			
	Streptococcus pyogenes	Scarlet fever			

BIOLOGY IS THE STUDY OF LIFE. Some forms of life cannot be seen without the aid of a microscope. Microbiology is the study of very small organisms, or microorganisms. This includes bacteria, some forms of fungus, and protists. Viruses are even smaller than bacteria. Virology is the study of viruses. Special microscopes and techniques are needed to view viruses because they are so small. An understanding of how microbes work is important in order to appreciate how antibiotics and other agents fight off infections and other conditions that affect the human species. To look into the world of microbes, we first must have some background on how life has been explained scientifically. From the dawn of humankind, human beings have tried to define what life is. To understand life, we must understand life forms and how they interact with each other.

As scientific techniques advance, so does our insight into the mysterious world of microbial life forms. Because of the strange and bizarre life forms that have been discovered on this planet, scientists believe now, more than ever, that life may exist on other planets. Microbes have been found in fossils dating back more than 3 billion years before the beginning of humankind. They have adapted to the drastic and harsh changes in the environment since the beginning of their existence. Microbes can live regardless of adverse conditions. Bacteria and other life forms have been a part of human evolution. Human beings benefit from bacteria in many ways. This chapter explores the positive and negative effects of bacteria on human beings.

Charles Darwin (Evolution)

In 1831, Charles Darwin traveled to the Galapagos Islands. There he studied the various species on each island. He discovered that evolution plays a key role in the survival of the fittest. It was his observations of the animals on the Galapagos Islands that made him question the theories of how species inhabited islands far from the mainland.

Darwin found that the species were not totally different nor were they the same as the species on the mainland. His research led him in another direction. From all his recorded notes and from previous research by animal researchers, Darwin found that tortoises, birds, insects, and even plants living on the many islands were similar to one another. However, even though they lived in proximity to one another, the species were different from one island to another. The reason for this major difference, Darwin believed, was that each species followed a different evolutionary path. The various animals and organisms living on each island developed into different species altogether. Only those species that survived the changes on each island would reproduce. Therefore, only the fittest survived. Darwin formed taxonomic categories based on the phylogenetic relationship between offspring from previous generations. He contributed to biology and is to this day considered the father of evolution.

The Golden Age of Microbiology

Until the discovery of the microscope in the 1600s, scientists did not know that organisms were made of cells nor did they know about microscopic organisms (see Chapter 1). An English eyeglass maker by the name of Robert Hooke invented the first microscope. His first observations, made with a crude type of microscope, were the cells of a simple cork. He described them as tiny boxes or cells. This was the beginning of the study of microscopic organisms. In 1674, Antoni van Leeuwenhoek invented a more sophisticated microscope and documented the observation of tiny microbes in a drop of water and teeth scrapings. He referred to these small organisms as "animalcules." Although many microbes

1900s			
	1953	Watson, Crick	Discovered the form of DNA
	1944	Avery, MacLeod, McCarty	Discovered that DNA is the genetic material
	1943	Delbruck, Luria	Discovered that bacteria could become infected with viruses
	1935	Stanley, Northrup, Summer	Gained the ability to crystallize viruses
	1928	Fleming, Chain, Florey	Credited with the discovery of penicillin
	1910	Ehrlich	Discovered syphilis
	1890	Ehrlich	Proved the theory of immunity
	1887	Petri	Created the Petri dish used for isolation of bacteria
	1884	Escherich	Discovered the bacteria *Escherichia coli*
	1884	Gram	Created the Gram staining process to determine bacterial cell wall
	1883	Koch	Discovered the bacteria *Vibrio cholerae*
	1882	Koch	Discovered the bacteria *Mycobacterium tuberculosis*
	1881	Koch	Created pure cultures
	1880	Pasteur	Began immunization techniques
	1879	Neisser	Found the microbe (named after him) *Neisseria gonorrhoeae*
	1876	Koch	Discovered the germ theory of disease
	1867	Lister	Proved that cleaning the hands between surgeries decreased the spread of infection from patient to patient
	1864	Pasteur	Created pasteurization
	1861	Pasteur	Proved spontaneous generation
1800s	1857	Pasteur	Discovered fermentation

FIGURE 29-1 The golden age of microbiology.

now were being discovered, there were many debates in the scientific world as to their origins.

In the beginning of microbiology, most scientists believed in spontaneous generation. The idea was that some organisms were generated from other organisms or their by-products. For example, it was believed that flies came from manure; maggots came from decaying corpses; and mice and snakes came from common soil. In the 100 years after the invention of the microscope, these inaccurate beliefs were disproved by scientific methods. They were replaced by the understanding that new life arises from preexisting living organisms. Scientific methods were set in place, and these methods are still used today to prove or disprove hypotheses.

Figure 29-1 gives a time line of major advances in the field of microbiology.

LOUIS PASTEUR

Louis Pasteur was a French scientist who devised experiments that would set the standards for scientific research in the future. He proved that unseen microorganisms exist in the air and in nonliving material such as broth. By using broth-filled glass beakers that were made to trap airborne microbes, he proved that the broth could be kept from contamination.

Many advances in scientific knowledge took place—from newly discovered bacteria to understanding the theory of evolution. It is no wonder that this time period was called the golden age of microbiology. Most of the discoveries made during this time extended human life. With the knowledge of bacteria and other microbes, scientists and doctors were able to fight infection. The average life span of an adult in the 1600s was 40 years; in contrast, midlife today is 40 years and many persons live into their 80s and 90s.

Classifications of Organisms (Taxonomy)

Scientists have classified organisms into seven different groups. These groups are based on structural similarities and clarify how different organisms survive and interact with each other. This knowledge serves to aid scientists in understanding evolutionary changes. The study of naming and classifying organisms is called taxonomy. Taxonomy is a difficult area of study because it can be hard to classify new organisms in a specific group when they may have similarities to more than one group.

ROBERT WHITTAKER (THE FIVE KINGDOMS)

The five kingdoms—Plantae, Animalia, Fungi, Protista, and Monera—were conceived by a scientist by the name of Robert Whittaker and are still in use today (Table 29-1). Four of the five kingdoms consist of eukaryotic organisms. Within each kingdom, the organisms are next divided into different phyla, followed by classes, orders, families, genera, and then finally species. These seven different classifications are used to organize all the known living organisms on planet Earth. Each kingdom, of course, contains many different types of organisms.

Viruses are not included in the five kingdoms. Scientists differ on the classification of viruses because they do not fit nicely into the characteristics of a "life form." Viruses are discussed at the end of this chapter.

Eukaryotic and prokaryotic organisms have different characteristics. The most obvious difference is that eukaryotes have a nucleus that binds DNA and prokaryotes do not. Also, eukaryotes do not have a cell wall structure as prokaryotes do. The cell wall allows antibiotics an attachment point that can break down the organism and kill it. Because eukaryotes do not have this wall, antibiotics cannot attach themselves. This difference makes it possible for antibiotics to kill microbes without harming the cells of the human body. Each eukaryotic kingdom is differentiated from the others by four main criteria:

1. Their individual pattern of development
2. Nutritional requirements
3. Tissue differentiation
4. Possession of flagella (form of locomotion)

TABLE 29-1 Kingdoms, Cell Characteristics, and Examples

Kingdoms	Characteristics	Examples
Plantae	Eukaryote	Pine trees, green algae, ferns, flowers
Animalia	Eukaryote	Sponges, worms, apes, starfishes, human beings
Protista	Eukaryote	Algae, water molds, amebae
Fungi	Eukaryote	Molds, yeasts, fungi
Monera	Prokaryote	Gram-positive and gram-negative bacteria

We briefly review each of the five kingdoms, isolating specific organisms that may have an adverse effect on human beings. In addition, a brief discussion of viruses covers their unique characteristics and abilities to harm and help us in the ever-growing fight against infection.

PLANTAE

The kingdom Plantae includes land (terrestrial) and water plants (aquatic). They are mainly multicellular and are classified further based on their photosynthetic pigmentation. Plants are eukaryotic organisms that obtain their food supply and energy from the sun through photosynthesis. They include mosses, ferns, flowers, conifers, and an array of other organisms. Human beings have a special relationship with plants; we need them for nutrition and protection from weather. We use parts of plants to build homes and make clothing and to treat various medical conditions. For example, digoxin is taken from the plant foxglove and is used to treat heart conditions. The bark from the ash tree *(Taxus brevifolia)* is used to treat ovarian cancer. More recently, *Ginkgo biloba* taken from the ginkgo tree has been used to increase memory (see Chapter 10).

Plant Cell Structure

Plant cells contain many of the same structures as animal cells. However, plant cells acquire energy differently than animal cells do. Figure 29-2 illustrates the differences between animal and plant cells. Plants have chloroplasts that are used to convert sunlight into energy, which then is stored. In addition, plants have a cell wall that is composed of cellulose that maintains cell shape. The vacuole of a plant cell also is much larger than those found in animal cells.

Not many diseases are transmitted easily by plants. Because plants are linked in many ways to animal cells, we have benefited from many plants, using them for food, flavorings, and colorings (dyes) and to treat various conditions.

Medically Relevant Conditions

Poison ivy and poison oak can cause a skin reaction when touched. Many plants can cause gastrointestinal upset or worse if eaten by persons or animals, and a few, such as digitalis, can cause death. Thus, it is wise never to ingest plants if you are not sure of the consequence. Many plants are used medicinally for treating various conditions that affect human beings. Some of these plants are discussed in Chapter 10. In addition to use as a medicinal product, plants also have nutritional and industrial value. Animals and human beings depend on plants for food.

ANIMALIA

The kingdom Animalia contains more species than any of the other kingdoms. Species in this kingdom are more complex physiologically than other species and rely on many motor skills and sensory organs. Ingested food must be broken down through a series of complicated steps before it can be used. More complex nervous systems may be necessary depending on the species of animal. The animal kingdom includes the more simplistic sponges, jellyfish, and clams and more complex organisms such as spiders, frogs, kangaroos, and mammals such as human beings.

Animal: Eukaryotic Cell Structure

Animal cells contain different structures than cells from plants and prokaryotes. The most obvious difference between animal cells and bacterial and plant cells is the lack of a cell wall. The cell composition for animal cells is shown in Figure 29-2.

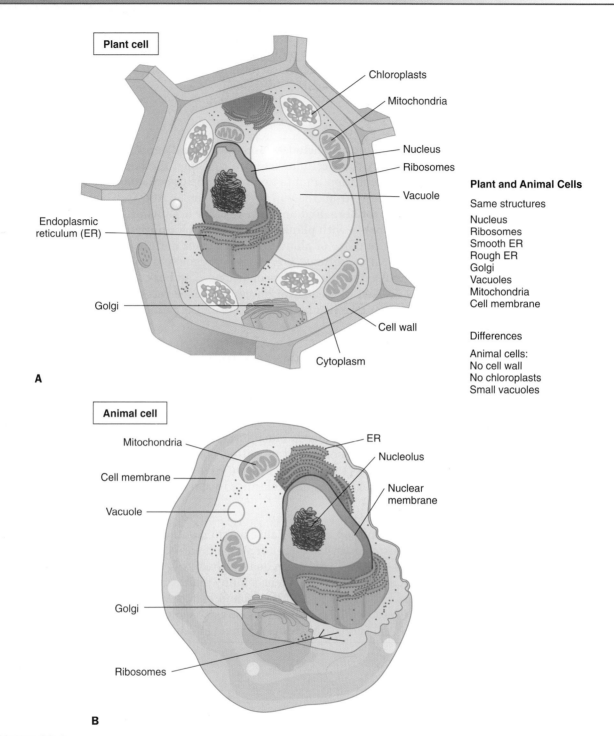

Plant cell

- Chloroplasts
- Mitochondria
- Nucleus
- Ribosomes
- Vacuole

Endoplasmic reticulum (ER)

Golgi

Cell wall

Cytoplasm

A

Plant and Animal Cells

Same structures

Nucleus
Ribosomes
Smooth ER
Rough ER
Golgi
Vacuoles
Mitochondria
Cell membrane

Differences

Animal cells:
No cell wall
No chloroplasts
Small vacuoles

Animal cell

- Mitochondria
- Cell membrane
- Vacuole
- Golgi
- Ribosomes
- ER
- Nucleolus
- Nuclear membrane

B

FIGURE 29-2 Major components of a plant cell **(A)**, an animal cell **(B)**, and a bacterial cell **(C)**. Animal cells do not have a cell wall, whereas bacterial cells are surrounded by a thin or thick barrier wall made of peptidoglycan.

Animal cells also lack the chloroplast that plant cells use to store energy from the sun. Animal cells get their energy from food rather than from the sun. Inside each animal cell are many structures that work in unison. The nucleus contains the DNA of the cell. This is the genetic code of the animal. Other structures in the cell include ribosomes, mitochondria, Golgi complex, plasma membrane, cytoplasm, vesicles, and rough and smooth endoplasmic reticulum. Table 29-2 outlines the functions of each structure.

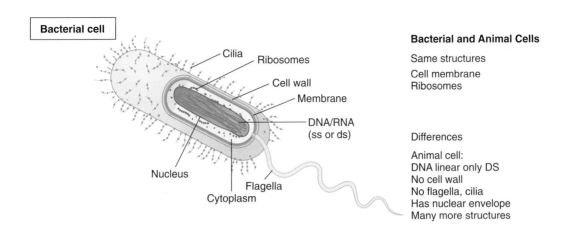

Bacterial cell

Bacterial and Animal Cells

Same structures
Cell membrane
Ribosomes

Differences

Animal cell:
DNA linear only DS
No cell wall
No flagella, cilia
Has nuclear envelope
Many more structures

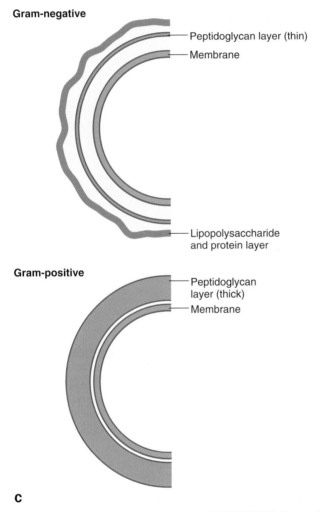

Gram-negative

Peptidoglycan layer (thin)
Membrane
Lipopolysaccharide and protein layer

Gram-positive

Peptidoglycan layer (thick)
Membrane

C

FIGURE 29-2, cont'd

Because four of the five kingdoms are made up of eukaryotic organisms, many types of species can cause human diseases. Various organisms in the animal kingdom can be transmitted to human beings from various vectors. Vectors are the carriers of disease organisms. How the organism moves through various environments throughout its life cycle ultimately reveals ways to avoid contact, as explained in the following.

TABLE 29-2 Characteristics and Structure of an Animal (Eukaryotic) Cell

Cell component	Structure	Description
Centrosomes	Rodlike structures	These contain centrioles, which are symmetrical in design; they are needed at the beginning of reproduction
DNA	Double helix	Genetic code responsible for many characteristics
Endoplasmic reticulum (ER)	Membranous network	Contained throughout the cytoplasm. Provides surface area for production and transportation and storage of molecules within cell. Attached ribosomes involved in lipid and protein synthesis.
Golgi complex	Flat membranous stacks of sacs	Serves as a transport system for enzymes and proteins and adds onto some products before they are sent out of the cell
Lysosomes	A single sac filled with digestive juices	Digestive sacs that dispose of unwanted particles within the cell. They then are emptied outside of the cell
Mitochondria	Cell-like structure with membranous material	Responsible for making adenosine triphosphate that then is carried to places within the cell where energy is needed to produce enzymes and so forth; cells contain many mitochondria that are located near production areas such as ER
Nucleus	Envelope containing DNA	Contains DNA and nucleolus; the nucleolus manufactures substances (such as ribosomes) used in the cytoplasm
Ribosomes	Small, dotlike structures	ER that contains ribosomes is referred to as rough ER; it produces proteins such as enzymes
RNA	Chain	A messenger for coding proteins
Smooth ER	Membranous network	Produces various lipid substances: has no ribosomes

Medically Relevant Conditions

The ameba *Entamoeba histolytica* is a parasitic organism that feeds on red blood cells. Its mode of transportation is from human being to human being via ingestion of cysts that are excreted in the feces. The vector or carrier of these disease-causing microorganisms includes human beings and mosquitoes.

Trichomonas vaginalis is another protozoan that causes infections in the male urinary tract and in the vagina of females. The organism is transferred mostly by sexual intercourse.

Dysentery is caused by another protozoan ciliate *Balantidium coli* and is transferred by feces to the mouth in a cyst form. When the cysts are ingested, they travel to the colon where they replicate.

Sporozoa, such as *Plasmodium vivax,* are responsible for the disease malaria. Their life cycle involves an infected female mosquito. The sporozoa in the salivary glands of the mosquito easily move into the human bloodstream once the mosquito bites the human being. From the bloodstream the sporozoa move to the liver, where they replicate and move into the bloodstream. As the parasites are released into the bloodstream, their toxic by-products cause the host to become sick. When an uninfected mosquito bites an infected human being, the cycle repeats (Figure 29-3).

Helminths (worms) are also protists but are categorized under different phyla (headings) than protozoa (single-celled organisms). Helminths are Platy-

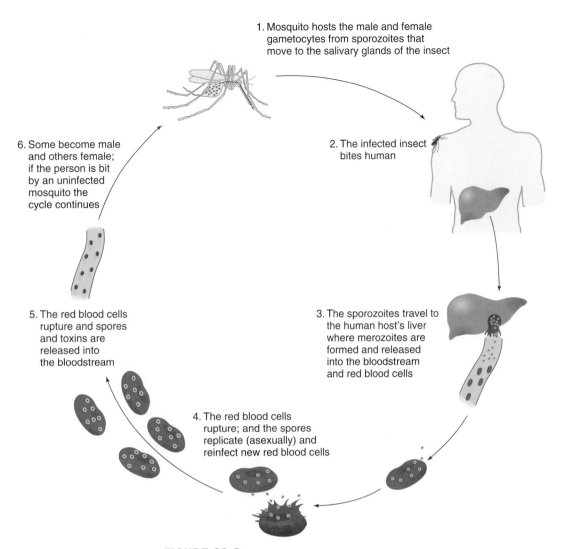

FIGURE 29-3 Life cycle of *Plasmodium vivax*.

1. Mosquito hosts the male and female gametocytes from sporozoites that move to the salivary glands of the insect

2. The infected insect bites human

3. The sporozoites travel to the human host's liver where merozoites are formed and released into the bloodstream and red blood cells

4. The red blood cells rupture; and the spores replicate (asexually) and reinfect new red blood cells

5. The red blood cells rupture and spores and toxins are released into the bloodstream

6. Some become male and others female; if the person is bit by an uninfected mosquito the cycle continues

helminthes (flatworms) or Aschelminthes (roundworms). These worms are multicellular eukaryotic organisms that have many of the same organs that human beings do. They have digestive, circulatory, nervous, excretory, and reproductive systems. These types of helminths live in soil and feed on organic material. Those that lack a digestive system remain parasitic. They must absorb digested nutrients from a host. Other differences between free-living and parasitic helminths are that the parasitic helminths may lack means of locomotion and their nervous system is simple because they do not have to be sensitive to their environment. The parasitic helminth life cycle is complex, which requires a more sophisticated reproductive system. Table 29-3 lists the human parasitic diseases. All forms of these parasites can be avoided by using a few precautions:

- Always cook meat thoroughly.
- Wear shoes when walking outside on soil.
- Never drink from stream water because it may be contaminated with feces from animals upstream.
- Wash your hands after playing with animals or after cleaning cat litter boxes.

TABLE 29-3 Parasitic Diseases Contracted by Human Beings

Organism	Species	Life cycle
Phylum: Platyhelminthes		
Trematodes (flukes)	*Paragonimus westermani*	Miracidium swims and imbeds in a snail and develops into the next form, cercaria, that invades lobster. A person eats lobster and contracts the adult fluke. Defecation into water continues the cycle.
Cestodes (tapeworms)	*Taenia saginata*	Proglottids containing eggs are found in feces defecated onto grass. Cattle ingest proglottids containing eggs. They hatch and bore into muscle and form a cyst. These are ingested by humans in uncooked meat, and the cycle continues
	Echinococcus granulosus	Human beings ingest eggs excreted in feces. Eggs hatch within the small intestine, and larvae migrate to liver or lungs. A cyst is formed. In the wild the host may be eaten by another animal, and the cycle continues.
Phylum: Aschelminthes		
Nematodes (roundworms)	*Enterobius vermicularis*	This species spends its entire life in the human host. Adult pinworms deposit eggs around the perianal region where they can be transferred via exposure to contaminated clothing.
	Ascaris lumbricoides	Adult form lives in small intestines of human host. Eggs are excreted and can survive in soil until another host ingests it. Eggs hatch in intestines, travel to lungs to mature stage, and then migrate to intestine to continue cycle.
	Necator americanus	Adult lives in small intestines of human beings; eggs are excreted and live in soil. Worm infects host by penetrating through the skin of the feet, from where it gets carried to the lungs via blood. It is coughed up and then ingested into the stomach, where it enters the intestine.
	Trichinella spiralis	Undercooked pork or beef containing cyst form enters the human digestive tract, where cysts reproduce live nematodes. They migrate to various muscles and tissues and remain to be parasites of the host.

PROTISTA

Most of the organisms in the kingdom Protista are unicellular, and all are eukaryotic. They are made up of five different plantlike and animal-like organisms. All are heterotrophic, which means they reproduce asexually. Some cause diseases in other organisms.

Protists include algae, water molds, amebae, and protozoans. Algae and water molds can be found in and around coastal waters. Certain forms of algae are macroscopic, reaching lengths from a few meters up to 50 m. From large brown kelp beds off the coast to algae found growing in trees, algae prefer moist to wet areas and need light to survive. They produce chlorophyll, which they use as a food source. Some protists, such as brown algae or lichens, anchor themselves to a surface. Other organisms such as euglenoids and green algae propel themselves by means of a flagellum, or a whiplike structure that moves them through water.

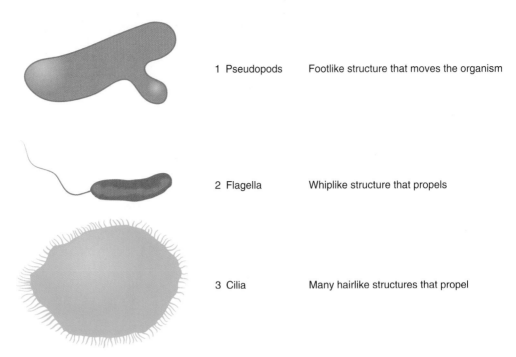

1 Pseudopods   Footlike structure that moves the organism

2 Flagella   Whiplike structure that propels

3 Cilia   Many hairlike structures that propel

FIGURE 29-4 Three forms of locomotion in protozoa.

Protozoans can live in water or soil, and they live off of bacteria and other organic particles. Protozoans can be a part of the "normal flora" of an animal, and most do not cause disease. Figure 29-4 shows their three modes of locomotion.

FUNGI

The Fungi kingdom is divided into true fungi and slime molds. Many have a complex reproductive cycle. Lichens are a specialized type of fungi that can grow in the most inhospitable environments.

Fungi are different from bacteria. The DNA of a fungus is contained within a nuclear membrane. Some of the organisms that belong in the kingdom Fungi include fleshy-type fungi, such as mushrooms, and also yeasts and certain types of molds. Fungi are aerobes (need air) or facultative anaerobes (partially need air). Yeasts are the only fungi that are not multicellular, but they too absorb nutrients from plants. They are round or oval and may be found on leaves of plants. Each single cell replicates by the process of budding or splitting into two (Figure 29-5).

Molds may have long filaments called hyphae and may form a mass large enough to be seen by the naked eye. Molds can infect and ultimately destroy (spoil) plants and food. Fungi play an important role in the environment because they are responsible for decomposing plant organisms. They use dead plants as a food source while cleaning the environment. Plants are more susceptible to fungal infections than are human beings. Many fungi do not cause illness; however, human beings can get some infections from specific species.

Medically Relevant Conditions

The species *Candida albicans* is a yeastlike organism that is part of the normal flora in the mouth and genitourinary tract of human beings. The organism is kept in check by the bacterial flora also present in the mouth and genitourinary areas. When antibiotics are taken that kill off the normal bacterial flora of these areas, the fungus *C. albicans* can proliferate and cause an infection. Other conditions caused by fungi are athlete's foot, lung and vaginal infections, and even

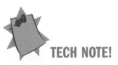

TECH NOTE!

Yeast (facultative anaerobe) usually is associated with baking bread and making beer. As the species *Saccharomyces cerevisiae* (baker's yeast) buds off, it expands and the bread dough rises. The yeast in beer gives off carbon dioxide as a by-product and gives beer its unique taste.

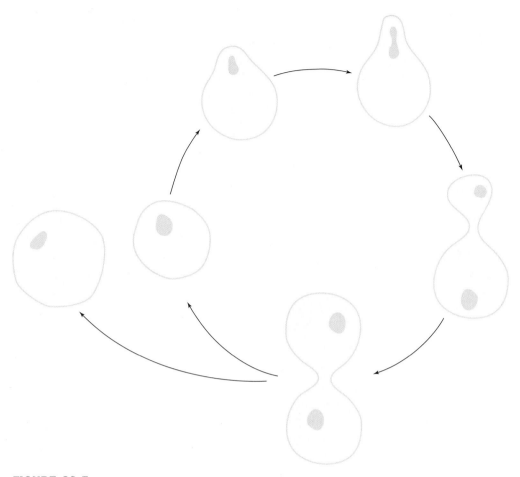

FIGURE 29-5 The budding process of replication of yeast cells. Yeast multiplies asexually by budding or sprouting a new cell that then breaks away from the mother cell.

BOX 29-1 CONDITIONS CAUSED BY FUNGI

Candida albicans	Multiple conditions
Tinea pedis	Athlete's foot
Pneumocystis carinii	Pneumonia
Tinea cruris	Jock itch
Tinea unguium	Cutaneous infection
Tinea capitis	Ringworm

sepsis. Fungus prefers warm moist environments; however, some species of fungi can grow under low-moisture conditions. A disease caused by a fungus is called mycosis. The types of agents used to kill fungi are referred to as antifungal agents (see Chapter 24). Many conditions are caused by fungi, as shown in Box 29-1.

The next section describes the characteristics of prokaryotic cells, the conditions caused by these organisms, and how antibiotics are used to treat them. Please refer to Chapter 24 for specific antimicrobial actions of antibiotics and their side effects.

MONERA

Monera, the smallest organisms (in size) of the seven kingdoms, may be the simplest in physiology but are the most abundant worldwide. Fossils of bacteria

Procaryotic cell size	Description of basic form		Description of basic cocci or bacilli shapes	
Coccus	oval or round	1. 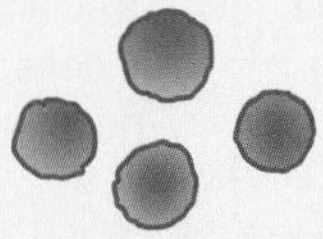	diplococcus diplobacilli	5. 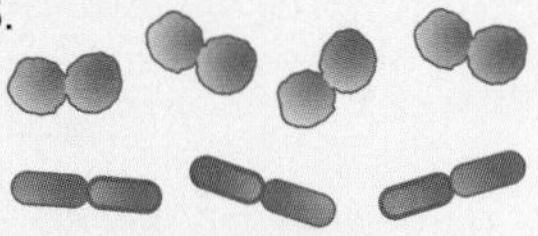
Bacillus	rectangular, rod shaped	2. 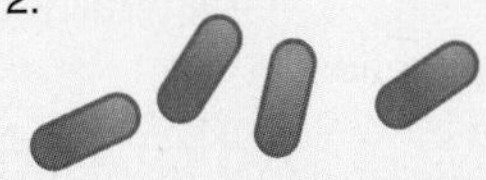	streptococcus streptobacilli	6. 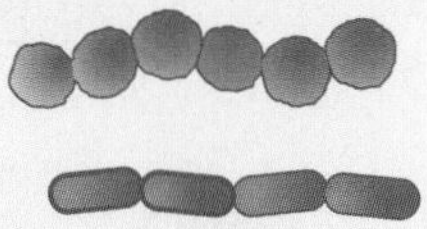
Spirilla	twisted, helical, corkscrew, spiral	3. 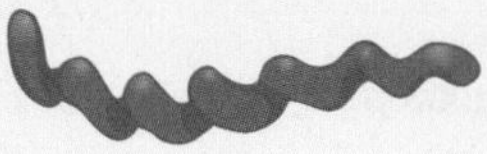	staphylococci staphylobacilli	7. 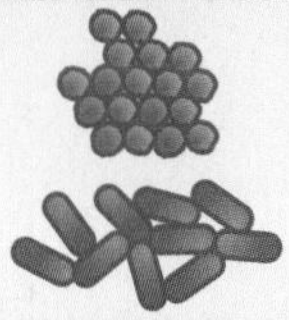
Vibrios	resemble commas	4. 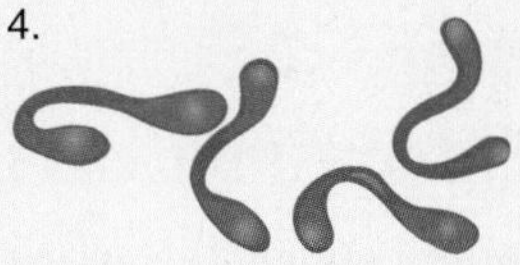		

FIGURE 29-6 Morphology of prokaryotic organisms. Pictures 1 to 6 show the various morphologies or shapes of microbes. The most common shapes include the following: *1*, coccus; *2*, bacilli; *3*, spirilla; *4*, vibrios. Picture 5 shows cocci microbes that are found in sets of two, called diplococci or diplobacilli. Those microbes found in strips are shown in picture 6: streptococci or streptobacilli. Picture 7 shows staphylococci and staphylobacilli, which are found in clusters.

have been dated back 3.5 billion years; in contrast, eukaryotic cells date back only 1.5 billion years. The cell structure of prokaryotes is less complicated than that of eukaryotic cells. Bacteria are classified further depending on how they derive their energy, as well as other characteristics.

Characteristics and Structure of Prokaryotes

Until now, we have explored a few of the many different types of eukaryotic cell organisms. Many basic differences exist between prokaryotic and eukaryotic cell structures. The visual characteristics of bacteria and other microbial organisms are used to describe the morphology or appearance of the organism (Figure 29-6).

Other characteristics specific to prokaryotes are that they can reproduce by binary fission (divide in two), they do not have a nuclear envelope, and amazingly, they have the ability to live in the most inhospitable environments, adding to their prevalence. Prokaryotes may be anaerobic or aerobic. Before the discovery of these minute life forms, the effects of bacteria were attributed to other causes, such as evil spirits.

Brief History of Antibiotics

In 1928, Alexander Fleming, a scientist who was studying crops plagued by infections, noticed that one of his agar plates was contaminated with a mold. This mold, later named *Penicillium notatum,* had a zone of clearance around it where no bacteria were growing because the mold had broken down the bacteria being grown on the agar plate. It took many years to isolate the active component within the mold—penicillin. Penicillin destroys bacteria by interacting with enzymes that are present within the bacterial cell wall.

TABLE 29-4 **Classes of Microorganisms within the Kingdom Monera**

Common name	Class	Characteristics
Wall-less prokaryotes	Mycoplasmata	Smallest known bacteria that can live outside host cells; lipid-type barrier helps protect them
Typical gram-positive cell wall	Rods, cocci	Thick walls made of peptidoglycan
	Actinomycetes	Thick walls made of peptidoglycan
Typical gram-negative cell wall	Anaerobic photosynthetic bacteria	Thin walls made of peptidoglycan
	Cyanobacteria	Thin walls made of peptidoglycan
	Nonphotosynthetic bacteria	Thin walls made of peptidoglycan
Altered cell wall type	Archaebacteria	Walls not composed of peptidoglycan but polysaccharides or proteins

STRUCTURE OF THE BACTERIAL CELL WALL

Because bacteria have many characteristics that are different from human body cells, certain drugs can be used to attack and kill bacteria without harming human cells. The bacteria cell has a wall or barrier made of peptidoglycan that protects it in the same way that our skin protects us from damage and intrusion (see Figure 29-2). Bacterial cell walls are made of a finely woven network of two forms of protective barriers. Penicillin disrupts the barrier and causes the bacteria to lyse or break open. Because human cells have a different type of membrane, and not a wall, surrounding them, they are not harmed.

Bacteria are determined to be either gram positive or gram negative. This basis is determined by a gram stain which differentiates the cell walls from one another due to their specific cell wall composition. There are several differences between characteristics between gram positive and gram negative bacteria. In gram-positive bacteria there are thick peptidoglycan layers linked by teichoic acids to the inner membrane. In contrast, a gram-negative cell wall has few peptidoglycan layers with no peptidoglycan layers. Gram-negative cells also differ in other aspects of their components such as an outer membrane, enabling them to withstand certain antibiotics, such as penicillin, as well as detergents, digestive enzymes, and certain dyes. In addition, gram-negative cell walls contain a lipid that becomes toxic when in the bloodstream of the host. Openings on the surface of the outer cell membrane of the gram-negative cell allow some chemicals to penetrate the cell. These openings are responsible for the difference shown between gram-negative and gram-positive bacteria on Gram stain; thus laboratory technicians can differentiate between the two types of organisms (Table 29-4).

Exterior of Bacterial Cell Walls

Glycocalyx is a sticky substance that surrounds many different types of bacteria. This thick layer is composed of different material depending on the species. The purpose of glycocalyx is to protect the bacteria from being destroyed by the immune system cells of the host. Bacteria can adhere better to surfaces because of their sticky surface. This increases the chance of bacterial survival.

ANTIBIOTIC SPECTRUM AND RESISTANCE

Antibiotics destroy bacteria by breaking down the cell walls of bacteria. To choose the right drug to destroy specific bacteria, the type of microbe must be

TABLE 29-5 Commonly Caused Bacterial Conditions

Organism	Disease	Morphology
Borrelia burgdorferi	Lyme disease	*Difficult to Gram stain
Clostridium botulinum	Botulism	Anaerobic, gram-positive rods
Clostridium tetani	Tetanus	Anaerobic, gram-positive rods
Escherichia coli	Cystitis (an opportunistic bacteria from the gastrointestinal tract)	Gram-negative rods
Haemophilus influenzae	Meningitis, respiratory infections, septicemia	Aerobic, gram-negative rods
Helicobacter pylori	Stomach ulcers	Aerobic, gram-negative rods
Mycobacterium leprae	Leprosy	*Difficult to Gram stain
Mycobacterium tuberculosis	Tuberculosis	*Difficult to Gram stain
Neisseria gonorrhoeae	Gonorrhea	Aerobic, gram-negative cocci
Staphylococcus aureus	Boils, carbuncles, abscesses	Aerobic, gram-positive cocci
Streptococcus pneumoniae	Pneumonia	Aerobic, gram-positive cocci
Streptococcus pyogenes	Scarlet fever	Aerobic, gram-positive cocci group A β-hemolytic

*For those microbial organisms that cannot be grown on artificial media agar plates, other means are used, such as acid-fast staining or an immunological test to determine whether the disease is present.

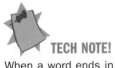

TECH NOTE!

When a word ends in *-ase,* it means that it is an enzyme.

determined. The first step in this process is to determine whether the bacteria are gram-positive or gram-negative.

Most penicillins are effective at breaking down the cell walls of gram-positive microbes. However, many forms of bacteria are not destroyed by penicillin because they secrete another type of enzyme that cuts the bond within the penicillin structure, thus rendering it useless against the bacteria. The name for this bacterial enzyme is penicillinase. Special additives can be included with penicillin-type agents to stop their destruction. Additives such as sulbactam added to ampicillin (Unasyn) allow the antibiotic to break the bacterial bonds, allowing the break in the cell wall to occur.

As the antibiotic spectrum broadens, so does the effectiveness against microbes; thus broad-spectrum antibiotics are effective against more microbes than narrow-spectrum antibiotics are. Narrow-spectrum antibiotics normally affect gram-positive microbes, whereas broad-spectrum antibiotics may affect gram-negative microbes. Broad-spectrum agents such as aminoglycosides are much more effective against gram-negative bacteria. Another important aspect of bacterial organisms is their ability to live with or without oxygen.

Some agents are specific, killing one type of bacteria. This is why it is important to choose the correct antibiotic. (Table 29-5 give examples of common types of conditions caused by bacteria.)

Bacteria reside just about everywhere in the world. Environments that contain bacteria include hot springs, the bottom of the ocean, deep in the earth's crust, and the mouths and intestinal systems of human beings. Bacteria that can live in the presence of air are called aerobic, whereas those that grow only in the absence of air are called anaerobic. Some bacteria called facultative anaerobes can live with a small amount of air or in airless environments. The relationship that some bacteria have with animals is mutually beneficial. This means that both organisms benefit from one another. For instance, various bacteria reside within the human gut, including *Escherichia coli* and *Lactobacillus,* that help break down food that can be absorbed into the body. The bacteria benefit by the nutrient-rich environment.

Viruses

One of the major disagreements in the scientific community is how to classify viruses. They do not fit nicely into any of the kingdoms outlined previously. In fact, viruses have their own field of study called virology (the study of viruses). Viruses not only infect animals but also infect plants and even bacteria. Plant viruses are responsible for destroying many food crops to the detriment of people and livestock.

CLASSIFICATION OF VIRUSES

Viruses can be categorized into three types:

1. Animal viruses
2. Plant viruses
3. Bacterial viruses

MORPHOLOGY AND CHARACTERISTICS OF VIRUSES

Viruses may have a double or single strand of DNA. They are different from other organisms because they also can have a double or single strand of RNA.

Basic classification of viruses includes determining their outer covering and any additional coating that they may contain, as shown in Figure 29-7.

Unenveloped viruses are covered by capsids; capsids are protective coverings made of proteins called capsomeres. Enveloped viruses have a capsid plus a covering of proteins, fats, and carbohydrates. Different viruses have different appearances; sometimes they resemble small space capsules.

Other ways to classify viruses or virions include determining their method of replication. This is probably one of the characteristics that is most different from the characteristics of organisms in any of the five kingdoms. As shown in Figure 29-8, viruses do not seem to replicate in any of the previously described methods; instead, they assemble themselves just as cars are assembled in a processing plant. In all living organisms except viruses, DNA is double stranded. RNA is replicated from the DNA information. Viruses invade a host cell and take over this replication to make more viral DNA.

Other differences between viruses and organisms of the other kingdoms include the way that viruses survive. Most organisms obtain nutrition from organic means or from the sun by photosynthesis and replicate by fission (splitting into two), sexual, or asexual means. Viruses do not fit any of these categories. They are closer to parasites, although most parasites do not kill their hosts as viruses do. Viruses assemble new virions by using the cell parts from their hosts. Some viruses can travel from host to host by way of blood, body fluids, or even the air. Thus, although they do have some similarities with other organisms, they do not behave as entities that can replicate without the components of the cells that they invade. All viruses are so small that they cannot be seen with a light microscope. To isolate and identify viruses, different methods must be used.

ANALYSIS OF VIRIONS

Viruses that infect bacteria (such as bacteriophages) can be grown on agar plates. However, those that cannot be grown on agar plates must be grown in animals, such as mice, rabbits, or other laboratory animals, to observe their

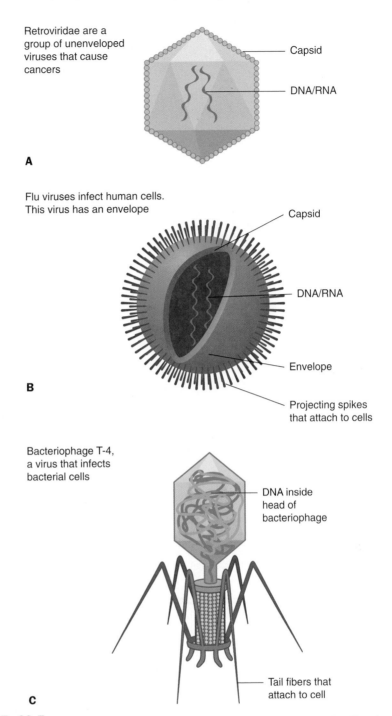

Retroviridae are a group of unenveloped viruses that cause cancers

Capsid

DNA/RNA

A

Flu viruses infect human cells. This virus has an envelope

Capsid

DNA/RNA

Envelope

Projecting spikes that attach to cells

B

Bacteriophage T-4, a virus that infects bacterial cells

DNA inside head of bacteriophage

Tail fibers that attach to cell

C

FIGURE 29-7 Viral composition. **A,** Unenveloped (capsomeres). **B,** Enveloped virus. **C,** Bacteriophage.

presence. Once the animal is infected, the tissue can be analyzed. To view the morphology of a virus an electron microscope (a very high-powered microscope) is used. The most common way to identify viruses is by their reaction with antibodies. When the human body comes into contact with a foreign substance, it makes antibodies in response to the antigen (foreign body), as shown in an experiment aimed at determining antibody formation in Figure 29-9.

Human viral diseases, such as human immunodeficiency virus (HIV), cannot be grown in laboratory animals. Although chimpanzees can be infected with one

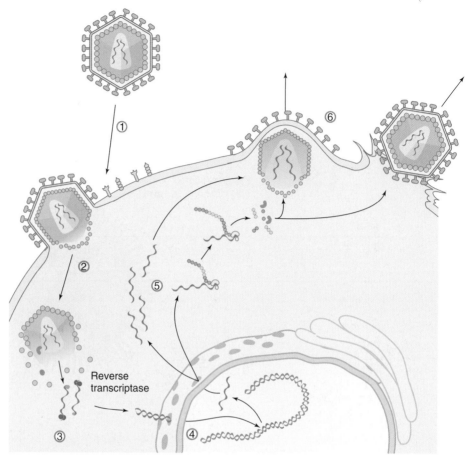

Reverse
transcriptase

① HIV virus attaches to host cell
② The capsid releases viral RNA into cytoplasm
③ The host's enzyme is used to replicate viral RNA into DNA
④ During latency period the viral DNA stays in the host cell's DNA
⑤ The virus's DNA is activated where it codes for proteins and RNA
   strands to be assembled
⑥ The newly formed viral cells either bud off or lyse out of the host
   cell releasing free HIV

FIGURE 29-8 Human immunodeficiency virus replication. Diagram of the replication process of viruses. Each component is made independently inside the host cell. All materials are made from the host cell. Once the parts are made, they are assembled.

FIGURE 29-9 Determination of antibody formation: antibody test using bacteriophages. This proves whether a person has formed antibodies against a certain antigen. **A,** A sample of blood (containing an antibody, O) is placed in a beaker. To this, two components are added: a complement (color when bound to antigen and antibody) and the antigen (A) to the antibody. **B,** The result would be that O and A bind together resulting in a color that makes this test positive. **C,** A sample of blood (with no antibody) is placed in a beaker. To this the two components are added. The result in this case is negative because there is no antibody present to complete the color change. Thus the blood has not come into contact with that specific antigen before.

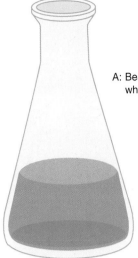

A: Beaker with solution that turns color when antigens are introduced

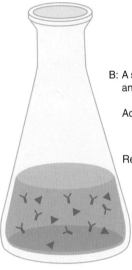

B: A sample of blood (containing antibodies) is placed in beaker

Add 1. Antigen
     2. Compound that turns color when/ if antigen binds to antibodies

Result: Positive: As the antigens ▲ bind to antibodies Y the solution turns color

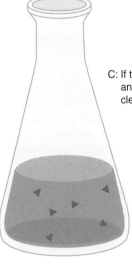

C: If the sample of blood does not contain any antibodies, the solution will remain clear, indicating a negative test

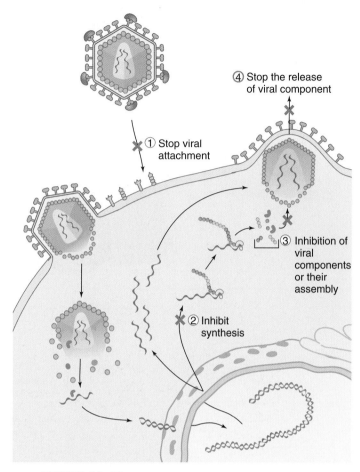

FIGURE 29-10 The four ways to stop viral infections.

strain of HIV, they do not show any symptoms. Thus viruses such as HIV are more difficult to learn about or perform tests on in the laboratory.

Another problem with the study of viruses is that viruses are made of the same components as their host. This means that they are more difficult to kill because the antibiotic will kill the healthy cells too, although researchers have discovered that viruses can be manipulated to work for them rather than against them. Examples of well-known viral diseases include the following:

Virus	Human Disease
Herpesvirus	Herpes
HIV retrovirus	Acquired immunodeficiency syndrome
HPV	Human papillomavirus
Poliovirus	Polio
Poxvirus	Chickenpox
Rabies virus	Rabies
Rhinovirus	Common cold

HOW VIRAL INFECTIONS ARE STOPPED

Many viral infections can be halted or delayed with the use of a variety of medications. Although more is being discovered concerning viruses, only a handful of agents currently are being used to treat various conditions caused by viruses. Each drug must be specific in its mechanism of action to lessen the adverse effects on normal human cells. The antivirals can succeed through one of four main mechanisms of action in overcoming viral synthesis and eventual spread. These mechanisms are shown in Figure 29-10 and are listed in Box 29-2. Most

BOX 29-2 METHODS OF VIRAL INHIBITION

1. Inhibit the ability of the virus to attach to the host cell. If an antibody can be made to fit the viral coating, then it may be possible to inhibit the attachment of the virion to a host cell.
2. Inhibit replication by suppressing synthesis of viral DNA/RNA. By interjecting an antiviral agent that attaches itself to the DNA of the host cell, it may disrupt the replication process that codes for important proteins and enzymes used by the virion. Other components include disruption of specific nucleic acids, DNA polymerase, and other critical enzymes necessary to the formation of viral DNA/RNA strands.
3. Inhibit the ability of the virus to assemble itself properly. If protein synthesis is disrupted, the virion may not be able to build a necessary component that is needed to continue infecting new hosts.
4. Inhibit the ability of the virus to break out of the host cell. If the assembly process is disrupted or altered, it may be possible to inhibit the virion from assembling its components in the proper order or manner. This faulty virion cannot attach itself to the cell wall of the host to move out of the cell where it can continue to reinfect new host cells.

agents are aimed at disruption of the DNA of the virus or a closely related component of the newly synthesized DNA viral strand. Drugs such as zidovudine cause inhibition of the viral replication of HIV. This drug moves into the DNA, where it halts continued synthesis of new viral DNA. Other agents, such as acyclovir, inhibit viral DNA polymerase, ultimately halting the synthesis of new viral DNA; acyclovir is used against herpes simplex and varicella-zoster viruses. Nonnucleoside reverse transcriptase inhibitors cause the premature termination of the growing viral DNA strand by interfering with specific enzymes of the virus.

USING VIRUSES TO FIGHT DISEASE

One of the most studied types of viruses is the bacteriophage. These viruses can be loaded with a vaccine and then used to immunize human beings. For example, by removing the DNA inside the capsid (head) of the bacteriophage, a non–disease-causing strain of poxvirus can be inserted. The virus then is injected into the human bloodstream, where the virus vaccine can attach easily to human cells and stimulate immunity to the poxvirus.

DO YOU REMEMBER THESE KEY POINTS?

- The names of the five kingdoms
- How the kingdoms are broken down
- Who was responsible for the theory of evolution
- The contributions of Louis Pasteur to microbiology
- How the golden age of microbiology changed history
- The characteristics of and differences between animal, plant, and bacterial cells
- The components of an animal cell and their functions
- The types of diseases/conditions spread by the organisms discussed in this chapter

- What morphological characteristics are used to distinguish between organisms
- The importance of the Gram stain in determining morphology of bacteria
- The composition of bacterial cell walls and how antibiotics affect them
- The types of environments in which bacteria can be found
- The differences between microorganisms and viruses
- How viruses replicate
- How viruses can be stopped from replicating and spreading
- The components of viruses

MULTIPLE CHOICE QUESTIONS

1. Charles Darwin is best known for _____.
  A. Evolution
  B. Genetics
  C. Taxonomy
  D. Classification

2. Of the groups of organisms listed, which one is not eukaryotic?
  A. Fungi
  B. Bacteria
  C. Animalia
  D. Plants

3. Of the five-kingdom classification system, which of those listed include bacteria?
  A. Plantae
  B. Animalia
  C. Protista
  D. Monera

4. Viruses can contain which of the following types of nucleic acids?
  A. Double-stranded DNA
  B. Single-stranded DNA
  C. Double- or single-stranded RNA
  D. All of the above

5. Which of the microbes listed is(are) part of a person's "normal flora"?
  A. *Candida albicans*
  B. *Borrelia burgdorferi*
  C. *Streptococcus pyogenes*
  D. Both A and C

6. Alexander Fleming is best known for the _____.
  A. Discovery of viruses
  B. Discovery of penicillin
  C. Classification of drugs
  D. Scientific method

7. The disease malaria is caused by the microbe _____.
  A. *Entamoeba histolytica*
  B. *Plasmodium vivax*
  C. *Trichomonas vaginalis*
  D. *Balantidium coli*

8. The function of the Golgi complex is to _____.
  A. Transport proteins through the cell membrane
  B. Tag proteins to aid them to reach their final destination
  C. Produce adenosine triphosphate; the power source for the cell
  D. Produce proteins

9. The main types of locomotion of protozoa are _____.
  A. Pseudopods
  B. Flagella
  C. Cilia
  D. All of the above

10. Some microbes can resist antibiotics because of specific enzymes that are called _____.
  A. Antimicrobials
  B. Penicillinase
  C. Antienzymes
  D. Antibiotics

TRUE/FALSE If the statement is false, then change it to make it true.

_____ **1.** Only animals can catch viruses.

_____ **2.** All cells have the same components.

_____ **3.** The mitochondria within each cell are analogous to a powerhouse.

_____ **4.** Gram-negative bacteria have a thicker layer of polypeptide bonds.

_____ **5.** The primary difference between smooth endoplasmic reticulum (ER) and rough ER is the absence of ribosomes on smooth ER.

_____ **6.** Protists include algae, water molds, and amebae.

_____ **7.** Plants use chloroplasts for the same purpose that animals use mitochondria.

_____ **8.** Spontaneous generation was believed to explain how life begins.

_____ **9.** Cocci, bacilli, and spirilla are the three main morphologies of bacteria.

_____ **10.** Animal and plant cells multiply by binary fission.

TECHNICIAN'S CORNER

Following the steps outlined in the workbook, perform a Gram stain of the cheek cells from inside your mouth. Locate and describe the morphology of the cells.

Compare your cells to those bacterial cells listed in the lab book.
To learn more about microbiology check out this website:
www.cellsalive.com

BIBLIOGRAPHY

Campbell N, Reece J: *Biology,* ed 7, Redwood City, Calif, 2004, Benjamin Cummings.

Greulach V, Chiappetta V: *Biology: The science of life,* Morristown, NJ, 1977, Silver Burdett.

Malarkey LM, McMorrow ME: *Nurse's manual of laboratory tests and diagnostic procedures,* ed 2, Philadelphia, 2000, Saunders.

Tortora G, Funke BR, Case CL: *Microbiology: an introduction,* ed 8, Redwood City, Calif, 2003, Benjamin Cummings.

Voet D, Voet J: *Biochemistry,* ed 3, New York, 2004, Wiley.

Chemistry

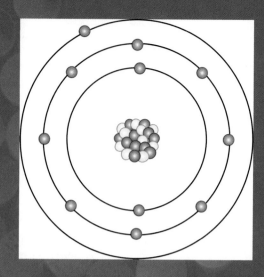

Objectives

UPON COMPLETING THIS CHAPTER, YOU SHOULD BE ABLE TO DO THE FOLLOWING:

- Name the 10 basic ions necessary for proper electrolyte balance and what each one contributes to the body.

- Define the terms *atom, molecule, proton, neutron,* and *electron.*

- Distinguish between ionic and covalent bonds.

- List the types of molecules that are formed from various nucleic acids.

- List the 20 amino acids necessary in a balanced diet.

- Distinguish between acids and bases.

- Distinguish between anions and cations.

- Describe how sodium bicarbonate balances pH.

- Explain how chemistry plays an important part in the action and reactions of drugs.

- Describe how enzymes and proteins are used in the body.

- Define the terms *inorganic* and *organic* as related to chemistry, giving an example of each.

- Define metabolism in terms of anabolism and catabolism.

AT FIRST, IT MAY NOT SEEM as though chemistry has much to do with the health care field. However, this is not true. Chemistry is at the heart of the discovery of new medicines and treatments and the understanding of chemical interactions in the body. For pharmacy technicians to become acquainted with the basic chemical reactions and interactions in the body is important. The goal of this chapter is to present the basics of chemistry and answer questions concerning why drugs interact with one another and the importance of these reactions within the body system.

Parts of an Atom

Atoms are made up of smaller particles called protons (positively charged), electrons (negatively charged), and neutrons (no charge). The center of the atom, the nucleus, contains the protons and neutrons. The electrons of a specific atom orbit around the nucleus in much the same way that the planets in our solar system orbit around the sun (Figure 30-1).

The nucleus of an atom is very small. Most of the atom is empty space. Most atoms have an equal number of positively charged protons and negatively charged electrons, giving them a net charge of zero. If an atom has more or fewer electrons than protons, it becomes charged and is called an ion. The structure of each atom is determined by the number of electrons that it has in the outer orbit.

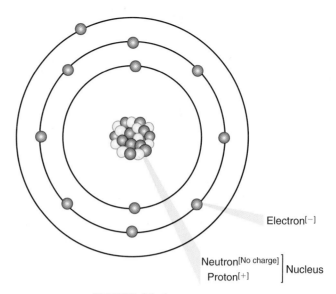

FIGURE 30-1 Electron orbit.

1	2	3	4	5	6	7	8	9	10	11	12	13	14	15	16	17	18
₁H																	₂He
₃Li	₄Be											₅B	₆C	₇N	₈O	₉F	₁₀Ne
₁₁Na	₁₂Mg											₁₃Al	₁₄Si	₁₅P	₁₆S	₁₇Cl	₁₈Ar
₁₉K	₂₀Ca	₂₁Sc	₂₂Ti	₂₃V	₂₄Cr	₂₅Mn	₂₆Fe	₂₇Co	₂₈Ni	₂₉Cu	₃₀Zn	₃₁Ga	₃₂Ge	₃₃As	₃₄Se	₃₅Br	₃₆Kr

FIGURE 30-2 Periodic table of elements. The elements K, Na, Cl, Mg, Se, and Cu are highlighted.

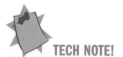

TECH NOTE!

A period refers to the row across the table, whereas a group indicates the vertical column. Each element is assigned a symbol; below the symbol is the atomic number.

Two types of bonding between atoms are ionic bonds and covalent bonds. When two atoms come into close contact with each other, the nucleus (positively charged) of the first atom is attracted to the electrons (negatively charged) of the other atom, and vice versa. These two atoms can exchange or transfer electrons, forming ionic bonds, or they can share the electrons, forming covalent bonds. Covalent bonds are stronger than ionic bonds because the electrons are held in a tighter arrangement. The joining of two or more different types of atoms can create different molecules, such as carbohydrates (sugars), lipids (fats), proteins (meat), and nucleic acids (DNA). Sometimes, when two oppositely charged ions come together, such as sodium (Na^+) and chloride (Cl^-), some of their charges are taken away because they form an ionic bond (NaCl). Not all charges are dropped when ions combine; in many cases there are charges left over, which usually are indicated at the right of the chemical name with a plus or minus sign.

The periodic table of elements has all of the known elements strategically placed according to their properties (Figure 30-2). The table has seven horizontal rows of elements. All of the elements are placed in a specific box next to other elements that are closely related to them; for example, across the top of the table are numbers 1 to 8. Looking down the first column of the chart, there are three important alkali metals: lithium, sodium, and potassium. They are in the same

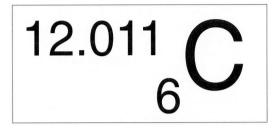

FIGURE 30-3 Carbon, represented by the letter *C.* Below the element is the atomic number. Above is the atomic weight.

column because of their similarities. They have one electron in their outer shell, and they are white, soft, and very reactive metals.

Elements also are listed in order based on the chemical property and size. As you can see, there are numbers assigned to each element. In Figure 30-3, carbon is the sixth element on the table, indicated with the number 6. Above the number 6 is 12.011, indicating the weight of the atom. The entire periodic table of elements categorizes elements by their elemental properties such as weight and types of bonds that they form. This makes it easier to learn their properties. Although the table lists each element by itself, in nature they are not necessarily found by themselves. For instance, the metal sodium by itself is highly reactive and would explode if it came into contact with oxygen. The same can be said of chloride. Even as a solid, chloride gives off deadly vapors when isolated. However, if you combine these two elements, you have NaCl, or sodium chloride (i.e., table salt). NaCl is also used in the hospital intravenous bags into which antibiotics and other medications are placed for administration to patients. Highlighted within the periodic table (Figure 30-2) are the elements most used in the pharmacy. These are also elements contained in the body that are measured in laboratory blood tests.

Charges are grouped in pairs: any excess of electrons appears as a − (negative sign), whereas any deficiency of electrons appears as a + (positive sign). For example, in a molecule of water, each hydrogen atom has one electron that can be shared or bonded. Oxygen has eight electrons. This number indicates the total number of electrons in oxygen. Oxygen has two electrons in its inner shell and six in its outer shell. Oxygen is able to accept another two electrons in its outer shell. When joined with two hydrogen molecules, there is no overall charge (neutral), as shown in Figure 30-4.

Some common atoms form tight bonds with other atoms to make substances such as water (oxygen and hydrogen) and common table salt (sodium chloride). Table 30-1 lists some of these compounds.

Molecules

Two distinct areas of study in chemistry are inorganic chemistry and organic chemistry. Inorganic chemistry is the study of all types of molecules that do not contain carbon atoms. Examples include some metals and gases such as iron (Fe) and oxygen (O). Together, the molecule FeO_2 makes ferric oxide, known as rust. Organic chemistry is the study of substances that contain carbon as one of the components of a molecule. What contains the most important carbon-based substances? The human body.

ENZYME ACTIVATORS AND INHIBITORS

Enzymes are proteins that can regulate the speed of reactions. They can speed up an action or inhibit (stop) reactions from taking place. They can be inactive

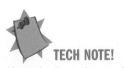

TECH NOTE!

If you look up the method of action of a specific drug and you read "unknown," it is because science still cannot answer the question of precisely how some drugs work in the human body.

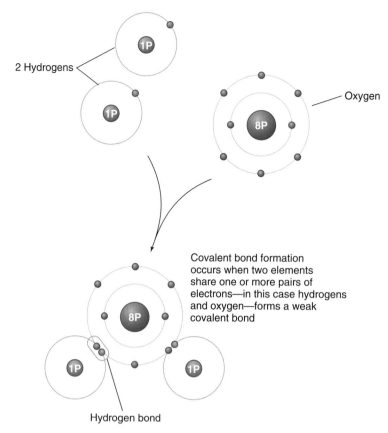

2 Hydrogens

Oxygen

Covalent bond formation occurs when two elements share one or more pairs of electrons—in this case hydrogens and oxygen—forms a weak covalent bond

Hydrogen bond

FIGURE 30-4 Water molecule formation. Water is one of the most important compounds on earth. Water composes approximately 65% to 75% of all living cells.

TABLE 30-1 Chemical Charges of Compounds

Substance	Positive charge	Negative charge	Chemical symbol
Acetate	2 C^{+4}, 3 H	O$_2^{-2}$	C$_2$H$_3$O$_2^-$
Ammonia	3 H	N^{-3}	NH$_3$
Bicarbonate	H$^+$, C^{+4}	O$_3^{-2}$	HCO$_3^-$
Ferrous sulfate	Fe^{+2}, S^{+4}	O$_4^{-2}$	FeSO$_4^-$
Hydrochloric acid	H$^+$	Cl$^-$	HCl
Magnesium hydroxide	Mg^{+2}, H	O^{-2}	MgOH
Potassium chloride	K$^+$	Cl$^-$	KCl
Potassium phosphate	K$^+$, P^{+4}	O$_4^{-2}$	KPO$_4^{-3}$
Sodium bicarbonate	Na$^+$, H$^+$, C^{+4}	O$_3^{-2}$	NaHCO$_3$
Sodium chloride	Na$^+$	Cl$^-$	NaCl
Water	2 H	O^{-2}	H$_2$O

TECH NOTE!

Hydrogen peroxide (H$_2$O$_2$) is used as an antiseptic. Have you poured hydrogen peroxide over an open wound? When it comes into contact with an enzyme (called catalase) present in living tissue, a reaction occurs that causes bubbles of oxygen to form. The oxygen helps remove foreign tissue debris.

until they come into contact with elements (called ions). For example, elements or ions such as chloride, zinc, iron, and magnesium can serve as activators of the digestive enzyme pepsin. Once pepsin is activated, it helps break down food to be absorbed by the intestines. Another enzymatic reaction is the reaction of hydrogen peroxide on a cut or scrape. Pharmacology includes the study of these types of reactions. An example of an inhibitory reaction occurs when a drug such as famotidine (Pepcid), which is taken for gastric secretion, inhibits specific histamine receptors. The result is that stomach acids are decreased.

Have you ever wondered how the human body can produce energy and perform other functions so quickly? It is because of catalysts (enzymes). These are protein molecules that speed up reactions by lowering the amount of energy needed to complete the reaction. Enzymatic reactions can speed up a reaction pathway.

Metabolism: Anabolism and Catabolism

The foods we eat must be broken down into usable molecules (catabolism) and built up into other new useful molecules (anabolism). Metabolism is comprised of all the processes that occur within the body are broken down into a series of steps or cycles. This cycle is the step-by-step process of the transformation of molecules, such as fatty acids, amino acids, and carbohydrates, into other molecules necessary to the body. A series of reactions are possible because of the interactions between ions and enzymatic reactions. This allows the body to break down and/or build up substances as needed. Metabolism is necessary for the control of hormones, protein synthesis, pH (acid/base), lipid (fat) levels, glucose (sugar) levels, and more. This area of study is called biochemistry and plays an important role in the study of pharmacology.

The human body needs certain nutrients daily. These are essential for proper growth and overall maintenance of the body. Diagnostic blood tests can reveal to a doctor and a pharmacist (when done in a hospital) any deficiencies of essential nutrients that may affect the health of a patient. Laboratory tests may help ensure that the proper dosage of medication and/or replacement therapy is given.

A pharmacist will look for specific values depending on the type of medication that the patient is taking. For instance, when a patient is receiving an aminoglycoside, such as gentamicin (antiinfective), the pharmacist will have clearance levels drawn (taken by blood sample) at certain times after the gentamicin has been administered intravenously. The results will tell the pharmacist how fast the patient's body is clearing the drug (excretion). The condition of the patient's kidneys affects the amount of drug that should be given. If a patient is older, he or she naturally will have a decrease in drug clearance. If an aminoglycoside is dosed at too high a level, it can build up in the kidneys. This adds an additional strain on the body system. Patients who may be at high risk are those with kidney failure, older adults, children, and those with an existing medical problem.

ELECTROLYTE REPLACEMENT

Electrolyte levels are another type of laboratory test result that pharmacists will receive in the pharmacy daily. Certain patients must be receiving 1-L intravenous bags that contain needed electrolytes or may require nutritional supplements by intraveneous methods, commonly known as hyperalimentation, or hyperal. These types of large-volume IVs are given as a total parenteral nutrition (administered through a large vein) or peripheral parenteral nutrition (given through a smaller vein; see Chapter 11). An intravenous bag is hung daily as a nutritional supplement if the patient cannot eat food, is healing from a stomach or intestine operation, or is about to undergo surgery to the stomach or intestines. Ingredients of a hyperalimentation bag include electrolyte, vitamin, and mineral replacement. This preparation is precalculated by the pharmacist after laboratory values have been sent to pharmacy.

In either case, the technician may be responsible for pulling the necessary electrolyte and/or parenteral medications to be placed in the hyperalimentation bag and for preparation of the bag. The size of the bags can range anywhere from 1 L up to 3 L. Regardless of the size of the hyperalimentation bag or the dosing, a new bag must be hung daily to ensure sterility. Electrolyte replacement consists of the ions potassium, sodium, chloride, phosphate, and magnesium. In addition, most hyperalimentation bags include an assortment of vitamins added daily. A standard preformulated hyperalimentation bag usually is given to patients until their laboratory results are received by the pharmacy. Except for the bag on the first day, each daily bag of hyperalimentation usually is tailor-made to the patient's specific needs.

Two types of ions are cations (those with a positive charge) and anions (those with a negative charge). Many cations and anions form bonds between one another, forming various molecules such as proteins, amino acids, and many different types of enzymes. Remember, enzymes are proteins that regulate reactions. What follows is a closer look at the role some of these important ions have in the human body:

K: Potassium is found mostly inside the cell, as opposed to the outside (extracellular fluid) where many other ions are found. Potassium is the principal cation of intracellular fluid and is necessary for homeostasis. Potassium plays a major role in the maintenance of muscles, such as the heart, and nerve impulses. A deficiency can cause a wide range of side effects, including cardiac irregularities. An excess of potassium can cause impaired conduction of heat.

Na: Sodium is a key component in the transfer of water between areas of the body and is found mostly in the extracellular fluid of the body. Sodium is the most abundant cation in extracellular fluid.

Cl: Chloride is found inside and outside the cells of the body. Chloride has a negative charge, which makes it an anion. Chloride is the most abundant anion in extracellular fluid. It also contributes to osmotic pressure. The combination of sodium (cation) and chloride (anion) makes up more than 65% of the acidic ions of the blood. Hydrogen and chloride (HCl) is another important combination in the body that works to help break down food in the stomach. Chloride is also important for the health of the heart muscle.

Mg: Magnesium is found in bones and the soft tissues of the body. Magnesium is used in the synthesis of adenosine triphosphate (ATP) and the release of energy from ATP. Magnesium plays a part in the overall maintenance of muscles of the heart and skeletal system and of the tissues of the nervous system. Magnesium is also a component in combination with other ions that helps proper bone growth.

Cu: Copper is a metal that the body uses in minute amounts. This ion helps keep the blood vessels, hair, and skin in a healthy state. Copper also is believed to play a role, along with iron, as a component of hemoglobin. Copper deficiency can affect the number of white blood cells. Too much copper can cause diarrhea, liver destruction, and even death.

P: Phosphorus is found mainly in the bones. Phosphorus participates in the making of certain enzymes, including ATP. This important enzyme is responsible for supplying the energy that human cells require. Phosphorus is always found in combination with alkalies.

Fe: When you think of iron, you may think of cast iron or you may think of good, healthy blood. The iron in the body is the same type of iron used in construction but in very small amounts. Iron is necessary to help hemoglobin bind to oxygen molecules as we breathe. If iron is deficient, anemia (iron deficiency anemia) may result. The amount of hemoglobin decreases, as well as the amount of oxygen carried by the blood. Iron is fat-soluble. Therefore an excessive iron intake can cause a toxic buildup, leading to severe side effects including brain damage, coma, or even death. This is especially true in children.

Ca: Calcium is important because it helps children grow big and strong, which is why it is important for children to drink enough milk. Calcium not only helps growing children's bones but also is important as we grow older. Calcium must be activated by vitamin D to be absorbed. Calcium is necessary to keep an acid/base balance and is a factor in blood coagulation. A decrease in calcium can cause cramping or twitching of the muscles. As we age, the body decreases its production of many necessary vitamins and minerals. Some drugs increase the absorption of calcium, whereas other drugs may decrease the absorption. This is one of the details that a pharmacist looks for when giving a patient consultation. For example, tetracycline should not be taken with calcium supplements because they decrease the effectiveness of the antibiotic. Not enough calcium in the body contributes to weak bones and muscles. This is especially true in older adults. Many older citizens have osteoporosis, which is related directly to many years of calcium deficiency. Too much calcium can contribute to heart and kidney disease. In addition to proper bone growth, calcium helps the muscles by increasing electrical impulses.

Zn: Zinc is only needed in minute amounts. Zinc is a vital component of the enzyme carbonic anhydrase found in hemoglobin. This enzyme helps in the stabilization of the pH of the blood. Zinc can never stand alone, it must be in combination with other chemicals.

Mn: Manganese is another important component of enzymes active in the Krebs cycle. Manganese is needed for proper growth, reproduction, and lactation. Mangansese is found in soft tissue, bone, and muscle.

I: Iodine is necessary for the proper functioning of the thyroid gland. A shortage of iodine can lead to goiter (enlargement of the thyroid gland). Because our salt is iodized, goiter often is not seen.

ACID-BASE REACTIONS

Acid-base reactions within the body are some of the most important reactions because they can make the difference between life and death. The pH scale is a representation of the amount of hydrogen in water. pH is a logarithmic function. This means that a tenfold increase in hydrogen is represented by one unit. The pH ranges from 1 (the most acidic) to 14 (the most basic). The normal pH of a blood is 7.4. If the pH of the blood changes by 0.4, such as to 7.8 or 7.0, life would end quickly for that person. The body works hard to maintain pH at a steady 7.4 by making buffers such as sodium bicarbonate. Remember, the ions that form molecules (as described previously) drive reactions that can change pH balance.

Amino Acids

Molecules form amino acids that perform different functions (see Figure 30-5). These amino acids include neurotransmitters (see Chapter 17) and metabolic intermediates. Each one of these amino acids can form long chains by linking the amino group of one to the carboxyl group of the next.

When this linking occurs, a reaction called dehydration takes place (the loss of a water molecule). When many amino acids join together, proteins are made. The overall molecule will not look like a straight chain. Amino acid chains can range from a few strung together (micromolecules) to more than a thousand (macromolecules). Their behavior is based on their shape, size, and chemical structure.

A hemoglobin molecule has 547 individual amino acids in its four amino acid chains. If one of these amino acids is in the wrong place or missing, a person

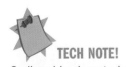

TECH NOTE!

Sodium bicarbonate is always kept on a crash cart for emergency situations, such as cardiac arrest. In cardiac arrest, the body is unable to keep the pH at 7.4 and becomes acidic (called acidosis), which can be fatal. Sodium bicarbonate is injected into the bloodstream where it can stabilize the blood pH.

The R groups represent the specific amino acid attached

FIGURE 30-5 Amino acid structure.

may have sickle cell anemia. Amino acids play an important role in everyday life because they are the components of proteins, many of which are enzymes. Enzymes are necessary for reactions to occur. Twenty main amino acids make up almost every protein known in the animal kingdom. They also make up many nutrients that the human body needs. The rings (called benzene rings) within amino acids (Figure 30-6) are a shortcut representation of a specific chemical arrangement as shown. Each corner of the ring represents a carbon atom and its adjoining hydrogen atom. The way in which the body breaks down various amino acids allows the body to produce energy to run bodily functions, such as moving about, working, and playing.

Mitochondria are the powerhouses of the human body; they produce power much the same way that a hydroelectric plant produces energy with the use of turbines and generators. The mitochondria (see Chapter 29) are contained within human cells and produce much of the power we use.

For instance, alanine, cysteine, glycine, serine, and threonine are turned into pyruvate. Pyruvate then enters the mitochondria (the cellular powerhouse). Pyruvate then is converted many times with the end result of three molecules of ATP, which powers the metabolism of the body with further reactions. ATP is essential for life, as are many other complex molecules.

The human body is composed of millions of molecules that form a complex series of actions and reactions within the body and with outside influences. Some of these influences are the food we eat, drugs we take, ambient temperature, stress, and even the air we breathe. The complexity of the human body is so great, researchers have only scratched the surface of how the body system works. Chemical reactions make life happen; thus the types of bonds, charges, reactions, and molecules formed are important in understanding life and how it relates to disease and other effects.

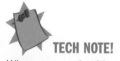

TECH NOTE!

When you work with certain chemicals, you will see the term *millimoles*. This is where the term comes from: 1 millimole is equal to 1/1000 mole. Phosphate is written in millimoles; the abbreviation is mM.

Amino acid base	R-side chain
COO^- $H-C-R$ NH_3	R-side chain
Basic Amino Acids	
Arginine	$-H_2C-H_2C-H_2C-NH$ $H_2^+N=C$ H_2N
Lysine	$-(H_2C)_3-H_2C-NH_3$
Histidine	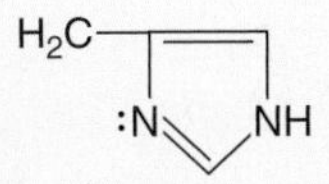 H_2C ... :N ... NH
Amino Acids with Aromatic Rings	
Phenylalanine	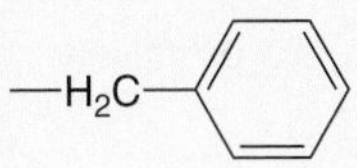 $-H_2C-$ (benzene ring)
Tyrosine	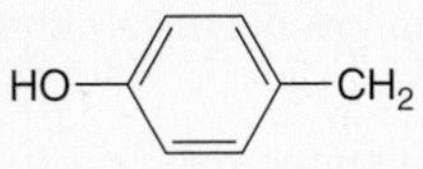 $HO-$ (ring) $-CH_2$
Tryptophan	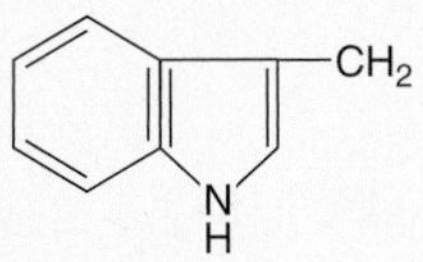 (indole ring) $-CH_2$
Acidic Amino Acids and their Amides	
Aspartic Acid	$-H_2C-COO^-$
Asparagine	$-H_2C-C-NH_2$ $\parallel$ O
Glutamic acid	$-H_2C-H_2C-COO^-$
Glutamine	$-H_2C-H_2C-C-NH_2$ $\parallel$ O

Amino acid	R-side chain
Amino Acids with Aliphatic R-Groups	
Glycine	$-H$
Alanine	$-CH_3$
Valine	$-H$ $\begin{array}{l}CH_3\\CH_3\end{array}$
Leucine	$-H_2C-HC$ $\begin{array}{l}CH_3\\CH_3\end{array}$
Isoleucine	$-HC$ $\begin{array}{l}H_2C-CH_3\\CH_3\end{array}$
Non-Aromatic Amino Acids with Hydroxyl R-Groups	
Serine	$-H_2C-OH$
Threonine	$-HC$ $\begin{array}{l}CH_3\\OH\end{array}$
Amino Acid with Sulfur-Containing R-Groups	
Cysteine	$-H_2C-SH$
Methionine	$-H_2C-CH_2$ S CH_3
Imino Acids	
Proline	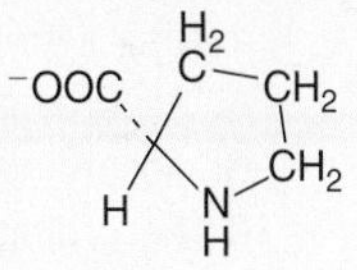 ^-OOC $\begin{array}{l}H_2\\C-CH_2\\CH_2\end{array}$ N ... H N ... H

FIGURE 30-6 Essential amino acids for human life. They are the basis for proteins which are responsible for normal body functions.

DO YOU
REMEMBER THESE
KEY POINTS?

- The major chemical elements that are essential to human beings
- The difference between ionic and covalent bonds
- The difference between an anion and a cation
- What makes up an element
- What makes up a molecule
- What an enzyme is and the importance of enzymatic reactions
- The measurements used in chemistry and in pharmacy
- The pH of the blood that is necessary for human life
- What makes a base or an acid

**MULTIPLE
CHOICE
QUESTIONS**

1. Organic chemistry is the study of _____.
   A. Metals
   B. Carbon-based matter
   C. Water
   D. All of the above

2. Which of the following statements is true concerning the parts of an atom?
   A. Protons are negatively charged, electrons are positively charged, and neutrons are neutral in charge
   B. Neutrons are negatively charged, electrons are positively charged, and protons are neutral in charge
   C. Protons are positively charged, neutrons are negatively charged, and electrons are neutral in charge
   D. Protons are positively charged, electrons are negatively charged, and neutrons are neutral in charge

3. Which of the following molecules is not essential to life?
   A. Carbohydrates
   B. Lipids
   C. Proteins
   D. All are important

4. The elements in the periodic table of elements are listed in order of all of the following criteria except _____.
   A. According to properties and number of protons
   B. According to size
   C. According to their shapes
   D. According to weight of the atoms

5. Which of the chemicals listed has no charge when combined into a compound?
   A. Sodium chloride   C. Ferrous sulfate
   B. Sodium bicarbonate   D. Both A and B

6. The best definition of the distinction between organic and inorganic chemistry is
   _____.
   A. Organic is about people, whereas inorganic is about all other life
   B. Organic is about carbon, whereas inorganic is not
   C. Organic is about human beings, whereas inorganic is about bacterial components
   D. Organic explains reactions, whereas inorganic does not

7. Of the elements listed, which is not monitored by the pharmacy when preparing hyperalimentation bags for patients?
   A. Potassium   C. Magnesium
   B. Sodium   D. Hydrogen

8. Which chemicals listed is (are) a component of the enzyme adenosine triphosphate?
   A. Fe   C. P
   B. K   D. Both B and C

9. A blood pH of 7.9 is considered _____.

    A. Acidic   C. Normal

    B. Basic   D. Buffered

10. Pyruvate is a key component is the making of _____.

    A. Amino acids   C. The citric acid cycle

    B. Sugar   D. ATP

TRUE/FALSE   **If the statement is false, then change it to make it true.**

_____ **1.** Proteins are made up of amino acids.

_____ **2.** Dehydration is the loss of a water molecule when amino acids combine.

_____ **3.** Sodium chloride is a buffer.

_____ **4.** Iron and zinc play key roles in the hemoglobin count of blood.

_____ **5.** A peripheral parenteral nutrition may be ordered for a person who is unable to eat.

_____ **6.** Most intravenous solutions are placed into isotonic solutions such as NaCl.

_____ **7.** Anions are positive, whereas cations are negative.

_____ **8.** Enzymes always make reactions move forward.

_____ **9.** Metabolism is the making of molecules.

_____ **10.** Ionic and covalent refer to the two types of bonds that atoms form.

TECHNICIAN'S CORNER

A customer comes into the pharmacy to get a prescription for ferrous sulfate tablets filled. She is taking the following drugs:

Tetracycline

Milk of magnesia

Cimetidine

The pharmacist will give a consultation to the patient, letting her know whether there is any problem, but you want to know for yourself whether there is any contraindication. What, if any, interactions are there between ferrous sulfate and the patient's current medications?

Look up the answer in the *Drug Facts and Comparisons*.

Starting Your Career as a Pharmacy Technician

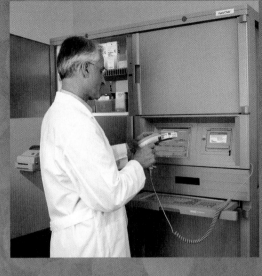

Review for the PTCB Examination

T HE FOLLOWING PRACTICE EXAM IS formatted in the same fashion as the PTCB exam with multiple choice questions (A, B, C, or D). Most of the questions are in the text, although the examination may ask questions that are geared more toward technicians who have worked in pharmacy for some time.

Section I: Assisting the Pharmacist and Other Duties

Section I of the PTCB practice exam includes assisting the pharmacist in serving patients and is 64% of the questions asked on the exam. This includes taking in new prescriptions, assisting the pharmacist, record keeping, and preparing controlled substances for delivery. Other tasks include understanding formulary, preparing and/or repackaging medications, calibrating equipment, and calculations. The first 80 questions cover these types of questions that may be asked on the exam.

1. When a prescription inhaler is dispensed, how often should a patient package insert be given to the patient?
   A. Only if the patient asks for one
   B. The first time the prescription is filled
   C. Every time the prescription is filled
   D. Every 6 months

2. Which of the following DEA numbers is correct for Dr. Paul J. Hanson?
   A. AH 1234575
   B. PH 1234567
   C. APH 8494783
   D. BH 1234631

3. A patient requests valid refills of a rabeprazole and albuterol inhaler. Which two medications should be filled?
   A. Accolate and Alupent
   B. Atenolol and Proventil
   C. Tapazole and Serevent
   D. Aciphex and Ventolin

4. Trace elements are used in the following solutions _____.
   A. Antibiotics
   B. Insulin drips
   C. Sterile water
   D. TPNs

5. Which of the following agents are sympathomimetic decongestants?
   A. Pseudoephedrine
   B. Benzonatate
   C. Metaproternol
   D. None of the above

6. A prescription with directions to instill iii qtts OS qod would require the label to read _____.
   A. Inject 3 mL into left side every day
   B. Instill three drops into the eyes twice daily
   C. Instill three drops into the left eye every other day
   D. Instill three drops into both eyes every other day

7. A prescription for APAP #4 contains how much codeine?
   A. 7.5 mg
   B. 15 mg
   C. 30 mg
   D. 60 mg

8. Which of the drugs listed below is not a cephalosporin?
   A. Ceftriaxone
   B. Zinacef
   C. Clarithromycin
   D. Cefazolin

9. Gentamicin can be given in which forms?
   A. Intravenous and ophthalmic
   B. Intravenous and orally
   C. Orally and rectally
   D. Orally and topically

10. How many doses of Zinacef 500 mg can be prepared from 10 gm bulk vial?
    A. 20 doses
    B. 50 doses
    C. 100 doses
    D. 200 doses

11. Estraderm is available in which type of dosage form?
    A. Oral tablets
    B. Implant
    C. Vaginal ring
    D. Topical patch

12. A prescription is written for Penicillin Vee K susp 500 mg PO qid for 10 days. What volume of a 250 mg/5 mL suspension will need to be dispensed to fill the order for 10 days?
    A. 100 mL
    B. 400 mL
    C. 500 mL
    D. 1000 mL

13. What volume of a 2% erythromycin solution can be made from 15 g of erythromycin powder?
    A. 250 mL
    B. 500 mL
    C. 750 mL
    D. 900 mL

14. You receive an order for 10 mEq of magnesium sulfate to be added to a TPN. You have a 50-mL vial of 4 mEq/mL of magnesium sulfate in stock. How much do you need to inject into the TPN?
    A. 1 mL
    B. 2.5 mL
    C. 5 mL
    D. 50 mL

15. If you have a 70% dextrose solution, how many grams are in 50 mL of solution?
    A. 5 mg
    B. 5 g
    C. 35 mg
    D. 35 g

16. Which of the following drugs needs to be prepared in a laminar horizontal flow hood?
    A. Nebcin
    B. Septra
    C. Cytoxan
    D. A and B

17. Of the drugs listed below, which one is not indicated to lower cholesterol?
    A. Pravachol
    B. Zaroxolyn
    C. Lipitor
    D. Zocor

18. Which auxiliary label(s) would need to be attached to the drug Orap?
    A. Do not take if you are breast-feeding
    B. Do not take with grapefruit juice
    C. Stay out of the sunlight
    D. Both A and B

19. The drug Prilosec is classified as a(n) _____.
    A. H_2 blocker
    B. NSAID
    C. Beta-blocker
    D. Proton pump inhibitor

20. The four middle numbers of the NDC represent _____.
   A. Package size
   B. Manufacturer
   C. The product, strength, and dosage form
   D. The package size, manufacturer, and dosage form

21. A prescription is given to you for a medication which has the following sig: Take I tab sl prn. This translates into _____.
   A. Take one tablet sublingually daily for pain
   B. Take one tablet as directed
   C. Take one tablet sublingually as needed
   D. Take one tablet at bedtime as needed for pain

22. The type of measuring device used to measure out 2.5 mL of solution would be _____.
   A. A 1-mL oral dropper
   B. A 5-mL teaspoon
   C. A 20-mL oral dose syringe
   D. A 10-mL oral dose syringe

23. When insulin is added to a TPN, which type is used?
   A. Lente
   B. Ultra Lente
   C. Regular
   D. All of the above

24. Syrup of ipecac is indicated for what type of result?
   A. Emesis
   B. Dilute poisons
   C. Add flavor to children's medications
   D. Antihistamine

25. A prescription is ordered for clindamycin suspension. You have 75 mg/5 mL in stock. How many milliliters are needed for a 300-mg dose for 7 days?
   A. 70 mL
   B. 140 mL
   C. 150 mL
   D. 450 mL

26. You have a vial of heparin 20,000 units/mL. How many milliliters are needed for a 12,500-unit dose?
   A. 0.025 mL
   B. 0.265 mL
   C. 0.625 mL
   D. 0.1 mL

27. The Roman numeral CL is equivalent to _____.
   A. 1050
   B. 150
   C. 50
   D. None of the above

28. How many ounces are contained in 1 pt?
   A. 8 oz
   B. 12 oz
   C. 16 oz
   D. 24 oz

29. Which of the following drugs is not a laxative?
   A. Metamucil
   B. Colace
   C. Bisacodyl
   D. Imodium

30. Which of the following drugs requires an auxiliary label stating that "This drug may cause discoloration of the urine"?
    A. Septra
    D. Sinemet
    C. Doxycycline
    D. Pyridium

31. How many grams of 0.45% normal saline and 5% dextrose are in a 1-L bag of IV solution?
    A. 4.5 g of 0.45% NS; 5.0 g of 5% dextrose
    B. 4.5 g of 0.45% NS; 50 g of 5% dextrose
    C. 0.45 g of 0.45% NS; 0.5 g of 5% dextrose
    D. None of the above

32. A prescription order for neomycin 0.75 g PO bid × 30 days is submitted. In stock you have 500-mg tablets. How many tablets will the patient use per day?
    A. ½ tablet daily
    B. 1½ tablets daily
    C. 3 tablets daily
    D. 3½ tablets daily

33. You need to prepare a dose of lidocaine 500 mg with your supply, which is a 10-mL vial of 2% lidocaine. How much should you draw up into a syringe?
    A. 2.5 mL
    B. 12.5 mL
    C. 25 mL
    D. 250 mL

34. There is an order for epinephrine 10 mg stat. How much will you draw into a syringe from a 10-mL vial of epinephrine 1:1000?
    A. 1 mL
    B. 10 mL
    C. 100 mL
    D. 1000 mL

35. A doctor prescribes his patient Vasotec 7.5 mg PO bid × 30 days. You have 5-mg tablets in stock. How many will it take to fill this script?
    A. 15 tablets
    B. 45 tablets
    C. 84 tablets
    D. 90 tablets

36. You receive an order for Demerol 20 mg IM. Your supply is Demerol 50 mg/mL. How much will you draw into a syringe?
    A. 0.64 mL
    B. 0.4 mL
    C. 4 mL
    D. 40 mL

37. Using your penicillin injectable stock of 125,000 units/mL, how many milliliters will it take to prepare 1 million units?
    A. 500 mL
    B. 125 mL
    C. 80 mL
    D. 8 mL

38. A doctor orders gentamicin 3 mg/kg/day for a 75-lb child. How many milligrams will the child receive per day? You have in stock gentamicin 80 mg/mL.
    A. 10.22 mg/day
    B. 22.5 mg/day
    C. 10.22 mg/day
    D. 102.3 mg/day

39. An oral suspension comes in 100 mg/5 mL. The doctor orders 0.25 g PO tid. How many milliliters will this patient receive daily?
    A. 0.04 mL
    B. 12.5 mL
    C. 25 mL
    D. 37.5 mL

40. You receive an order for 1500 mL of 5% dextrose over 12 hours. The drop factor is 15 gtt/mL. What will the drops be per minute on this order?
    A. 0.3 gtt/min
    B. 1.5 gtt/min
    C. 8.3 gtt/min
    D. 31.2 gtt/min

41. To prepare 500 mL of a 5% dextrose solution, you must use your available stock of 2% and 10% dextrose. How much of each will you need to prepare the order?
    A. 187 mL of 2%; 312.5 mL of 10 %
    B. 312.5 mL of 2%; 187.5 mL of 10%
    C. 340.9 mL of 2%; 159.1 of 10%; then qs with water to equal 1000 mL
    D. 250 mL of 2%; 250 mL of 10%

42. How many milliliters of 35% acetic acid must be mixed with 15% acetic acid to give 1000 mL of 10% acetic acid?
    A. 166.7 mL of 35%; 833.3 mL of 15%
    B. 833.3 mL of 35%: 166.7 mL of 15%
    C. 357.1 mL of 35%; 642.9 mL of 15%
    D. 642.9 mL of 35%; 357.1 mL of 15%

43. How many grams of drug are in 500 mL of solution if it is a 40% solution?
    A. 20 g
    B. 125 mg
    C. 200 mg
    D. 200 g

44. How many drams are in 16 oz of solution?
    A. 4 drams
    B. 80 drams
    C. 120 drams
    D. 264 drams

45. If the infusion rate of an IV is 1000 mL over 10 hours and the drop factor is 15 gtt/mL, what is the drops per minute?
    A. 2 gtt/min
    B. 20 gtt/min
    C. 22 gtt/min
    D. 25 gtt/min

46. The medication that needs to be protected from light in a special container is _____.
    A. Nitroglycerin
    B. Prozac
    C. Phenytoin
    D. Cardura

47. The amount of hydrocortisone powder needed to prepare 8 oz of 2% hydrocortisone cream is _____.
    A. 0.24 g
    B. 0.48 g
    C. 2.4 g
    D. 4.8 g

48. You receive a prescription for a 5-year-old patient for Cipro 500-mg tablets with instructions take 1 tab bid × 10 days. You would bring this to the attention of the pharmacist because _____.
 A. This medication does not come in this dosage form.
 B. The strength of drug written is very high for a child. Notify the registered pharmacist.
 C. The strength of this drug is not written for a long enough time.
 D. Nothing is wrong with this prescription.

49. KCl is an abbreviation for: _____.
 A. Sodium chloride
 B. Iodine chloride
 C. Phosphate chloride
 D. Potassium chloride

50. If a patient is allergic to penicillin and comes in with a prescription for Keflex, what should you know?
 A. The patient will have a severe allergy to this medication as well. Notify the registered pharmacist.
 B. The patient might have sensitivity to this medication as well. Notify the registered pharmacist.
 C. The patient most likely will not have an allergic reaction. Do not notify the registered pharmacist.
 D. The patient will not have an allergy to this medication. Do not notify the registered pharmacist.

51. Which of the books listed below is related most closely to the information contained in patient package inserts?
 A. *PDR*
 B. *Drug Facts and Comparisons*
 C. *Drug Topics Red Book*
 D. None of the above

52. The trade name for glyburide is _____.
 A. Phenytoin
 B. Glucophage
 C. Micronase
 D. Glucotrol

53. The trade name for fluvastatin is _____.
 A. Eulexin
 B. Mevacor
 C. Lithium
 D. Lescol

54. The drug metronidazole comes in which dosage forms?
 A. Tablets and capsules
 B. Injectable
 C. Lotion, cream, and gel
 D. All of the above

55. The drug Betagan would be used _____.
 A. In the ear
 B. In the eye
 C. On the face
 D. On an infection anywhere on the body

56. Which of the following drugs is an H$_2$ antagonist?
   A. Tums
   B. Loratadine
   C. Tagamet
   D. Milk of magnesia

57. The abbreviation *Rx* means _____.
   A. Pharmacy
   B. Drug
   C. Narcotic
   D. Prescription

58. The abbreviation *ac* means _____.
   A. At meals
   B. Before meals
   C. After meals
   D. At bedtime

59. The main indication for the drug phenytoin is _____.
   A. Anticonvulsant
   B. Antidepressant
   C. Antianxiety
   D. Diabetes

60. The main indication for the drug triamterene/HCTZ is _____.
   A. Antibiotic
   B. Antihypertensive
   C. Anticoagulant
   D. Diuretic

61. Which of the drugs listed below is an SSRI?
   A. Nabumetone
   B. Ketorolac
   C. Celexa
   D. Lopressor

62. Which drug listed below is an antiviral?
   A. Cisplatin
   B. Biaxin
   C. Zovirax
   D. Neurontin

63. Which drug listed below is not an SSRI?
   A. Elavil
   B. Prozac
   C. Zoloft
   D. Paxil

64. Extemporaneous compounding is when _____.
   A. Stock solutions are prepared
   B. When a mortar and pestle is used to mix medication
   C. When medications are made in a laminar flow hood
   D. When medications are made in a vertical flow hood

65. If nitroglycerin sl 1/200 grains was ordered, what strength would you take from the shelf to fill this order?
   A. 0.2 mg
   B. 0.3 mg
   C. 0.4 mg
   D. 0.6 mg

66. Of the following drug combinations, which would be a drug-drug interaction?
    A. Aspirin and codeine
    B. Digoxin and penicillin
    C. Coumadin and aspirin
    D. Estrogen and Mobic

67. Of the diagnostic devices listed below, which one is used for urinalysis?
    A. One Touch
    B. First Choice
    C. Glucostix
    D. Diastix

68. The term *prophylaxis* means _____.
    A. A weak immune system
    B. To treat with medications at home
    C. Preventive treatment
    D. To treat after a condition has been determined

69. The term *half-life* refers to _____.
    A. The life of a medication on the shelf
    B. The amount of time it takes a chemical to be decreased by half
    C. The amount of time it takes a chemical to begin to be effective
    D. Certain medications only last half as long in the body system

70. If a dose of medication is to be given at 0600, 1400, and 2200, the doses are given at what times?
    A. 6 AM, 4 PM, and 2 AM
    B. 6 AM, 2 PM, and 2 AM
    C. 6 AM, 4 PM, and 2:20 PM
    D. 6 AM, 2 PM, and 10 PM

71. Which of the drugs listed below is a scheduled IV drug?
    A. Codeine
    B. Oxycodone/ASA
    C. Ativan
    D. Percocet

72. Nosocomial infections are found to originate in _____.
    A. The nose
    B. Third World countries
    C. In hospitals
    D. In laboratories

73. How many milliliters are contained in $1\frac{1}{2}$ tbsp of liquid?
    A. 15 mL
    B. 22.5 mL
    C. 37.5 mL
    D. 45 mL

74. Of the solutions listed below, which ones should not be stored at 10°C?
    A. Promethazine suppositories
    B. Mannitol solution
    C. Opened antibiotics
    D. Amoxicillin suspension

75. An order of insulin is added to a TPN bag. The directions are to add 100 units of insulin NPH. You draw up 10 mL of insulin, to push it into the bag. Is there anything wrong with this scenario?
    A. Only a pharmacist can add insulin.
    B. You cannot add insulin after a TPN is made.
    C. You have added 10 times more insulin than ordered.
    D. You have not added enough insulin to the bag.

76. A prescription for a buccal tablet would be labeled _____.
  A. Place in the rectum
  B. Chew the tablet
  C. Place under the tongue
  D. Place against the inside of the check

77. A person weighing 67 kg is how many pounds?
  A. 30.5 lb
  B. 147.4 lb
  C. 134 lb
  D. None of the above

78. Cyanocobalamin is what type of vitamin?
  A. Vitamin A
  B. Vitamin B_6
  C. Vitamin K
  D. Vitamin B_{12}

79. Of the needles listed below, which is in order from smallest to largest that are used in pharmacy?
  A. 14 gauge; 16 gauge; 18 gauge; 20 gauge
  B. 27 gauge; 19 gauge; 18 gauge; 16 gauge
  C. 1 gauge; 2 gauge; 3 gauge; 4 gauge
  D. None of the above is used in pharmacy.

80. Of the following intravenous medications, which cannot be mixed with NS?
  A. Cefazolin
  B. Ampicillin
  C. Primaxin
  D. All of these can be mixed with NS.

Section II: Maintaining Medication and Inventory Control Systems

This section, which accounts for 25% of the exam, is testing your knowledge on inventory such as proper storage of medications, compounding, repackaging, how to handle recalls, and hazardous wastes. Also tested are record keeping, understanding policies and procedures, and performing quality assurance tests on compounded medications.

81. The recommended storage temperature for unopened Xalantin is _____.
  A. Room temperature
  B. 2°C to 8°C (36°F to 46°F)
  C. 15°C to 30°C (59°F to 86°F)
  D. −20°C to −10°C (−4°F to 14°F)

82. When an investigational drug expires, you should _____.
  A. Do nothing; only a pharmacist can handle investigational drugs
  B. Remove the drug from the shelf and place it in the hazardous waste bin
  C. Record the quantity and lot number, and return it to the manufacturer
  D. Record the quantity and lot number, and return to the FDA

83. Which of the following forms is needed for pharmacy to dispense controlled substances _____.
    A. Form 222
    B. Form 224
    C. Form 225
    D. Form 363

84. When unit dosing a tablet, what is the necessary labeling for each unit dose label?
    A. Trade name of drug, strength, color, expiration date
    B. Trade and generic name of drug, strength, manufacturer lot number, and expiration date
    C. Generic and trade name of drug, dosage form, strength, pharmacy lot number, and expiration date
    D. Name of drug, dosage form, color, strength, lot number, and expiration date

85. A glass compounding slab is used for _____.
    A. A hard clean surface to mix all compounding products
    B. A smooth surface to mix ointments
    C. A smooth surface to mix ointments and creams
    D. A smooth surface to mix all topical medications

86. An empty capsule number 5 will hold how many milligrams of powder?
    A. 1000 mg
    B. 500 mg
    C. 100 mg
    D. 50 mg

87. When adding weights to a Class A balance, you should use tweezers because _____.
    A. The weights are irregularly shaped and hard to pick up
    B. The tweezers have a better grip than your fingers
    C. The oils from your skin will dirty and alter the actual weights
    D. You do not need to use tweezers

88. A compounding prescription says to prepare a medication and qs solution to 100 mL. This means _____.
    A. Make enough solution to equal 100 mL
    B. Add the appropriate solution to the medication to equal 100 mL
    C. To pour off any medication over 100 mL
    D. None of the above

89. Which of the following drugs should not be stocked on an adult crash cart?
    A. Nitroglycerin patches
    B. Sodium bicarbonate PFS
    C. Valium injectable vial
    D. Atropine PFS

90. A PCA is used to _____.
    A. Administer antibiotics for children
    B. Administer analgesics
    C. Administer controlled analgesics
    D. Administer anticonvulsants

91. Lipids should be stored _____.
    A. At room temperature
    B. In the refrigerator
    C. In the freezer
    D. In a fireproof cabinet

92. When stocking shelves with new stock, you should _____.
   A. Remove all outdated stock first
   B. Rotate stock, placing the longer expiration dates to the back
   C. Place new stock in a different container next to the older stock
   D. Both A and B

93. Which of the following explanations best defines formulary?
   A. A set of rules and guidelines for pharmacy personnel
   B. A list of drugs that are approved by the pharmacy management
   C. A list of drugs that are approved by the P and T committee
   D. A set of guidelines for nurses on how to use medications

94. Which drug below is not available in the dosage form described?
   A. Heparin injectable
   B. Warfarin 2.5-mg tablets
   C. Prednisone 1 mg/mL suspension
   D. Morphine sulfate 15 mg CR tablets

95. A prescription calls for amoxicillin suspension to be compounded. What auxiliary label(s) will you place on the container?
   A. Keep refrigerated after opening
   B. Keep refrigerated; take until gone
   C. Keep refrigerated; take until gone; shake well before using
   D. Keep refrigerated; shake well before using; expiration date

96. Of the medications listed below, which one is a C-II drug?
   A. Clonazepam
   B. Valium
   C. Meperidine
   D. Lortab

97. A C-II drug can be refilled _____.
   A. As many times as the refill indicates
   B. A maximum of 5 times or within 6 months from the original order, whichever comes first
   C. Only twice
   D. A new prescription is needed for each prescription fill

98. When a drug is recalled and is considered a Class 1, this means _____.
   A. This is the lowest level used for products that may have a minor defect
   B. This is when the drug may cause serious but reversible harm
   C. This is the highest level of recall for products that could cause serious illness or may even be fatal
   D. None of the above

99. When repackaging medications into unit dose containers, which of the listed required information does not need to be recorded in a logbook?
   A. The dosage form
   B. The person who repackaged the medication
   C. The date the medication was prepared
   D. The patient's name and medical record number

100. Within the policies and procedures manual, the requirement for pharmacists to counsel patients on medications they have not taken before is listed under which law?
   A. Durham-Humphrey Amendment
   B. Kefauver-Harris Amendment
   C. The Prescription Drug Marketing Act
   D. OBRA '90

101. The program under the FDA that allows health care professionals to report any adverse reactions is _____.
   A. DEA Form 222
   B. MedWatch
   C. Pharmacist in charge
   D. AARP

102. As new stock arrives at the pharmacy, the technician should check the following information on the stock against the invoice: _____.
   A. Name, strength, and quantity
   B. Name, strength, dosage form, and quantity
   C. Name, strength, dosage form, quantity, and expiration date
   D. Name, strength, dosage form, quantity, expiration date, and delivery person's name

103. Which of the following automated systems is used specifically in hospitals to stock PAR levels of medications on nursing floors?
   A. Baker Cell systems
   B. Pyxis
   C. Robot systems
   D. All of the above

104. A drug manufacturer is required by law to recall any product that has been found to violate any of the following guidelines except _____.
   A. Labeling is wrong
   B. Drug batch was contaminated
   C. Any change occurring that causes the drug to fall outside the FDA or manufacturer's guidelines
   D. The drugs sent to the pharmacy were damaged in transit

105. Where would be the "best" place to store phenol?
   A. In the refrigerator
   B. On a shelf at room temperature
   C. On the bottom shelf behind cabinet doors
   D. Locked in the narcotics room

106. Grinding tablets into a fine powder in a porcelain mortar is an example of _____.
   A. Flocculation
   B. Emulsification
   C. Levigation
   D. Trituration

107. Which drug agency is responsible for regulating medical devices?
   A. FDA
   B. DEA
   C. EPA
   D. OSHA

108. Which of the following medications is available as an inhaler for asthma?
   A. Propranolol
   B. Albuterol
   C. Nasonex
   D. Both B and C

109. Transdermal nitroglycerin would be kept in which section of the pharmacy?
   A. The topicals
   B. The oral medications
   C. The liquids
   D. In the refrigerator

110. A pregnant patient arrives with a prescription for temazepam 15 mg q hs. What do you do?
A. Fill the prescription.
B. Label the medication with "take at bedtime" and "may cause drowsiness."
C. Alert the pharmacist because this is a pregnancy category X.
D. Alert the pharmacist because this is a pregnancy category A.

111. A stat order is called into the pharmacy by a nurse in the hospital unit. What do you do?
A. You can take the order orally, and then let the pharmacist know about it.
B. You should tell the nurse that she must send the order in writing.
C. You should give the phone to the pharmacist alerting him or her to a stat order.
D. You should fill the order immediately because it is a stat order.

Section III: Participating in the Administration and Management of Pharmacy Practice

Section III, which is 11% of the exam, covers information on refills, insurance claims, tracking how many scripts are filled, and audits. Other areas involve the law, Joint Commission on Accreditation of Healthcare Organizations standards, and knowing procedures for laminar flow hoods, equipment maintenance, automated systems, and computer software information.

112. What is the proper procedure for cleaning a laminar flow hood?
A. Spray the whole inside and wipe out all areas.
B. Clean the hood starting from the front working toward the back.
C. Clean the hood starting from the back side to side, top to bottom toward the front.
D. Wash the whole hood using a circular motion

113. Which of the agencies listed below is responsible for accreditation of an institutional facility?
A. APhA
B. DEA
C. JCAHO
D. ASHP

114. The main purpose of OSHA is to _____.
A. Ensure the safety of the patients
B. Ensure the safety of the drugs
C. Ensure the safety of air quality
D. Ensure the safety of the workplace

115. The MSDS contains what type of information?
A. Drug ingredients
B. How to clean up hazardous wastes
C. How to file a complaint about an incident
D. The ingredients and specifics of all types of products

116. A computer program used for dispensing medication in the pharmacy setting is referred to as _____.
A. Hardware
B. Software
C. Medware
D. Disks

117. Materials management refers to _____.
A. Inventory control
B. Drug storage
C. The drug procurement process
D. All of the above

118. If a pharmacy pricing formulary is the AWP plus 4.5 and the AWP is $90 for 100 tablets, what is the charge to the customer for a prescription of 30 tablets?
A. $27.50
B. $30.50
C. $31.50
D. $94.50

119. The cost of 100 tablets of a bottle of aspirin is $1.50. What would the dispensing charge be to yield a 50% gross profit?
A. $2.00
B. $2.10
C. $2.25
D. $2.50

120. Which of the programs listed below is administered by individual states?
A. Medicare
B. Medicaid
C. Med plan part A
D. Med plan part D

121. AWP can be found in which book?
A. *Drug Topics Red Book*
B. *PDR*
C. *American Drug Index*
D. *United States Pharmacopoeia*

122. If a manufacturer's invoice totals $520.00 with the terms 2% net, what amount should be remitted if it is paid within 30 days?
A. $490.00
B. $509.60
C. $520.00
D. $530.40

123. When choosing between state and federal requirements, which take precedence?
A. The state
B. The federal government
C. The institution you work for
D. The most stringent

124. A person who is over 65 years of age, who is disabled, or who has kidney failure would be covered by _____ insurance.
A. Medicaid
B. HMO
C. Medicare
D. PPO

125. Online processing of a third-party claim to determine payment is called _____.
A. Reconciliation
B. Processing degree
C. Adjudication
D. Authorization

Answer Key

1. B. The first time the prescription is filled (Chapter 18)
2. A. PH 1234575 (Chapter 2)

3. D. Aciphex (Chapter 20) and Ventolin (Chapter 18)

4. D. TPNs (Chapter 13)

5. A. Pseudoephedrine (Chapter 18)

6. C. Instill three drops into the left eye every other day (Chapter 5)

7. D. 60 mg (Chapter 4)

8. C. Clarithromycin (Chapter 24)

9. A. Intravenous and ophthalmic (Chapters 24 and 19)

10. A. 20 doses (Chapter 4)

11. D. Topical patch (Chapter 23)

12. B. 400 mL (Chapter 4)

13. C. 750 mL (Chapter 4)

14. B. 2.5 mL (Chapter 4)

15. D. 35 g (Chapter 4)

16. D. A and B (Chapter 16)

17. B. Zaroxolyn (Chapter 22)

18. D. Both A and B (Chapter 15)

19. D. Proton pump inhibitor (Chapter 20)

20. C. The product, strength, and dosage form (Chapters 2 and 14)

21. C. Take one tablet sublingually as needed (Chapter 5)

22. D. A 10-mL oral dose syringe (Chapter 2)

23. C. Regular (Chapter 13)

24. A. Emesis (Chapter 9)

25. B. 140 mL (Chapter 4)

26. C. 0.625 mL (Chapter 4)

27. B. 150 (Chapter 4)

28. C. 16 oz (Chapter 4)

29. D. Imodium (Chapter 20)

30. D. Pyridium (Chapter 20)

31. B. 4.5 g of 0.45% NS; 50 g of 5% dextrose (Chapter 4)

32. C. 3 tablets daily (Chapter 4)

33. A. 2.5 mL (Chapter 4)

34. B. 10 mL (Chapter 4)

35. D. 90 tablets (Chapter 4)

36. B. 0.4 mL (Chapter 4)

37. D. 8 mL (Chapter 4)

38. D. 102.3 mg/day (Chapter 4)

39. B. 12.5 mL (Chapter 4)

40. D. 31.2 gtt/min (Chapter 4)

41. B. 312.5 mL of 2%; 187.5 mL of 10% (Chapter 4)

42. A. 166.7 mL 35%; 833.3 mL of 15% (Chapter 4)

43. D. 200 g (Chapter 4)

44. C. 120 drams (Chapter 4)

45. D. 25 gtt/min (Chapter 4)

46. A. Nitroglycerin (Chapter 22)

47. D. 4.8 g (Chapter 4)

48. B. The strength of drug written is very high for a child. Notify the registered pharmacist. (Chapter 24)

49. D. Potassium (Chapter 30)

50. B. The patient might have sensitivity to this medication as well. Notify the registered pharmacist. (Chapter 24)

51. A. *PDR* (Chapter 6)

52. C. Micronase (Chapter 16)

53. D. Lescol (Chapter 22)

54. D. All of the above (Chapter 24)

55. B. In the eye (Chapter 19)

56. C. Tagamet (Chapter 20)

57. D. Prescription (Chapter 5)

58. B. Before meals (Chapter 5)

59. A. Anticonvulsant (Chapter 17)

60. D. Diuretic (Chapter 21)

61. C. Celexa (Chapter 15)

62. C. Zovirax (Chapter 28)

63. A. Elavil (Chapter 15)

64. B. When a mortar and pestle is used to mix medication (Chapter 12)

65. B. 0.3 mg (Chapter 4)

66. C. Coumadin and aspirin (Chapter 8)

67. D. Diastix (Chapter 16)

68. C. Preventive treatment (Chapter 5)

69. B. The amount of time it takes a chemical to be decreased by half of its strength (Chapter 5)

70. D. 6 AM, 2 PM, and 10 PM (Chapter 4)

71. C. Ativan (Chapter 2)

72. C. In hospitals (Chapter 11)

73. B. 22.5 mL (Chapter 4)

74. B. Mannitol solution (Chapter 21)

75. C. You have added 10 times too much insulin (Chapters 4, 7, and 13)

76. D. Place against the inside of the cheek (Chapter 5)

77. B. 147.4 lb (Chapter 4)

78. D. Vitamin B_{12} (Chapter 26)

79. B. 27 gauge; 19 gauge; 18 gauge; 16 gauge (Chapter 13)

80. D. All of these can be mixed with NS (Chapter 24)

81. B. 2°C to 8°C (36°F to 46°F) (Chapters 14 and 19)

82. C. Record the quantity and lot number, and return it to the manufacturer (Chapter 4)

83. B. Form 224 (Chapter 2)

84. C. Generic and trade name of drug, dosage form, strength, lot number, and expiration date (Chapter 12)

85. C. A smooth surface to mix ointments and creams (Chapter 12)

86. C. 100 mg (Chapter 12)

87. C. The oils from your skin will dirty and alter the actual weights (Chapter 12)

88. B. Add the appropriate solution to the medication to equal 100 mL (Chapter 4)

89. A. Nitroglycerin patches (Chapter 11)

90. C. Administer controlled analgesics (Chapter 2)

91. A. At room temperature (Chapter 14)

92. D. Both A and B (Chapter 14)

93. C. A list of drugs that are approved by the P and T committee (Chapter 11)

94. C. Prednisone 1 mg/mL solution (Chapter 25)

95. D. Keep refrigerated; shake well before using; expiration date (Chapter 8)

96. C. Meperidine (Chapter 2)

97. D. A new prescription is needed for each prescription fill. (Chapter 2)

98. C. This is the highest level of recall for products that could cause serious illness or may even be fatal. (Chapter 2)

99. D. The patient's name and medical record number (Chapter 12)

100. D. OBRA '90 (Chapter 2)

101. B. MedWatch (Chapter 2)

102. C. Name, strength, dosage form, quantity, and expiration date (Chapter 12)

103. B. Pyxis (Chapters 11 and 14)

104. D. The drugs sent to the pharmacy were damaged in transit (Chapter 14)

105. C. On the bottom shelf behind cabinet doors (Chapter 14)

106. D. Trituration (Chapter 12)

107. A. FDA (Chapter 2)

108. B. Albuterol (Chapter 18)

109. A. The topicals (Chapter 22)

110. C. Alert the pharmacist because this is a pregnancy category X (Chapter 7)

111. C. You should give the phone to the pharmacist. (Chapter 7)

112. C. Clean the hood starting from the back side to side, top to bottom toward the front. (Chapter 13)

113. C. JCAHO (Chapter 11)

114. D. Ensure the safety of the workplace (Chapter 2)

115. D. The ingredients and specifics of all types of products (Chapter 6)

116. B. Software (Chapter 6)

117. D. All of the above (Chapter 14)

118. C. $31.50 (Chapter 4)

119. C. $2.25 (Chapter 4)

120. B. Medicaid (Chapter 14)

121. A. *Drug Topics Red Book* (Chapter 6)

122. B. $509.60 (Chapter 4)

123. D. The most stringent (Chapter 2)

124. A. Medicaid (Chapter 14)

125. C. Adjudication (Chapter 14)

Appendixes

A

Abbreviations

DISEASE STATES

AIDS	acquired immunodeficiency syndrome
ARDS	adult respiratory distress syndrome
ARF	acute renal failure
ASHD	arteriosclerotic heart disease
CA	cancer
CAD	coronary artery disease
CF	cystic fibrosis
CHD	coronary heart disease
CHF	congestive heart failure
COPD	chronic obstructive pulmonary disease
CRD	chronic respiratory distress
CVA	cerebrovascular accident
DVT	deep venous thrombosis
GERD	gastroesophageal reflux disease
HIV	human immunodeficiency virus
HTN	hypertension
MI	myocardial infarction (heart attack)
MS	multiple sclerosis
NIDDM	non-insulin dependent diabetes mellitus (type 2)
STD	sexually transmitted disease
TB	tuberculosis
TIA	transient ischemic attack
URI	upper respiratory infection
UTI	urinary tract infection

DRUG AND SOLUTION ABBREVIATIONS

ABVD	Adriamycin (doxorubicin), bleomycin, vinblastine, and dacarbazine
ACE	angiotensin-converting enzyme
ACEI	angiotensin-converting enzyme inhibitor
Ach	acetylcholine
ADH	antidiuretic hormone
APAP	acetaminophen
aq	water
ASA	aspirin, acetylsalicylic acid
AZT	zidovudine
BDZ	benzodiazepine
CCB	calcium channel blocker
D5	5% dextrose
D5/ 0.9 NS	5% dextrose and 0.9% sodium chloride
DDAVP	desmopressin acetate
DES	diethylstilbestrol
DIG	digoxin
DTP	diphtheria, tetanus toxoids & pertussis vaccine
HCTZ	hydrochlorothiazide
IgG	immunoglobulin G
INH	isoniazid
LR	lactated ringers
MAOI	monoamine oxidase inhibitors
MOM	milk of magnesia
MS, MSO$_4$	morphine sulfate
MVI	multivitamin
NPH	neutral protamine Hagedorn (insulin)
NSAID	nonsteroidal antiinflammatory drug
NTG	nitroglycerin
PB	phenobarbital
PCN	penicillin
PNV	prenatal vitamins
PPN	peripheral parenteral nutrition
SSRI	selective serotonin reuptake inhibitors
T$_3$	triiodothyronine
T$_4$	levothyroxine
TCN	tetracycline
TMP	trimethoprim
TMP/ SMX	trimethoprim/ sulfamethoxazole
t-PA	tissue plasminogen activator
TPN	total parenteral nutrition
ZnO	zinc oxide

MEASUREMENTS

amt	amount
BSA	body surface area
C	centigrade
c	cup
cc	cubic centimeter
cm	centimeter
dr, Z	dram
F	Fahrenheit
fl	fluid
g	gram
gtt	drops
H, hr	hour
IU	International Unit
kcal	kilocalorie
kg	kilogram
L	liter
lb, #	pound
liq	liquid
m	micron, microgram
m, Â	minim
mcg	microgram
MDI	metered dose inhaler
mEq	milliequivalent
Mg	magnesium
mg	milligram
min	minute
mixt	mixture
ml	milliliter
mm	millimeter
mmol	millimole
mo	month
no	number
oz,	ounce
pt	pint
qt	quart
qty	quantity
gr	grain

675

ss—	one-half	**noc**	in the night
temp	temperature	**Non**	do not repeat; no
trit	triturate	**rep**	refills
tsp	teaspoonful	**non rep**	do not repeat
vol	volume	**NPO**	nothing by mouth
x	times	**OD**	right eye
y	year	**oint**	ointment
<	less than	**OS**	left eye
=	equal to	**OU**	each eye
>	greater than	**p̄**	after
↑	increase	**pc**	after meals
↓	decrease	**per**	by
		PM	after noon

DRUG DOSE INTERVALS, FORMS, AND INSTRUCTIONS

a.d.	right ear	**po**	by mouth
a.s.	left ear	**pr**	per rectum
aa—	of each	**prn**	whenever necessary
ac	before meals	**pulv**	powder
Adhib	to be administered	**q**	every
ad lib	as needed or desired	**q12h**	every 12 hours
ad us.	Ext for external use	**q2h**	every 2 hours
ad	up to	**q4h**	every 4 hours
Aer	aerosol	**q6h**	every 6 hours
AM	before noon	**q8h**	every 8 hours
am	morning	**qam**	every morning
amp	ampule	**qd**	every day
asap	as soon as possible	**qh**	every hour
au	both ears	**qhs**	every bedtime
AWP	average wholesale price	**qid**	four times a day
bid	twice a day	**qod**	every other day
c̄	with	**Qs ad**	a sufficient quantity to make
cap	capsule	**qs**	quantity sufficient
d	day	**rep**	repeat
D/C	discharge	**Rx**	prescription only; take; a recipe
d/c	discontinue	**s̄**	without
det	give	**SC, sq, subQ**	subcutaneous
dict	as directed	**Sig**	label, let it be printed
dil	dilute	**sl, subling**	sublingual
disp	dispense	**sol**	solution
EC	enteric coated	**solv**	dissolve
elix	elixir	**stat**	immediately
emul	emulsion	**supp**	suppository
ext	extrac	**syr**	syrup
gtt	drops	**tabs**	tablets
hs	bedtime, hour of sleep	**tbsp**	tablespoonful
IM	intramuscular	**tid**	three times a day
inj	injection	**tr, tinc**	tincture
IT	intrathecal	**u.d., u.dict**	as directed
IV	intravenous	**ud**	unit dose
		ung	ointment
		vag	vaginal

VO	verbal order
wa	while awake

ORGANIZATIONS

AACP	American Association of Clinical Pharmacy; American Assoication of Colleges of Pharmacy
AAPT	American Association of Pharmacy Technicians
ACPE	American Council on Pharmaceutical Education
APhA	American Pharmaceutical Association
ASHP	American Society of Health-Systems Pharmacists
CDC	Centers for Disease Control and Prevention
DEA	Drug Enforcement Administration
FDA	Food and Drug Administration
HCFA	Health Care Financing Administration
JCAHO	Joint Commission on Accreditation of Healthcare Organizations
NABP	National Association of the Boards of Pharmacy
NHA	National Healthcareer Association
P&T	Pharmacy and Therapeutics Committee
PTCB	Pharmacy Technician Certification Board
PTEC	Pharmacy Technician Education Council

PHARMACY CHEMICAL ABBREVIATIONS & TERMS

Ca	calcium
Cl	chlorine

CO_2	carbon dioxide
DNA	deoxyribonucleic acid
Etoh	alcohol
Fe	iron
$FeSO_4$	ferrous sulfate
H_2O	water
HCl	hydrochloric acid
K	potassium
KCl	potassium chloride
$MgSO_4$	magnesium sulfate
Mn	manganese
MVI	multivitamin
Na	sodium
NaCl	sodium chloride
$NaHCO_3$	sodium bicarbonate
NS	normal saline
O_2	oxygen
RPh	registered pharmacist
PharmD	Doctor of Pharmacy
PPI	patient package insert
PPO	preferred provider organization
Se	selenium
SWI	sterile water for injection
Zn zinc	

MEDICAL TERMS

Ab	antibody
ABGs	arterial blood gases
ACLS	advanced cardiac life support
ADE	adverse drug experience
ADR	adverse drug reaction
BBB	blood brain barrier
Bib	drink
bm	bowel movement
BP	blood pressure
BSN	Bachelor of Science in Nursing
BUN	blood urea nitrogen
c/o	complaint of
CBC	complete blood count
CNS	central nervous system
comp	compound

CS	cesarean section	**EENT**	eye, ear, nose, throat	**NPO**	nothing by mouth	**syr**	syringe
CSF	cerebrospinal fluid			**OD**	Doctor of Optometry; overdose	**UTI**	urinary tract infection
CT	clotting time	**exp**	expired			**VS**	vital signs
DNR	do not resuscitate	**GI**	gastrointestinal				
DO	Doctor of Osteopathy	**Hx**	history	**OR**	operating room		
		LVN	Licensed Practical Nurse	**OTC**	over the counter		
DP	Doctor of Podiatry			**PCA**	patient-controlled analgesia	**REFERENCE BOOK ABBREVIATIONS**	
DPM	Doctor of PodiatryMedicine	**MRI**	magnetic resonance imaging				
				pt	patient	**AJHP**	American Journey of Health-Systems of Pharmacy
DR, MD	Doctor; Doctor of medicine	**N & V**	nausea and vomiting	**R/O**	rule out		
				RN	registered nurse	**NF**	National Formulary
DVM	Doctor of Veterinary Medicine	**neg**	negative	**RR**	Recovery Room		
		NKA	no known allergies	**S&S**	signs and symptoms	**USAN**	United States adopted names
Dx	diagnosis			**sat**	saturated		
ECG, EKG	electrocardiogram	**NKDA**	no known drug allergies	**SOB**	shortness of breath	**USP**	United States Pharmacopeia

Trade name	Generic name	Indication (Main condition used for)	Trade name	Generic name	Indication (Main condition used for)
Abilify	aripiprazole	Psychosis	Astelin	azelastine	Allergies (ophthalmic)
Accupril	quinapril	Hypertension			
AcipHex	rabeprazole	Gastroesophageal reflux disease (GERD)	Atacand	candesartan cilexetil	Hypertension
			Atarax	hydroxyzine	Anxiety
			Ativan	lorazepam	Anxiety/sedation
Actonel	risedronate	Paget's disease/ osteoporosis	Augmentin	amoxicillin, potassium clavulanate	Infection (antibiotic)
Actos	pioglitazone	Diabetes	Avalide	hydrochlorothiazide(HCTZ)/ irbesartan	Hypertension
Adderall	amphetamine mixed salts	Narcolepsy, attention-deficit disorder (CII)	Avandia	rosiglitazone maleate	Diabetes
			Avapro	irbesartan	Hypertension
Advair Diskus	salmeterol, fluticasone	Asthma	Avelox (antibiotic)	moxifloxacin	Infection
Aldactone	spironolactone	Edema	Azmacort, Nasacort	triamcinolone	Allergies (corticosteroids)
Allegra	fexofenadine	Allergies			
Alphagan P	brimonidine tartrate	Glaucoma	Bactroban (antibiotic)	mupirocin	Infection
Altace	ramiril	Hypertension			
Amaryl	glimepiride	Diabetes type 2	Benicar HCT	olmesartan medoxomil/ HCTZ	Hypertension
Ambien	zolpidem	Insomnia			
Amoxil	amoxicillin	Infection (antibiotic)	Bentyl	dicyclomine hydrochloride	Irritable bowel syndrome
Anaspaz, Cystospaz	hyoscyamine sulfate	Peptic ulcer, spasms			
			Bextra	valdecoxib	Pain, inflammation
Antivert	meclizine	Motion sickness, vertigo	Biaxin XL	clarithromycin	Infection (antibiotic)
			BuSpar	buspirone	Depression
Apri, Aviane	ethinyl estradiol, desorgestrel; ethinyl estradiol, levonorgestrel	Contraceptive	Calan,	verapamil SR	Hypertension, angina
			Capex,	fluocinolone acetonide	Psoriasis, dermatitis
Aricept	donepezil	Alzheimer's disease/dementia	Capoten	captopril	Hypertension
Armour Thyroid	thyroid	Hormonal replacement	Cardura	doxazosin mesylate	Hypertension
			Cartia XT	diltiazem	Angina
Arthrotec	diclofenac, misoprostol	Arthritis	Catapres	clonidine	Hypertension

Trade name	Generic name	Indication (Main condition used for)	Trade name	Generic name	Indication (Main condition used for)
Cefzil	cefprozil	Infection (antibiotic)	Flomax	tamsulosin	Benign prostatic hypertrophy
Celebrex	celecoxib	Pain, inflammation			
Celexa	citalopram	Antidepressant	Flonase	fluticasone	Seasonal allergic rhinitis
Cialis	tadalafil	Impotence			
Clarinex	desloratadine	Allergies	Floxin	ofloxacin	Infection (antibiotic)
Cleocin	clindamycin	Infection (antibiotic)	Folvite	folic acid	Folate deficiency/ pernicious anemia
Cogentin	benztropine	Parkinson's disease			
No trade name	colchicine	Gout			
			Fosamax	alendronate	Osteoporosis
Combivent	ipratropium/albuterol	Asthma	Glucophage	metformin	Diabetes
Concerta	methylphenidate	Attention-deficit disorder/ narcolepsy	Glucotrol	glipizide	Diabetes type 2
			Glucovance	glyburide/metformin	Diabetes
			GoLYTELY	polyethylene glycolectrolyte solution	Constipation, bowel cleansing (pre-op)
Cordarone	amiodarone	Cerebrovascular accident			
Coreg	carvedilol	Hypertension	No trade name	insulin	Diabetes type 1
Cosopt	dorzolamide, timolol	Glaucoma			
Coumadin	warfarin	Blood clots (prophylaxis)	Hytrin	terazosin	Hypertension
			Hyzaar	losartan, HCTZ	Hypertension, edema
Cozaar	losartan	Hypertension			
Crestor	rosuvastatin	High cholesterol	Imitrex	Sumatriptan	Migraine
Cymbalta	duloxetine	Depression, diabetic peripheral neuropathy	Inderal	propranolol	Arrhythmia, myocardial infarction, angina pectoris
Cytotec	misoprostol	Gastric ulcers			
Darvocet-N	propoxyphene napsylate, acetaminophen (APAP)	Moderate to severe pain (CIV)	Isordil	isosorbide	Acute angina
			Keflex	cephalexin	Infection (antibiotic)
Deltasone	prednisone	Inflammation (steroid)			
			Klonopin	clonazepam	Convulsions
Depakote	divalproex sodium	Seizures	Klor-Con	potassium chloride	Potassium replacement
Desyrel	trazodone	Depression			
Detrol LA	tolterodine	Incontinence	Lamictal	lamotrigene	Infection (antifungal)
Diflucan	fluconazole	Infection (antifungal)			
Dilantin	phenytoin	Convulsions	Lanoxin,	digoxin	Arrhythmia, myocardial infarction
Diovan	valsartan	Hypertension			
Ditropan XL	oxybutynin	Reflex neurogenic bladder			
			Lantus	insulin glargine	Diabetes type 1 and 2
Duragesic	fentanyl citrate	Narcotic analgesia and sedation (CII)			
			Lasix	furosemide	Edema
Dyazide	triamterene, HCTZ	Hypertension, edema	Lescol	fluvastatin	High cholesterol
			Levaquin	levofloxacin	Infection (antibiotic)
Dynacin	minocycline	Infection (antibiotic)	Lexapro	escitalopram	Depression
Effexor XR	venlafaxine	Depression	Lioresal	baclofen	Muscle spasms
Elavil	amitriptyline	Depression	Lipitor	atorvastatin	High cholesterol
Elidel	pimecrolimus	Atopic dermatitis (topical)	Lopid	gemfibrozil	High cholesterol
			Lopressor	metoprolol tartrate, metoprolol succinate	Hypertension
Esidrix	HCTZ	Edema			
Estrace	estradiol	Hormonal replacement	Lotensin	benazepril hydrochloride	Hypertension
			Lotrel	amlodipine, benazepril	Hypertension
Evista	raloxifene	Osteoporosis	Lunesta	eszopiclone	Insomnia
Femiron	ferrous fumarate	Iron deficiency	Macrobid, Macrodantin	nitrofurantoin	Infection (antibiotic)
Fioricet	butalbital, APAP, caffeine	Pain (nonnarcotic)			
Flagyl	metronidazole	Infection (antiprotozoal)	Mevacor	lovastatin	High cholesterol
			Micronase	glyburide	Diabetes
Flexeril	cyclobenzaprine	Muscle pain, spasms	Monopril	fosinopril	Hypertension
			Motrin	ibuprofen	Pain, inflammation

Trade name	Generic name	Indication (Main condition used for)	Trade name	Generic name	Indication (Main condition used for)
Naprosyn	naproxen	Pain, inflammation	SMZ/TMP	trimethoprim-sulfamethoxazole	Infection
Nasonex	mometasone furoate	Inflammation (topical corticosteroid)	Solu-Medrol	methylprednisolone	Inflammation (steroid)
Neurontin	gabapentin	Convulsions	Soma	carisoprodol	Acute painful musculoskeletal conditions
Nexium	esomeprazole	GERD			
Niaspan	niacin	High cholesterol			
Norvasc	amlodipine	Hypertension	Strattera	atomoxetine	Attention-deficit/hyperactivity disorder
Omnicef	cefdinir	Infection (antibiotic)			
Ortho Tri-Cyclen Lo	ethinyl estradiol, norgestimate	Contraceptive	Synthroid	levothyroxine	Hormonal replacement
Ortho-Evra	ethinyl estradiol, norelgestromin	Contraceptive	Tylenol with codeine	APAP, codeine	Moderate to severe pain (CIII)
OxyContin	oxycodone hydrochloride	Moderate to severe pain (CII)	Tegretol	carbamazepine	Seizures
Patanol	olopatadine hydrochloride	Allergies (opthalmic)	Temovate	clobetasol	Leprosy
Paxil	paroxetine	Depression	Tenoretic	atenolol, chlorthalidone	Hypertension
No trade name	penicillin V potassium	Infection (antibiotic)	Tenormin	atenolol	Hypertension
Pepcid	famotidine	GERD	Tessalon Perles	benzonatate	Coughing
Percocet	oxycodone, APAP	Moderate to severe pain (CII)	Topamax	topiramate	Seizures
			Tricor	fenofibrate	High cholesterol
Phenergan	promethazine	Allergies, nausea	Ultracet	tramadol, APAP	Pain, fever
Plavix	clopidogrel	Atherosclerosis	Ultram	tramadol	Moderate to severe pain
Pravachol	pravastatin	High cholesterol			
Premarin	conjugated estrogens	Hormone replacement	Valium	diazepam	Anxiety, convulsions
Prempro	conjugated estrogens/ medroxyprogesterone	Hormonal replacement	Valtrex	valacyclovir	Infection (antiviral)
			Vasotec	enalapril	Hypertension
			Viagra	sildenafil citrate	Erectile dysfunction
			Vibramycin	doxycycline	Infection (antibiotic)
Prevacid	lansoprazole	Ulcers/GERD	Vicodin	hydrocodone, APAP	Moderate to severe pain (CIII)
Prilosec	omeprazole	Ulcers/GERD			
Protonix	pantoprazole	GERD	Vioxx	rofecoxib	Pain and inflammation
Proventil	albuterol	Asthma			
Prozac	fluoxetine	Depression	Viracept	nelfinavir	Acquired immunodeficiency syndrome
Pulmicort		Acute asthma, prophylaxis for asthma			
			Vistaril	hydroxyzine pamoate	Anxiety
Quinamm	quinine sulfate	Malaria	Wellbutrin SR	bupropion hydrochloride	Depression
Reglan	metoclopramide	Diabetic gastric stasis/antiemetic	Xalatan	latanoprost	Glaucoma
			Xanax	alprazolam	Anxiety
Remeron	mirtazapine	Depression	Zantac	ranitidine	Ulcer
Restoril	temazepam	Insomnia	Zestoretic	lisinopril, HCTZ	Hypertension
Rhinocort Aqua,	budesonide	Allergies, rhinitis	Zestril	lisinopril	Hypertension
			Zetia	ezetimibe	High cholesterol
Risperdal	risperidone	Psychosis	Ziac	bisoprolol fumarate, HCTZ	Hypertension
Seroquel	quetiapine fumarate	Psychotic/bipolar disorders	Zinacef	cefuroxime	Infection (antibiotic)
			Zithromax	azithromycin	Infection (antibiotic)
Sinemet	carbidopa, levodopa	Parkinson's disease	Zocor	simvastatin	High cholesterol
Sinequan	doxepin	Anxiety, convulsions	Zoloft	sertraline	Depression
Singulair	montelukast	Asthma	Zovirax	acyclovir	Infection (antiviral)
Skelaxin	metaxalone	Acute painful musculoskeletal conditions	Zyloprim	allopurinol	Gout
			Zyprexa	olanzapine	Psychosis
			Zyrtec	cetirizine	Allergies

*Modified for technician students; placed in generic to trade and trade to generic format.

Top 30 Herbal Remedies

Karen Snipe			Karen Snipe		
Common name	**Scientific name**	**Reported uses**	**Common name**	**Scientific name**	**Reported uses**
Aloe vera (leaf)	*Aloe* spp.	Wound and burn healing	Ginger (root)	*Zingiber officinale*	Antiemetic, antiinflammatory, gastrointestinal distress, dyspepsia
American ginseng (root)	*Panax quinquefolius*	Energy, stress, immune system builder			
Bilberry (berry)	*Vaccinium myrtillus*	Eye and vascular disorders	Ginkgo (root)	*Ginkgo biloba*	Memory, increased blood flow, dementia, asthma
Cascara sagrada (aged bark)	*Rhamnus purshiana*	Laxative	Ginseng	*Panax quinquefolius, Panax ginseng*	Increase physical endurance and concentration. Lessens fatigue and stress
Cat's claw (root, bark)	*Uncaria tomentosa*	Antiinflammatory, antimicrobial, antioxidant, immunosupportive			
Chondroitin	Nutriceutical	Osteoarthritis	Glucosamine	Nutriceutical	Osteoarthritis and rheumatoid arthritis
Cranberry (berry)	*Vaccinium macrocarpon*	Urinary tract infection			
Echinacea (flower, root)	*Echinacea purpurea* *Echinacea angustifolia*	Antiviral, arthritis, immunostimulant	Goldenseal (root)	*Hydrastis canadensis*	Antimicrobial, gastritis, bronchitis, cystitis
Evening primrose (seed oil)	*Oenothera biennis*	ADD, diabetes, skin disorders, endometriosis, hyperglycemia, multiple sclerosis, PMS, menopause, arthritis	Grapeseed (seed, skin)	*Vitis vinifera*	Antioxidant, allergies, circulation, asthma
			Green tea (leaf)	*Camellia sinensis*	Anticancer, antioxidant, lower cholesterol
Feverfew (leaf)	*Tanacetum parthenium*	Antiinflammatory, rheumatoid arthritis, migraines	Isoflavones (soy)	Nutriceutical	Cancer prevention, decreased bone loss, lower cholesterol, menopausal symptoms
Garlic (bulb)	*Allium sativum*	Antimicrobial, high blood pressure, cholesterol			

683

Karen Snipe			Karen Snipe		
Common name	**Scientific name**	**Reported uses**	**Common name**	**Scientific name**	**Reported uses**
Kava (root)	*Piper methysticum*	ADD, ADHD, anxiety, sedation	Wild yam (tuber)	*Dioscorea villosa*	Female vitality
Milk thistle (seed)	*Silybum marianum*	Antioxidant, liver diseases	Black cohosh (root)	*Cimicifuga racemosa*	Menopause, PMS, mild depression, arthritis
Saw palmetto (berry)	*Serenoa repens*	Benign prostatic hyperplasia	Fish oils	Nutriceutical	Diabetes, dysmenorrhea, high blood pressure, memory, psoriasis
Siberian ginseng (root)	*Eleutherococcus senticosus*	Athletic performance, stress, immune builder			
St. John's wort (flowering buds)	*Hypericum perforatum*	Depression, anxiety, antiviral, antibacterial, antiinflammatory	Melatonin	Nutriceutical	Insomnia
			Dong quai (root)	*Angelica sinensis*	Anemia, high blood pressure, energy (females), menopause, dysmenorrhea, PMS
Valerian (root)	*Valeriana officinalis*	Sedative, PMS, menopause, muscle spasms			

ADD, Attention-deficit disorder; *ADHD,* attention-deficit/hyperactivity disorder; *PMS,* premenstrual syndrome.

D

Math Review for Pharmacy Technicians

James J. Mizner, Jr.

PROPORTIONS

A ratio is a relationship between two parts of a whole or between one part and the whole. A ratio can be written as 1/2 or 1:2. A proportion is a relationship between two ratios. A proportion may be written as 1/2 = 2/4 or 1:2::2:4. Most pharmaceutical calculations performed in retail or institutional settings can be accomplished by using proportions.

Proportion problems can be solved in two ways. The first involves cross multiplying and dividing, and the second is described as comparing the means and extremes. Both methods yield the same answer if set up correctly. The following problem is solved using both methods.

$$\frac{4}{7} = \frac{x}{28}$$

where x is the unknown.

METHOD 1: CROSS MULTIPLY AND DIVIDE

$$\frac{4}{7} = \frac{x}{28}$$

1. Multiply the numerator on the left-hand side of the equation by the denominator on the right-hand side.

$$4 \times 28 = 112$$

2. Multiply the denominator of the left-hand side of the equation by the numerator on the right-hand side of the equation.

$$7 \times x = 7x$$

3. Divide both sides of the equation by the denominator that is on the side where a number is multiplied by x.

$$\frac{112}{7} = \frac{7x}{7}$$

$$16 = x$$

4. Always make sure that measurement units (such as *mg* or *units*) in the numerators correspond with one another and that the units in the denominators are the same as one another. If they are not, the likelihood of an incorrect answer increases.

METHOD 2: MEANS AND EXTREMES

1. $4:7::x:28$, where the first and last number in the series are considered the extremes and the two numbers in the middle are considered the means. In this situation the 4 and the 28 represent the extremes and the 7 and x represent the means. One multiplies the extremes (4×28) and then multiplies the means ($7 \times x$).

$$4 \times 28 = 7 \times x$$

$$112 = 7x$$

2. Divide both sides of the equation by the number that is on the side where a number is multiplied by x.

$$112 \div 7 = 7x \div 7$$

$$16 = x$$

3. Always make sure that the measurement units (such as *mg* or *units*) in the first and third positions are the same and that the units in the second and fourth positions are the same. If they are not, the likelihood of an incorrect answer increases.

QUESTIONS

1. If you have a cephalexin suspension of 250 mg/5 mL and need a dose of 375 mg, how many milliliters do you need?
2. If you have an albuterol liquid of 2 mg/5 mL and need a dose of 6 mg, how many milliliters do you need?
3. If you have atenolol 50 mg per tablet and need a dose of 25 mg, how many tablets do you need?
4. If you have warfarin 5 mg per tablet and need a dose of 17.5 mg, how many tablets do you need?
5. If you have aspirin 5 gr per tablet and need a dose of 7.5 gr, how many tablets do you need?

PERCENTS

Percents are another method of showing a relationship between parts and the whole. Percent means "parts per 100." A number less than 1 is considered less than 100%, and a number greater than 1 is greater than 100%. A percent can be calculated using ratios, fractions, or decimals.

RULES

1. To convert a decimal to percent, multiply the number by 100 and add a percent sign (%).
2. To convert a percent to a decimal, remove the percent sign and divide by 100.
3. To convert a fraction to a percent, divide the numerator by the denominator, multiply by 100, and add a percent sign.
4. To convert a percent to a fraction, drop the percent sign, write the value of the number as the numerator, place it over a denominator of 100, and reduce it to its lowest terms.
5. To convert a ratio to a percent, divide the first number by the second number, multiply by 100, and add a percent sign.

Percents can be calculated by setting up a proportion. The numerator represents parts and the denominator wholes. The left hand side of the equation can be expressed as follows:

$$\frac{\text{Parts of the whole}}{\text{Whole}}$$

The right hand side of the equation is expressed in a percent form, where the numerator is a percent of the whole (the denominator is considered 100%).

$$\frac{\text{Percent}}{100\%}$$

The equation would look like this:

$$\frac{\text{Parts of the whole}}{\text{Whole}} = \frac{\text{Percent}}{100\%}$$

To solve this type of problem, one must know two of the three variables: parts of the whole, the whole, or percent. One must identify the term as a part of the whole, the whole, or a percent. After identifying them and placing them in the equation, one cross multiplies and divides to find the missing term.

QUESTIONS
1. What is 25% of 60?
2. What is 9% of 70?
3. What percent is 14 of 30?
4. What percent is 17 of 85?
5. What number is 105% of 95?
6. What number is 75% of 75?

METRIC, HOUSEHOLD, AND APOTHECARY CONVERSIONS
The practice of pharmacy uses the metric system, the household system, and the apothecary system for the calculation of dosage and doses. A pharmacy technician must be able to calculate doses of medication in any of these systems and to convert them from one system to another system. Memorization of the basic conversions is essential. By using proportions, one can solve any conversion.

METRIC SYSTEM
Weight (gram)
1000 microgram (mcg) = 1 milligram (mg)
1000 mg = 1 gram (g)
1000 g = 1 kilogram (kg)
Volume (liter)
1000 mL = 1 liter (L)

HOUSEHOLD SYSTEM
Weight
2.2 lb = 1 kg
Volume
5 mL = 1 teaspoon (tsp)
3 tsp = 1 tablespoon (tbsp)
2 tbsp = 1 fluid ounce (fl oz)
8 fl oz = 1 cup
2 cups = 1 pint (pt)
2 pt = 1 quart (qt)
4 qt = 1 gallon (gal)

APOTHECARY SYSTEM
Weight
20 grains (gr) = 1 scruple
3 scruples = 1 dram
8 drams = 1 ounce
12 ounces = 1 pound
Volume
60 minims = 1 fluid dram
8 fluid dram = 1 fluid ounce

Apothecary	Metric
16.23 minims	= 1 mL
1 fl dram	= 4 mL
1 fl oz	= 29.57 mL (30 mL)
1 g	= 15.432 gr
1 gr	= 65 mg
1 lb (avoirdupois)	= 454 g
1 oz (apothecary)	= 31.1 g
1 oz (avoirdupois)	= 28.35 g

QUESTIONS
1. How many milligrams are in 25 g?
2. How many grams is 1.5 kg?
3. How many milliliters are in 2.5 fl oz?
4. How many teaspoons are in 4 fl oz?
5. How many tablespoons are in 1 fl pt?
6. How many milliliters are in 1.75 L?
7. How many milligrams are in 7.5 gr?
8. How many grains are in 200 mg?
9. How many grams are in 4 oz (weight)?
10. How many micrograms are in 0.5 mg?
11. How many pounds does a 60-kg person weigh?
12. You have a pint solution containing 5 mg/mL. How many milligrams does the pint contain?
13. A dose of an antacid is 1 tbsp. How many doses are in an 8-oz bottle?
14. You are to prepare a dose containing 5 gr of active ingredient. How many 65-mg tablets will be used?
15. A physician orders diphenhydramine elixir 2 tsp 4 times a day. A 4-oz bottle containing 12.5 mg/tsp is supplied. How many milligrams will the patient receive in each dose?
16. You are told to dispense 1 cup of medication. The dose is 1 tbsp, and the concentration is 20 mg/mL. How many grams of medication are being dispensed?
17. If there are 25 mg in a tablespoon, how many grams are in 1 L of solution?
18. A 6-fl oz bottle of cough syrup is given as 1 tsp 4 times a day. How many doses are in the bottle?
19. A patient is to receive one tablet of Nitrostat 1/200 gr. How many milligrams are in one tablet?
20. A medication has 150 mg in 480 mL. How many milligrams are in 1.5 fl oz?
21. How many grains are found in 0.4 mg?
22. There are 100 mg in a teaspoon. How many grams are in 1 gal?
23. One pint of a product contains 500 mg. How many milligrams are found in 5 mL?
24. There are 250 mcg in 1 tsp. How many milligrams are in 4 fl oz?
25. How many grains are found in a teaspoon of medication if it contains 125 mg/tsp?

UNITS

Several pharmaceutical products made from biological products are expressed as "units" or international units. Examples of these products include insulin, heparin, and vitamin E. Units represent an amount of activity within a particular system. Each pharmaceutical product is unique in determining the amount of activity of that product. Units represent a concentration and may be expressed as units/tablet or units/milliliter.

QUESTIONS

1. A patient is to receive Humulin insulin (100 units/mL) at a dose of 65 units at 7:30 AM. How many milliliters should be drawn into the insulin syringe?
2. You are to prepare a minibag of intravenous fluids and must put 1000 units of heparin in 100 mL of normal saline. You have a multidose vial that has 10,000 units/10 mL. How many milliliters must be put in the intravenous minibag?
3. A physician's hospital medication order calls for isophane insulin suspension to be administered to a 150-lb patient on the basis of 1 unit/kg per 24 hours. How many units of isophane insulin suspension should be administered daily?
4. Pertussis vaccine contains 4 protective units per 0.5 mL. How many protective units would be contained in a 7.5-mL multiple-dose vial?
5. If 1 mg of penicillin V represents 1520 penicillin V units, how many micrograms represent 1 unit?

MILLIEQUIVALENTS

Certain pharmaceutical products contain dissolved mineral salts and are capable of carrying an electrical charge through the solution. These substances are measured in milliequivalents (mEq) and are important when working with intravenous fluids. Sodium chloride and potassium chloride are two of the more common products expressed in milliequivalents.

QUESTIONS

1. An order requires 30 mEq of potassium phosphate. You have available 4.4 mEq/mL of potassium. How many milliliters will you put in the intravenous bag? (Hint: 4.4 mEq:1 mL::30 mEq:x)
2. A 20% potassium chloride solution has a strength of 40 mEq in 15 mL. You receive an order for 20 mEq. How many milliliters are needed?

PEDIATRIC DOSAGES

Children require different amounts of medication from adults. These doses are affected by the individual's age, weight, body surface area, organ development, sex, and disease state. Age in children is broken down into the following general categories:

Neonate: birth to 1 month
Infant: 1 month to 1 year
Early childhood: 1 year to 5 years
Late childhood: 6 years to 12 years
Adolescence: 13 years to 17 years

To calculate the appropriate dosage for children, one of several methods may be used. Young's rule uses age as a guide for children 1 to 12 years old; Clark's rule uses weight as the determining factor; milligrams per kilogram uses the patient's weight in kilograms; and body surface area uses height and weight as the basis for choosing a dose.

$$\text{Young's rule} = \frac{\text{Age of child (expressed in years)} \times \text{Adult dose}}{\text{Age of child (years)}}$$

$$\text{Clark's rule} = \frac{\text{Weight of child (expressed in pounds)}}{150\,\text{lbs}} \times \text{Adult dose}$$

All four of the previously mentioned methods require the use of the adult dose for drug calculation, and the given parameter desired by each method should be provided so that the practitioner can calculate the appropriate pediatric dose. The adult dose may be measured in milligrams, milliliters, units, milliequivalents, grains, or tablets.

QUESTIONS

1. How much medication should be given to a 5-year-old child if the adult dose is 500 mg?
2. How much medication should be given to a child weighing 60 lb if the adult dose is 100 mg?
3. How much medication should be give to a child weighing 40 lb if the adult dose is 2 mg/kg/day?
4. How much medication should be given in one dose to a child weighing 70 lb if the adult dose is 10 mg/kg/day and the patient is to receive four doses a day?
5. How much medication should be given to a child who is 30 months old if the adult dose is 100 mg?

CONCENTRATION/DILUTION

A concentration is a strength. A concentration can be expressed as a fraction (e.g., mg/mL, mEq/mL, units/mL), a ratio (e.g., 1:100, 1:1000, 1:10,000), or a percent (e.g., 10%, 25%, 50%). Percents are found in solids (%w/w) and in solutions (%w/v or %v/v).

The %w/w is the number of grams per 100 g, %w/v is the number of grams per 100 mL, and %v/v is the number of milliliters per 100 mL.

More than 90% of all problems involving concentrations result in a dilution or in compounding a final product in which the final concentration is less than the initial strength. In daily application a pharmacist receives an order to prepare a product of a given strength and volume (weight). This is known as the final strength (FS) and final volume (FV). The pharmacist must go to the shelf, choose the product of a given strength [initial strength (IS)] and determine the amount [initial volume (IV)] needed to prepare the compound. The same process is done in preparing solids, except an initial weight (IW) and final weight (FW) are substituted for initial and final volumes.

One can use the following equation for this situation:

$$\text{Initial volume} \times \text{Initial strength} = \text{Final volume} \times \text{Final strength}$$

or

$$\text{IV} \times \text{IS} = \text{FV} \times \text{FS}$$

THREE HINTS TO PREVENT ERRORS IN SOLVING DILUTION PROBLEMS

1. Initial strength must be larger than final strength.
2. Initial volume must be less than final volume.
3. Final volume minus initial volume equals amount of diluent (inert substance) to be added to make the final volume.

QUESTIONS

1. A 20% solution has been diluted to 480 mL and is now a 5% solution. What was the initial volume?

2. A 12.5% (w/v) topical antiseptic is available to the pharmacy. The pharmacist receives an order for 100 mL of a 1:4000 solution. How much of the original solution is necessary to fill the order?

3. A pharmacy receives an order for 4 oz of 5% solution. How much active ingredient is required to make the solution?

4. A pharmacist has weighed out 3 g of coal tar and has given it to the technician to compound a 1% ointment. What is the final weight of the correctly compounded prescription?

5. How many 600-mg ibuprofen tablets are needed to make 4 oz of a 15% ibuprofen ointment?

6. One tablespoon of 85% boric acid solution is diluted to 10%. How many 2-oz bottles can be prepared from the final solution?

7. A drug is supplied as a 40 mg/mL in a 50-mL vial. You have been asked to make 10 mL of a 10 mg/mL solution. How much concentrate and diluent are needed?

8. The pharmacy has 8 oz of a 40% solution, and 120 mL of water is added to decrease the concentration. What is the new concentration?

9. A technician is asked to weigh out 10 g of menthol and is told to dissolve it in distilled water to make a 5% solution. An order is received from a physician, and the technician is asked to make a 2.5% solution. What is the final volume?

10. How many milliliters of water must be added to make a 20% solution from 1 L of a 50% solution?

ALLIGATION

Alligations are used in pharmacy when a pharmacist or pharmacy technician is compounding a solution or solid. The strength being prepared is different from what is available on the shelf. In this situation, there are at least two different concentrations on the shelf—one that is greater than the desired concentration and one that is less than the desired concentration.

For example a pharmacist receives an order to prepare 4 oz of a 10% solution using a 25% and 5% solution. How much of each these should the pharmacist use?

Step 1: Draw a tic-tac-toe table.

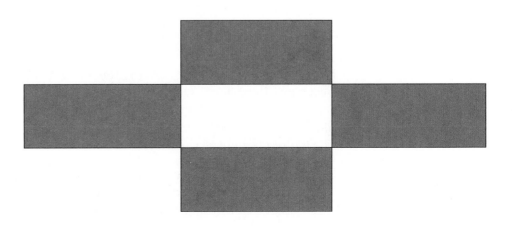

Step 2: Place the highest concentration in the upper left hand corner, the lowest concentration in the lower left hand corner, and the desired concentration in the middle.

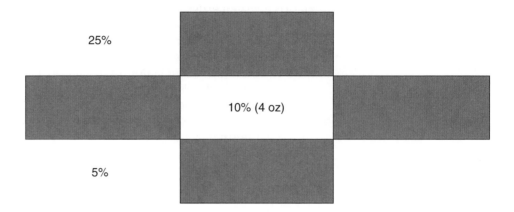

Step 3: Subtract the desired concentration from the highest concentration and place that number in the lower right hand corner and express the answer as parts. Next subtract the lowest concentration from the desired concentration and place that number in the upper right hand corner and label it as parts.

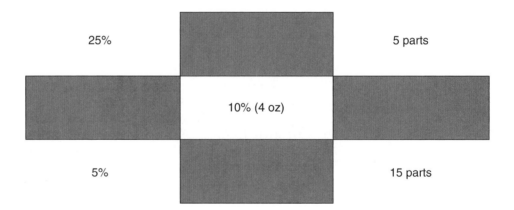

Step 4: Total the number of parts: 5 parts + 15 parts = 20 parts.
Step 5: Set up a proportion using the parts of the highest and lowest concentration and the total quantity to be prepared.

$$25: \frac{5 \text{ parts}}{20 \text{ parts}} \times 40 \text{ oz} = 1 \text{ oz of } 25\% \text{ needed}$$

$$25: \frac{15 \text{ parts}}{20 \text{ parts}} \times 40 \text{ oz} = 3 \text{ oz of } 5\% \text{ needed}$$

Step 6: Check your work by adding the amounts of each concentration to see if they equal the amount to be compounded.

QUESTIONS

1. You receive a prescription to make 4 oz of a 10% solution. On your shelf you find 25% and 5% solutions. What proportions of each will you use?
2. The pharmacy receives a medication order to prepare a 15% ointment weighing 2 oz. Your pharmacy stocks a 50% ointment and a 10% ointment. How much of each is required to make this compound?

3. A physician calls in a prescription requiring 1 oz of a 1% ointment for a patient. The pharmacy carries only a 2.5% ointment. How much of the 2.5% ointment and an inert base must be incorporated to make this product?

4. A hospital pharmacy compounds a 25% soaking solution for patients. The solution is prepared by combining 10% and 30% solutions. How much of each is required to make 1 L?

5. A pharmacy is to prepare 500 mL of D_5W. How much of $D_{10}W$ and SWFI (Sterile Water for Injection) are required to compound this solution?

6. A pharmacy is asked to make $D_{7.5}W$ using SWFI, D_5W, $D_{10}W$, and $D_{20}W$. What are the possible combinations to make this product?

7. A pharmacy is to prepare 500 mL of D_8W. The pharmacy stocks SWFI, D_5W, and $D_{10}W$. How much of these ingredients should be used to make this solution?

8. A physician orders a prescription of 4 oz of 1.5% hydrocortisone cream. The pharmacy stocks 0.5% and 2.5% cream. How much of each should be used to make this compound?

9. What proportions of a 10% ointment and 75% ointment should be used in preparing a 50% ointment?

10. What amounts of 90% alcohol and distilled water are needed to make 1 L of 25% alcohol?

FLOW RATES

Calculation of flow rates is used in the preparation of intravenous medications. A pharmacist may need to calculate the amount of fluid to be administered over time, calculate the flow rate of intravenous fluids, and control the amount of medication that the patient is to receive. One of the variables a pharmacist may face is the number of drops of a medication in 1 mL. The viscosity of the solution affects the number of drops. Several intravenous sets are available, including the following:

10 gtt/mL
15 gtt/mL
60 gtt/mL (which is known as a minidrip or microdrip set)

A flow rate is the same as infusion rate and rate of infusion and can be calculated using the following equation:

$$\text{Rate of infusion} = \frac{\text{Volume of fluid (or amount of drug, i.e., mg, mEq, or units)}}{\text{Time of infusion}}$$

A pharmacist may need to determine when an intravenous bag may need to be changed. This can be calculated using the following equation:

$$\text{Time of infusion} = \frac{\text{Volume of fluid (or amount of drug)}}{\text{Rate of infusion}}$$

An infusion pump may be used to deliver an exact amount of medication to the patient. In this situation the pharmacist may need to know how many drops per minute are to be administered. This may be calculated by using the following equation:

$$\frac{\text{Drops}}{\text{minute}} = \frac{\text{Number of mL}}{\text{hour}} \times \frac{\text{Number of drops}}{\text{mL}} \times \frac{\text{1 hour}}{60}$$

QUESTIONS

1. How many milliliters would a patient receive in 1 hour if it takes 45 minutes for 100 mL to be infused?

2. If a patient is given 1 L of an intravenous solution and the infusion rate is 125 mL/hr, how long will the intravenous bag last?

3. If a 1000-mL intravenous bag is hung at 9 <u>am</u> and the infusion rate is 100 mL/hr, when will the next bag need to be hung?

4. An intravenous solution is to flow at 100 mL/hr using a 10-drop set. How many drops per minute are administered?

5. A 1-L intravenous solution is to flow at 75 mL/hr using a 15-drop set. How many drops per minute are administered?

6. If 250 mL at 30 gtt/min is administered using a minidrip set. What is the flow rate in milliliters per hour?

7. If 2 g in 50 mL is administered over 60 minutes using a 10-drop set, how many drops per minute will the patient receive?

8. A 220-lb male is to receive 1 L of a medication dosed at 10 mcg/kg/min. How many milligrams per hour will he receive?

9. A patient is to receive 100 mL over 45 minutes using a 10-drop set. How should the pump be set?

10. A patient is to receive 2 L of normal saline infused over 24 hours using a 10-drop kit.
    A. How many milliliters per hour is this?
    B. How many milliliters per minute is this?
    C. How many drops per minute is this?

TEMPERATURE CONVERSIONS

To solve math problems converting Fahrenheit to Celsius or Celsius to Fahrenheit, the following formula can be used:

$$9°C = 5°F - 160$$

where C represents the temperature in Celsius and F represents the temperature in Fahrenheit. Only one of the two variables must be known to solve this problem. For example, if one was given a temperature of 75° F, one would multiply 75° by 5, subtract 160 from the answer, and then divide it by 9. The answer would be 23.8° C. On the other hand, if one is told that the temperature is 20° Celsius, one would multiply the 20 by 9, add 160 to it, and then divide it by 5, resulting in an answer of 68° F.

QUESTIONS

1. Convert the following temperatures to Celsius:
   A. 25° F
   B. 35° F
   C. 65° F
   D. 50° F

2. Convert the following temperatures to Fahrenheit:
   A. 45° C
   B. 30° C
   C. 25° C
   D. 38° C

E

Health Insurance Portability and Accountability Act of 1996 (HIPAA)

Robert M. Fulcher and Eugenia M. Fulcher

The Health Insurance Portability and Accountability Act of 1996 is better known as HIPAA. Although it was written in the later part of the twentieth century, it was not placed in effect until April 14, 2003, because of problems encountered in setting rates and with computerizing parts of the system. HIPAA requires that all forms used in connection with medical information must be standardized. This means that all medical bills, laboratory reports, hospital records, and medication records must be formatted in the same manner. Every insurance company is required to use the same forms. More importantly for the pharmacy, it sets boundaries on the use and the disclosure of protected health information and requires that patients be informed of how their protected information will be used.

HIPAA legislation is divided into two sections. The first section, or Title I, protects insurance coverage for workers and their families when workers move from job to job or when terminated from a job. The second part of the legislation, or Title II, protects patient rights. The Department of Health and Human Services has established national standards for electronic health care transactions. Another provision is that all electronic patient information must be secured to protect the privacy of patients. The Centers for Disease Control and Prevention also has joined the act by stating that health information can be disclosed without authorization from the patient "for the purpose of preventing or controlling disease, injury, or disability," including "public health surveillance, investigation, and intervention."

When a patient is treated by a health care provider, a record is made of the treatment. The record typically contains information about the diagnosis, treatment, and future plan of treatment for the patient. Statistical data or data taken without identification of the patient are not covered by the privacy rules of the HIPAA legislation. However, any disclosure that could be identified with the patient must have a signed consent form before it is released. The forms are provided to the patient in a hospital setting, in a physician's office, or when a prescription is filled in the pharmacy of his or her choice. Any provider that will use a third party in the treatment process must obtain the written consent of the patient before sharing any protected health information with the third party. This written consent must be obtained only once, but the consent form must be written in plain language and must inform the patient that the information may be used and disclosed to the third party. Also, consent must state that the patient's right to review the privacy notice is available and that the patient has a right to request restrictions to or revoke consent. The form must be dated and signed by the individual, although the signature does not require verification.

The information that HIPAA protects includes the following:

1. Any information related to past, present, or future physical and mental health
2. Past, present, or future payments for health services received
3. Specific care the patient received, is receiving, or is willing to receive
4. Any information that can identify the patient as the individual receiving the care
5. Any information that someone reasonably could use to identify a patient as receiving care

This information is referred to as protected health information.

A limited number of scenarios do not require a specific authorization from the patient. Some of these special cases include local agencies, such as power, gas, and phone companies, or emergency medical assistance during an emergency, such as hurricanes or floods, when life-sustaining equipment is involved. When this scenario arises, the pharmacist should make the decision about whether to provide the information. If a patient designates a family member or another person for the release of information, the requirements of HIPAA do not apply. When law enforcement needs information to protect citizens or in response to court orders or subpoenas, the privacy of the information may be superseded by the need to protect the public.

Under the HIPAA statutes, a hospital is allowed to continue to give callers basic information about a patient, as long as the caller meets specific criteria. The caller must ask for a specific patient by name. The information relayed about the patient may be a one- or two-word description of the patient's condition, the patient's hospital phone number, and the patient's room number, unless the patient requests that this information not be released.

The rulings for the physician's office are stringent on identification of patients. The area for signing in for an appointment must be private, and the patient's name must be removed from the list immediately after signing in. This requirement is one reason that many physician's offices are using an electronic method of signature as a means of signing patients in for treatment. Under all conditions, the patient's privacy must be protected from other patients and visitors in the office.

Confidentiality is a major tenet of the HIPAA regulations. Because medical professionals and allied health professionals have dealings with patients, conversations with the patient must take place in an area where other patients cannot overhear what is being said. This tenet presents a major problem in pharmacy because in most states, counseling of each patient is required by insurance companies. The patient counseling and education must be done in an area where privacy is ensured, such as a counseling room; but if this area is not available, the pharmacist must use professional judgment to ensure that the patients' rights are not violated.

Because patients with third-party payment obtain medication at checkout, the signature ledger should be protected. This means that the ledger should be out of sight except when a patient is signing, and the previous signatures should be covered before a new signature is obtained.

Handling medication bottles that have been brought back to the pharmacy for refills poses another problem. Any identification of the patient on the bottle, such as prescription number or name, must be obliterated using a black marker or by stripping the label from the bottle before disposal. Some pharmacies are even separating old prescription bottles from other waste for special disposal. In addition, the label on any medication that is returned to the pharmacy for whatever reason must be removed from the bottle, and the medication must be placed with damaged merchandise to be destroyed. The patient's privacy must always be protected.

HIPAA provides a set of standards for patient privacy and requires that all health care providers implement the policies and procedures to limit access to protected health information. In addition, health care professionals must remember that patients have rights. The rights of patients include the following:

- The right to obtain a written copy of the notice of privacy practices of the pharmacy where they obtain their medications
- The right to obtain a copy of their designated record set of protected health information
- The right to request an amendment to their health record
- The right to obtain an accounting of any disclosures of their protected health information
- The right to file a complaint regarding the handling of their protected health information
- The right to authorize that protected health information be used or disclosed for purposes other than treatment, payment, or health care operation

Because we live in an electronic age, there is a growing need for the protection of patient privacy. With HIPAA, this privacy is protected and the patient has control of what medical information is relayed to entities, both in the medical field and out of the medical field.

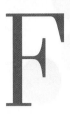 F

Proper Hand Care for Medical Asepsis in Pharmacy

Robert M. Fulcher and Eugenia M. Fulcher

Hand cleansing is a routine procedure for medical asepsis in the medical arena, including pharmacy, whether in an inpatient or community pharmacy. Hand washing has long been the cornerstone of infection control, but compliance with this procedure has not always been easy. Beginning in the 1960s, the Centers for Disease Control and Prevention issued guidelines for how health care workers should cleanse their hands properly to prevent transmission of transient flora found on the hands.

Resident flora live and grow in the epidermis (outer layer of the skin) and the dermis (deeper layer of the skin). Resident flora are for the most part nonpathogenic. Transient flora live and grow only on the epidermis. These bacteria adhere to the skin during the daily activities of touching persons, objects, and supplies. Transient flora tend to be more pathogenic and are passed easily to others through contact. However, these bacteria can be removed easily from the skin by washing hands. Therefore, it is of utmost importance for the pharmacy technician to adhere to the guidelines for hand sanitization as issued by the Centers for Disease Control and Prevention.

Hands should be washed carefully each day on arrival in the pharmacy area, when the hands are obviously soiled, after using the restroom, and after eating. These are basically the times that were taught to us as children, but compliance is difficult. In 2002 the Centers for Disease Control and Prevention changed the guidelines to call for medical aseptic hand sanitization during the day to keep bacteria to a minimum while handling medications. The new cleansing requirements still applied to those times listed previously, but hands may be sanitized with an alcohol-based hand rub between hand washing. Using an alcohol-based hand rub is faster, does not require rinsing, is more effective in removing transient flora, and prevents drying of the pharmacy technician's hands from constant hand washing. The drying of skin leads to chapped, irritated, and cracked skin that in turn leads to dermatitis. The procedure for sanitizing hands takes only 20 to 30 seconds, whereas hand washing requires 1 to 2 minutes.

The disadvantages of alcohol-based hand rubs are the stinging sensation if the skin is cut or scraped, and they are more expensive than soap and water. Furthermore, if the hands are grossly contaminated or dirty, alcohol-based hand rubs are not effective.

The amount of hand rub required depends on the manufacturer and is indicated in the instructions for use. The appropriate amount of hand rub should be placed in the center of the palm of the hand, and then the hands should be rubbed together, ensuring that the hand rub reaches all parts of the hands, including between the fingers. The rubbing motion should continue until the entire rub is absorbed.

Because the hand rub is alcohol-based, the fluid will be flammable and should be handled in the same manner as all flammable substances. The bottles should be placed safely to prevent spillage, and the hands should be rubbed together with enough friction to perform the task but should not be rubbed so vigorously that it may cause static electricity.

As with all medical personnel, the pharmacy technician should perform hand sanitization for medical asepsis and for prevention of transmission of transient flora. Keeping the hands clean is important for the technician and for patients who are receiving medications. If the pharmacy technician is preparing intravenous fluids, the hand-washing techniques are more stringent and should be followed according to the policies and procedures of the medical facility.

G
Answer Key to Odd-Numbered Review Exercises

Chapter 1
History of Medicine and Pharmacy

Multiple Choice
1. C
3. A
5. B
7. D
9. A

True/False
1. F: Minerals and animals were used by shaman in their practice. Incisions were also used as remedies.
3. T
5. F: The role of technicians in pharmacy has expanded and is continuing to expand.
7. F: Pharmacists have more contact with patients than ever. Laws such as OBRA90 require patient consultations.
9. F: Because of the responsibilities in pharmacy, the technician's job description requires more experience and education.

Chapter 2
Law and Ethics of Pharmacy

Multiple Choice
1. A
3. A
5. B
7. D
9. C

True/False
1. F: Thalidomide was not allowed to be sold in the United States.
3. F: CI drugs are not prescribed because there is no medicinal use indicated for them.

5. F: Contraindicated means that the agent should not be used by people with certain conditions.
7. F: Only a pharmacist can take an oral prescription over the phone.
9. T

Chapter 3
Pharmacy Associations, Certification, and Settings for Technicians

Multiple Choice
1. A
3. D
5. D
7. B
9. C

True/False
1. F: Each state's Board of Pharmacy determines their state's regulations.
3. T
5. T
7. F: 15 minutes maximum
9. F: Although there are only a few at this time that require certification, there are more that are in the planning stages of requiring some type of certification.

Chapter 4
Conversions and Calculations Used by Pharmacy Technicians

1. 20%
3. 40%
5. 0.2
7. XX
9. C
11. II
13. 90
15. 19
17. 1
19. 6
21. 4.4
23. 1
25. 250
27. 240 tab
29. 15 ml
31. 215.28 ml of 70% solution mixed with 285.71 ml of the water
33. 1 mg epinephrine
35. 4.16 gtts/min (this would be rounded to 4 gtts/min)

Chapter 5
Dosage Forms, Abbreviations, and Routes of Administration

Multiple Choice
1. B
3. D
5. A
7. D
9. C

True/False
1. F: Eye medications are sterile; therefore, they can be used in both eye and ear. Ear medications are not sterile; therefore, these agents cannot be used in the eye.
3. F: Diabetics use injectable medications at home. Also, many patients receive home health care and receive their IV treatments at home.
5. F: Phenol is used to increase the shelf life of products.
7. T
9. T

Chapter 6
Referencing

Multiple Choice
1. D
3. C
5. D
7. B
9. A

True/False
1. F: Classification is the type of drug based on its chemical structure, whereas indication is a list of the types of conditions that the agents are used for.
3. F: Monographs must be submitted before approval of FDA.
5. F: A technician can attain continuing education via seminars, online, and through journals made especially for technicians.
7. F: All technicians use reference books if they want to be well informed. A technician should also look into continuing education, reading articles, and asking pharmacists about specific drug questions.
9. T

Chapter 7
Competency, Communication, and Ethics

Multiple Choice
1. C
3. C
5. C
7. D
9. D

True/False
1. F: Required by board, certified by Pharmacy Technician Training Board (PTCB)
3. T
5. F: Your actions determine this, as well as title.
7. F: Morals are rights and wrongs, whereas ethics are the actions on morals.
9. T

Chapter 8
Prescription Processing

Multiple Choice
1. E
3. D
5. B

7. C
9. C

True/False
1. T
3. T
5. T
7. T
9. F: OBRA 90 is the consultation act.

Chapter 9
Over-the-Counter Medications and Skin Care Products

Multiple Choice
1. C
3. B
5. D
7. B
9. C
11. B

True/False
1. T
3. T
5. F: Fungus
7. F: The dermis contains the nerves and blood vessels.
9. F: Not infections

Chapter 10
Complementary Alternative Medicine

Multiple Choice
1. D
3. D
5. D
7. A
9. A

True/False
1. F: It is still nontraditional.
3. F: Still popular in other countries
5. F: They are still drugs and may interact and cause illness.
7. F: Punctures use needles rather than pressure.
9. T

Chapter 11
Hospital Pharmacy

Multiple Choice
1. A
3. D
5. D
7. D
9. D

True/False
1. F: By committee
3. T
5. F: Technicians can enter orders and fill them although the pharmacist must verify the computer orders and the medication by visual check.
7. F: It is the level of stock that must be kept at all times.
9. F: They can answer many (nondiscretionary) types of questions.

Chapter 12
Repackaging and Compounding

Multiple Choice
1. B
3. D
5. B
7. B
9. D

True/False
1. F: It is a set of standards for manufacturers.
3. T
5. T
7. F: All ingredients used in compounding must show an expiration date, including sterile water.
9. F: When preparing a topical, tapping the jar only removes the bubbles trapped inside the cream. The compounder should then smooth out the top with a spatula.

Chapter 13
Aseptic Technique

Multiple Choice
1. A
3. D
5. D
7. D
9. D

True/False
1. F: Stocking should be done daily or as needed.
3. F: They should be wiped back to front.
5. T
7. F: They should be checked yearly.
9. F: Goggles do not have to be worn if a shield is present.

Chapter 14
Pharmacy Stock and Billing

Multiple Choice
1. D
3. D
5. D
7. D
9. C

True/False
1. F: Generic is less expensive.
3. T
5. F: Everyone is responsible.
7. T
9. F: Material Safety Data Sheet

Chapter 15
Psychopharmacology

Multiple Choice
1. D
3. D
5. C
7. B
9. A

True/False
1. F: It is a physical side effect of involuntary movements of the extremities.
3. T
5. F: SSRIs are most commonly used.
7. F: "Dizzy/Drowsy" and "Do not drink alcohol"
9. T

Chapter 16
Endocrine System

Multiple Choice
1. B
3. C
5. B
7. D
9. C

True/False
1. F: This disease occurs in adulthood.
3. F: Hormones are secreted from the primary glands and sent into the bloodstream where they will then reach the target tissue.
5. T
7. T
9. T

Chapter 17
Nervous System

Multiple Choice
1. C
3. D
5. D
7. A
9. A
11. D
13. D
15. D
17. D
19. D

True/False
1. F: Both white and gray matter make up various areas of the brain and spinal cord.
3. T
5. T
7. F: ALS is a degenerative disease of the motor cells within the CNS.
9. F: Blocking agents only block muscle movement, not pain perception.

Chapter 18
Respiratory System

Multiple Choice
1. B
3. B
5. C
7. D
9. D

True/False
1. F: Nitrogen
3. F: Viruses
5. F: Can be due to environmental conditions as well.
7. F: Smokers are more at risk.
9. F: TB is very contagious.

Chapter 19
Visual and Auditory Systems

Multiple Choice
1. D
3. C
5. D
7. C
9. D

True/False
1. F: The orbit
3. T
5. F: Otics may not be placed in the eye because they are not sterile.
7. T
9. F: Otitis media is infection of the middle ear.

Chapter 20
Gastrointestinal System

Multiple Choice
1. E
3. C
5. D
7. B
9. D

True/False
1. T
3. T

5. F: Simethicone is an antiflatulent agent.
7. T
9. F: Constipation is the most common side effect of aluminum.

Chapter 21
Urinary System

Multiple Choice
1. B
3. A
5. C
7. C
9. C

True/False
1. F: The renal fascia
3. F: It may be necessary due to loss of potassium.
5. T
7. T
9. T

Chapter 22
Cardiovascular System

Multiple Choice
1. B
3. A
5. D
7. C
9. D
11. D
13. C
15. C

True/False
1. F: The heart pumps both oxygenated and deoxygenated blood.
3. T
5. F: VLDL and LDL
7. F: Cholesterol is a component of steroids.
9. F: CHF is managed by medication.
11. F: Cause vasodilation
13. F: First line of treatment are nitrates.
15. F: Aspirin has the least of the three.
17. F: They lower blood pressure.
19. F: Not potassium-sparing agents

Chapter 23
Reproductive System

Multiple Choice
1. D
3. A
5. C
7. D
9. D

True/False
1. F: Females are born with all of the ova, whereas males produce sperm throughout life after puberty.
3. T
5. F: In biphasic contraceptives, the progestins are increased in the second half of the cycle.
7. F: Barrier methods are contraceptives, especially condoms; are effective against sexually transmitted disease.
9. F: Sildenafil is not safe for use with a history of cardiac disease, hypertension, or use of nitrates and should not be used more than once a day.

Chapter 24
Antiinfectives

Multiple Choice
1. A
3. D
5. D
7. D
9. A
11. D
13. D
15. D

True/False
1. F: Some microbes make up the human normal flora.
3. F: Anaerobic organisms do not survive in oxygen, aerobic organisms need oxygen.
5. F: Fungal infection
7. T
9. T
11. F: All herpes viruses are contagious.

Chapter 25
Antiinflammatories and Antihistamines

Multiple Choice
1. B
3. D
5. D
7. C
9. C

True/False
1. F: There are many OTC agents, such as aspirin or ibuprofen.
3. F: Suppositories are commonly used for nausea and vomiting when an oral agent cannot be tolerated.
5. F: Aspirin 975 mg is by prescription only.
7. F: Steroids can be used for pain and inflammation.
9. F: Other causes include allergies, stress, or colds or flu.

Chapter 26
Vitamins and Minerals

Multiple Choice
1. B
3. D

5. D
7. A
9. C

True/False
1. T
3. F: Federal Drug Administration
5. T
7. F: The lack of iodine
9. T

Chapter 27
Vaccines

Multiple Choice
1. D
3. D
5. D
7. A
9. C

True/False
1. T
3. T
5. F: The liver
7. T
9. T

Chapter 28
Oncology Agents

Multiple Choice
1. D
3. D
5. C
7. D
9. D

True/False
1. T
3. F: Trained technicians can prepare them.
5. T
7. F: Vesicant refers to the ability of the agent to cause damage to the epithelial tissue.
9. F: Make red blood cells.

Chapter 29
Microbiology

Multiple Choice
1. A
3. D
5. D
7. B
9. D

True/False
1. F: Plants and bacteria can also be infected.
3. T
5. T
7. T
9. T

Chapter 30
Chemistry

Multiple Choice
1. B
3. D
5. D
7. D
9. A

True/False
1. T
3. F: Sodium bicarbonate
5. T
7. F: Anions are negative, and cations are positive.
9. T

Glossary

Abortifacient   Any treatment that causes abortion of a fetus

Abortivo   Cualquier tratamiento que causa el aborto de un feto

Absorption   The taking in of nutrients from food and liquids

Absorción   La toma de nutrientes de alimentos y líquidos

Accommodation   The change that occurs in the ocular lens when it focuses at various distances

Acomodación   El cambio que ocurre en el lente del ojo cuando éste enfoca a varias distancias

Acidification   The conversion to an acidic environment

Acidificación   La conversión a un ambiente ácido

Acidosis   The increase of acid content of the blood resulting from the accumulation of acid or loss of bicarbonate; the pH of blood is lowered

Acidosis   El aumento del contenido ácido en la sangre como resultado de la acumulación de ácido o de la pérdida de bicarbonato; la disminución del pH de la sangre

Acoustic nerve   The cranial nerve that controls the senses of hearing and equilibrium and eventually leads to the cerebellum and medulla

Nervio acústico   El nervio craneal que controla los sentidos del oído y del equilibrio y que eventualmente llega hasta el cerebelo y la médula

Acquired immunity   Immunity that has been acquired through exposure to an antigen or infectious agent

Inmunidad adquirida   Inmunidad que se adquiere por medio de la exposición a un antígeno o a un agente infeccioso

Addison's disease   Condition resulting in a decrease in adrenocortical hormones, such as mineralocorticoids and glucocorticoids, that causes symptoms including muscle weakness and weight loss

Enfermedad de Addison   Enfermedad que da como resultado una disminución de las hormonas adrenocorticoides, como mineralocorticoides y glucocorticoides, y que causa síntomas que incluyen debilidad muscular y pérdida de peso

Adjudication   Electronic insurance billing for medication payment

Adjudicación   Facturación electrónica del seguro para el pago de medicamentos

Aerobic   A term that describes organisms that need oxygen to survive

Aeróbico   Organismos que necesitan oxígeno para sobrevivir

Afferent   The direction of the neuronal impulse from the body toward the central nervous system

Aferente   La dirección del impulso neuronal desde el cuerpo hasta el sistema nervioso central

Alkalosis   The increase of alkalinity of the blood resulting from the accumulation of alkali or reduction of acid content; the pH of blood is raised

Alcalosis   El aumento de la alcalinidad de la sangre como resultado de la acumulación de álcali o de la reducción del contenido ácido; el pH de la sangre es elevado

Alligation   A method of determining the needed amounts of two different concentrations to prepare a needed concentration

Aligación Un método para determinar las cantidades necesarias de dos concentraciones diferentes para preparar una concentración dada

Amenorrhea Absence or suppression of menses

Amenorrea Ausencia o falta de menstruación

Amino acids Macromolecules that make up proteins

Aminoácidos Macromoléculas que forman las proteínas

Anabolism To build up; the constructive phase of metabolism

Anabolismo Acumular; la fase constructiva del metabolismo

Anaerobic A term that describes organisms that live in the absence of oxygen

Anaeróbico Organismos que viven en ausencia de oxígeno

Analgesic A drug that relieves pain by reducing the perception of pain

Analgésico Una medicina que alivia el dolor al reducir la percepción del dolor

Anaphylactic shock A severe allergic reaction that causes blood pressure to decrease rapidly, the heart to go into ventricular tachycardia, and airways to close; a medical emergency that will cause death if not treated immediately

Choque anafiláctico Una reacción alérgica severa que causa una rápida disminución de la presión sanguínea, taquicardia ventricular y cierre completo de las vías respiratorias; una emergencia médica que causa la muerte si no se trata inmediatamente

Androgen Male hormone

Andrógeno Hormona masculina

Anemia A deficiency of circulating red blood cells; a symptom of disease, not a disease

Anemia Una deficiencia de los glóbulos rojos en la sangre; un síntoma de enfermedad, no una enfermedad

Angina A severe, often constricting pain affecting the pectoris, or chest region, caused by lack of oxygen to the heart cells

Antibiotic Chemical agent produced by organisms and used to treat infections

Antibióticos Agentes químicos producidos por organismos y que se utilizan para tratar infecciones

Antibiotic spectrum The variety of microbes that a particular antibiotic can treat. Broad-spectrum agents can treat many different types of organisms, whereas narrow-spectrum agents treat only a select few.

Espectro de un antibiótico La variedad de microbios que un antibiótico específico puede tratar. Los agentes de espectro amplio pueden tratar muchos tipos de organismos diferentes, mientras que los agentes de espectro reducido pueden tratar sólo unos pocos.

Antibodies Proteins contained within plasma cells that neutralize or destroy antigens; also known as immunoglobulins

Anticuerpos Proteínas que se hallan en las células plasmáticas que neutralizan o destruyen los antígenos; también conocidas como inmunoglobulinas

Antiemetic Agent that stops nausea and vomiting

Antiemético Agente que hace parar la náusea y el vómito

Antigen The marker on cell surfaces that marks the cell as a "self-cell"; it stimulates the production of antibodies

Antígeno El marcador en la superficie celular que marca la célula como "auto-célula"; estimula la producción de anticuerpos

Antihypertensive Agent that decreases blood pressure

Antihipertensivo Agente que disminuye la presión sanguínea

Antiinflammatory A drug that reduces swelling, redness, and pain and that promotes healing

Antiinflamatorio Una medicina que reduce la hinchazón, el enrojecimiento y el dolor y facilita la curación

Antimicrobial Chemical agent produced by scientists to prevent growth of or kill microorganisms

Antimicrobiano Agentes químicos producidos por los científicos para impedir el crecimiento de microorganismos o para matarlos

Antineoplastic An agent used to prevent the development, proliferation, or growth of neoplastic cells; a medication used in treatment of abnormal cells

Antineoplástico Un agente que se usa para impedir el desarrollo, proliferación o crecimiento de las células neoplásticas; medicamento que se usa en el tratamiento de células anómalas

Antipruritic A drug that relieves itching, usually an antihistamine or an antiinflammatory drug

Antipruriginoso Una medicina que alivia la picazón, por lo general un antihistamínico o un antiinflamatorio

Antipyretic Medication that reduces fever

Antiseptic A substance that slows or stops growth of microorganisms on surfaces such as skin

Antiséptico   Una sustancia que retarda o detiene el crecimiento de microorganismos en superficies como la piel

Antitussive   A drug that can decrease the coughing reflex of the central nervous system

Antitusivo   Una medicina que puede disminuir el reflejo tusígeno (de tos) del sistema nervioso central

Anxiety   Feelings of apprehension, dread, and fear, with characteristics including tension, restlessness, tachycardia, dyspnea, and a sense of hopelessness

Ansiedad   Sentimientos de aprensión, miedo y temor, con características que incluyen tensión, falta de descanso, taquicardia, disnea y una sensación de desesperanza

Apothecary   Latin term for pharmacist

Apotecario   Término latín para farmacéutico

Apothecary system   A system of measurement used in pharmacy

Appendicitis   Inflammation of the appendix

Apendicitis   Inflamación del apéndice

Aqueous humor   A fluid that is found in the anterior and posterior chambers of the eye

Humor acuoso   Un fluido que se halla en las cámaras anterior y posterior del ojo

Arrhythmia   Irregular rhythm of the heart

Aritmia   Ritmo irregular del corazón

Artery   A vessel that carries oxygenated blood from the heart to the tissues of the body

Arteria   Un vaso sanguíneo que transporta sangre con oxígeno desde el corazón hasta los tejidos del cuerpo

ASA   Acetylsalicylic acid (aspirin)

ASA   Ácido acetilsalicílico (aspirina)

Aseptic technique   The procedures used to eliminate the possibility of a drug becoming contaminated with microbes or particles

Técnica aséptica   Los procedimientos que se usan para eliminar la posibilidad de que una medicina se contamine con microbios o partículas

Asthma   A condition in which narrowing of the airways impedes breathing

Asma   Una enfermedad en la cual el estrechamiento de las vías respiratorias impide el respirar

Atom   The smallest unit of an element

Átomo   La unidad más pequeña de un elemento

Atomic mass   The mass (mostly referred to as weight) of an atom expressed in the units 1660×10^{-24}

Masa atómica   La masa (la mayoría de las veces llamada peso) de un átomo expresada en unidades de 1660×10^{-24}

Attenuated   An altered or weakened live vaccine made from the disease organism against which the vaccine protects

Atenuado   Una vacuna de microorganismo vivo, modificado o debilitado, hecha del organismo de la enfermedad contra la cual protege dicha vacuna

Auditory canal   A 1-inch segment of tube that runs from the external ear to the middle ear

Canal auditivo   Segmento tubular de una pulgada de largo que va desde el oído externo hasta el oído medio

Auditory ossicles   The set of three small bony structures in the ear: malleus, incus, and stapes

Huesecillos del oído   La serie de tres pequeñas estructuras óseas en el oído: martillo, yunque y estribo

Autocrine   Denoting a mode of hormone action in which a hormone binds to receptors on and affects the function of the cell type that produced it

Autoimmune disease   Condition in which a person's tissues are attacked by his or her immune system; abnormal antigen-antibody reaction

Enfermedad autoinmunitaria   Enfermedad en la cual los tejidos de una persona son atacados por su propio sistema inmunológico; reacción anómala de antígeno-anticuerpo

Autonomic   Self-controlling or involuntary

Autónomo   Que se controla solo o de modo involuntario

Autonomic nervous system   Division of the nervous system that controls the involuntary body functions; consists of sympathetic and parasympathetic divisions

Sistema nervioso autónomo   Parte del sistema nervioso que controla las funciones corporales involuntarias, está formada del sistema simpático y del sistema parasimpático

Auxiliary label   An adhesive label that is attached to a container with specific instructions or information pertaining to the medication inside

Etiqueta auxiliary   Una etiqueta adhesiva que se pone en un envase con instrucciones específicas o información relativa al medicamento que hay en su interior

Avitaminosis   Vitamin deficiency

Avitaminosis   Deficiencia de vitaminas

Avoirdupois system A system of measurement used for determination of weight

Axon The part of a nerve cell that conducts impulses away from a cell body

Axón La parte de una célula nerviosa que conduce los impulsos nerviosos hacia el exterior de la célula

Ayurveda A holistic medical system originating in India

Ayurveda Un sistema de medicina holístico originario de India

Bacteria Unicellular organisms

Bacterias Organismos unicelulares

Bactericidal Agent that kills bacteria

Bactericida Agentes que matan bacterias

Bacteriostatic Agent that prevents the growth of bacteria but does not kill the microbe

Bacteriostático Agentes que impiden el crecimiento de las bacterias pero que no mata el microbio

Benign A nonmalignant neoplasm

Benigno Un neoplasma no maligno

Benign prostatic hypertrophy Nonmalignant enlargement of prostate gland

Hipertrofia prostática benigna Agrandamiento no maligno de la próstata

Binary fission The method of reproduction by which a single cell divides into two separate cells

División binaria El método de reproducción por el cual una célula simple se divide en dos células individuales

Bioavailability The amount of drug that reaches its intended destination by being absorbed into the bloodstream

Bioequivalence The difference between a drug that is manufactured in a different dosage form or by a different company; includes the rate of absorption, distribution, metabolism, and excretion

Biology The study of life

Biología El estudio de la vida

Biopsy A procedure in which a piece of tissue is removed from a patient for examination and diagnosis; the tissue is a sample of the whole

Biopsia Un procedimiento en el cual se extrae una porción de tejido del cuerpo de un paciente para analizarlo y hacer un diagnóstico; el tejido es una muestra del todo

Bipolar disorder Depressive psychosis, alternating between excessive phases of mania and depression; formerly known as manic-depressive

Trastorno bipolar Psicosis depresiva en la que se alternan fases exageradas de manía y de depresión; antes se conocía como psicosis maníaco-depresiva

Blister pack Container usually made of plastic that holds a single-dose tablet or capsule

Envase–ampolla Envase por lo general hecho de plástico que contiene una tableta o cápsula de una dosis unitaria

Blood urea nitrogen A test that measures the nitrogen in the blood in the form of urea

Nitrógeno ureico en la sangre Un análisis que mide el nitrógeno que hay en la sangre en forma de urea

Blood–brain barrier A barrier formed by special characteristics of capillaries to prevent certain chemicals from moving into the brain

Barrera hematoencefálica Una barrera formada por características especiales que poseen los capilares para impedir que ciertas sustancias químicas lleguen al cerebro

Board of Pharmacy State board that regulates pharmaceutical practice

Junta de Farmacia Junta estatal que regula la práctica farmacéutica

Bolus A single dose of drug

Bradykinins Chemicals produced by the body and responsible for inflammation and pain

Bradykinins Agentes químicos que produce el cuerpo y que originan inflamación y dolor

Brand/trade name Trademark of a drug or device created by the originating manufacturing company

Marca/denominación commercial Marca registrada de una medicina o de un aparato creado por la compañía fabricante original

Bulk compounding A larger quantity of medication that can fill a large order at one time or several smaller orders in the future

Compuesto al por mayor Una gran cantidad de medicamento que puede cubrir una cantidad grande de medicina recetada de una sola vez o varias cantidades pequeñas en el futuro

Bulk forming Fiber used as a stimulant to the intestines or to cause a feeling of fullness to decrease appetite

Formadores de masa Fibra que se utiliza como estimulante de los intestinos o para crear una sensación de saciedad a fin de disminuir el apetito

Calibration The markings on a measuring device

Calibración Las marcas (la escala) de un aparato de medida

Cancer A general term used to describe malignant neoplasms

Cáncer Un término general usado para describir neoplasmas malignos

Capillary Extremely small vessel that connects the ends of the smallest arteries (arterioles) to the smallest veins (venules), where exchanges of nutrients and wastes, O_2 and CO_2 can occur; blood vessels at cellular level

Capilar Vaso sanguíneo extremadamente pequeño que une las terminaciones de las arterias más pequeñas (arteriolas) a las venas más pequeñas (vénulas), en el que pueden producirse intercambios de nutrientes y sustancias de desecho, O_2 y CO_2 pueden ocurrir; vasos sanguíneos en los niveles celulares

Carbohydrates Chemical substances that include sugars, glycogen, starches, and cellulose with only a carbon, hydrogen, and oxygen makeup

Carbohidratos o hidratos de carbono Sustancias químicas en las que se incluyen azúcares, glucógenos, almidones y celulosas, y que están formadas sólo por carbono, hidrógeno y oxígeno.

Carcinogen A substance or chemical that can increase the risk of developing cancer

Carcinógeno Una sustancia o agente químico que puede aumentar el riesgo de desarrollar cáncer

Catabolism To break down; the destructive phase of metabolism

Catabolismo Descomponer; la fase destructiva del metabolismo

Catalyst A molecule that allows chemical reactions to take place rapidly but is not altered in the reaction

Catalítico Una molécula que permite que una reacción química se produzca con mayor rapidez pero sin que la molécula misma sufra modificaciones

Cataract Loss of transparency of the lens of the eye

Catarata Pérdida de transparencia del lente del ojo

Cell body The main part of a neuron from which axons and dendrites extend

Cuerpo celular La parte principal de una neurona de la cual se extienden los axones y las dendritas

Central nervous system Brain and spinal cord

Cerebrospinal fluid A fluid that fills the ventricles of the brain and also lies in the spaces of the brain or spinal cord and the arachnoid layer of the meninges

Fluido cerebrospinal Un fluido que llena los ventrículos del cerebro y que también se halla en los espacios de la capa aracnoidea de las meninges y del cerebro o de la médula espinal

Certified pharmacy technician A technician who has passed the National Certification Examination; the technician can use the abbreviation CPhT after his or her name

Cervical Neck region

Cervical Región del cuello

Chemical structure The shape of molecules and their location to one another

Estructura química La forma de las moléculas y su ubicación respectiva

Chemotherapy The treatment of a disease with toxic chemical substances to slow the disease process or to kill cells

Quimioterapia El tratamiento de una enfermedad por medio del uso de sustancias químicas tóxicas para retardar el proceso de la enfermedad o matar ciertas células

Chiropractic Manual manipulation of the joints and muscles

Quiropráctica Manipulación manual de las articulaciones y los músculos

Chloasma Hyperpigmentation of skin, limited or confined to a certain area

Cloasma Hiperpigmentación de la piel, limitada o confinada a una cierta área

Chronic obstructive pulmonary disease A disease process in which the lungs have decreased ability for gas exchange; also known as emphysema and chronic bronchitis

Enfermedad pulmonar obstructiva crónica Proceso patológico en el cual disminuye la capacidad de los pulmones para inhalar y exhalar; también conocido como enfisema y bronquitis crónica

Chyme The soupy consistency of food after mixing with stomach acids as it passes into small intestines

Quimo La consistencia espesa en que se transforman los alimentos al mezclarse con los ácidos gástricos al pasar al intestino delgado

Clinical pharmacist Pharmacist who monitors patient medications in inpatient and some retail settings

Farmacéutico clínico Farmacéutico que controla los medicamentos de los pacientes en hospitales y algunas farmacias de venta al por menor

Coagulate To solidify or change from a fluid state to a solid state

Coagular Solidificar o cambiar del estado fluido al estado sólido

Code blue A coded message to indicate an emergency in a hospital situation

Código azul Un mensaje codificado para indicar una emergencia en un hospital

Coenzyme A compound that activates an enzyme

Coenzima Un compuesto que hace que se active una encima

Cofactor A factor that must be present for other factors to be active

Cofactor Un factor que debe estar presente para que otros factores sean activos

Communication The ability to express oneself in such a way that one is readily and clearly understood

Comunicación La capacidad de expresarse de modo que se produzca una comprensión clara e inmediata

Competency The capability or proficiency to perform a function

Competencia La capacidad o aptitud para cumplir una función

Compounding The act of mixing, reconstituting, and packaging a drug

Composición El acto de mezclar, reconstituir y empaquetar una medicina

Cones Photoreceptors responsible for color (daylight vision)

Conos Elementos fotorreceptores responsables de la visión en color (visión diurna)

Confidentiality To keep privileged customer information from being disclosed without the customer's consent

Confidencialidad Acto de no revelar información confidencial sobre un cliente o paciente sin el consentimiento del interesado

Congestive heart failure Accumulation of blood in the circulatory system caused by the inability of the heart to pump efficiently

Insuficiencia cardiaca congestiva Acumulación de sangre en el sistema circulatorio debido a la incapacidad del corazón de bombearla de manera eficaz

Constipation Dry, hard stools that may be decreased in frequency

Estreñimiento Deposiciones fecales secas y duras que pueden presentarse con menor frecuencia de la normal

Continuing education Education beyond the basic technical education, usually required for license renewal

Educación continua Educación que va más allá de la educación técnica básica, usualmente necesaria para renovar una licencia

Controlled substance Any substance that is similar to the structures of drugs in schedule I or II, primarily stimulants, depressants, and hallucinogens.

Cornea The transparent tissue covering the anterior portion of the eye

Córnea El tejido transparente que recubre la parte anterior del ojo

Coronary artery disease Coronary artery disease which is defined by a set of conditions affecting the heart caused by atherosclerosis and angina pectoris

Corticosteroid A steroid produced by the adrenal cortex

Cough reflex Response of the body to clear air passages of foreign substances and mucus by a forceful expiration

Tos refleja Respuesta del cuerpo para limpiar las vías respiratorias de sustancias extrañas y mucosidades por medio de una expiración vigorosa

Covalent bond The sharing of electrons between two atoms

Unión covalente El tipo de unión en el cual dos átomos comparten electrones

Cream A hydrophilic base

Crema Una base hidrófila

Cretinism Condition in which the development of the brain and body is inhibited by congenital lack of thyroid secretion

Cretinismo Enfermedad en la cual se inhibe el desarrollo cerebral y corporal debido a una carencia congénita de secreciones tiroideas

Cushing's disease Syndrome causing an increase in secretion of the adrenal cortex that includes symptoms such as a moon face and deposits of fat (buffalo hump)

Enfermedad de Cushing Síndrome que produce un incremento en la secreción de la corteza adrenal y que incluye síntomas como redondez del rostro y depósitos de grasa (joroba de búfalo)

Cycloplegia Paralysis of the ciliary muscle in the eye

Cicloplegia Parálisis del músculo ciliar en el ojo

Cystic fibrosis An inherited disorder that causes production of very thick mucus in the respiratory tract and affects the pancreas and sweat glands; the patient experiences difficulty breathing and has frequent respiratory infections

Fibrosis quística Un trastorno hereditario que causa la producción de mucosidades muy espesas en el tracto respiratorio; afecta el páncreas y las glándulas sudoríparas; el paciente experimenta dificultad para respirar y padece infecciones respiratorias frecuentes

Débride To remove dead or damaged tissue

Desbridar Eliminar tejidos muertos o deteriorados

Decongestants Drugs that reduce swelling of the mucous membranes by constricting dilated blood vessels; they reduce blood flow to nasal tissues, thus reducing nasal congestion

Descongestionantes Medicinas que reducen la hinchazón de las membranas mucosas al contraer los vasos sanguíneos dilatados; reduciendo el flujo sanguíneo a los tejidos nasales y la congestión nasal

Dendrite The part of a neuron that branches out to bring impulses to the cell body

Dendrita La parte de la neurona que se ramifica hacia el exterior para llevar los impulsos al cuerpo célula

Deoxyribonucleic acid (DNA) The complex nucleic acids that are bases for genetic continuance

Ácido desoxirribonucleico (AND) Los ácidos nucleicos complejos que son la base de la continuidad genética

Depot An area of the body where a substance can accumulate or be stored for later distribution

Depósito Una área del cuerpo en la cual se puede acumular o almacenar una sustancia para su distribución posterior

Depression A mental state characterized by sadness, feelings of loss and grief, and loss of appetite and that may include suicidal thoughts

Depresión Un estado mental caracterizado por tristeza, sentimientos de pérdida y pena, pérdida de apetito y puede incluir ideas de suicidio

Dermatitis Inflammation of the skin associated with itching and burning

Dermatitis Inflamación de la piel asociada con picazón y ardor

Desquamation A normal process of shedding the top layer of the skin, also known as exfoliation

Descamación Un proceso normal de desprendimiento de la capa superior de la piel, también se conoce como exfoliación

Diagnosis A doctor's assessment of the cause of a condition

Diagnóstico Una declaración de un médico sobre la causa de una enfermedad

Dialysis The passage of a solute through a semipermeable membrane to remove toxic materials and to maintain fluid, electrolyte, and pH levels of the body system when the kidneys no longer work

Diálisis El paso de un soluto a través de una membrana semipermeable para eliminar materiales tóxicos y para mantener el fluido, el electrolito y el pH del sistema corporal cuando los riñones no funcionan

Diarrhea Frequent, watery, loose stools

Diarrea Deposiciones fecales, frecuentes, aguadas y poco espesas

Digestion The mechanical, chemical, and enzymatic action of breaking food into molecules that can be used in metabolism

Digestión La descomposición mecánica, química y enzimática de los alimentos para convertirlos en moléculas utilizables en el metabolismo

Distribution The ability of a drug to pass into the bloodstream

Diuresis The secretion and passage of large amounts of urine from the body

Diuresis La secreción de grandes cantidades de orina y su expulsión del cuerpo

Diuretic An agent that increases urine output and diuresis

Diurético Un agente que aumenta la expulsión de orina y la diuresis

Dogma Code of beliefs based on tradition rather than fact

Dogma Código de creencias basado en tradiciones más bien que en hechos

Drug classification Categorization based on the action of a drug and its usage

Clasificación de medicinas Se basa en el método de acción y en el uso de la medicina

Drug education coordinator Pharmacist who helps set protocol in a hospital setting

Coordinador de educación sobre medicinas Farmacéutico que ayuda a establecer un protocolo en el ámbito hospitalario

Drug Enforcement Administration Federal agency within the Department of Justice that enforces laws against the misuse of controlled substances

Agencia para el cumplimiento de las leyes anti–droga Agencia federal del Departamento de Justicia que regula la mala utilización de las sustancias controladas

Drug Facts and Comparisons Reference book found in all pharmacies containing detailed information on all medications

"Drug Facts and Comparisons" Libro de referencia que se encuentra en todas las farmacias y que contiene información detallada sobre todos los medicamentos

Dysmenorrhea Painful menstruation

Dismenorrea Menstruación dolorosa

Dyspepsia Heartburn, indigestion, epigastric discomfort

Dystonia Symptoms that include twisting, repeated jerking movements, and/or abnormal posture

Distonía Síntomas que incluyen torsiones, contracciones involuntarias repetidas y/o posturas anómalas

Edema A local or generalized condition in which body tissues retain an excessive amount of tissue fluid

Edema Una enfermedad localizada o generalizada en la cual los tejidos corporales retienen una cantidad excesiva de fluido tisular

Efferent The conduction of electrical impulses away from the central nervous system to the body

Eferencia La conducción de impulsos eléctricos desde el sistema nervioso central al resto del cuerpo

Electrolytes Charged elements called cations (which have positive charges) and anions (which have negative charges)

Electrolitos Elementos cargados eléctricamente que se denominan cationes (con carga positiva) y aniones (con carga negativa)

Electron The smallest subset of an atom that contains a negative charge

Electrón La división más pequeña de un átomo que tiene carga negativa

Elixir A base solution that is a mixture of alcohol and water

Elixir Una solución de base que es una mezcla de alcohol y agua

Emesis Vomiting

Emesis Vómito

Emulsification To make into a emulsion, or bind together

Endometriosis Condition in which tissue resembling endometrium is found outside the uterine cavity, usually in the pelvic area

Endometriosis Enfermedad en la cual un tejido similar al endometrio se encuentra fuera de la cavidad uterina, usualmente en la región pélvica

Endometrium Mucous membrane lining of the uterus

Endometrio Membrana mucosa que recubre el útero

Enzyme A protein that speeds up a reaction by reducing the amount of energy required to initiate a reaction; also called a biological catalyst

Enzima Una proteína que acelera una reacción al reducir la cantidad de energía requerida para iniciar dicha reacción; se denomina también un catalítico biológico

Erythema Redness of the skin resulting from capillary dilation

Eritrema Enrojecimiento de la piel producido por la dilatación de los capilares sanguíneos

ESBLs Extended-spectrum beta-lactamases

Ethics The values and morals that are used within a profession

Ética Los valores y principios morales vigentes en una profesión

Eustachian tube A tubular structure within the middle ear that runs to the nasopharynx (throat)

Trompa de Eustaquio Una estructura tubular en el interior del oído medio que llega hasta la nasofaringe (garganta)

Euthyroid Normal-functioning thyroid gland

Eutiroidismo Funcionamiento normal de la glándula tiroides

Excretion Elimination of waste products through stools and urine

Excreción Eliminación de productos de desecho a través de las heces y la orina

Exophthalmos Prominence of the eyeball because of increase thyroid hormone

Exoftalmos Prominencia del globo ocular debido a un incremento de la hormona tiroidea

Expectorant Chemical that causes the removal of mucous secretions from the respiratory system; it loosens and thins sputum and bronchial secretions for ease of expectoration

Expectorante Sustancia química que causa la expulsión de secreciones mucosas del sistema respiratorio; los expectorantes hacen menos espesos los esputos y secreciones bronquiales para facilitar su expulsión

Extrapyramidal Symptoms of taking antipsychotic medications that include parkinsonism, dystonia, and tremors

Extrapiramidal Síntomas de la toma de medicamentos antisicóticos, los cuales incluyen parkinsonismo, distonías y temblores

Facultative anaerobe A microorganism that can live with or without oxygen

Anaeróbico facultative Un microorganismo que puede vivir con o sin oxígeno

Fallopian tubes Narrow passage between the ovary and the uterus

Trompas de Falopio Pasaje estrecho entre los ovarios y el útero

Fat–soluble Drugs that are absorbed into the fat layer of the body
Liposoluble Medicinas que se absorben en la capa de grasa corporal

Fat–soluble vitamin Vitamin that is soluble in fat and therefore is stored in body fat; vitamins A, D, E, and K are fat-soluble
Vitamina liposoluble Vitamina que es soluble en grasa, y que por tanto se almacena en la grasa corporal; las vitaminas A, D, E y K son liposolubles

FDA Food and Drug Administration
FDA Administración de Drogas y Alimentos

Fertilization The process by which the sperm unites with the ovum to create a new life
Fertilización El proceso por medio de cual el espermatozoide se une con el óvulo para crear una nueva vida

Flocculation The process by which a solute comes out of a solution in the form of flakes or precipitation; the solute then can be filtered out of the solution

Floor stock Supplies kept on hand in different units of a hospital
Almacén de planta Suministros que se tienen a mano en las distintas unidades de un hospital

Food and Drug Administration Federal agency within the Department of Health and Human Services that regulates the manufacture and safeguarding of medications
Administración de Drogas y Alimentos Agencia federal del Departamento de Salud y Servicios Humanos que regula la fabricación y el control de calidad de los medicamentos

Formulary A list of preferred drugs to be stocked by the pharmacy; also a list of drugs covered by an insurance company
Formulario Una lista de medicinas prioritarias para tener almacenadas en la farmacia; también, una lista de medicinas cubiertas por una compañía de seguros

Fungicide Agent that kills fungus
Funguicida Agentes que matan hongos

Gametes Sex cells, or ova and sperm
Gametos Células sexuales; es decir, óvulos y espermatozoides

Gastritis Inflammation of the stomach lining
Gastritis Inflamación de los tejidos que recubren el estómago

Gauge The size of the needle opening
Calibre El tamaño de la abertura de la aguja

Generic name Name assigned to a medication by the Food and Drug Administration; nonproprietary name of a drug
Nombre genérico Nombre que la Administración de Drogas y Alimentos le asigna a un medicamento; nombre común de una medicina

Globulin Protein that is insoluble in water; immune globulins protect against diseases
Globulina Proteínas no solubles en agua; las inmunoglobulinas protegen contra las enfermedades

Glucose Simple sugar
Glucosa Azúcar simple

Goiter Condition in which the thyroid gland is enlarged because of lack of iodine, known as simple goiter, or because of a tumor, known as toxic goiter
Bocio Enfermedad en la cual la tiroides aumenta de tamaño debido a una carencia de yodo, se conoce como bocio simple; si es causado por un tumor, se conoce como bocio tóxico

Government insurance Medicaid and Medicare
Seguro del gobierno Medicaid y Medicare

Gram A basic unit of weight (mass) of the metric system equal to the weight of a cubic centimeter (cc) or a milliliter (mL) of water
Gramo Unidad básica de peso (masa) del sistema métrico y que es igual al peso de un centímetro cúbico (cc) o un mililitro (ml) de agua

Gram–negative bacteria Bacteria that are unable to keep crystal violet stain when washed in acid alcohol
Bacteria gram negativa Bacteria que no pueden mantener el colorante cristal violeta cuando se tratan con ácido alcohol

Gram–positive bacteria Bacteria that are able to keep crystal violet stain when washed in acid alcohol
Bacteria gram positiva Bacteria que mantienen el colorante cristal violeta cuando se tratan con ácido-alcohol

Graves' disease Condition caused by hypersecretion of thyroid with diffuse goiter, exophthalmos, and skin changes
Enfermedad de Graves Enfermedad originada por una secreción excesiva de la tiroides; esta enfermedad se presenta con bocio difuso, exoftalmos y cambios en la piel

Half–life **1.** The amount of time it takes a chemical to be decreased by one half.
2. The time required for half the amount of a substance such as a drug in a living system to be eliminated or disintegrated by natural

processes. **3.** The time required for a concentration of a substance in a body fluid (blood plasma) to decrease by half.

Hard copy The original prescription
Copia en papel La receta original

Health Insurance Portability and Accountability Act of 1996 Federal act for protecting patients' rights
Ley de Responsabilidad y Transferibilidad del Seguro de Salud de 1996 Ley federal para proteger los derechos de los pacientes

Helminth Multicellular worm
Helminto Gusano pluricelular

Hemoglobin The iron-containing pigment on red blood cells that carries oxygen to the tissues
Hemoglobina El pigmento de los glóbulos rojos que contiene hierro y que transporta oxígeno a los tejidos

Herb Any herbaceous plant consisting of fleshy stems
Hierba Cualquier planta herbácea de tallos tiernos

Heterotrophic The ability to reproduce asexually
Heterotrópica La capacidad de reproducción asexual

Histamine A substance that interacts with tissues, producing an allergic reaction
Histamina Una sustancia que interactúa con los tejidos produciendo una reacción alérgica

HMO Health Maintenance Organization
HMO Organización para el mantenimiento de la salud

Homeopathy A system of therapy based on the belief that medicinal substances that cause a specific symptom can be used to treat an illness that yields the same symptoms
Homeopatía Un sistema terapéutico basado en la creencia de que las sustancias medicinales que causan un síntoma específico pueden usarse para tratar una enfermedad que presente los mismos síntomas

Homeostasis The equilibrium pertaining to the balance of the body with respect to fluid levels, pH level, and chemicals
Homeóstasis El equilibrio relativo al balance del cuerpo con respeto a los niveles de fluidos, pH y sustancias químicas

Horizontal flow hood Environment for the preparation of sterile products that uses air originating from the back of the hood moving forward across the hood out into the room

Campana de flujo horizontal Medio para la preparación de productos estériles en el que se utiliza una corriente de aire que tiene su origen en la parte posterior de la campana y que continua hacia delante a través de la campana para después salir en la habitación

Hormones Chemical substances produced and secreted into the bloodstream or duct by an endocrine gland that result in a physiologic response at a specific target tissue
Hormonas Sustancias químicas producidas y secretadas en la corriente sanguínea o en los conductos por una glándula endocrina y que provocan una respuesta fisiológica en un tejido objetivo específico

Household system A system of measurement commonly used for weight, volume, and length in the United States
Sistema nacional Un sistema de medidas comúnmente usado para medir peso, volumen y largo en los Estados Unidos

Hydrophilic Water loving; any substance that easily goes into water
Hidrófilo Que le gusta el agua; cualquier sustancia que se disuelve fácilmente en agua

Hydrophobic Water hating; any substance that does not go into or mix in water
Hidrófobo Que rechaza el agua; cualquier sustancia que no se disuelve en el agua o que no se mezcla con ella

Hyperalimentation Parenteral nutrition for patients who are unable to eat solids or liquids
Hiperalimentación Nutrición parenteral para pacientes que no pueden ingerir alimentos sólidos o líquidos

Hypercalcemia Unusually high concentration of calcium in the blood
Hipercalcemia Concentración de calcio en la corriente sanguínea más alta de lo normal

Hyperglycemia Abnormally high glucose content circulating in the bloodstream
Hiperglicemia Contenido de glucosa en la sangre más alto de lo normal

Hyperkalemia An excessive amount of potassium in the blood

Hyperlipidemia Abnormally high concentration of lipids in the circulatory system

Hypertension High blood pressure

Hypervitaminosis A disorder caused by the intake of too many vitamins; more common with fat-soluble vitamins
Hipervitaminosis Un trastorno causado por la toma de una cantidad excesiva de vitaminas; es más común con las vitaminas liposolubles

Hypocalcemia Low concentration of calcium in the blood

Hipocalcemia Baja concentración de calcio en la sangre

Hypoglycemia Abnormally low glucose content circulating in the bloodstream

Hipoglicemia Contenido de glucosa en la corriente sanguínea más bajo de lo normal

Hypokalemia An abnormally low concentration of potassium in the blood

Hypotension Low blood pressure

Immunity A type of resistance to infection resulting from an immune response from the body or from agents such as vaccinations

Inmunidad Un tipo de resistencia a una infección que es el resultado de una respuesta inmunológica del cuerpo o de agentes como las vacunas

Immunosuppressive 1. A substance or procedure which prohibits a normal immune response by the body to fight off such an attack. 2. Agents used to prevent organ rejection.

Incontinence Loss of control over excretion of urine or feces

Inert ingredient An ingredient that has little or no effect on body functions

Ingrediente inactivo Un ingrediente que tiene muy poco o ningún efecto en las funciones corporales

Influenza A respiratory tract infection caused by an influenza virus

Influenza Una infección del tracto respiratorio causada por un virus

Ingestion The act of taking in food or liquid

Ingestión Acto de tomar alimentos o líquidos

Inhale To breathe in; directions used for an inhaler

Inhibit To stop or hold back; to keep a reaction from taking place

Inhibir Detener o impedir una reacción; prevenir que ésta tenga lugar

Inpatient A hospitalized patient

Interno Paciente hospitalizado

Inpatient or in-house pharmacy Hospital pharmacy

Farmacia interna Farmacia de un hospital

Inpatient pharmacy A pharmacy in a hospital or institutional setting

Farmacia interna Una farmacia dentro de un hospital u otra institución

Insomnia Difficulty falling or staying asleep

Insomnio Dificultad para dormir o conciliar el sueño

Instill To place into; instructions used for ophthalmic or otic drugs

International time A 24-hour method of keeping time in which hours are not distinguished between AM and PM, but are counted continuously and consecutively through the entire day

Tiempo internacional Un método de 24 horas para contar el tiempo en el cual las horas no se diferencian en a.m. y p.m., sino que se cuentan de forma continua y consecutiva a lo largo de todo el día

Intrinsic factor A naturally produced protein that is necessary for the absorption of vitamin B_{12}

Factor intrínseco Una proteína producida de forma natural y que es necesaria para la absorción de la vitamina B_{12}

Invasive The tendency for a tumor or mass to move into tissues and/or organs in proximity

Invasiva La tendencia de un tumor o una masa a desplazarse hacia el interior de los tejidos y/o órganos que se hallan en sus proximidades inmediatas

Ion An atom or a group of atoms with a leftover unbalanced charge

Ión Un átomo o un grupo de átomos con un resto de carga sin equilibrar

Ionic bond The transfer of electrons between two atoms

Enlace iónico La transferencia de electrones entre dos átomos

Keratolytic A drug that causes shedding of the outer layer of the skin

Queratolítico Una medicina que ocasiona el desprendimiento de la capa externa de la piel

Kilocalorie A measurement of energy or heat expended or used up in a chemical activity; the amount of heat needed to change the temperature of 1 kg of water 1°C; abbreviated kcal.

Kilocaloría Una medida de energía o calor que se desprende o se gasta durante una actividad química; la cantidad de calor que se necesita para cambiar la temperatura de 1 Kg de agua un grado Celsìus

Labyrinth A bony maze composed of the vestibule, cochlea, and semicircular canals of the inner ear

Laberinto Un conjunto óseo formado por el vestíbulo, la clóquea y los canales semicirculares del oído interno

Laminar flow hood Environment for the preparation of sterile products

Campana de flujo laminar Medio para la preparación de productos estériles

Legend drug   Drug that requires a prescription for dispensing

Medicina de venta con receta   Medicina que no puede venderse sin una receta

Leukemia   A progressive disease marked by malignancy of the blood-forming cells found in the hemopoietic tissues, organs, and bloodstream, causing the circulation of abnormal blood cells

Leucemia   Una enfermedad progresiva caracterizada por la malignidad de las células sanguíneas que se hallan en los tejidos hemopoyéticos, en los órganos y en la corriente sanguínea, causando origen a la circulación de células sanguíneas anómalas

Levigate   To make into a smooth paste or into a fine powder depending on the agent used

Lipids   Fats and fatty acids

Lípidos   Grasas y ácidos grasos

Lumbar   The region of the back that includes the area between the ribs and the pelvis; the area around the waist

Lumbar   La región de la espalda que incluye el área entre las costillas y la pelvis; la zona alrededor de la cintura

Lymphoma   A term used to describe a malignant disorder of lymphoid tissue

Linfoma   Un término que se usa para describir un trastorno maligno del tejido linfático

Macro   Large

Macro   Grande

Malignant   An invasive and destructive pattern of rapid, abnormal cell growth; often fatal

Maligno   Un patrón invasivo y destructivo de crecimiento celular rápido y anómalo; con frecuencia mortal

Mania   A form of psychosis characterized by excessive excitement, elevated mood, and exalted feelings

Manía   Una forma de psicosis que se caracteriza por una agitación excesiva, estado de ánimo elevado y sentimientos exaltados

MAR   Medication administration record

MAR   Registro de administración de medicación

Melanoma   A malignant neoplasm of the pigmented cells of skin; it may metastasize to other organs

Melanoma   Un neoplasma maligno de las células pigmentadas de la piel; se puede metastatizar a otros órganos

Menopause   Cessation of menstruation; a natural phenomenon in which the woman passes from a reproductive state to a nonreproductive state

Menopausia   Cese de la menstruación; un fenómeno natural por el cual la mujer pasa de un estado reproductivo a otro no reproductivo

Metabolism   The physical and chemical changes that take place within an organism

Metabolismo   Los cambios físicos y químicos que tienen lugar dentro de un organismo

Metastasis   The movement or spread of cancerous cells through the body to organs in distant areas

Metástasis   El movimiento o la expansión de células cancerosas a través del cuerpo hasta órganos distantes

Meter   Basic measurement of length in the metric system

Metro   Medida básica de longitud del sistema métrico

Metered dose inhaler   A device for supplying medications to the lungs through inhalation

Inhalador dosificador   Un método de administración de medicamentos a los pulmones por medio de inhalación

Metric system   A system of measurement based on multiples of 10

Micro   Small

Micro   Pequeño

Microbial   Refers to microorganisms (very small organisms) not visible without a microscope

Microbiano   Referente a microorganismos (muy pequeños) que no son visibles sin un microscopio

Microbiology   The study of microscopic organisms

Microbiología   El estudio de los organismos microscópicos

Microgram   One thousandth of a milligram; metric unit of measure

Microgramo   Milésima parte de un miligramo; unidad de medida métrica

Micturition   Urination

Milligram   One thousandth of a gram; metric unit of measure

Miligramo   Milésima parte de un gramo; unidad de medida métrica

Miosis   Contraction of the pupil

Miosis   Contracción de la pupila

Misbranding   Deceptive or misleading labeling of a product that may lead the consumer to believe that the product will cure an illness

Mitosis   Cellular reproduction that creates two identical daughter cells from the DNA of the parent cell

Mitosis Reproducción celular que da origen a dos células hijas idénticas a partir del ADN de la célula madre

Mole Avogadro's number: 6.02×10^{23} atoms, molecules, or ions

Mol Número de Avogrado: 6.02×10^{23} átomos, moléculas o iones

Molecular biosynthesis The making of chemical compounds within a living organism

Biosíntesis molecular La producción de compuestos químicos en el interior de un organismo vivo

Molecule The smallest particle of a compound

Molécula La partícula más pequeña de un compuesto

Monoamine oxidase An enzyme (includes MAO-A and MAO-B) found in the nerve terminals, the neurons, and liver cells; inactivates chemicals such as tyramine, catecholamines, serotonin, and certain medications

Monoaminooxidosa Una enzima (incluye MAO-A y MAO-B) que se halla en las células de las terminales nerviosas, las neuronas y el hígado; esta enzima inactiva sustancias químicas como la tiramina, las catecolaminas, la serotonina y ciertos medicamentos

Monograph Medication information sheet provided by the manufacturer that includes side effects, dosage forms, indications, and other important information

Monografía Hoja de información sobre un medicamento proporcionada por el fabricante y que incluye efectos secundarios, formas de dosificación, indicaciones y otra información importante

Morals Ethics; honorable beliefs

Moral Ética; creencias honorables

Morphology Appearance, including shape, size, structure, and Gram stain characteristics of organisms; study of organisms without studying the function of organisms

Morfología Apariencia de los organismos incluyendo características de forma, tamaño, estructura y coloración del gram de los organismos; estudio de los organismos sin estudiar sus funciones

Mortar and pestle A bowl and rounded knob used to grind substances into fine powder

Mortero Un tazón y mazo redondeado que se usan para moler sustancias hasta convertirlas en polvo fino

MRSA Methicillin-resistant *Staphylococcus aureus*

Mutation An unexpected change in the molecular structure within the DNA, causing a permanent change in cells

Mutación Un cambio inesperado en la estructura molecular del ADN que causa un cambio permanente en las células

Mycosis Fungal disease

Micosis Infección por hongos

Mydriasis Dilation of the pupil

Midriasis Dilatación de la pupila

Myocardial infarction Death of the heart muscle

Myopia Nearsightedness

Miopía Vista corta

Myxedema Condition associated with a decrease in overall thyroid function in adults; also known as hypothyroidism

Mixedema Enfermedad relacionada con una disminución de la función tiroidea general en los adultos; se conoce también como hipotiroidismo

Narcotic A drug (such as opium) that in moderate doses dulls the senses, relieves pain, and induces profound sleep but in excessive doses causes stupor, coma, or convulsions. This may include drugs such as marijuana or LSD (lysergic acid diethylamide). Opium, opiates (derivatives of opium) and opioids are included.

National Association of Boards of Pharmacy National organization for members of state boards of pharmacy

Asociación Nacional de Juntas Farmacéuticas Organización nacional para miembros de juntas farmacéuticas estatales

Nationally Certified Technician One who is proficient in minimum standards set by the Pharmacy Technician Certification Board

Técnico con Certificación Nacional Individuo competente dentro de los estándares mínimos establecidos por la Junta de Certificación de Técnicos Farmacéuticos

Negative feedback A self-regulating mechanism in which the output of a system has input or control on the process; a factor within a system that causes a corrective action to return the system to normal range

Retrocontrol negativo Un mecanismo autorregulado en el cual el resultado de un sistema tiene entrada o control en el proceso; un factor dentro de un sistema que produce una acción correctiva para que el sistema vuelva a su ámbito normal

Neoplasm An abnormal tissue growth

Neoplasma Un crecimiento anómalo de un tejido

Nerve terminal   The end portion of the neuron where nerve impulses cause chemicals to be released; these cross a small space, called a synaptic cleft, and carry the impulse to another neuron

Terminal nerviosa   El extremo final de la neurona en donde los impulsos nerviosos causan que se liberen sustancias químicas; estas cruzan un espacio pequeño, denominado hendidura sináptica, y llevan el impulso a otra neurona

Neuroblastomas   Cancerous tumors that originate from the embryonic stage of life

Neuron   The functional unit of the nervous system, which includes the cell body, dendrites, axon, and terminals

Neurona   La unidad funcional del sistema nervioso, compuesta por el cuerpo celular, las dendritas, el axón y las terminales nerviosas

Neurosis   Mental illness arising from stress or anxiety in the patient's environment without loss of contact with reality; phobias can be listed in this category

Neurosis   Enfermedad mental que surge del estrés o la ansiedad en el entorno del paciente, sin que haya una pérdida de contacto con la realidad, las fobias pueden encuadrarse en esta categoría

Neutron   A subset of an atom that does not contain a charge

Neutrón   Una subdivisión de un átomo la cual no tiene carga

NIDDM   Non–insulin-dependent diabetes mellitus

NKDA   No known drug allergy

NKDA   No se le conocen alergias a medicamentos

Nocturia   Having to urinate excessively at night

Nonproductive cough   Cough that does not produce mucous secretions from the respiratory tract

Tos improductiva   Tos que no produce secreciones mucosas del tracto respiratorio (tos seca)

Normal flora   Microorganisms that reside harmlessly in the body and do not cause disease but may aid the host organism

Flora normal   Microorganismos que se hallan en el cuerpo y que no causan enfermedades, sino que pueden ser beneficiosos para el organismo en el que se encuentran

Nosocomial infection   An infection acquired during hospitalization

Infección nosocomial   Una infección adquirida durante una hospitalización

NSAIDs   Nonsteroidal antiinflammatory drugs

NSAID   Medicamentos antiinflamatorios no esteroides

Nucleic acid   The bases contained within DNA

Ácido nucleico   Las bases que se hallan en el ácido desoxirribonucleico (ADN)

Ointment   A hydrophobic product such as petroleum jelly

Ungüento   Un producto hidrófobo como la vaselina

On–call   A medication to be administered when directed, usually for preanesthesia

A petición   Un medicina que se administra cuando se ordena, normalmente como preanestesia

Oncogene   A previously normal gene that may be affected adversely by infection, such as a retrovirus, which causes a mutation and may produce cancer

Oncógeno   Un gen que era normal pero que puede haber sido afectado de forma adversa por una infección, como un retrovirus, que causa una mutación y puede producir cáncer

Oocyte or ova   The female reproductive germ cell

Oocito u óvulo   La célula germinal femenina

Ophthalmic   Pertaining to the eye

Oftálmico   Perteneciente al ojo

Opioid   A synthetic analgesic that is similar to opium

Opium   An analgesic that is made from the poppy plant

Orbit   The rotation of electrons around the nucleus

Órbita   La rotación de los electrones alrededor del núcleo

Osteoarthritis   Also known as degenerative joint disease

Osteoporosis   Condition associated with the decrease of bone mass and the softening of the bones, resulting in the increased possibility of bone fractures

Osteoporosis   Enfermedad relacionada con una disminución de la densidad ósea y el ablandamiento de los huesos, que da como resultado un aumento en la posibilidad de fracturas óseas

OTC   Over-the-counter

OTC   De venta libre (sin receta)

Otic   Pertaining to the ear

Ótico   Perteneciente al oído

Outpatient pharmacy   Pharmacy that serves patients in their communities; a pharmacy that is not in inpatient facilities

Farmacia externa   Farmacias que sirven a los pacientes en sus comunidades; farmacias que no están en instalaciones en la que hay pacientes internos

Over–the–counter medication   Medication that can be purchased without a prescription; nonlegend medications

Medicamento de venta libre   Medicamento que se puede comprar sin receta; medicamentos de venta sin receta

Paget's disease   Condition that affects older adults in which the density of the bones decreases, resulting in softening and weakening

Enfermedad de Paget   Enfermedad que afecta a adultos de edad avanzada en la cual disminuye la densidad de los huesos, dando como resultado su ablandamiento y debilitamiento

Palliative   That which brings relief but does not cure

Paliativo   Proporciona alivio, pero no cura

PAR   Periodic automatic replacement

PAR   Reemplazo automático periódico

Paracrine   Denoting a type of hormone function in which hormone synthesized in and released from endocrine cells binds to its receptor

Parasite   Organism that requires a host for nourishment and reproduction

Parásito   Organismo que necesita un organismo huésped para alimentarse y reproducirse

Parasympathetic nervous system   Division of the autonomic nervous system that functions during restful situations; "breed or feed" part of autonomic nervous system

Sistema nervioso parasimpático   División del sistema nervioso autónomo que funciona durante los momentos de descanso; parte del sistema nervioso autónomo encargada de "criar o alimentar"

Parenteral medications   Medication administered by injection, such as intravenously or intramuscularly

Parenteral   Medicamento que se administra por inyección, como el que se administra por vía intravenosa o intramuscular

Passive immunity   Resistance that has been acquired through a transfer of antibodies from another person or animal, or from mother to child

Inmunidad pasiva   Resistencia que ha sido adquirida a través de una transferencia de anticuerpos de otra persona o animal, o de la madre al hijo

PCA   Patient-controlled analgesia

Peptic ulcer   An ulcerative condition of the lower esophagus, stomach, or duodenum, usually resulting from the bacterium *Helicobacter pylori*

Úlcera péptica   Enfermedad ulcerativa del esófago inferior, estómago o duodeno; por lo general, es producida por la bacteria *Helicobacter pylori*

Peptidoglycan   The substance that comprises bacterial cell walls, specifically of gram-negative and gram-positive microbes

Peptidoglicano   La sustancia que posee barreras de células bacterianas, específicamente de microbios gram negativos y gram positivos

Peripheral nervous system   The division of the nervous system outside the brain and spinal cord

Sistema nervioso periférico   La parte del sistema nervioso que está fuera del cerebro y la médula espinal

Peripheral parenteral   Injection of a medication into the veins located on the periphery of the body system instead of a central vein or artery

Parenteral periférica   Inyección de un medicamento en las venas localizadas en la periferia del sistema corporal, y no en una vena o arteria central

Peristalsis   The contraction and relaxation of the tubular muscles of the esophagus, stomach, and intestines that move food substances from the mouth to the anus

Peristalsis   La contracción y relajación de los músculos tubulares del esófago y los intestinos que llevan las sustancias alimenticias desde la boca hasta el ano

Pharmacist   Person who dispenses drugs and counsels patients on medication use, side effects and possible interactions with other drugs and/or food

Farmacéutico   Persona que dispensa medicamentos y aconseja a los pacientes

Pharmacokinetics   The life of the drug, which includes absorption, metabolism, distribution, and excretion

Pharmacology   The study of drugs and their effects on the body

Farmacología   El estudio de las medicinas, las drogas, y sus efectos en el cuerpo

Pharmacy clerk   Person who assists the pharmacist at the front counter of the pharmacy; the person who accepts payment for medications

Dependiente de farmacia   Persona que ayuda al farmacéutico en el mostrador de la farmacia; la persona que cobra por los medicamentos

Pharmacy technician   Person who assists a pharmacist by filling prescriptions and performing other nondispensing tasks

Técnico farmacéutico   Persona que ayuda al farmacéutico preparando recetas y realizando otras tareas, excepto despachar medicinas a los pacientes

Pharmacy Technician Certification Board   National board for the certification of pharmacy technicians

Junta de Certificación de Técnicos Farmacéuticos   Junta nacional para la certificación de técnicos de farmacia

Pheochromocytomas   Tumors of the adrenal gland that produce excess adrenaline

Physician's Desk Reference   Reference book of medications

"Physicians' Desk Reference"   Libro de referencia sobre los medicamentos

Placebo   Inert compound thought to be an active agent

Placebo   Componente inactivo del que se piensa que puede ser un agente real

POS   Point of sale

POS   Punto de venta

PPO   Preferred provider prganization

PPO   Organización de proveedores preferidos

Precipitate   To separate from solution or suspension

Pre–op   A drug ordered to be given before surgery

Pre–operatoria   Una medicina que se receta para administrarla antes de una cirugía

PRN   Latin term *(pro re nata)* meaning "as needed"

Productive cough   Cough that expectorates mucous secretions from respiratory tract

Tos productiva   Tos que arrastra secreciones mucosas del tracto respiratorio

Professionalism   Conforming to right principles of conduct (work ethics) as accepted by others in the profession

Profesionalismo   Conducta que está en conformidad con los principios correctos (ética laboral) tal como los aceptan las otras personas de la profesión

Prophylaxis   Treatment given before an event to prevent the event from happening

Profilaxis   Tratamiento que se da antes de que ocurra un hecho para impedir que dicho hecho tenga lugar

Protectant   A substance that acts as a barrier between the skin and an irritant

Protector   Una sustancia que actúa como una barrera entre la piel y un agente irritante

Protocol   A set of standards and guidelines within which a facility works

Protocolo   Una serie de estándares y pautas de trabajo por las que se rige un establecimiento

Proton   A subatomic particle of an atom that holds a positive charge

Protón   Una partícula subatómica de un átomo que tiene carga positiva

Protozoa   Kingdom Protista; unicellular organisms that are parasites

Protozoos   Reino Protista; organismo unicelulares parasitarios

PRSP   Penicillin-resistant *Streptococcus pneumoniae*

Pruritus   Itching

Prurito   Picazón

Psychosis   A mental illness characterized by loss of contact with reality

Psicosis   Una enfermedad mental caracterizada por la pérdida de contacto con la realidad

PTH   Parathyroid hormone

Punch method   Filling of capsules by hand with powdered medication premeasured

Pyelonephritis   Inflammation of the kidney and renal pelvis

Recall   When a drug or device must be returned to the manufacturer because of failure to meet Food and Drug Administration standards

Devolución   Cuando hay que devolver una medicina o un aparato al fabricante porque no cumple los estándares de la Administración de Drogas y Alimentos

Reconstitution   To mix a liquid and a powder to form a suspension or solution

Reconstitución   Acción de mezclar un líquido con una sustancia en polvo para formar una suspensión o una solución

Remission   The span of time during which a disease, such as cancer, is not spreading; this may be permanent or temporary

Remisión   El lapso de tiempo durante el cual una enfermedad, como el cáncer, no se propaga; puede ser permanente o temporal

Repackaging   The act of reducing the amount of medication taken from a bulk bottle; unit dosing is a form of repackaging

Re–envasado   El acto de reducir la cantidad de medicamento que se toma de un envase grande; la dosis unitaria es una forma de re-envasado

Rheumatoid arthritis   A progressive degenerative and crippling immune disease

Rhinitis Inflammation of the lining of the nose; runny nose

Rinitis Inflamación de los tejidos que recubren la nariz; nariz que gotea

ROA Route of administration

ROA Vía de administración

Rods Photoreceptors that respond to dim light and are responsible for black and white color (night vision)

Bastoncillos Elementos fotorreceptores que responden ante la luz atenuada y son responsables para la visión en blanco y negro (visión nocturna)

RTS Return to stock

RTS Devolver al almacén

Rx Latin abbreviation for "recipe," commonly used to mean "prescription"; legend drug; prescription drug

Rx Término latín para "receta," se usa con frecuencia para indicar "receta," medicina de venta con receta

Sarcoma A malignant neoplastic growth arising from the connective tissue

Sarcoma Un crecimiento neoplástico maligno que surge del tejido connectivo

Schizophrenia A group of mental disorders characterized by inappropriate emotions and unrealistic thinking

Esquizofrenia Un grupo de trastornos mentales que se caracterizan por emociones inapropiadas y pensamientos irreales

Script A prescription

Escrito Una receta

Shaman Medicine person who holds a high place of honor in a tribe

Chamán Curandero que tiene un puesto de honor en una tribu

Sig Medication directions written in pharmacy terms on a prescription

Sig (Signatura) Instrucciones escritas para la medicación en términos farmacéuticos en una receta

Simmonds' disease A pituitary disorder that is a form of hypopituitarism in which all pituitary secretions are deficient

Solute The ingredient that is dissolved into a solution

Soluto En una solución, el ingrediente que se disuelve

Solution A water base in which the ingredient or ingredients dissolve completely

Solución Una base de agua en la cual el ingrediente o los ingredientes se disuelven completamente

Solvent The greater part of a solution

Solvente La mayor parte de una solución

Somatic The motor neurons that control voluntary actions of the skeletal muscles

Somáticas Las neuronas motoras que controlan las acciones voluntarias de los músculos esqueletales

Species Of Latin origin meaning "kind"

Especies Palabra de origen latín que significa "tipo"

Spermatogenesis The process of producing sperm with half the number of chromosomes

Sputum Fluid coughed up from the lungs and bronchial tissues

Esputo Fluido expulsado por la tos desde los pulmones y los tejidos bronquiales

Stat order A medication order that must be filled as soon as possible, usually within 5 to 15 minutes

Receta stat Una receta que debe despacharse lo antes posible, por lo general en 5 a 15 minutos

Steroid Messenger chemical produced by the body that helps fight inflammation and pain

Esteroides Sustancias químicas que actúan como mensajeros y que son producidas por el cuerpo para ayudar a combatir la infamación y el dolor

Stroke Impaired cerebral blood flow caused by thrombosis, hemorrhage, or embolism

Sunscreen A substance that protects the skin from ultraviolet light, which causes sunburns; skin protection factor (SPF) rates effectiveness

Filtro solar Una sustancia que protege la piel de los rayos ultravioletas, los cuales causan quemaduras solares; el factor de protección de la piel (SPD) se usa para clasificar la eficacia de estos filtros

Suspension A solution in which the powder does not dissolve into the base and which must be shaken before using

Suspensión Una solución en la cual el polvo no se disuelve en la base y debe agitarse antes de ser usada

Symbiotic A close relationship between two species

Simbiótica Una estrecha relación entre dos especies

Sympathetic nervous system Division of the autonomic nervous system that functions during stressful situations; "fight or flight" part of autonomic nervous system

Sistema nervioso simpático División del sistema nervioso autónomo que funciona durante situaciones de estrés; la parte del sistema nervioso autónomo encargada de "luchar o huir"

Synthesis   The formation of chemical components within the body system
Síntesis   La formación de compuestos químicos dentro del sistema corporal

Synthetic   Medication made in a laboratory
Sintético   Medicamento hecho en un laboratorio

Syrup   A sugar-based liquid
Jarabe   Un líquido con base de azúcar

Systemic   Pertaining to the entire body rather than to individual body parts
Sistémico   Perteneciente a todo el cuerpo más bien que a partes individuales del mismo

Tardive dyskinesia   Unwanted side effects of taking phenothiazines that include slow, rhythmical involuntary movements that are generalized or specific to one muscle group
Discinesia tardía   Efectos secundarios negativos de la toma de fenotiazinas y que incluyen movimientos involuntarios lentos y rítmicos que pueden ser generalizadores o afectar a un grupo muscular específico

Taxonomy   The science of classification and nomenclature of organisms
Taxonomía   La ciencia de la clasificación y nomenclatura de organismos

Therapeutic   Curative, treatment that is effective
Terapéutico   Curativo, tratamiento que es efectivo

Thoracic   Relates to the thorax or the chest
Torácico   Relativo al tórax o al pecho

Thrombin   An enzyme that is formed in coagulating blood from prothrombin; this enzyme reacts with fibrinogen, converting it into fibrin, which is essential in the formation of blood clots; tested by performing a prothrombin time or partial thromboplastin time blood test
Trombina   Una enzima que se forma a partir de la protombrina para coagular la sangre. Ésta reacciona con el fibrinógeno, que se convierte en fibrina, la cual es fundamental en la formación de los coágulos de sangre. Se analiza realizando análisis de sangre de tiempo de protrombina o de tiempo parcial de protrombina

Thrombolytic   Medication used to break up a thrombus or blood clot
Trombolítico   Medicamento que se usa para deshacer un trombo o coágulo de sangre

Thyroxine   Known as T_4; contains four ions of iodine
Tiroxina   Conocida como T_4, tiene cuatro iones de yodo

Tincture   A base solution of alcohol
Tintura   Una solución con base de alcohol

Total parenteral nutrition   Large-volume intravenous nutrition administered through the central vein (subclavian vein), which allows for a higher concentration of solutions
Nutrición parenteral total   Nutrición intravenosa de gran volumen administrada a través de la vena central (vena subclaviana), lo cual permite usar soluciones con concentraciones elevadas

Tourette's syndrome   A disorder characterized by multiple motor tics, lack of muscle coordination, and involuntary, purposeless movements that are accompanied by grunts and barks
Síndrome de Tourette   Un trastorno que se caracteriza por múltiples tics motores, incluyendo falta de coordinación muscular y movimientos involuntarios y sin sentido acompañados de gruñidos y rugidos

Toxoid   A toxin that has been rendered harmless but still invokes an antigenic response
Anatoxina   Una toxina que se ha vuelto inofensiva pero que todavía produce una respuesta antígena

Trace elements   Elements that are needed by the body in very small amounts
Elementos traza   Elementos que el cuerpo necesita en cantidades muy pequeñas

Trade name   Brand-name drug; the company that first applies for a patent on the chemical structure of a medication or generic name is allowed to name the product with a patented name
Denominación commercial   Medicamento de marca; la compañía que primero solicita una patente de la estructura química de un medicamento o un nombre genérico se le permite darle un nombre a ese producto con una marca patentada

Transient ischemic attacks   A temporary reduction of oxygen and blood in the brain

Triiodothyronine   Known as T_3; contains three ions of iodine
Triodotironina   Conocida como T_3, tiene tres iones de yodo

Triturate   To grind or crush powder such as a tablet into fine particles

Tympanic membrane   A membranous skin that separates the external ear from the middle ear
Membrana del tímpano   Una piel membranosa que separa el oído externo del oído medio

Ulcer   A lesion on a mucous surface of the gastrointestinal tract
Úlcera   Una lesión estomacal en la superficie mucosa del tracto gastrointestinal

Unit dose   A single dose of a drug
Dosis unitaria   Una sola dosis de una medicina

Universal precautions A set of standards that lowers the possibility of contamination; used to prepare medications

Precauciones universals Una serie de estándares que reducen la posibilidad de contaminación; se usan en la preparación de medicamentos

Urinary retention The inability to empty the bladder completely

Urinary tract infection Infection of the kidney, bladder, prostate gland, or the urethra

Urolithiasis Kidney stones

Urticaria A skin eruption of itching wheals

Urticaria Erupción cutánea de ampollas que producen picazón

Vaccine Toxoids or attenuated viral components that are given to create a response from the body that results in immunity

Vacunas Toxides o componentes virales atenuados que se administran para crear una respuesta del cuerpo que tiene como resultado la inmunidad

Valence The number of electrons gained, lost, or shared when an atom bonds with another atom; determined by the electrons in the outer orbit

Valencia El número de electrones que un átomo gana, pierde o comparte cuando se une con otro átomo; está determinada por los electrones que hay en la órbita más externa.

Vasodilation Widening of the blood vessels that allows for increased blood flow

Vasodilatación Ensanchamiento de los vasos sanguíneos que permite una mayor circulación de sangre

Vector An entity by which infections are transferred, but the entity of transference does not have the disease and does not need to be living. For example, a mosquito bite transfers malaria. In this case, the mosquito is the vector.

Vector Una entidad que transmite infecciones, pero la entidad transmisora no padece la enfermedad. Por ejemplo, la picadura de un mosquito transmite la malaria. En este caso, el mosquito es el vector

Vein A vessel that carries deoxygenated blood to or toward the heart

Vena Un vaso sanguíneo que transporta la sangre sin oxígeno hasta el corazón

Vertical flow hood Environment for preparation of chemotherapy treatments that uses air originating from the roof of the hood moving downward that is captured in a vent located on the floor of the hood

Campana de flujo vertical Medio para la preparación de tratamientos de quimioterapia en el que se utiliza una corriente de aire que parte del techo de la campana y que se mueve hacia abajo, hasta entrar en un hueco de ventilación que se halla en el suelo de la campana

Villus A projection from the surface of a mucous membrane; in the gastric tract, these projections increase the surface area for absorption of nutrients and liquids in the small intestines

Vellosidad Una proyección de la superficie de una membrana mucosa en el tracto gástrico, estas proyecciones aumentan el área de superficie para la absorción de nutrientes y líquidos en el intestino delgado

Virology The study of viruses

Virología El estudio de los virus

Virus An organism that replicates by using the host's cell parts, including DNA, ribosomes, and proteins

Virus Un organismo que se reproduce utilizando partes de las células del organismo huésped, incluyendo el ADN, ribosomas y proteínas

Viscosity The thickness of a solution or fluid (e.g., corn syrup is very viscous)

Viscosidad El espesor de una solución o fluido (ej.: el jarabe de maíz es muy viscoso)

Volume The amount of liquid enclosed within a container

Volumen La cantidad de liquido que puede contener un envase

VRE Vancomycin-resistant enterococci

Water–soluble vitamin Vitamin that is soluble in water and is not readily stored by the body; these are excreted continually in the urine and must be replaced constantly

Vitamina soluble en agua Vitamina que se disuelve en el agua y que por lo tanto no se almacena fácilmente en el cuerpo; se excreta continuamente en la orina, por lo cual tiene que reemplazarse constantemente.

Compensación laboral Una cobertura de seguro que el gobierno exige y hace cumplir, destinada a trabajadores que se lesionan en el trabajo

Illustration Credits

CHAPTER 2

Figures 2-1, 2-3: Courtesy of Drug Enforcement Administration.
Figure 2-2: Potter PA, Perry AG: *Fundamentals of nursing*, ed 5, St. Louis, 2001, Elsevier.

CHAPTER 4

Figure 4-1: Gray Morris D: *Calculate with confidence*, ed 4, St. Louis, 2005, Elsevier.
p 65: Cleocin. Courtesy of Pfizer.
P 67: Cimetidine. Courtesy of Zenith-Ivax Goldline Pharmaceuticals.
P 68: Tegretol. Courtesy of Basel Pharmaceuticals.
P 70: Amoxil. Courtesy of GlaxoSmithKline.
P 72: Potassium chloride. Courtesy of American Pharmaceutical Partners.

CHAPTER 5

Figures 5-5, 5-6, 5-11: Clayton B, Stock Y: *Basic pharmacology for nurses*, ed 12, St. Louis, 2003, Elsevier.
Figure 5-7: Potter PA, Perry AG: *Fundamentals of nursing*, ed 5, St. Louis, 2001, Elsevier.

CHAPTER 8

Figure 8-5: Courtesy of Cardinal Health, San Diego, California.

CHAPTER 9

Figure 9-3: *Mosby's medical, nursing, & allied health dictionary*, ed 6, St. Louis, 2005, Elsevier.
Figures 9-4, 9-5, 9-6, 9-8: Barkauskas V et al: *Health and physical assessment*, ed 3, St. Louis, 2002, Elsevier.
Figure 9-7: Gerdin J: *Health careers today*, ed 4, St. Louis, 2007, Elsevier.

CHAPTER 10

Figures 10-1, 10-2, 10-3: Potter PA, Perry AG: *Fundamentals of nursing*, ed 5, St Louis, 2001, Elsevier.

CHAPTER 11

Figure 11-2: Elkin MK, Perry AG, Potter PA: *Nursing interventions and clinical skills*, ed 4, St. Louis, 2007, Elsevier.

CHAPTER 13

Figures 13-3, 13-5, 13-7, 13-8, 13-15: Potter PA, Perry AG: *Fundamentals of nursing*, ed 5, St. Louis, 2001, Elsevier.
Figure 13-10: Gray Morris D, *Calculate with confidence*, ed 4, St. Louis, 2005, Elsevier.
Figures 13-12, 13-16: Elkin MK, Perry AG, Potter PA: *Nursing interventions and clinical skills*, ed 4, St. Louis, 2007, Elsevier.

Figure 13-13: Courtesy of NuAire PharmaGard Systems, Plymouth, Minnesota.

Figure 13-19: Barkauskas V et al: *Health and physical assessment*, ed 3, St. Louis, 2002, Elsevier.

CHAPTER 15

All illustrations of pills courtesy of Multum Information Services, Inc.

CHAPTER 17

All illustrations of pills courtesy of Multum Information Services, Inc.

Figure 17-8: Applegate E: *The anatomy and physiology learning system*, ed 2, St. Louis, 2006, Elsevier.

CHAPTER 18

All illustrations of pills courtesy of Multum Information Services, Inc.

Figure 18-4: *Mosby's medical, nursing, & allied health dictionary*, ed 6, St. Louis, 2005, Elsevier.

Figure 18-5: Elkin MK, Perry AG, Potter PA: *Nursing interventions and clinical skills*, ed 4, St. Louis, 2007, Elsevier.

CHAPTER 20

All illustrations of pills courtesy of Multum Information Services, Inc.

CHAPTER 21

All illustrations of pills courtesy of Multum Information Services, Inc.

Figures 21-6, 21-7: *Mosby's medical, nursing, & allied health dictionary*, ed 6, St. Louis, 2005, Elsevier.

CHAPTER 22

All illustrations of pills courtesy of Multum Information Services, Inc.

CHAPTER 23

All illustrations of pills courtesy of Multum Information Services, Inc.

CHAPTER 24

All illustrations of pills courtesy of Multum Information Services, Inc.

CHAPTER 25

All illustrations of pills courtesy of Multum Information Services, Inc.

Figures 25-1, 25-3, 25-5, 25-7: *Mosby's medical, nursing, & allied health dictionary*, ed 6, St. Louis, 2005, Elsevier.

Figure 25-2: Barkauskas V et al: *Health and physical assessment*, ed 3, St. Louis, 2002, Elsevier.

CHAPTER 27

Figures 27-2, 27-3, 27-4, 27-5: *Mosby's medical, nursing, & allied health dictionary*, ed 6, St. Louis, 2005, Elsevier.

Index

Page numbers followed by b indicate box(es); f, figure(s); t, table(s).

A

Abbokinase. *See* Urokinase.
Abbreviations
  for dosage forms, 81, 84, 92t
  in *Drug Topics Red Book,* 108, 110t
  origination and function of, 82
  for primary units and clinics, 211b
  for routes of administration, 93t
Abortion pill. *See* Mifepristone.
Absinthe, 7
Absorption, 97, 97f, 414-416, 416t, 436
Abstinence, 501t
Acarbose, 306, 323
Accolate. *See* Zafirlukast.
Accutane. *See* Isotretinoin.
ACE inhibitors. *See* Angiotensin-converting
    enzyme (ACE) inhibitors.
Acebutolol, 457, 477
Acellular vaccines, 587b
Acetaminophen
  for children, 82-83, 548
  overdoses of, 159b, 374
  for pain, 153t, 214, 295
Acetaminophen/caffeine, 162t
Acetaminophen/codeine, 26t
Acetaminophen/hydrocodone, 26t, 555
Acetaminophen/oxycodone, 555
Acetate, 644t
Acetazolamide, 449, 450, 472
Acetic acid, 405t
Acetohexamide, 323t
Acetylcholine, 334t, 343, 343b, 351, 353,
    393-394
Acetylcholinesterase, 344
Acetylcysteine, 374
Acetylsalicylic acid. *See* Aspirin.
Achromycin. *See* Tetracycline.
Acid-base reactions, 647
Acidosis, 647b
AcipHex. *See* Rabeprazole sodium.
Acne, 158t, 165, 166-168, 168t
Acoustic nerve, 403b
Acquired immunodeficiency syndrome (AIDS),
    273, 515t, 532, 534, 534b
Acromegaly, 313, 314t
Activase. *See* Alteplase.
Activated charcoal, 429
Active immunity, 534, 585
Actonel. *See* Risedronate.
Actos. *See* Pioglitazone.
Acupressure, 182, 183t, 184f
Acupuncture, 182, 183t, 184f

Acyclovir, 531, 532t, 592, 637
Adalat. *See* Nifedipine.
Addiction, treatment of, 182, 286
Addison's disease, 314t, 319-321
Additives, 99, 99t, 156b, 230, 231t, 258
Add-O-Vial, 90, 91f, 92
ADD-Vantage system, 247, 248f
Adenosine, 212t
Adenosine triphosphate (ATP), 646
Adipose tissue, 164f
Adrenal cortex, 311, 312t, 319, 319t, 542
Adrenal glands
  conditions and their treatments, 319-321,
    319t
  functions of the, 307f, 308, 311-312, 312t,
    319-321, 542
Adrenal medulla, 311, 321, 642t
Adrenalin. *See* Epinephrine.
Adrenergic agents, 330, 340b, 342-343, 342t.
    See also individual adrenergic agents.
Adrenergic antagonists, 487
Adrenergic blockers, 340b
Adrenocoricotropic hormone, 310t, 314t, 319
Advair Diskus. *See* Fluticasone
    propionate/salmeterol.
Adverse medication reactions, 28
  reporting of, 21-22, 22f
Advil. *See* Ibuprofen.
Aerobic microbes, 514
AeroBid. *See* Flunisolide.
Aerosols, 88, 88f, 93t, 96
Aerosporin. *See* Polymyxin B sulfate.
Aesculapius, 3, 4, 5
Afferent neurons, 331-332, 337, 337f
Afrin. *See* Oxymetazoline.
Aftate. *See* Tolnaftate.
Agency for Healthcare Research and Quality,
    127b
Agitation, 191, 288
AK-Pred. *See* Prednisolone.
Albuterol, 99b, 375, 376
Alcohol, 7, 7b, 159t, 188, 297, 298
Alcoholics Anonymous, 286
Aldactazide. *See*
    Spironolactone/hydrochlorothiazide.
Aldactone. *See* Spironolactone.
Aldosterone, 312t
Alendronate, 318
Aleve. *See* Naproxen sodium.
Alkylating agents, 608
Alkylation, 608
Allegra. *See* Fexofenadine.

Allergic vasculitis, 547, 547f
Allergies
  prevalence of, 560
  reaction cycle, 545, 546f, 547
  treatments for
    antihistamines, 160, 160t, 373, 397, 547,
      548t, 560-562
    decongestants, 160, 160t, 363, 374-375,
      397
    goldenseal, 184
    metered dose inhalers, 88
    nasal sprays, 95-96
  types of, 369, 560b
Alligation, 73-75
Allopathy, 188
Aloe vera, 189
Alpha-adrenergic agents, 330
Alpha-adrenergic blocking agents, 330, 491,
    493
Alpha-receptors, 333f, 340, 342, 642t
Alprazolam, 298
Alprostadil, 491t
ALS. *See* Amyotrophic lateral sclerosis
    (ALS).
Alteplase, 481-482
Alternative medicine, 180, 181, 182. *See also*
    Complementary alternative medicine.
Aluminum, 419
Alupent. *See* Metaproterenol.
Alveolar sacs, 363, 365f, 366
Alveolar walls, 369
Alzheimer's disease, 330, 351, 357t, 569
Amantadine, 354
Amaryl. *See* Glimepiride.
Ambien. *See* Zolpidem.
Amebiasis, 527
Amenorrhea, 497, 498
Amerge. *See* Naratriptan.
Americaine. *See* Benxocaine.
American Association of Pharmacy
    Technicians, 48, 49t, 113, 113t
American Drug Index, 111
American Hospital Formulary Service Drug
    Information, 109-110, 111t
American Journal of Health-System
    Pharmacy, 113t
American Medical Association, 127b
American Pharmacists Association, 43, 44b,
    48, 50t, 113, 114
American Society of Health-System
    Pharmacists (ASHP), 43, 44b, 48, 49t,
    113, 114, 127b